Understanding Arthritis

Understanding Arthritis

Edited by Jerry Larson

hayle
medical

New York

Hayle Medical,
750 Third Avenue, 9th Floor,
New York, NY 10017, USA

Visit us on the World Wide Web at:
www.haylemedical.com

ISBN: 978-1-63241-722-0

Cataloging-in-Publication Data

Understanding arthritis / edited by Jerry Larson.
    p. cm.
Includes bibliographical references and index.
ISBN 978-1-63241-722-0
1. Arthritis. 2. Joints--Diseases. I. Larson, Jerry.
RC933 .U53 2019
616.722--dc23

Contents

Chapter 22

Chapter 23

Chapter 24

Preface

This book aims to highlight the current researches and provides a platform to further the scope of innovations in this area. This book is a product of the combined efforts of many researchers and scientists, after going through thorough studies and analysis from different parts of the world. The objective of this book is to provide the readers with the latest information of the field.

All disorders which affect the joints can be termed as arthritis. The common symptoms of arthritis include swelling, redness, joint pain and reduced movement of the affected joints. Osteoarthritis and rheumatoid arthritis are the most common forms of arthritis. Osteoarthritis is a disease of the joints that results in the breakdown of joint cartilage and underlying bone. Rheumatoid arthritis is a disorder which results in warm, swollen, and painful joints. There is no known cure for rheumatoid arthritis and osteoarthritis. However, physical therapy, orthopedic bracing, lifestyle changes and medications can help in the management of pain. This book unfolds the innovative aspects of arthritis which will be crucial for the progress of evaluation and management of this disorder. It includes some of the vital pieces of work being conducted across the world, on various topics related to it. For all those who are interested in arthritis, this book can prove to be an essential guide.

I would like to express my sincere thanks to the authors for their dedicated efforts in the completion of this book. I acknowledge the efforts of the publisher for providing constant support. Lastly, I would like to thank my family for their support in all academic endeavors.

Editor

Control of cytokine mRNA degradation by the histone deacetylase inhibitor ITF2357 in rheumatoid arthritis fibroblast-like synoviocytes: beyond transcriptional regulation

Chiara Angiolilli[1,2*] (ID), Pawel A. Kabala[1,2†], Aleksander M. Grabiec[2,3†], Marzia Rossato[1,4], Wi S. Lai[5], Gianluca Fossati[6], Paolo Mascagni[6], Christian Steinkühler[6], Perry J. Blackshear[5], Kris A. Reedquist[1,2], Dominique L. Baeten[2†] and Timothy R. D. J. Radstake[1†]

Abstract

Background: Histone deacetylase inhibitors (HDACi) suppress cytokine production in immune and stromal cells of patients with rheumatoid arthritis (RA). Here, we investigated the effects of the HDACi givinostat (ITF2357) on the transcriptional and post-transcriptional regulation of inflammatory markers in RA fibroblast-like synoviocytes (FLS).

Methods: The effects of ITF2357 on the expression and messenger RNA (mRNA) stability of IL-1β-inducible genes in FLS were analyzed using array-based qPCR and Luminex. The expression of primary and mature cytokine transcripts, the mRNA levels of tristetraprolin (TTP, or ZFP36) and other AU-rich element binding proteins (ARE-BP) and the cytokine profile of fibroblasts derived from $ZFP36^{+/+}$ and $ZFP36^{-/-}$ mice was measured by qPCR. ARE-BP silencing was performed by small interfering RNA (siRNA)-mediated knockdown, and TTP post-translational modifications were analyzed by immunoblotting.

Results: ITF2357 reduced the expression of 85% of the analyzed IL-1β-inducible transcripts, including cytokines (*IL6*, *IL8*), chemokines (*CXCL2*, *CXCL5*, *CXCL6*, *CXCL10*), matrix-degrading enzymes (*MMP1*, *ADAMTS1*) and other inflammatory mediators. Analyses of mRNA stability demonstrated that ITF2357 accelerates *IL6*, *IL8*, *PTGS2* and *CXCL2* mRNA degradation, a phenomenon associated with the enhanced transcription of TTP, but not other ARE-BP, and the altered post-translational status of TTP protein. TTP knockdown potentiated cytokine production in RA FLS and murine fibroblasts, which in the latter case was insensitive to inhibition by ITF2357 treatment.

(Continued on next page)

* Correspondence: c.angiolilli@umcutrecht.nl
†Pawl Kabala and Aleksander Grabiec contributed equally to this work.
†Dominique Baeten and Timothy Radstake contributed equally to this work.
[1]Laboratory of Translational Immunology and Department of Rheumatology and Clinical Immunology, University Medical Center Utrecht, Utrecht, The Netherlands
[2]Amsterdam Rheumatology and Immunology Center, Department of Clinical Immunology and Rheumatology and Department of Experimental Immunology, Academic Medical Center/University of Amsterdam, Amsterdam, The Netherlands
Full list of author information is available at the end of the article

(Continued from previous page)

Conclusions: Our study identifies that regulation of cytokine mRNA stability is a predominant mechanism underlying ITF2357 anti-inflammatory properties, occurring via regulation of TTP. These results highlight the therapeutic potential of ITF2357 in the treatment of RA.

Keywords: Rheumatoid arthritis, Fibroblast-like synoviocytes, Inflammation, mRNA stability, Tristetraprolin, Histone deacetylase inhibitor, ITF2357

Background

Rheumatoid arthritis (RA) is a chronic immune-mediated inflammatory disease, characterized by the excessive activation of the immune system and the uncontrolled production of cytokines and other inflammatory mediators in synovial joints. Cytokines such as tumor necrosis factor (TNF) and interleukin (IL)-1β produced by macrophages and lymphocytes infiltrating the synovial tissue lead to the abnormal activation of fibroblast-like synoviocytes (FLS), which in turn causes bone and cartilage deterioration [1]. Regulation of inflammatory cytokines occurs at multiple levels and results from the intricate modulation of epigenetic regulatory mechanisms, activation of intracellular signaling pathways, control of messenger RNA (mRNA) stability and protein translation. The correct regulation of mRNA decay is critical for immune homeostasis, as it allows cells to quickly adjust the expression of inflammatory mediators, the overproduction of which could adversely affect the organism [2]. Conditions that interfere with stability of mRNA are associated with diverse diseases, including chronic inflammation and cancer [3].

Adenosine uridine (AU)-rich elements (AREs) represent one of the largest and most important groups of *cis*-acting mRNA stability determinants. AREs allow the recruitment of *trans*-acting ARE binding proteins (ARE-BP), which in turn mediate mRNA degradation [4]. Several human ARE-BP have been identified, such as tristetraprolin (TTP, or ZFP36), TTP family members BRF1 (ZFP36L1) and BRF2 (ZFP36L2), AU-rich binding factor-1 (AUF1, or HNRNPD), KH-type splicing regulatory protein (KHSRP), and Hu antigen R (HuR, or ELAVL1). The majority of ARE-BP promote the recruitment of ARE-containing mRNAs to the exosomes for eventual degradation, although some, such as HuR and Hu family members, act as mRNA stabilizing factors [5].

The expression of several ARE-BP was found to be dysregulated in RA, and their silencing shown to affect key regulatory mechanisms in arthritis pathogenesis, both in vitro and in vivo [6–10]. To date, TTP is the ARE-BP that has been best characterized and associated with RA development and disease progression [11, 12]. TTP expression is altered in patients with synovium affected by RA [11] and TTP-deficient mice display a severe inflammatory phenotype that includes synovial pannus formation and erosive arthritis [10]. Remarkably,

overexpression of endogenous TTP or mutations at TTP phosphorylation sites protect mice in experimental models of arthritis [11, 13].

Growing interest in the modulation of ARE-BP in RA pathology has thus promoted the search for novel inhibitory compounds that can reverse the aberrant expression and function of ARE-BP. Inhibitors of the mitogen-activated protein kinase (MAPK) p38, a critical regulator of the phosphorylation status and activity of multiple ARE-BP, have been extensively used to dampen uncontrolled production of pro-inflammatory cytokines resulting from dysregulated mRNA decay [14]. However, p38 inhibitors are currently not approved for RA treatment due to molecule-related adverse events, such as cutaneous toxicity, and limited clinical efficacy [15, 16]. HDACi represent a novel class of small molecule drugs that have shown promising results in vitro and in vivo in models of RA and immune-related diseases [17, 18] and have demonstrated initial clinical efficacy in the treatment of systemic-onset juvenile idiopathic arthritis [19]. Although the primary mechanism of action of HDACi is proposed to rely on the regulation of chromatin opening and transcription, studies have reported that HDACi can impair cytokine mRNA expression despite favoring their transcriptional activation [20, 21]. We previously reported that pan-specific HDACi ITF2357 (Givinostat) and trichostatin A (TSA) prevented IL-6 production in RA FLS and macrophages by promoting accelerated degradation of *IL6* mRNA [22].

In this study, we aimed to dissect the transcriptional and post-transcriptional regulation of cytokine mRNA expression by ITF2357, and to identify whether, and through which mechanisms, HDACi can restore the balance in mRNA-stability mechanisms that are deregulated in RA.

Methods

Patient material and FLS isolation

FLS were derived from synovial tissue specimens obtained from patients with RA by needle arthroscopy, as previously described [23], cultured in medium supplemented with 10% fetal bovine serum (FBS, Invitrogen), and used between passages 4 and 10. All patients fulfilled the criteria for the classification of RA and had active disease including clinical arthritis of the joint from which the synovial biopsies were obtained [24].

FLS treatment and stimulation

FLS were cultured overnight in Dulbecco's Modified Eagle Medium (DMEM, Life Technologies) containing 1% FBS prior to incubation with cytokines. Cells were pre-incubated for 30 min with either 250 nM pan-HDAC inhibitor ITF2357 (Italfarmaco) or 5 µM p38 inhibitor (SB202190, Sigma) and stimulated with 1 ng/ml IL-1β (R&D Systems). Information about the specificity of the HDACi is published [25].

RNA extraction and gene expression profiling

RNeasy Micro Kit (Qiagen) was used for RNA extraction. Quantity and purity of RNA was assessed using a Nanodrop spectrophotometer (Nanodrop Technologies). RNA was reverse-transcribed using a First-Strand complementary DNA (cDNA) synthesis kit (Thermo Scientific) and quantitative (q)PCR was performed using Sybr Select PCR Master Mix (Applied Biosystems). For qPCR array analysis, RNA was reverse-transcribed using an RT^2 HT First Strand Kit (Qiagen), cDNA was mixed with Sybr Green qPCR Master Mix (Qiagen) and expression of 83 genes involved in FLS activation was analyzed using RT^2 Profiler customized qPCRarrays. qPCR reactions were performed on a StepOnePlus Real-Time PCR System (Applied Biosystems) and relative mRNA expression was calculated using StepOne Software V.2.1 (Applied Biosystems). Sequences of the primers used are listed in Additional file 4. The ratio between the gene of interest and the expression of human *GAPDH* or murine *ACTB* housekeeping genes, or the expression of five housekeeping genes (*B2M*, *HPRT1*, *RPL13A*, *GAPDH* and *ACTB*) was calculated for qPCR and qPCR arrays, respectively.

Protein extraction and immunoblotting

FLS were lysed in Laemmli's buffer and protein content was quantified with a BCA Protein Assay Kit (Pierce). Equivalent amounts of total protein lysate were then mixed with loading buffer and boiled at 95 °C for 5 min. Proteins were resolved by electrophoresis on either 4–12% Bis-Tris SDS NuPAGE gels (Invitrogen) for 1 h at constant 200 V, or on 10% SDS-PAGE gels for 5 h at constant 70 V for better separation of immunoreactive bands ranging between 26 and 55 kDa. Gels were transferred to polyvinylidene difluoride (PVDF) membranes (Bio-Rad Laboratories), membranes were blocked in Tris-buffered saline (pH 8.0) containing 0.05% Tween-20 (Bio-Rad) and 4% milk (Bio-Rad), washed and probed overnight at 4 °C with antibodies recognizing TTP (Cell Signaling), histone 3 (H3) (Cell Signaling) or tubulin (Sigma-Aldrich). After washing, membranes were incubated with horseradish peroxidase (HRP)-conjugated swine anti-rabbit or goat anti-mouse immunoglobulin secondary antibody (Dako), and protein visualization was performed using a ChemiDoc MP system (Bio-Rad).

Luminex assay

RA FLS were left unstimulated or were treated with 250 nM ITF2357 for 30 min prior to stimulation with 1 ng/ml IL-1β for 24 h. Supernatants were harvested and IL-8, matrix metalloproteinase (MMP)-3, CXCL-10, CXCL-5 and CXCL-6 protein secretion determined by Luminex (BioRad) according to the manufacturer's instructions at the core facility of the Academic Medical Center (AMC).

Analysis of mRNA stability

FLS were left unstimulated or were treated with 250 nM ITF2357 for 30 min prior to stimulation with 1 ng/ml IL-1β. After 2 h of stimulation culture medium was discarded, cells were washed and fresh medium containing 10 µg/ml actinomycin D (ActD) (Sigma-Aldrich) was added. Cells were then harvested at 0, 2 and 5 h following the addition of ActD, RNA was isolated, and the rates of mRNA degradation in the presence or absence of HDACi assessed using a customized RT^2 Profiler™ PCR Array set (SABiosciences) as described above. Transcripts displaying at least 1.5-fold change in the rate of degradation, compared to IL-1β-stimulated controls were analyzed.

Lambda phosphatase treatment

FLS were lysed in 1 × NEBuffer (New England Biolabs) supplemented with 1 mM $MnCl_2$. Cell lysate was incubated on ice for 20 min, spun down, and supernatant was collected and incubated with 10,000 U/ml lambda (λ) phosphatase (New England Biolabs) at 30 °C for 30 min. Protein lysate was added to loading buffer and boiled at 95 °C for 5 min, and further processed for immunoblotting as described above.

siRNA transfection

RA FLS were transfected using DharmaFECT1 (Thermo Scientific). The day before transfection, cells were incubated with DMEM containing 10% FBS which was then replaced with OPTI-MEM serum-reduced medium. AUF1, BRF1, BRF2, KHSRP, HuR and TTP specific small interfering RNA (siRNA) (20 nM) and control non-targeting siRNA (20 nM), (Thermo Scientific) were mixed with DharmaFECT1 and incubated for 20 min at room temperature prior to transfection; 24 h after transfection, medium was replaced with DMEM containing 10% FBS and this was left for another 24 h.

TTP wild-type and knockout MEF

Mouse embryonic fibroblasts (MEF) were derived from littermate E14.5 *Zfp36 (TTP) +/+* and *Zfp36 (TTP)– /–* embryos, as previously described [10]. *Zfp36–/–* mice were generated by inserting a targeting vector containing a neomycin resistance gene (neo) in the TTP protein-coding region, which generated multiple stop codons and precluded synthesis of the functional protein. MEFs were maintained in medium containing 10% FBS, 100 U/ml penicillin, 100 µg/ml streptomycin, and 2mM L-glutamine. Zfp36−/− cells were regularly maintained for one passage in feeding medium containing 0.3 mg/ml of the selection antibiotic Geneticin (G418, Thermo Fisher Scientific).

Statistical analysis

Data are presented as mean ± SEM unless otherwise indicated. One-way analysis of variance (ANOVA) was used for analyzing sets of data requiring multiple comparisons. Wilcoxon matched pairs test and the ratio t test was used for all other paired comparisons. Data were analyzed using GraphPad software 7 with p values < 0.05 considered statistically significant.

Results

ITF2357 rapidly suppresses the expression of IL-1β-induced inflammatory genes

We and others have shown that the pan-HDACi ITF2357 is a potent suppressor of genes regulating inflammatory activation, adhesion, angiogenesis, cell survival and extracellular matrix degradation [25–27]. Specifically, by screening a broad subset of genes relevant to disease pathology in RA, we found that treatment with ITF2357 reduced the expression of the majority of genes responsive to IL-1β stimulation in RA FLS [26]. To gain more insight into temporal changes in gene expression in the presence of the HDACi, we analyzed the kinetics of mRNA regulation of 83 selected genes using customized qPCR arrays (Fig. 1a and Additional file 1). ITF2357 reduced the expression of 85% of the analyzed transcripts, regardless of the kinetics of gene induction after IL-1β stimulation. As earlier shown for IL6 [22], the reduction observed in cytokine mRNA accumulation after ITF2357 treatment corresponded to changes at the protein level (Fig. 1b).

Reduced expression of a subset of ITF2357-regulated genes is associated with mRNA decay

In a previous study we demonstrated that both the pan-HDACi ITF2357 and trichostatin A (TSA) accelerate the mRNA decay of IL6 in RA FLS and healthy donor macrophages [22]. To test whether this observation could be extended to other inflammatory mediators, we analyzed mRNA stability of the genes screened in our mRNA kinetics experiment. In addition to IL6 mRNA, the stability of other transcripts, such as IL8, CXCL2, PTGS2, ADAMTS1, and BCL2L1, was reduced after ITF2357 treatment (Additional file 2). In contrast, other genes including MMP1, MMP3, CXCL5, CXCL6, CXCL10, FoxO1 and ADAMTS1 were not affected by ITF2357 at the post-transcriptional level, even though their mRNA expression was reproducibly regulated by ITF2357 (Additional files 1 and 2). Independent qPCR

assays confirmed reduced mRNA stability of IL6, IL8, CXCL2 and PTGS2 transcripts after ITF2357 treatment (Fig. 2a).

In order to further dissect the transcriptional and post-transcriptional effects of ITF2357 on mRNA expression, we quantified unspliced primary transcripts of the genes that were either affected (IL6, IL8 and PTGS2) or unaffected (MMP1) by ITF2357 at the level OF mRNA decay, and compared them with their respective mature transcripts (Fig. 2b). The difference between primary and mature transcript expression of IL6, IL8 and PTGS2 after 4 h treatment with ITF2357 was modest; however, it became more prominent at 8 h and marked a pronounced reduction in the expression of the mature transcript. Conversely, MMP1 primary and mature transcript rates were similar. These results confirmed that genes found unaffected by ITF2357 in terms of mRNA decay (e.g. MMP1) are predominantly regulated at the transcriptional level, while those destabilized by ITF2357 treatment are post-transcriptionally regulated.

ITF2357 leads to TTP transcriptional and post-translational changes

Early studies in cancer cells indicated that HDACi modulate ARE-BP function [28, 29]. Therefore, we investigated the expression of both destabilizing (TTP, AUF1, BRF1, BRF2, KHRSP) and stabilizing (HuR) ARE-BP after short treatment with ITF2357 in RA FLS. We found that TTP was induced by IL-1β and further upregulated by ITF2357. Conversely, other ARE-BP were either not induced by IL-1β or did not exhibit a specific regulation pattern in combination with the HDACi (Fig. 3a). We confirmed that ITF2357 led to sustained TTP mRNA expression at later time points (Fig. 3b), while not inducing any of the other ARE-BP (data not shown). We thus investigated whether induction of TTP mRNA expression by ITF2357 could also derive from the enhanced stability of the transcript. Surprisingly, ITF2357 rather acted as a destabilizing factor of TTP mRNA (Fig. 3c), while enhancing TTP primary transcript at all time points (Fig. 3d).

Following inflammatory or growth factor-driven p38 MAPK activation, TTP protein is phosphorylated on different amino acid residues, becoming inactivated [30]. We therefore examined whether ITF2357 could also affect TTP activity by altering its post-translational status. After 2 h IL-1β stimulation, we observed increased intensity of an immunoreactive band (45 kDa) at the expected mobility for TTP (Fig. 3e). A band with higher molecular weight of approximately 47 kDa was detected after 4 h, and confirmed by higher immunoblot resolution (Additional file 3A), suggesting phosphorylation of the protein [31]. ITF2357 significantly reduced the intensity of the higher band (Fig. 3e and Additional file 3A), similarly

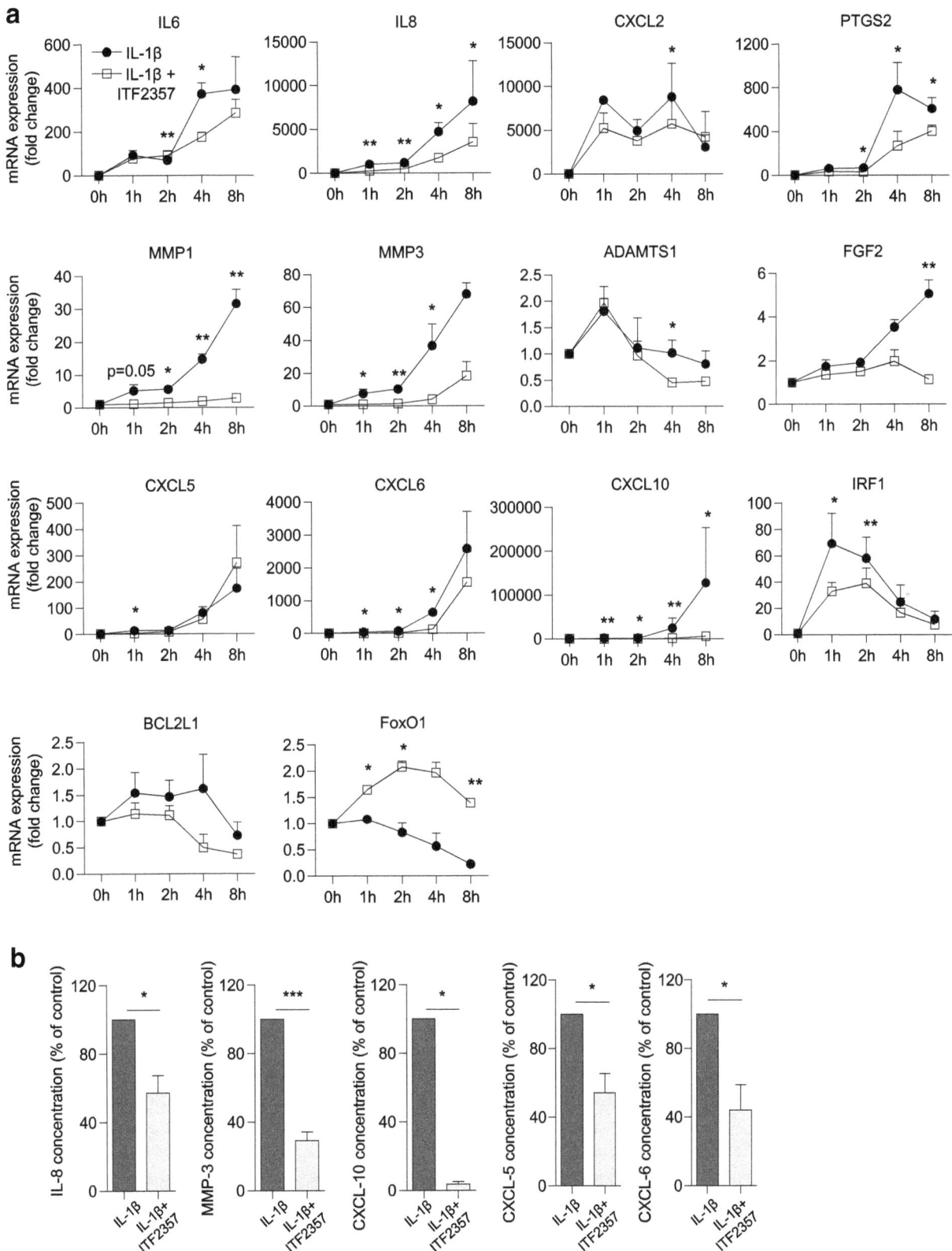

Fig. 1 (See legend on next page.)

(See figure on previous page.)
Fig. 1 ITF2357 suppresses the expression of IL-1β-responsive genes. **a** Rheumatoid arthritis (RA) fibroblast-like synoviocytes (FLS) ($n = 3$) were either left untreated or were treated with ITF2357 prior to incubation with IL-1β for the indicated time. Temporal changes in mRNA accumulation of IL-1β-inducible genes were monitored using a customized qPCR array system. Data are presented as fold changes in mRNA levels compared to unstimulated cells in the presence or absence of ITF2357 Differences in fold changes between IL-1β and IL-1β + ITF2357 conditions, for each time point, were analyzed by ratio t test: *$p < 0.05$, **$p < 0.01$. **b** RA FLS were either left untreated or were treated with ITF2357 prior to incubation with IL-1β for 24 h. FLS supernatant was harvested and levels of IL-8, matrix metalloproteinase (MMP)-3, CXCL-10 ($n = 6$) CXCL-5 and CXCL-6 ($n = 5$) were measured by Luminex. Protein concentrations were normalized to 100% in each experiment for samples not treated with histone deacetylase inhibitor and expressed as the percentage of control:*$p < 0.05$, ***$p < 0.001$, ratio t test

to p38 MAPK inhibition (Additional file 3B). Additionally, protein lysate treatment with λ-phosphatase reduced the intensity of TTP band upon IL-1β stimulation but did not further reduce TTP signal in samples treated with either ITF2357 or p38 inhibitor (Additional file 3C). Together, these results suggest that ITF2357 has a dual role in the regulation of TTP, by inducing mRNA expression at the transcriptional level, and by preventing TTP phosphorylation and subsequent inactivation.

ITF2357 suppresses cytokine production independently of AUF1, BRF1, BRF2, KHSRP and HuR

Despite the prevalent effect of ITF2357 on TTP mRNA induction, we could not exclude the possibility that ITF2357 may impact other ARE-BP by different mechanisms of action, e.g. by modifying their post-translational state. To investigate whether any of the other ARE-BP included in our study would be required for ITF2357 effects on *IL6*, *IL8*, *CXCL2* or *PTGS2* mRNA expression, we performed knockdown of AUF1, BRF1, BRF2, KHSRP and HuR in RA FLS, achieving 80–95% silencing efficiency (Fig. 4a). We observed that knockdown of these genes led to minor changes in cytokine gene expression (Fig. 4b) and that ITF2357 similarly suppressed cytokine production in both control and ARE-BP knockdown conditions. A trend towards downregulation of *IL6* and *PTGS2* mRNA expression was noticeable upon KH-type splicing regulatory protein (KHSRP) knockdown, possibly indicating alternative mechanisms of regulation by this ARE-BP, which go beyond direct control of mRNA stability [32]. Overall, these results indicate that, despite potential post-translational modifications occurring on other ARE-BP after ITF2357 treatment, these would not be sufficient to mediate changes in the expression of the inflammatory mediators considered in our study.

TTP silencing causes pro-inflammatory responses in RA FLS and is required to prevent ITF2357-dependent *IL6* suppression in murine fibroblasts

We next investigated the effects of TTP silencing on cytokine expression in RA FLS. TTP siRNA-mediated knockdown resulted in 50% reduction of TTP mRNA expression (Fig. 5a, left panel), confirmed at the protein level (Fig. 5a, right panel), which was sufficient to cause

increased cytokine expression of *IL6*, *IL8*, *CXCL2* and *PTGS2* (Fig. 5b), but not *MMP1* (data not shown) both in unstimulated (*IL6*, *IL8*) and IL-1β-stimulated conditions (*IL6*, *IL8*, *PTGS2*). Although not statistically significant ($p = 0.05$), induction of *CXCL2* after TTP knockdown was also observed. ITF2357 still mediated cytokine suppression in the presence or absence of TTP (Fig. 5c), possibly because TTP silencing only reduced the steady-state levels of TTP mRNA but was unable to fully prevent its upregulation by ITF2357 (Fig. 5c, right panel). In line with this hypothesis, recent studies indicated that, even when minimal, TTP expression is sufficient to suppress inflammatory responses [30].

Because TTP protein domains are remarkably conserved within vertebrates, and share a common regulatory mechanism [33, 34], we made use of fibroblasts derived from wild-type ($ZFP36^{+/+}$) and TTP knockout ($ZFP36^{-/-}$) mice [35], and stimulated them with IL-1β to mimic experimental conditions used in RA FLS. Higher expression of *IL6*, *CXCL2* and *PTGS2* mRNA in $ZFP36^{-/-}$ fibroblasts indicated that these cytokines are TTP targets, as previously described [36–38]. In addition, while in wild-type fibroblasts *IL6* mRNA expression was significantly reduced by ITF2357, no significant suppression was observed in $ZFP36^{-/-}$ fibroblasts (Fig. 5d). A similar trend was also observed for *CXCL2*, while *PTGS2* was not reduced by ITF2357 in wild-type fibroblasts. Our findings indicate that TTP is an important regulator of cytokine mRNA expression in RA FLS, and suggest that this ARE-BP is responsible for mediating part of the anti-inflammatory properties of ITF2357.

Discussion

In RA and in other immune-mediated inflammatory diseases (IMIDs), the excessive production and accumulation of cytokines and chemokines contributes to the perpetuation of chronic inflammation and immune responses [1]. Continuous exposure to pro-inflammatory stimuli drives RA FLS to develop an epigenetically imprinted, aggressive phenotype and inflammatory memory that promotes the degradation of synovial joints [39]. Development of immunomodulatory epigenetic inhibitors has emerged in recent years. Among these, HDACi comprise a class of small anti-inflammatory molecules that showed pre-clinical

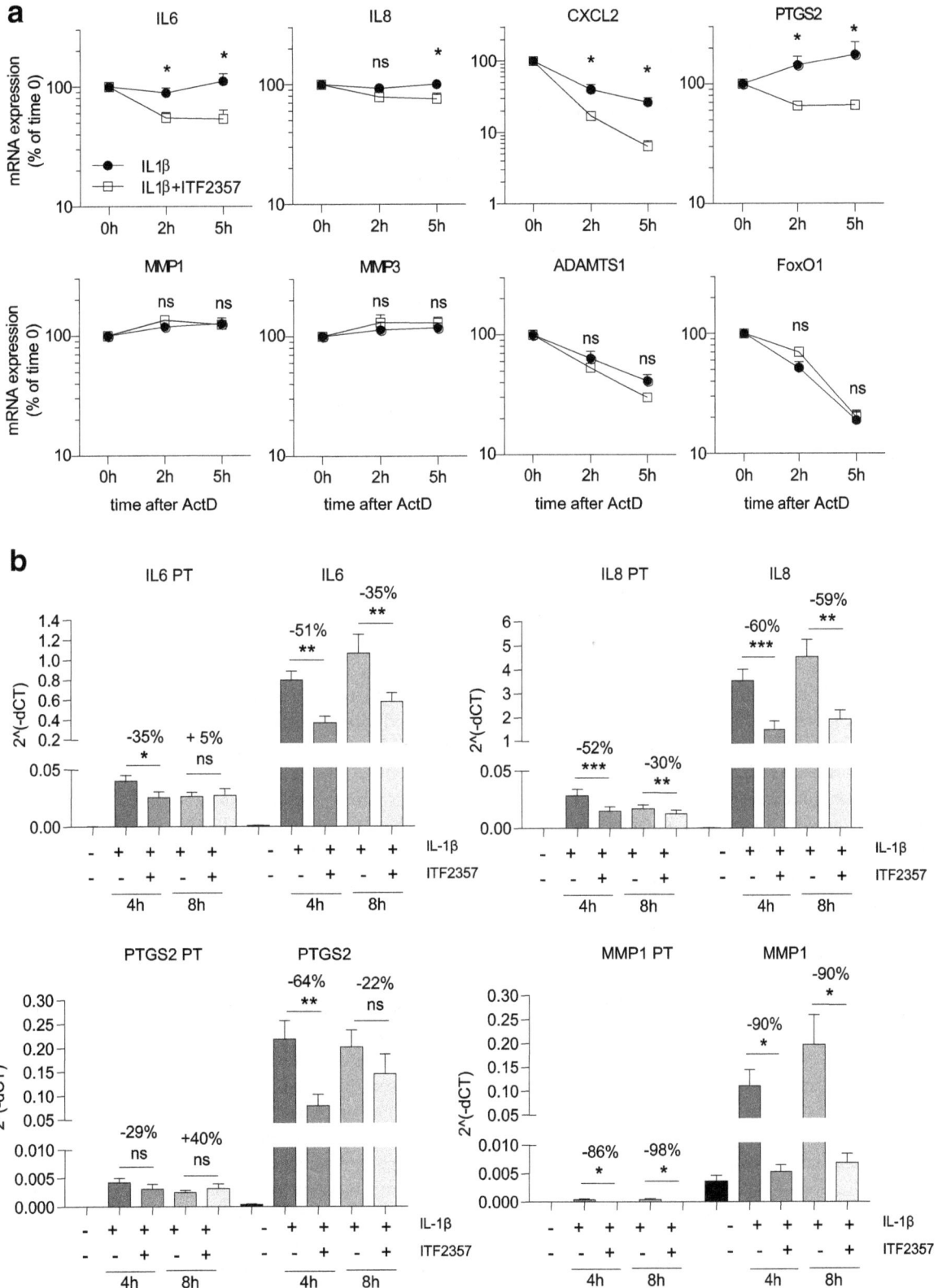

Fig. 2 (See legend on next page.)

(See figure on previous page.)

Fig. 2 ITF2357 accelerates the mRNA decay of inflammatory markers. **a** Rheumatoid arthritis (RA) fibroblast-like synoviocytes (FLS) ($n = 6$) were left untreated or were treated with ITF2357 prior to incubation with IL-1β for 2 h. Transcription was blocked with actinomycin D (ActD) and RNA extracted at the indicated time points. Graphs show representative genes with enhanced mRNA degradation in the presence of ITF2357 (top panel), and examples of genes that were not regulated by ITF2357 at the level of transcript stability (bottom panel): *$p < 0.05$, Wilcoxon matched pairs test. **b** RA FLS ($n = 7$) were left untreated or were treated with ITF2357 prior to incubation with IL-1β for 4 and 8 h. The expression of primary transcripts (PT) and mature transcripts of *IL6, IL8, PTGS2* and *MMP1* were assessed by qPCR. Results are presented as $2^{\wedge(-\Delta CT)}$ of the targets of interest normalized to *GAPDH* housekeeping gene. Percentages indicate the average suppression caused by the presence of ITF2357 in the 7 independent experiments: *$p < 0.05$, **$p < 0.01$, ***$p < 0.001$, one-way analysis of variance with Greenhouse-Geisser correction followed by Fisher's least significant difference test

potential for the treatment of RA [18]. Despite extensive research in recent years, the mode of action of these compounds remains largely unknown.

Here we show that in RA FLS, pan-HDACi ITF2357 efficiently suppresses cytokine production independently of the kinetics of gene induction by IL-1β. As we previously found that IL-6, a key cytokine contributing to RA pathobiology, was suppressed by ITF2357 via acceleration of *IL6* mRNA decay [22], we aimed to investigate whether post-transcriptional, rather than transcriptional, regulatory events could be the key factor explaining the broad anti-inflammatory effects of ITF2357. Of note, recent reports indicate that prolonged exposure to TNF leads to a gradual reshaping of the FLS transcriptome, which is largely dependent on mRNA stability processes [14], highlighting the importance of post-transcriptional regulatory mechanisms in maintaining the chronicity of inflammation in RA. We extended our analysis to additional IL-1β-induced cytokines (*IL8, CXCL2*) and mediators of inflammatory responses, matrix degradation, and cell survival (*PTGS2, ADAMTS1,* and *BCL2L1*). We confirmed that a subset of these genes, specifically *IL8, CXCL2* and *PTGS2*, were subject to mRNA stability regulation by ITF2357. On the contrary, some targets displayed sustained stability (*MMP1–3, CXCL10, CXCL5–6)*, while others rapidly decayed over time but were not further destabilized by ITF2357 (*IRF1, FoxO1*). More intriguingly, kinetics played an important role in the transcriptional or post-transcriptional regulation of genes affected by ITF2357. Indeed, while mostly affected at the transcriptional level after shorter exposure to ITF2357, the mRNA expression of *IL6, IL8* and *PTGS2* was post-transcriptionally regulated at later time points. These results indicate that the initial anti-inflammatory events mediated by ITF2357 occur by suppressing the nascent production of cytokine mRNA, while subsequent immune suppressive functions are related to the destabilization of their transcripts.

A key mechanism responsible for the post-transcriptional regulation of gene expression is ARE-BP-mediated mRNA decay [4]. We evaluated whether ARE-BP could mediate the effects of ITF2357 on cytokine mRNA stability in RA FLS and found that TTP mRNA expression rapidly increased after short exposure to IL-1β. After treatment with ITF2357, TTP mRNA was not stabilized despite being

induced at all time-points, implying that a transcriptional component is responsible for the regulation of this ARE-BP by HDACi. To date, the mRNA-destabilizing TTP has been best described as a regulator of inflammatory processes [40]. TTP expression is significantly increased in the synovial joints in RA compared to non-inflamed joints, and it is abundant in macrophages and synovial fibroblasts [41], possibly indicating a relevant role for this ARE-BP in these cells. Studies of peripheral blood mononuclear cells in RA have reported a global reduction of TTP expression, compared to healthy controls and patients with osteoarthritis (OA) [12, 42]. In animal studies, knockout of TTP has been shown as sufficient to the development of a complex inflammatory phenotype, characterized by auto-immunity and polyarthritis [10] On the contrary, induction of TTP expression is protective in collagen-induced arthritis (CIA) [13].

In our study, we observed that besides affecting the transcriptional regulation of TTP, ITF2357 additionally reduced the abundance of a higher molecular-weight form of TTP. Treatment with phosphatase confirmed this as the phosphorylated form of the protein. The destabilizing effects of ITF2357 on TTP mRNA decay further support this finding, as dephosphorylated and active TTP would also cause its own mRNA to be degraded [13]. The equilibrium between the phosphorylated and the dephosphorylated pools of TTP has frequently been reported to be a critical feature in the determination of the inflammatory response [30]. Mice expressing a phosphorylation-deficient form of TTP, in which serines 52 and178 are converted to arginine residues, are protected from CIA, as a consequence of increased functionality of the protein [11, 30]. Also, activation or depletion of phosphatases that revert TTP to its dephosphorylated form, such as PP2A and Dusp1, reduce the production of cytokines such as *IL6, IL8* and *TNF*, and increase broad pro-inflammatory gene expression, respectively [11, 43, 44].

Phosphorylation is the most common post-translational modification of TTP and other ARE-BP, but other modifications have been reported [45, 46]. Thus, it remains possible that ITF2357 may enhance the acetylation levels of TTP and subsequently reduce its phosphorylation. Indirect regulation of TTP phosphorylation by HDACi is

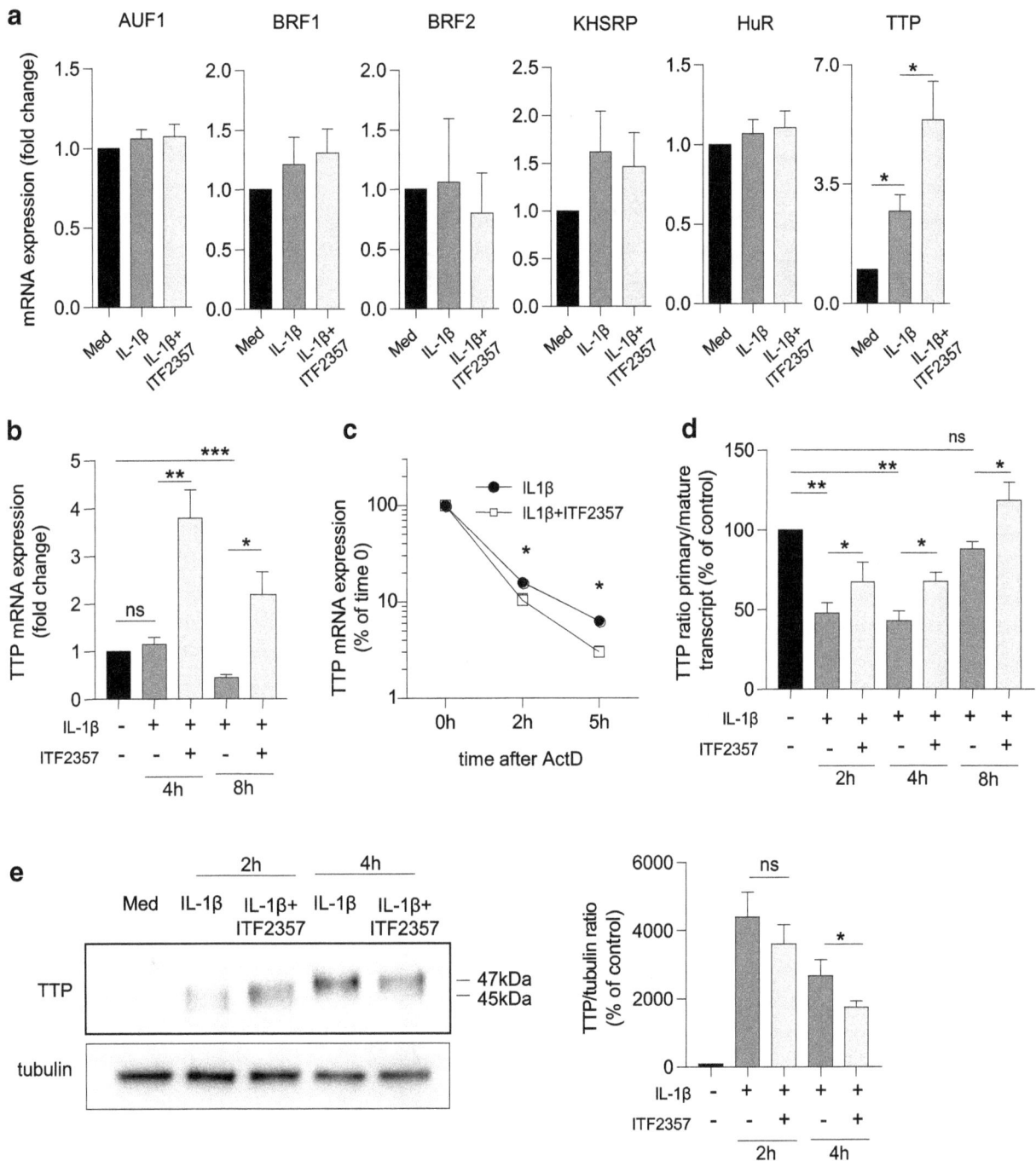

Fig. 3 Tristetraprolin (TTP) expression and activity are induced by ITF2357. **a, b** Rheumatoid arthritis (RA) fibroblast-like synoviocytes (FLS) were left untreated or were treated with ITF2357 before incubation with IL-1β for either 2 h (**a**, $n = 4$) or for 4 and 8 h (**b**, $n = 6$). The mRNA expression of the Adenosine uridine-rich elements (ARE) binding proteins (ARE-BP) was analyzed by qPCR. **c** RA FLS ($n = 6$) were subject to mRNA stability analysis as specified in Fig. 2a and TTP expression was analyzed by qPCR: *$p < 0.05$, Wilcoxon matched pairs test. **d** RA FLS ($n = 4$) were treated with ITF2357 before incubation with IL-1β for either 2 h, 4 h or 8 h and the expression levels of TTP primary and mature transcript were analyzed by qPCR. Graph shows the $2^{(-\Delta CT)}$ ratio of the primary/mature transcript normalized to *GAPDH* housekeeping gene. **e** RA FLS were left untreated or were treated with ITF2357 before incubation with IL-1β for 2 and 4 h. Protein lysates were processed for immunoblotting with antibodies recognizing TTP and tubulin (left panel) and signal intensity ($n = 8$) was subsequently quantified by densitometry analysis (right panel). Band with higher apparent molecular mass corresponds to the post-translationally modified protein. **d, e** *$p < 0.05$, **$p < 0.01$, one-way analysis of variance with Greenhouse-Geisser correction followed by Fisher's least significant difference test. ActD, actinomycin D; AUF, AU-rich binding factor; KHSRP, KH-type splicing regulatory protein; HuR, Hu antigen R

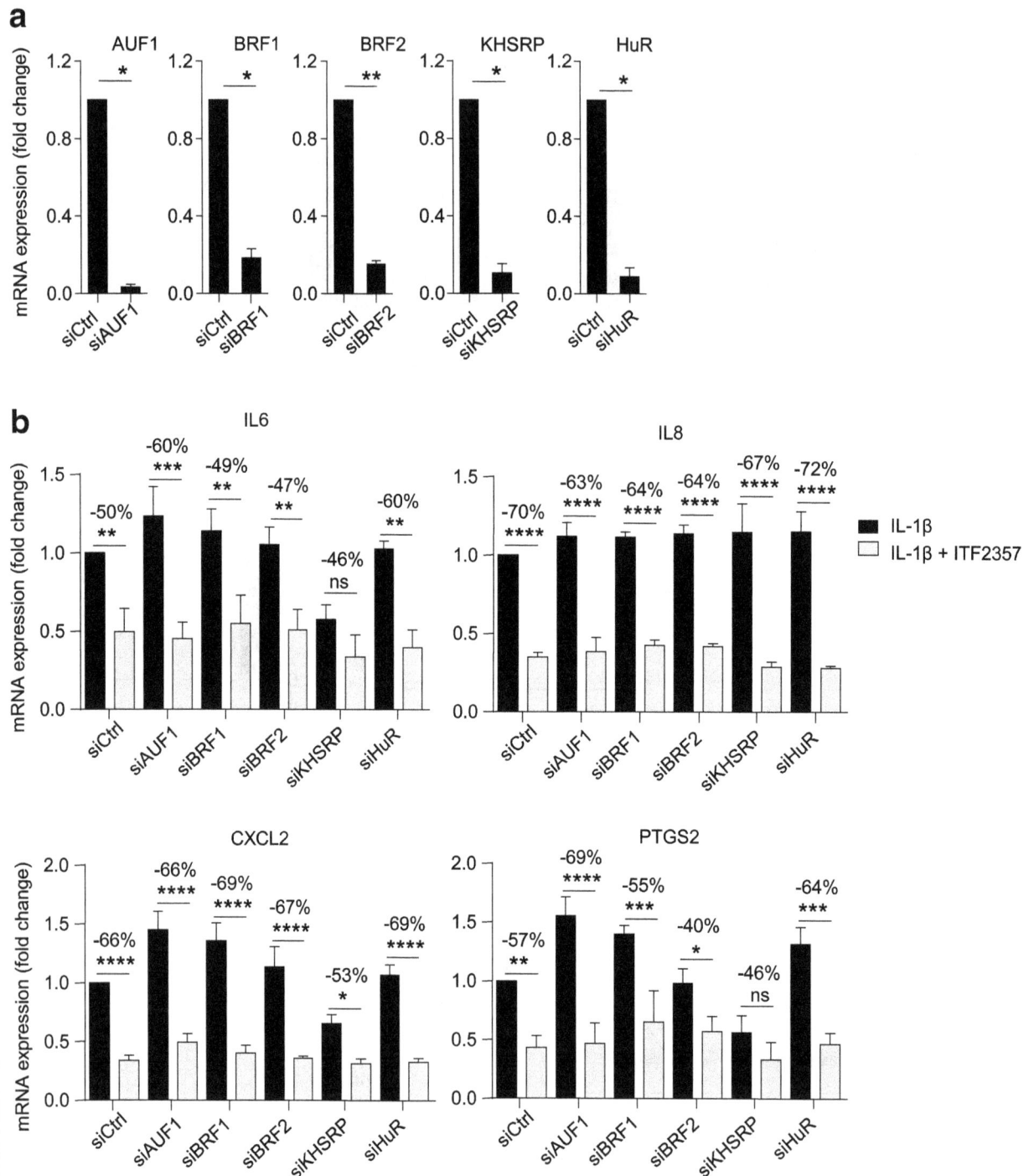

Fig. 4 Knockdown of adenosine uridine-rich elements binding proteins does not cause changes in the expression of inflammatory mediators. **a** Rheumatoid arthritis (RA) fibroblast-like synoviocytes (FLS) (*n* = 3) were left untransfected or were transfected for 72 h with 20 nM control non-targeting siRNA (siCtrl) or 20 nM specific siRNA targeting *AUF1* (siAUF1), *BRF1* (siBRF1), *BRF2* (siBRF2), *KHSRP* (siKHSRP) and *HuR* (siHuR). Knockdown efficiency was verified at the mRNA level by qPCR. Data are presented as fold expression of mRNA compared to siCtrl transfected cells:*p < 0.05, **p < 0.01, ratio *t* test. **b** RA FLS (n = 3) were transfected as in **a** and further left untreated or treated with ITF2357, prior to stimulation with IL-1β for 8 h. *IL6*, *IL8*, *CXCL2* and *PTGS2* expression were determined by qPCR. Data are presented as fold expression of mRNA compared to siCtrl-treated IL-1β stimulated cells: *p < 0.05, **p < 0.01, ***p < 0.001, ****p < 0.0001, one-way analysis of variance followed by Fisher's least significant difference test

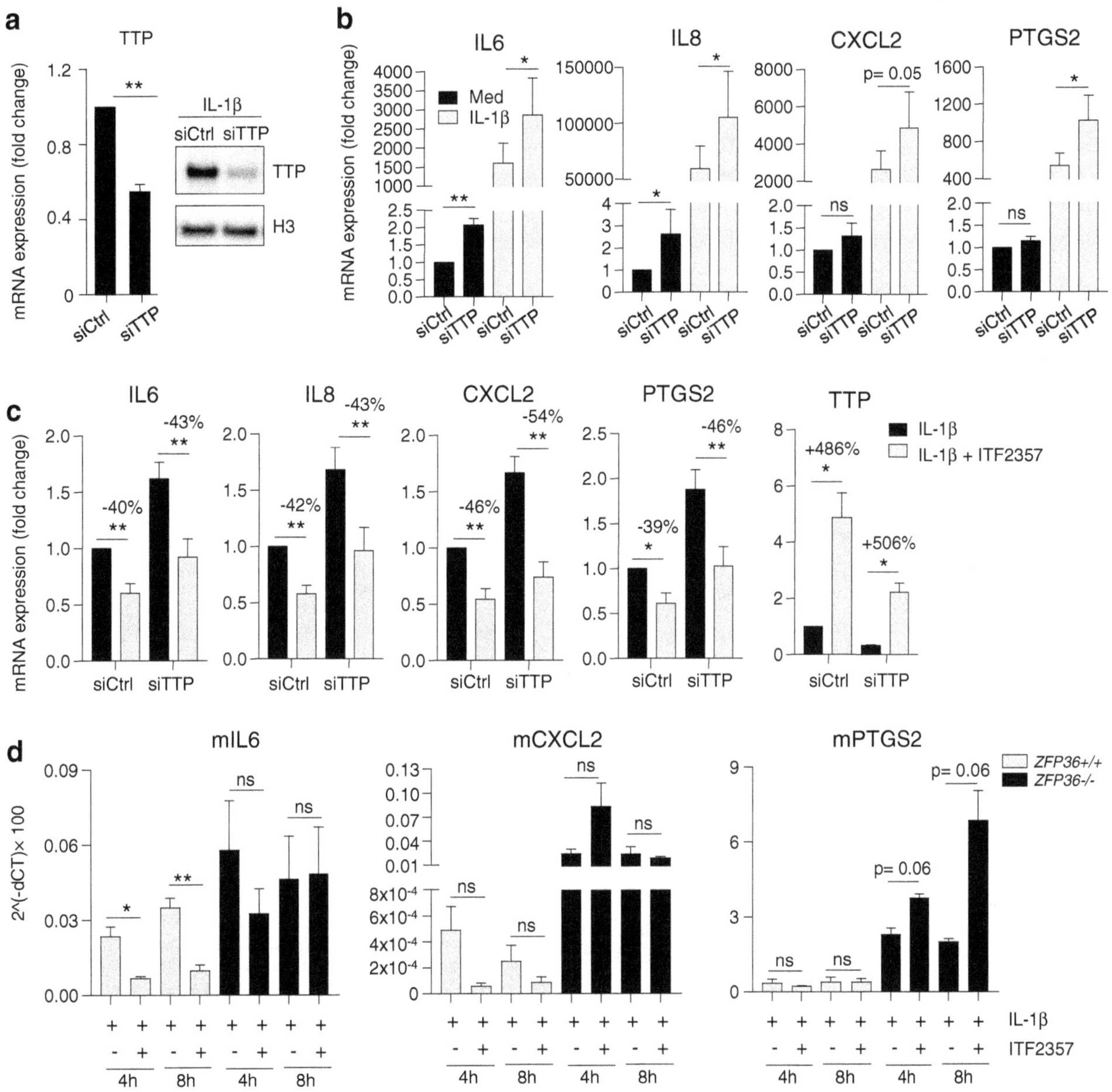

Fig. 5 Tristetraprolin (TTP) silencing in rheumatoid arthritis (RA) fibroblast-like synoviocytes (FLS) and murine fibroblasts induces cytokine expression. **a** RA FLS (n = 4) were left untransfected or were transfected with control non-targeting siRNA (siCtrl) or specific siRNA targeting TTP (siTTP). Knockdown efficiency was verified at the mRNA level by qPCR (left panel) and by immunoblotting (right panel). For immunoblot samples, cells were stimulated with IL-1β for 2 h. Protein lysate was analyzed with antibodies recognizing TTP or control H3: **p < 0.01, ratio t-test. **b** RA FLS (n = 7) were transfected as in **a**, and further left untreated or treated with ITF2357, prior to stimulation with IL-1β for 8 h. Gene expression was determined by qPCR. Data are presented as fold change in mRNA expression compared to siCtrl conditions. **c** RA FLS were processed as in **b**, IL6, IL8, CXCL2 and PTGS2 (n = 7) and TTP expression (n = 3) was determined by qPCR. Data presented as fold change in mRNA expression compared to siCtrl-IL-1β stimulated conditions. **d** Wild-type (ZFP36+/+) or TTP knockout (ZFP36−/−) murine fibroblasts (n = 4) were either left untreated or treated with ITF2357 and were further stimulated with IL-1β. Gene expression was determined by qPCR. Results are presented as $2^{(-\Delta CT)} \times 100$ of the target of interest normalized to ACTB housekeeping gene. **b-d** *p < 0.05, **p < 0.01, one-way analysis of variance with Greenhouse-Geisser correction followed by Fisher's least significant difference test

yet another possibility. In fact, evidence from the literature suggests that HDAC1,2 and 3 can bind to and acetylate Dusp1 [47]. On the contrary, direct effects of HDACi on p38 activation are likely to be excluded, as we found pan-HDACi to leave p38 phosphorylation unaltered in IL-1β-stimulated FLS [22]. Similarly, ITF2357 may affect mRNA stability independently of the c-Jun N-terminal kinase (JNK) signaling pathway, as FoxO1 mRNA stability, previously shown to be mediated by JNK inhibition [48] was not affected by ITF2357.

We tested whether single silencing of multiple ARE-BP could result in the differential regulation of *IL6*, *IL8*, *CXCL2* and *PTGS2*. Unlike other ARE-BP, TTP silencing caused increased expression of inflammatory mediators and proved to be a critical regulatory factor in RA FLS. Additionally, ITF2357 reduced *IL6* and *CXCL2* production in *ZFP36*$^{+/+}$ but not *ZFP36*$^{-/-}$ murine fibroblasts, overall demonstrating crucial involvement of TTP in *IL6* regulation by HDACi.

Conclusions

Recent studies suggested that the induced expression and the reduced phosphorylation of TTP could be beneficial in dampening inflammatory responses in arthritis [11]. Our results indicate that ITF2357 functions as an activator of TTP function and transcription in RA FLS, and provide novel understanding of how HDACi dictate not only the transcriptional, but also the post-transcriptional regulation of inflammatory genes. These findings provide rationale for further evaluation of HDACi as a therapeutic tool in RA and other chronic inflammatory diseases.

Abbreviations

ActD: Actinomycin D; ARE: Adenosine uridine-rich elements; ARE-BP: ARE-binding proteins; AUF1: AU-rich binding factor-1; DMEM: Dulbecco's Modified Eagle Medium; FBS: Fetal bovine serum; FLS: Fibroblast-like synoviocytes; HDACi: Histone deacetylase inhibitor; HuR: Hu antigen R; IL: Interleukin; JNK: c-Jun N-terminal kinase; kDa: KilotDalton; KHSRP: KH-type splicing regulatory protein; MAPK: Mitogen-activated protein kinase; MMP: Matrix metalloproteinase; mRNA: messenger RNA; PT: Primary transcripts; RA: Rheumatoid arthritis; TNF: Tumor necrosis factor; TSA: Trichostatin A; TTP: Tristetraprolin

Acknowledgements

The authors would like to thank Dr R Lutter and the Luminex core facility (Academic Medical Center, University of Amsterdam) for performing the measurement of soluble proteins in RA FLS supernatants.

Funding

AM Grabiec is currently supported by the National Science Center, Poland (POLONEZ fellowship UMO-2015/19/P/NZ7/03659); this project has received funding from the European Union's Horizon 2020 research and innovation program under the Marie Skłodowska-Curie (grant agreement number 665778KA). WS Lai and PJ Blackshear are supported by the Intramural Research Program of the NIEHS, NIH. Reedquist is supported by the Dutch Arthritis Association (NR 11–1–403); TR Radstake is supported by a grant from the European Research Council (ERC); DL Baeten is supported by a VICI grant from the Netherlands Scientific Organization (NWO) and a Consolidator grant from the ERC.

Authors' contributions

CA, PAK and AMG contributed to research design, performed experiments, analyzed data and contributed to writing the paper; WSL, GF, PM, CS and PJB interpreted data and contributed to writing the manuscript. MR, KAR, DLB and TRDJR designed the research, interpreted data and contributed to writing the manuscript. All authors read and approved the final version of the manuscript.

Consent for publication

Not applicable.

Competing interests

The authors declare that they have no competing interests.

Author details

[1]Laboratory of Translational Immunology and Department of Rheumatology and Clinical Immunology, University Medical Center Utrecht, Utrecht, The Netherlands. [2]Amsterdam Rheumatology and Immunology Center, Department of Clinical Immunology and Rheumatology and Department of Experimental Immunology, Academic Medical Center/University of Amsterdam, Amsterdam, The Netherlands. [3]Department of Microbiology, Faculty of Biochemistry, Biophysics and Biotechnology, Jagiellonian University, Kraków, Poland. [4]Functional Genomics Center, University of Verona, Verona, Italy. [5]Signal Transduction Laboratory, National Institute of Environmental Health Sciences, Research Triangle Park, NC 27709, USA. [6]Italfarmaco Research and Development, Cinisello Balsamo, Italy.

References

1. Smolen JS, Aletaha D, Mcinnes IB. Rheumatoid arthritis. Lancet. 2016; 388:2023–38.
2. Turner M, Diaz-Munoz MD. Rna-binding proteins control gene expression and cell fate in the immune system. Nat Immunol. 2018;19:120–9.
3. Khabar KS. Post-transcriptional control during chronic inflammation and cancer: a focus on AU-rich elements. Cell Mol Life Sci. 2010;67:2937–55.
4. Carpenter S, Ricci EP, Mercier BC, Moore MJ, Fitzgerald KA. Post-transcriptional regulation of gene expression in innate immunity. Nat Rev Immunol. 2014;14:361–76.
5. Schoenberg DR, Maquat LE. Regulation of cytoplasmic mRNA decay. Nat Rev Genet. 2012;13:246–59.
6. Schmidt N, Pautz A, Art J, Rauschkolb P, Jung M, Erkel G, Goldring MB, Kleinert H. Transcriptional and post-transcriptional regulation of iNOS expression in human chondrocytes. Biochem Pharmacol. 2010;79:722–32.
7. Nieminen R, Vuolteenaho K, Riutta A, Kankaanranta H, Van Der Kraan PM, Moilanen T, Moilanen E. Aurothiomalate inhibits Cox-2 expression in chondrocytes and in human cartilage possibly through its effects on Cox-2 mRNA stability. Eur J Pharmacol. 2008;587:309–16.
8. Chen J, Cascio J, Magee JD, Techasintana P, Gubin MM, Dahm GM, Calaluce R, Yu S, Atasoy U. Posttranscriptional gene regulation of Il-17 by the RNA-binding protein Hur is required for initiation of experimental autoimmune encephalomyelitis. J Immunol. 2013;191:5441–50.
9. Wang KT, Wang HH, Wu YY, Su YL, Chiang PY, Lin NY, Wang SC, Chang GD, Chang CJ. Functional regulation of Zfp36l1 and Zfp36l2 in response to lipopolysaccharide in mouse Raw264.7 macrophages. J Inflamm (Lond). 2015;12:42.
10. Taylor GA, Carballo E, Lee DM, Lai WS, Thompson MJ, Patel DD, Schenkman DI, Gilkeson GS, Broxmeyer HE, Haynes BF, et al. A pathogenetic role for TNF alpha in the syndrome of cachexia, arthritis, and autoimmunity resulting from tristetraprolin (TTP) deficiency. Immunity. 1996;4:445–54.
11. Ross EA, Naylor AJ, O'neil JD, Crowley T, Ridley ML, Crowe J, Smallie T, Tang TJ, Turner JD, Norling LV, et al. Treatment of inflammatory arthritis via targeting of tristetraprolin, a master regulator of pro-inflammatory gene expression. Ann Rheum Dis. 2017;76:612–9.
12. Fabris M, Tolusso B, Di Poi E, Tomietto P, Sacco S, Gremese E, Ferraccioli G. Mononuclear cell response to lipopolysaccharide in patients with rheumatoid arthritis: relationship with tristetraprolin expression. J Rheumatol. 2005;32:998–1005.
13. Patial S, Curtis AD 2nd, Lai WS, Stumpo DJ, Hill GD, Flake GP, Mannie MD, Blackshear PJ. Enhanced stability of tristetraprolin mRNA protects mice against immune-mediated inflammatory pathologies. Proc Natl Acad Sci U S A. 2016;113:1865–70.
14. Loupasakis K, Kuo D, Sokhi UK, Sohn C, Syracuse B, Giannopoulou EG, Park SH, Kang H, Ratsch G, Ivashkiv LB, et al. Tumor necrosis factor dynamically regulates the mRNA stabilome in rheumatoid arthritis fibroblast-like synoviocytes. PLoS One. 2017;12:E0179762.
15. Cohen SB, Cheng TT, Chindalore V, Damjanov N, Burgos-Vargas R, Delora P, Zimany K, Travers H, Caulfield JP. Evaluation of the efficacy and safety of pamapimod, a P38 map kinase inhibitor, in a double-blind, methotrexate-controlled study of patients with active rheumatoid arthritis. Arthritis Rheum. 2009;60:335–44.
16. Salgado E, Maneiro JR, Carmona L, Gomez-Reino JJ. Safety profile of protein kinase inhibitors in rheumatoid arthritis: systematic review and meta-analysis. Ann Rheum Dis. 2014;73:871–82.
17. Angiolilli C, Baeten DL, Radstake TR, Reedquist KA. The acetyl code in rheumatoid arthritis and other rheumatic diseases. Epigenomics. 2017; 9:447 61.

18. Joosten LA, Leoni F, Meghji S, Mascagni P. Inhibition of Hdac activity by Itf2357 ameliorates joint inflammation and prevents cartilage and bone destruction in experimental arthritis. Mol Med. 2011;17:391–6.

19. Vojinovic J, Damjanov N, D'urzo C, Furlan A, Susic G, Pasic S, Iagaru N, Stefan M, Dinarello CA. Safety and efficacy of an oral histone deacetylase inhibitor in systemic-onset juvenile idiopathic arthritis. Arthritis Rheum. 2011;63:1452–8.

20. Fukae J, Amasaki Y, Yamashita Y, Bohgaki T, Yasuda S, Jodo S, Atsumi T, Koike T. Butyrate suppresses tumor necrosis factor alpha production by regulating specific messenger RNA degradation mediated through a cis-acting au-rich element. Arthritis Rheum. 2005;52:2697–707.

21. Roger T, Lugrin J, Le Roy D, Goy G, Mombelli M, Koessler T, Ding XC, Chanson AL, Reymond MK, Miconnet I, et al. Histone deacetylase inhibitors impair innate immune responses to toll-like receptor agonists and to infection. Blood. 2011;117:1205–17.

22. Grabiec AM, Korchynskyi O, Tak PP, Reedquist KA. Histone deacetylase inhibitors suppress rheumatoid arthritis fibroblast-like synoviocyte and macrophage Il-6 production by accelerating mRNA decay. Ann Rheum Dis. 2012;71:424–31.

23. Van De Sande MG, Dm G, Lodde BM, Van Baarsen LG, Alivernini S, Codullo V, Felea I, Vieira-Sousa E, Fearon U, Reece R, et al. Evaluating antirheumatic treatments using synovial biopsy: a recommendation for standardisation to be used in clinical trials. Ann Rheum Dis. 2011;70:423–7.

24. Aletaha D, Neogi T, Silman AJ, Funovits J, Felson DT, Bingham CO 3rd, Birnbaum NS, Burmester GR, Bykerk VP, Cohen MD, et al. 2010 Rheumatoid arthritis classification criteria: an American College of Rheumatology/European League Against Rheumatism collaborative initiative. Arthritis Rheum. 2010;62:2569–81.

25. Li S, Fossati G, Marchetti C, Modena D, Pozzi P, Reznikov LL, Moras ML, Azam T, Abbate A, Mascagni P, et al. Specific inhibition of histone deacetylase 8 reduces gene expression and production of proinflammatory cytokines in vitro and in vivo. J Biol Chem. 2015;290:2368–78.

26. Angiolilli C, Kabala PA, Grabiec AM, Van Baarsen IM, Ferguson BS, Garcia S, Malvar Fernandez B, Mckinsey TA, Tak PP, Fossati G, et al. Histone deacetylase 3 regulates the inflammatory gene expression programme of rheumatoid arthritis fibroblast-like synoviocytes. Ann Rheum Dis. 2016.

27. Golay J, Cuppini L, Leoni F, Mico C, Barbui V, Domenghini M, Lombardi L, Neri A, Barbui AM, Salvi A, et al. The histone deacetylase inhibitor Itf2357 has anti-leukemic activity in vitro and in vivo and inhibits Il-6 and VEGF production by stromal cells. Leukemia. 2007;21:1892–900.

28. Sobolewski C, Sanduja S, Blanco FF, Hu L, Dixon DA. Histone deacetylase inhibitors activate tristetraprolin expression through induction of early growth response protein 1 (EGR1) in colorectal cancer cells. Biomol Ther. 2015;5:2035–55.

29. Li C, Tang C, He G. Tristetraprolin: a novel mediator of the anticancer properties of resveratrol. Genet Mol Res. 2016;15.

30. Ross EA, Smallie T, Ding Q, O'neil JD, Cunliffe HE, Tang T, Rosner DR, Klevernic I, Morrice NA, Monaco C, et al. Dominant suppression of inflammation via targeted mutation of the mRNA destabilizing protein tristetraprolin. J Immunol. 2015;195:265–76.

31. Clark AR, Dean JL. The control of inflammation via the phosphorylation and dephosphorylation of tristetraprolin: a tale of two phosphatases. Biochem Soc Trans. 2016;44:1321–37.

32. Briata P, Bordo D, Puppo M, Gorlero F, Rossi M, Perrone-Bizzozero N, Gherzi R. Diverse roles of the nucleic acid-binding protein KHSRP in cell differentiation and disease. Wiley Interdiscip Rev RNA. 2016;7:227–40.

33. Blackshear PJ, Perera L. Phylogenetic distribution and evolution of the linked RNA-binding and NOT1-binding domains in the tristetraprolin family of tandem CCCH zinc finger proteins. J Interf Cytokine Res. 2014;34:297–306.

34. Cao H, Deterding LJ, Blackshear PJ. Phosphorylation site analysis of the anti-inflammatory and mRNA-destabilizing protein tristetraprolin. Expert Rev Proteomics. 2007;4:711–26.

35. Lai WS, Parker JS, Grissom SF, Stumpo DJ, Blackshear PJ. Novel Mrna targets for tristetraprolin (TTP) identified by global analysis of stabilized transcripts in TTP-deficient fibroblasts. Mol Cell Biol. 2006;26:9196–208.

36. Tang T, Scambler TE, Smallie T, Cunliffe HE, Ross EA, Rosner DR, O'neil JD, Clark AR. Macrophage responses to lipopolysaccharide are modulated by a feedback loop involving prostaglandin E2, dual specificity phosphatase 1 and tristetraprolin. Sci Rep. 2017;7:4350.

37. Qiu LQ, Lai WS, Bradbury A, Zeldin DC, Blackshear PJ. Tristetraprolin (TTP) coordinately regulates primary and secondary cellular responses to proinflammatory stimuli. J Leukoc Biol. 2015;97:723–36.

38. Zhao W, Liu M, D'silva NJ, Kirkwood KL. Tristetraprolin regulates interleukin-6 expression through P38 MAPK-dependent affinity changes with mRNA 3' untranslated region. J Interf Cytokine Res. 2011;31:629–37.

39. Bottini N, Firestein GS. Duality of fibroblast-like synoviocytes in RA: passive responders and imprinted aggressors. Nat Rev Rheumatol. 2013;9:24–33.

40. Newman R, Mchugh J, Turner M. RNA binding proteins as regulators of immune cell biology. Clin Exp Immunol. 2016;183:37–49.

41. Brooks SA, Connolly JE, Diegel RJ, Fava RA, Rigby WF. Analysis of the function, expression, and subcellular distribution of human tristetraprolin. Arthritis Rheum. 2002;46:1362–70.

42. Sugihara M, Tsutsumi A, Suzuki E, Wakamatsu E, Suzuki T, Ogishima H, Hayashi T, Chino Y, Ishii W, Mamura M, et al. Effects of infliximab therapy on gene expression levels of tumor necrosis factor alpha, tristetraprolin, T cell intracellular antigen 1, and Hu antigen R in patients with rheumatoid arthritis. Arthritis Rheum. 2007;56:2160–9.

43. Smallie T, Ross EA, Ammit AJ, Cunliffe HE, Tang T, Rosner DR, Ridley ML, Buckley CD, Saklatvala J, Dean JL, et al. Dual-specificity phosphatase 1 and tristetraprolin cooperate to regulate macrophage responses to lipopolysaccharide. J Immunol. 2015;195:277–88.

44. Rahman MM, Rumzhum NN, Hansbro PM, Morris JC, Clark AR, Verrills NM, Ammit AJ. Activating protein phosphatase 2a (Pp2a) enhances tristetraprolin (TTP) anti-inflammatory function in A549 lung epithelial cells. Cell Signal. 2016;28:325–34.

45. Blackwell E, Ceman S. Arginine methylation of RNA-binding proteins regulates cell function and differentiation. Mol Reprod Dev. 2012;79:163–75.

46. Huang L, Yu Z, Zhang Z, Ma W, Song S, Huang G. Interaction with pyruvate kinase M2 destabilizes tristetraprolin by proteasome degradation and regulates cell proliferation in breast Cancer. Sci Rep. 2016;6:22449.

47. Jeong Y, Du R, Zhu X, Yin S, Wang J, Cui H, Cao W, CJ L. Histone deacetylase isoforms regulate innate immune responses by deacetylating mitogen-activated protein kinase phosphatase-1. J Leukoc Biol. 2014;95:651–9.

48. Grabiec AM, Angiolilli C, Hartkamp LM, Van Baarsen LG, Tak PP, Reedquist KA. JNK-dependent downregulation of Foxo1 is required to promote the survival of fibroblast-like synoviocytes in rheumatoid arthritis. Ann Rheum Dis. 2015;74:1763–71.

2

Enhanced IL-6/phosphorylated STAT3 signaling is related to the imbalance of circulating T follicular helper/T follicular regulatory cells in patients with rheumatoid arthritis

Qian Niu, Zhuo-chun Huang, Xiao-juan Wu, Ya-xiong Jin, Yun-fei An, Ya-mei Li, Huan Xu, Bin Yang[*] and Lan-lan Wang[*] [iD]

Abstract

Background: Follicular helper T (Tfh) cells are specialized in helping B lymphocytes, which play a central role in autoimmune diseases that have a major B cell component, such as in rheumatoid arthritis (RA). Follicular regulatory T (Tfr) cells control the over-activation of Tfh and B cells in germinal centers. Dysregulation of Tfh cells and Tfr cells has been reported to be involved in the pathogenesis of some autoimmune diseases. However, the balance of Tfh and Tfr cells, and their roles in the development and progression of RA are still not clear.

Methods: In this study, we enrolled 44 patients with RA (20 patients with active RA and 24 patients with inactive RA) and 20 healthy controls, and analyzed the frequencies of circulating Tfh and Tfr cells, expression of programmed death-1 (PD-1), inducible co-stimulator (ICOS), intracellular IL-21, and pSTAT3 in Tfh cells, and serum levels of IL-6. The correlation among these parameters and that of Tfh or Tfr cells with disease activity were also analyzed.

Results: Patients with RA (especially active RA) had higher frequencies of Tfh cells, but lower percentages of Tfr cells, thereby resulting in elevated ratios of Tfh/Tfr. Expression levels of PD-1 and IL-21 in Tfh cells were higher in patients with RA than in healthy subjects, while no difference in ICOS expression was observed between patients and controls. Both pSTAT3 expression and serum IL-6 levels increased in patients with RA, and positive correlation between them was observed. Additionally, pSTAT3 expression was positively correlated with Tfh cell frequency. The Disease Activity Score in 28 joints based on C-reactive protein (DAS28-CRP) was negatively correlated with Tfr cell frequency, but was positively correlated with both Tfh/Tfr ratio and PD-1 expression.

Conclusions: Results demonstrated that enhanced IL-6/pSTAT3 signaling may contribute to promotion of Tfh cells, consequently skewing the ratio of Tfh to Tfr cells, which may be crucial for disease progression in RA.

Keywords: Rheumatoid arthritis, Follicular helper T cells, Follicular regulatory T cells, PD-1, ICOS, IL-21, IL-6, STAT3, DAS28-CRP

* Correspondence: yangbinhx@scu.edu.cn; wanglanlanhx@163.com
Department of Laboratory Medicine, West China Hospital, Sichuan University,
37#, Guoxue Alley, Chengdu 610041, China

Background

Rheumatoid arthritis (RA) is a chronic inflammatory autoimmune disease, characterized by symmetrical inflammation of synovium, which mainly affects the peripheral diarthrodial joints, leading to progressive destruction of articular cartilage and bones, culminating in severe pain and disability [1]. The pathogenesis of RA is complicated and not yet fully elucidated; however, both innate mechanism and highly evolved adaptive immune functions seem to operate simultaneously to create and propagate the inflammatory reactions attacking the joints [2, 3]. The robust production of autoantibodies, including rheumatoid factor (RF) and anti-cyclic citrullinated peptides antibodies (ACPA), is a crucial factor in RA pathophysiology, that can lead to immune-complex deposition and the subsequent recruitment and activation of inflammatory leukocytes in the joints [4]. Usually, it is preceded by activation, somatic diversification, and affinity maturation of auto-reactive B lymphocytes, which occur in the germinal centers (GC) [5]. In these processes, follicular helper T (Tfh) cells are the principal CD4$^+$ T helper cell subpopulation, providing essential help to B cells [6], whereas regulatory T cells (Tregs) function to control B cell responses and play a critical role in the establishment of self-tolerance.

Tfh cells occur predominantly in the B cell follicles, playing a key role in GC formation, B cell development and maturation, and immunoglobulin class switching. They can be distinguished from other subsets of differentiated CD4$^+$ T cell lineages by the high expression of C-X-C chemokine receptor type 5 (CXCR5), programmed death-1 (PD-1), inducible co-stimulator (ICOS), CD40 ligand (CD40L), and secretion of interleukin-21 (IL-21) [7, 8]. Accumulating evidence has shown that dysregulation of Tfh cells and IL-21 could result in disordered autoimmunity, contributing to various autoimmune diseases, such as systemic lupus erythematosus (SLE) and ankylosing spondylitis (AS) [9, 10]. The high frequency of circulating Tfh cells (which could imply enhanced cell differentiation) is also reported to correlate with disease activity in patients with new-onset RA [11]. Tfh cells are localized in lymphoid follicles, making it difficult to study these cells. However, a recent study has shown that human peripheral blood CD4$^+$CXCR5$^+$ cells have functional properties similar to Tfh cells [12]. Circulating CXCR5$^+$ T cells, which secrete high levels of IL-21 to promote B cell differentiation into plasma cells, are more capable of facilitating B cell maturation and humoral responses than CXCR5$^-$ T cells [13]. Thus, circulating Tfh cells are crucial for the pathogenesis of autoimmune diseases [14].

Tfh cell differentiation involves multiple micro-environmental factors; one clinical study showed that secretion of IL-6 by plasmablasts resulted in Tfh cell differentiation [15]. IL-6 is involved in human Tfh cell differentiation; after binding to its receptor, it phosphorylates the signal transducer and activator of transcription 3 (STAT3), which is essential for dimerization and nuclear translocation [16]. IL-6 is an inflammatory cytokine with an important role in the pathogenesis of RA and our previous study [17] had shown that serum IL-6 level obviously increased in patients with RA. In this study, we hypothesized that the circulating Tfh cells may be elevated via the IL-6/STAT3 signal pathway.

Enhanced GC reactions must be regulated to prevent the excessive production of auto-antibodies, and an increasing number of studies have found that follicular regulatory T (Tfr) cells—a specialized population of Tregs that are primarily located in germinal centers—can specifically suppress Tfh and B cells to control the GC reaction [18, 19]. Tfr cells share the phenotypic characteristics of both Tfh cells and classical Tregs, simultaneously expressing Foxp3 and CXCR5, as well as PD-1 and ICOS [18–20], thereby playing an opposing role with Tfh cells in the regulation of humoral immunity [21]. The immune homeostasis of Tfh and Tfr cells is reported to be disrupted in the peripheral blood of patients with autoimmune diseases such as SLE, myasthenia gravis (MG), and multiple sclerosis (MS) [22–24]. However, few studies have investigated the role of Tfh/Tfr imbalance in the pathogenesis of RA in detail. The role of Tfr cells and their relationship with other T cell subsets in the abnormal immune responses of RA remain to be elucidated.

Therefore, we determined the frequencies of circulating CD4$^+$CXCR5$^+$Foxp3$^-$ Tfh and CD4$^+$CXCR5$^+$Foxp3$^+$ Tfr cells, and the expression of PD-1, ICOS, intracellular IL-21 and phosphorylated STAT3 (pSTAT3) in Tfh cells in patients with RA and corresponding healthy controls (HCs). The correlation of Tfh and Tfr cells with disease activity in RA was investigated.

Methods

This prospective study was performed in accordance with a protocol approved by the Ethics Committees of West China Hospital. Written informed consent was obtained from all participants.

Participants

Forty-four patients with RA were enrolled in this study. All patients met the American College of Rheumatology (ACR)/European League Against Rheumatism (EULAR) classification criteria (2010) [25]. The exclusion criteria were as follows: subjects with other autoimmune diseases or tumors, plasma exchanges or thymectomy prior to the study, and with acute inflammation in the preceding 4 weeks. Disease activity was assessed by the Disease Activity Score in 28 joints based on C-reactive protein (DAS28-CRP). Routine measurements were made of CRP, RF, and ACPA (screened by electro-chemiluminescence

Table 1 Characteristics of the patients with RA and the healthy controls

Characteristics	Active RA (n = 20)	Inactive RA (n = 24)	HCs (n = 20)	P value
Age (years)[a]	46 (38–57)	47 (40–53)	48 (39–55)	> 0.05
Female (n (%))	16 (80.0)	18 (75.0)	15 (75.0)	> 0.05
Symptom duration (months)[a]	10 (5–60)	15 (8–70)	ND	0.015[b]
Swollen joint count (out of 28)[a]	5 (3–8)	2 (1–5)	ND	0.039[b]
Tender joint count (out of 28)[a]	6 (2–9)	4 (1–7)	ND	0.027[b]
CRP (mg/L)[a]	6.5 (2.1–13.8)	4.0 (1.4–9.2)	ND	0.031[b]
DAS28-CRP (3)[a]	4.2 (3.5–5.6)	1.8 (1.0–2.8)	ND	0.001[b]
ACPA (IU/ml)[a]	451.9 (222.2–1208.0)	129.6 (6.0–322.6)	ND	0.006[b]
RF (IU/ml)[a]	132.0 (30.73–267.3)	23.8 (19.0–75.1)	ND	0.027[b]
ACPA ≥ 17 IU/ml (n (%))	18 (90.0)	17 (70.8)	ND	> 0.05[b]
RF ≥ 20 IU/ml (n (%))	15 (75.0)	17 (70.8)	ND	> 0.05[b]
ACPA ≥ 17 IU/ml + RF ≥ 20 IU/ml (n (%))	14 (70.0)	16 (66.7)	ND	> 0.05[b]
ACPA ≤ 17 IU/ml + RF ≤ 20 IU/ml (n (%))	3 (15.0)	4 (16.7)	ND	> 0.05[b]

RA rheumatoid arthritis, *HC* healthy controls, *CRP* C-reactive protein, *DAS28* Disease Activity Score 28, *ACPA* anti-cyclic citrullinated peptide antibody, *RF* rheumatoid factor, *ND* not determined
[a]Data are presented as median (IQR)
[b]Patients with active RA vs. patients with inactive RA, Mann–Whitney *U* test

immunoassay (ECLIA) using the Cobas e601, Roche Pharma ltd., Reinach, Switzerland). The patient group was compared to a group of 20 age-matched and sex-matched HCs. The characteristics of the patients and HCs are shown in Table 1.

Cell preparation

The experiments were carried out within 1 hour of obtaining the heparinized venous blood samples from the participants. For analysis of intracellular IL-21, 500 μl of whole blood from every sample was cultured in a complete culture medium (Roswell Park Memorial Institute (RPMI) 1640 supplemented with 10% heat-inactivated fetal calf serum) for 5 h, in the presence of phorbol 12-myristate 13-acetate (PMA, 50 ng/ml, Sigma-Aldrich, St. Louis, MO, USA), ionomycin, calcium salt (1 μg/ml, Sigma-Aldrich), and monensin (BD GolgiStop™, 1 μg/ml, BD Biosciences, San Diego, CA, USA). The incubators were set at 37 °C under a 5% CO_2 environment. The remaining unstimulated whole blood was aliquoted into tubes (50 μl each) for further analysis of PD-1, ICOS, Tfr, and pSTAT3.

Flow cytometry

The monoclonal antibodies targeting human CD3 (clone SP34–2, peridin chlorophyll protein (PerCP)), CD4 (clone SK3, fluorescein isothiocyanate (FITC)), IL-21 (clone 3A3-N2.1, phycoerythrin (PE)), and pSTAT3 (clone 4/ P-STAT3, PE) were all purchased from BD Biosciences; PD-1 (clone MIH4, PE), ICOS (clone ISA-3, PE), and Foxp3 (clone 236A/E7, PE) were all from eBioscience (San Diego, CA, USA); and CXCR5 (clone J252D4, APC) was from BioLegend (San Diego, CA, USA). Appropriate isotype controls were used to enable correct compensation and confirm antibody specificity. For PD-1 and ICOS analysis, 50 μl of unstimulated cells were incubated with surface-staining antibodies (CD3-PerCP, CD4-FITC, CXCR5- allophycocyanin (APC), and PD-1-PE or ICOS-PE) at 4 °C for 30 min in the dark. To detect intracellular IL-21 and Tfr cells (defined as $CD4^+$ $CXCR5^+Foxp3^+$ T cells), 50 μl stimulated (for IL-21 detection) and 50 μl unstimulated cells (for Tfr detection) were incubated with surface-staining antibodies (CD3-PerCP, CD4-FITC, and CXCR5-APC) at 4 °C for 30 min in the dark. Surface-stained cells were fixed and permeabilized with a Foxp3 Staining Set (eBioscience) and stained with PE-conjugated IL-21 or PE-conjugated Foxp3. For pSTAT3 analysis, 50 μl of unstimulated cells were incubated with surface-staining antibodies (CD4-FITC and CXCR5-APC) at 4 °C for 30 min in the dark. Then, 20 μg/ml recombinant human (rh) IL-6 (MN 550071) was added to stimulate the 50-μl surface-stained whole blood for 30 min at 37 °C in the dark. Stimulated cells were lysed and fixed with Lyse/ Fix buffer (BD Biosciences) at 37 °C for 10 min and then permeabilized in Perm Buffer III (BD Biosciences) for 30 min on ice. Finally, the cells were stained with PE-conjugated pSTAT3 (pY705) and PerCP-conjugated CD3 at 4 °C for 30 min in the dark, after washing twice with BD Pharmingen stain BSA buffer (BD Biosciences).

Stained cells were run on a FACSCanto II cytometer (BD Biosciences), and the data were analyzed using FACSDiva software (BD Biosciences).

Determination of serum IL-6

Serum samples were collected on the day of flow cytometry and stored at – 80 °C before detection. The concentration of serum IL-6 was quantified by ECLIA using the Cobas e601 (Roche) instrument, following the standard operating procedure (SOP) of the Department of Laboratory Medicine in West China Hospital of Sichuan University. Results are expressed as picograms per milliliter.

Statistical analysis

Summary statistics (number and percentage or median and interquartile range (IQR)) were used to describe the participants' baseline characteristics. Numerical results were expressed as mean ± SEM or median (IQR), and analyzed using the IBM SPSS software (version 22.0; IBM Corp., Armonk, NY, USA). The significance level was set at 0.05 for all statistical tests. The data were initially analyzed using analysis of variance or the Kruskal-Wallis H test. If a significant result was observed, Holm-Sidak's test or Dunn's test was used to detect inter-group differences. Spearman's correlation coefficient with the two-tailed P value was calculated to test for correlation between pairs of continuous variables.

Results

Frequencies of circulating Tfh and Tfr cells in patients with RA and the HCs

To investigate the status of circulating Tfh and Tfr cells, we detected the frequencies of CD4$^+$CXCR5$^+$Foxp3$^-$ Tfh and CD4$^+$CXCR5$^+$Foxp3$^+$ Tfr cells, which were gated from CD3$^+$CD4$^+$ T cells in a flow cytometry analysis of patients with RA and HCs (Additional file 1: Figure S1A, B). According to the DAS28-CRP score, patients with RA were divided into two groups: the active RA group ($n = 20$) with DAS28-CRP > 3.2 and the inactive RA group ($n = 24$) with DAS28-CRP ≤ 3.2.

Frequencies of circulating Tfh cells in patients with active RA (25.0 ± 1.6%) were significantly higher than those either in patients with inactive RA (18.4 ± 1.1%) or in HCs (18.2 ± 1.3%) ($P < 0.01$, Fig. 1a). Compared to the HC group (2.0 ± 0.2%), frequencies of peripheral Tfr cells were significantly lower in both the active RA (0.9 ± 0.1%) and inactive RA groups (1.2 ± 0.2%) ($P < 0.05$). However, there was no obvious difference between the two RA groups ($P > 0.05$) (Fig. 1b). In addition, the active RA group had the highest ratios of Tfh cells to Tfr cells (36.5 ± 5.6%), followed by the inactive RA group (23.6 ± 3.2%) and the control group (10.2 ± 0.8%) ($P < 0.05$, Fig. 1c).

Expression of PD-1, ICOS, intracellular IL-21 or pSTAT3 in circulating Tfh cells of patients with RA and the HCs

CD4$^+$CXCR5$^+$ T cell gating allowed us to investigate the expression of PD-1, ICOS, IL-21, or pSTAT3 (Additional file 2: Figure S2A-D). As shown in Fig. 2, the expression of PD-1 and IL-21 in either the active RA group (31.5 ± 2.1% and 4.9 ± 0.6%, respectively) or inactive RA group (26.5 ± 2.5% and 4.5 ± 0.5%, respectively) was significantly higher than that in the HCs (13.4 ± 0.8% and 2.7 ± 0.3%, respectively) ($P < 0.05$, Fig. 2a and c), while there was no difference observed in ICOS expression in circulating CD4$^+$CXCR5$^+$ T cells among the three groups (active RA, 15.5 ± 2.3%; inactive RA, 13.2 ± 1.2%; HCs, 12.3 ± 1.0%; $P > 0.05$, Fig. 2b). The expression of pSTAT3 in CD4$^+$CXCR5$^+$ Tfh cells was highest in the active RA group (51.3 ± 3.4%), followed by that in the inactive RA group (39.3 ± 1.9%) and the control group (29.7 ± 1.7%) ($P < 0.05$, Fig. 2d).

Concentration of serum IL-6 in patients with RA and the HCs

Significantly elevated serum IL-6 levels were observed in patients with RA compared with the control group (1.7 (1.6–2.6) pg/ml, $P < 0.001$), and the difference in levels in the two RA groups (active RA group, 27.6

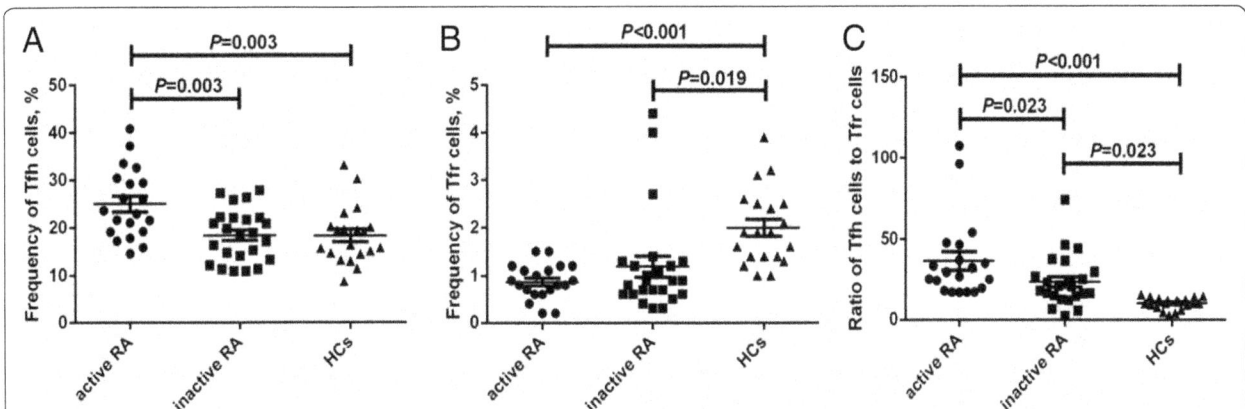

Fig. 1 Frequencies of circulating follicular helper T (Tfh) and follicular regulatory T (Tfr) cells in patients with rheumatoid arthritis (RA) and the healthy controls (HCs). Horizontal bars indicate the mean and error bars represent the SEM. The frequencies of circulating CD4$^+$CXCR5$^+$Foxp3$^-$ Tfh cells (**a**) and CD4$^+$CXCR5$^+$Foxp3$^+$ Tfr cells (**b**) were investigated gating on CD4$^+$ T cells in patients with active RA (circles), patients with inactive RA (squares), and the HCs (triangles). **c** Ratios of Tfh to Tfr cells in patients with active RA (circles), patients with inactive RA (squares), and the HCs (triangles)

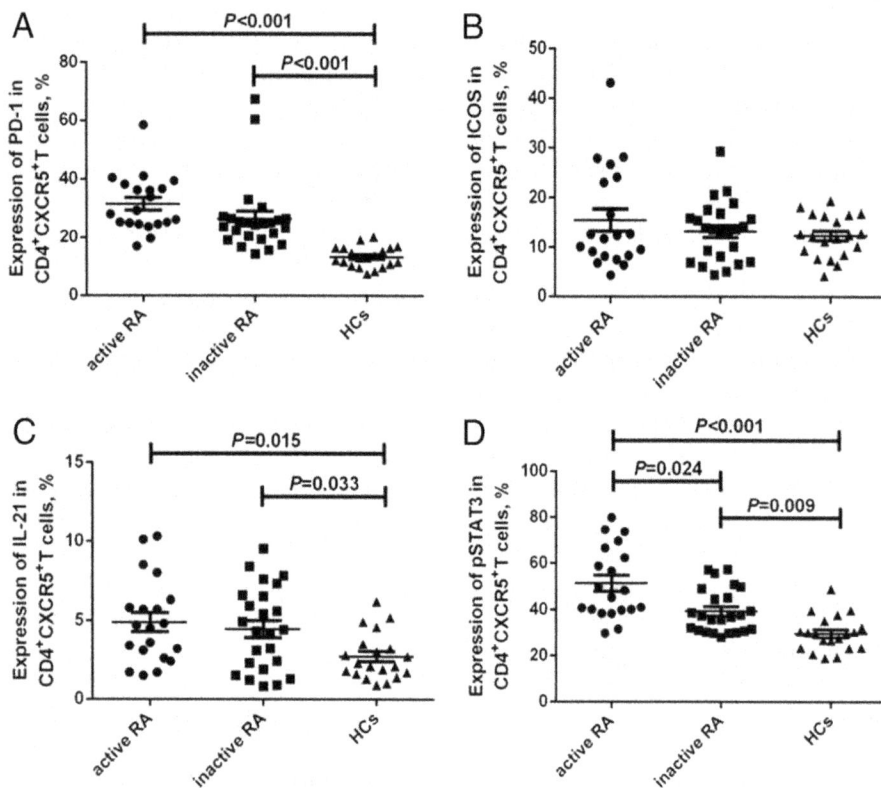

Fig. 2 Expression of programmed death-1 (PD-1), ICOS, intracellular IL-21 or pSTAT3 in circulating CD4⁺CXCR5⁺ follicular helper T (Tfh) cells of patients with rheumatoid arthritis (RA) and the healthy controls (HCs). Horizontal bars indicate the mean and error bars represent the SEM. The expression of PD-1 (**a**), inducible co-stimulator (ICOS) (**b**), intracellular IL-21 (**c**) or phosphorylated STAT3 (pSTAT3) (**d**) was investigated gating on CD4⁺CXCR5⁺ T cells in patients with active RA (circles), patients with inactive RA (squares), and the HCs (triangles)

(12.0–51.4) pg/ml; inactive RA group, 7.7 (3.2–15.0) pg/ml) was also significant ($P < 0.01$) (Fig. 3, IL-6 levels are shown on a logarithmic scale).

Correlation between pSTAT3 expression and serum IL-6 level
There was positive correlation between pSTAT3 expression and serum IL-6 level ($r = 0.425$, $P = 0.005$, Fig. 4).

Correlation between pSTAT3 expression and circulating Tfh or Tfr cell frequency
As shown in Fig. 5, there was positive correlation between pSTAT3 expression and circulating Tfh cell frequency ($r = 0.477$, $P = 0.001$). However, there was no correlation between pSTAT3 expression and either Tfr frequency or Tfh/Tfr ratio ($P > 0.05$).

Correlation between the frequencies of circulating Tfh or Tfr cells and the DAS28-CRP
The frequency of circulating Tfr cells was negatively correlated with the DAS28-CRP ($r = -0.337$, $P = 0.025$, Fig. 6a), while the ratio of Tfh cells to Tfr cells was positively correlated with the DAS28-CRP ($r = 0.510$, $P < 0.001$, Fig. 6b). However, there was no correlation between Tfh frequency and the DAS28-CRP ($P > 0.05$).

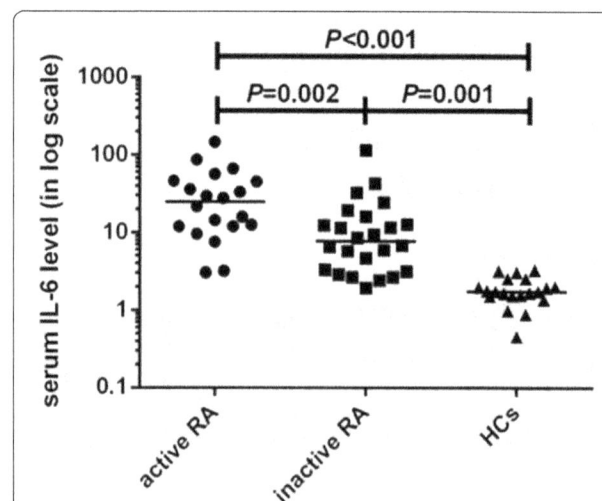

Fig. 3 Serum IL-6 levels in patients with active rheumatoid arthritis (RA) (circles), patients with inactive RA (squares), and the healthy controls (HCs) (triangles). IL-6 levels (pg/ml) are shown in a log scale. Horizontal bars indicate the median

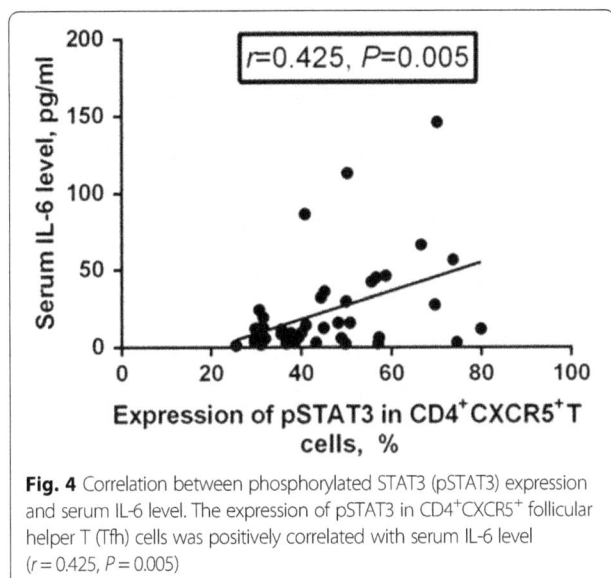

Fig. 4 Correlation between phosphorylated STAT3 (pSTAT3) expression and serum IL-6 level. The expression of pSTAT3 in CD4+CXCR5+ follicular helper T (Tfh) cells was positively correlated with serum IL-6 level ($r = 0.425$, $P = 0.005$)

Correlation between PD-1, ICOS, or IL-21 expression and the DAS28-CRP

PD-1 expression was positively correlated with the DAS28-CRP ($r = 0.323$, $P = 0.033$, Fig. 7), while neither ICOS expression nor IL-21 expression were correlated with the DAS28-CRP ($P > 0.05$).

Discussion

Blood CD4+CXCR5+ T cells may, to some extent, represent the circulating counter-part of memory Tfh cells [13], and additional molecular markers, i.e., PD-1 and ICOS, could be used to identify the activation status of Tfh cells [6]. PD-1 supports the survival of B cells and formation of plasma cells by interacting with PD-L1 and

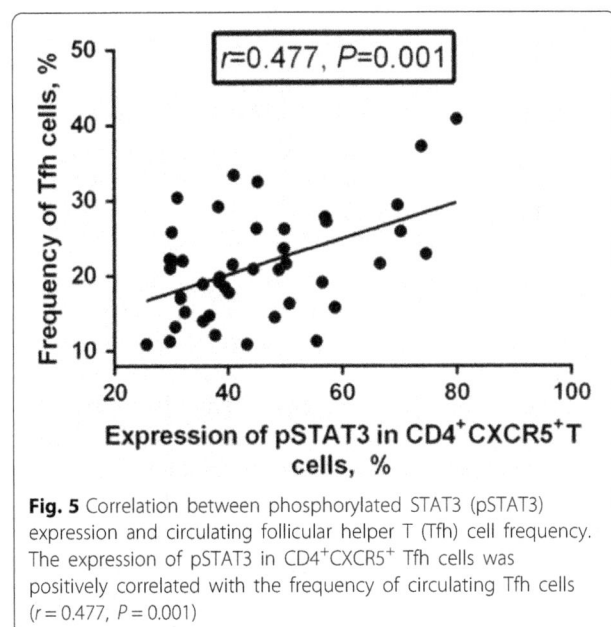

Fig. 5 Correlation between phosphorylated STAT3 (pSTAT3) expression and circulating follicular helper T (Tfh) cell frequency. The expression of pSTAT3 in CD4+CXCR5+ Tfh cells was positively correlated with the frequency of circulating Tfh cells ($r = 0.477$, $P = 0.001$)

PD-L2 on GC B cells [26], whereas ICOS can positively regulate humoral responses and IL-21 production [27]. In this study, we revealed that in both the active and inactive RA groups, the expression of PD-1 in Tfh cells was significantly higher than that in the HC group, and was positively correlated with the DAS28-CRP score. Although the expression of ICOS in Tfh cells was a little higher in patients with RA than in HCs, the difference was not significant. These findings suggest that enhanced expression of PD-1, but not ICOS, in Tfh cells might be involved in the development and progression of RA, and be of potential value as an indicator and therapeutic target of RA.

However, the inhibitory function of PD-1 on T cells and B cells, which is important in peripheral tolerance, cannot be ignored [28]. The up-regulated expression of PD-1 in Tfh cells in patients with RA, as observed in this study, might result from spontaneous compensatory regulation of the immune system so that PD-1+ Tfh cells can negatively regulate autoimmune responses in patients with RA. Actually, increased expression of PD-1 has been detected in human synovial tissue and fluid in RA, which might reflect the negative feedback regulation of inflammation in the joints [29]. Therefore, elucidation of the influence of enhanced PD-1 expression in Tfh cells in the development of RA would require further study.

Tfh cells secrete IL-21, a cytokine that has been found to not only promote naive T cell differentiation into potent B helper cells, but also to promote GC B cell responses through CD-40 L/CD-40 interaction [14]. Moreover, Tfh cells regulate B cell proliferation, differentiation, and antibody production via the secretion of IL-21 [13, 30]. To further understand the ability of peripheral Tfh cells to produce IL-21, we detected the expression of intracellular IL-21 in Tfh cells in patients with RA. The results showed that the expression of IL-21 in Tfh cells was significantly higher in patients with RA than in HCs, but was not correlated with the DAS28-CRP, indicating the augmented capacity of circulating Tfh cells to secrete IL-21 in patients with RA and increased potency to promote B cell proliferation, differentiation, and antibody production. Reportedly, exposure of CD4+ T cells to IL-21 drives them to differentiate into a Tfh cell subset partly through modulation of the expression of CXCR5 and CCR7 by IL-21 in an autocrine manner [31, 32]. However, there was no correlation between IL-21 expression with Tfh cell frequency in the present study. Actually, in addition to IL-21, numerous other cytokines, including IL-6, IL-12, and TGF-β, also reportedly contribute to Tfh cell differentiation [33].

Tfr cells express Foxp3 and have been identified to be involved in regulating the GC reaction [19]. Given that Tfh and Tfr cells have opposite roles in regulating GC responses, balance of their activities is critical for

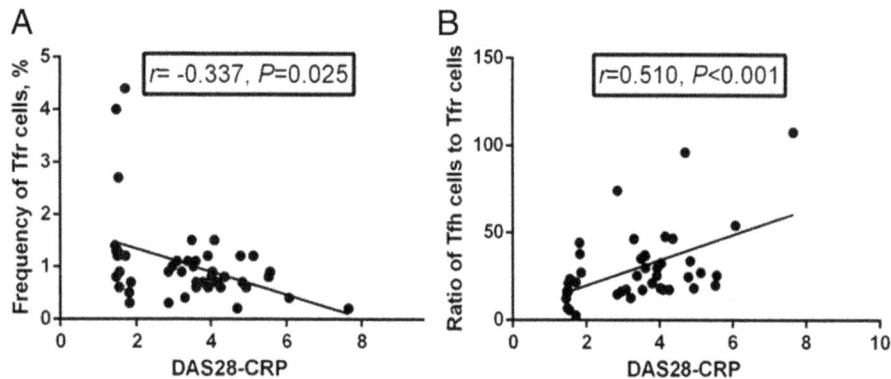

Fig. 6 Correlation between circulating follicular helper T (Tfh) or follicular regulatory T (Tfr) cell frequency and the Disease Activity Score in 28 joints based on C-reactive protein (DAS28-CRP). The circulating Tfr cell frequency was negatively correlated with DAS28-CRP ($r = -0.337$, $P = 0.025$) (**a**), while the Tfh/Tfr ratio was positively correlated with DAS28-CRP ($r = 0.510$, $P < 0.001$) (**b**)

immune homeostasis. An impaired Tfr compartment could enhance Tfh activity, resulting in the expansion of auto-reactive B cells and autoantibody production [34]. The dysregulation of Tfh and Tfr cells has been reported to contribute to the development of many autoimmune diseases, including experimental autoimmune myasthenia gravis (EAMG) [35] and multiple sclerosis [24]. In this study, we presented evidence of imbalances between the circulating Tfh cell subsets and Tfr cells in patients with RA. Inconsistent with the report by Pandya JM et al. [36], we found a significant decrease in Tfr cell frequency in patients with RA, while Pandya JM et al. did not identify a significant difference in Tfr cell frequency between patients with early RA and HCs. The inconsistency between the results of Pandya JM et al. and ours might be attributed to the different symptom duration in the patients with RA enrolled in this study compared to

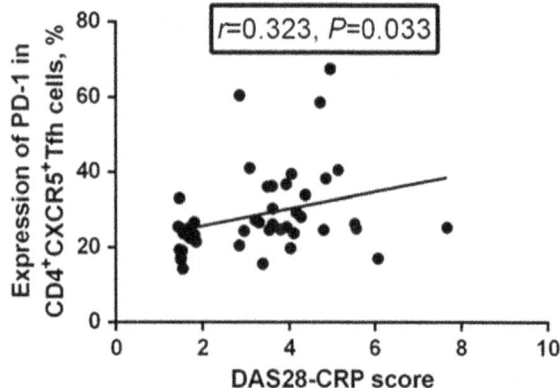

Fig. 7 Correlation between programmed death-1 (PD-1) expression and the Disease Activity Score in 28 joints based on C-reactive protein (DAS28-CRP). The expression of PD-1 in $CD4^+CXCR5^+$ follicular helper T (Tfh) cells was positively correlated with DAS28-CRP ($r = 0.323$, $P = 0.033$)

those in the previous study. The median symptom duration in all included patients with RA was 13 months in this study, whereas it was 6 months (suggesting a very early stage of RA) in Pandya's study.

Patients with active RA had marginally lower Tfr cell frequency than patients with inactive RA, but the difference was not significant. In spite of this, negative correlation was identified between the frequency of circulating Tfr cells and disease activity (DAS28-CRP). With the increased proportion of Tfh subsets and decreased percentage of Tfr cells, ratios of Tfh/Tfr were significantly increased in patients with RA, although no differences in the ratios were found between patients with active RA and those with inactive RA. In addition, Tfh/Tfr ratio was positively correlated with the DAS28-CRP. These results suggested that the imbalance of Tfh and Tfr cells might contribute to the breakdown of self-tolerance in RA, thus serving as a potential target for therapy and a meaningful tool for disease evaluation.

STAT3 has been reported as a positive regulator of Tfh cell differentiation. Mice with STAT3 deficiency or humans with functional STAT3 impairment have been reported to have reduced numbers of Tfh cells and an attenuated B cell response [37, 38]. Phosphorylation of STAT3, a marker of the activation of STAT3 pathways, has been reported to be activated mainly by IL-6, which induces Tfh differentiation and IL-21 production [38, 39]. In the present study, we observed significantly up-regulated expression of pSTAT3 in peripheral Tfh cells, as expected after being stimulated with IL-6, and significantly increased serum IL-6, especially in patients with active RA. Meanwhile, there was positive correlation between pSTAT3 expression and serum IL-6, which was consistent with the research of Deng et al. [40]. Further analysis revealed that pSTAT3 expression was positively correlated with circulating Tfh cell frequency, but there was no correlation between pSTAT3 expression and Tfh/Tfr ratio. Taken together, these results demonstrated that elevated serum IL-6 might be pivotal in promoting the imbalance of Tfh and Tfr cells in patients with RA, via activation of the STAT3 signaling pathway by induction of pSTAT3, so as to participate in the development and progression of RA.

Of note, although positive correlation was identified between the expression of pSTAT3 and circulating Tfh cell frequency, there was no correlation between pSTAT3 expression and PD-1, ICOS, or IL-21 expression. These results suggested that the up-regulated expression of pSTAT3 might mainly contribute to the increase in Tfh cell frequency but had no obvious effects on the expression of PD-1, ICOS, or IL-21 in Tfh cells in RA.

Despite all the important findings of this study, there are some limitations as well. In addition to PD-1 and ICOS, the chemokine receptors CXCR3 and CCR6 are also commonly used markers that define Tfh subsets, namely Tfh1, Tfh2, and Tfh17 [41]. These Tfh subsets are reported to exert different helper functions to B cells, which makes their exploration highly significant; these will be pursued in our future studies.

Conclusions
To the best of our knowledge, this is the first report to demonstrate the imbalance of Tfh subsets and Tfr cells in patients with RA. Increased Tfh cell percentages and decreased Tfr cell frequencies resulted in elevated Tfh/Tfr ratios. Augmented capacity of the circulating Tfh cells to secrete IL-21 and imbalance of Tfh/Tfr cells might contribute to the breakdown of self-tolerance in RA, and thus serve as a potential target for therapy and a meaningful tool for disease evaluation. Enhanced IL-6/pSTAT3 signaling might be potent in promoting the Tfh/Tfr imbalance, mainly via promotion of Tfh cells, and the immunopathogenesis of RA.

Abbreviations
ACPA: anti-citrullinated peptide antibodies; ACR: American College of Rheumatology; AS: Ankylosing spondylitis; CD40L: CD40 ligand; CRP: C-reactive protein; CXCR5: C-X-C chemokine receptor type 5; DAS28: Disease Activity Score in 28 joints; EAMG: Experimental autoimmune myasthenia gravis; EULAR: European League Against Rheumatism; GC: Germinal centers; HCs: Healthy controls; ICOS: Inducible co-stimulator; IL-21: Interleukin-21; IQR: Interquartile range; MG: Myasthenia gravis; MS: Multiple sclerosis; PD-1: Programmed death-1; pSTAT3: Phosphorylated signal transducer and activator of transcription; RA: Rheumatoid arthritis; RF: Rheumatoid factor; SLE: Systemic lupus erythematosus; Tfh cell: Follicular helper T cell; Tfr cell: Follicular regulatory T cell; Tregs: Regulatory T cells

Acknowledgements
We thank the patients for donating samples, and the hospital staff for making the study possible. This research was sponsored by the National Natural Science Foundation of China (number 81501816, 81772258, 81301496, 81601830).

Funding
This research was sponsored by the National Natural Science Foundation of China (number 81501816, 81772258, 81601830, 81301496). The funders had no role in study design, data collection and analysis, decision to publish, or preparation of the manuscript.

Authors' contributions
QN participated in the design of the study, data analysis and interpretation, statistical analysis, and writing of the manuscript. ZCH participated in the design of the research, statistical analysis, and writing of the manuscript. XJW participated in the performance of the research and revising of the manuscript. YXJ and YFA participated in the performance of the research and statistical analysis. YML and HX participated in the collection of samples and clinical data. BY and LLW participated in study design and revising of the manuscript. All authors have approved the final version of the manuscript.

Consent for publication
Not applicable.

Competing interests
The authors declare that they have no competing interests.

References
1. McInnes IB, Schett G. The pathogenesis of rheumatoid arthritis. N Engl J Med. 2011;365(23):2205–19.
2. Klareskog L, Catrina AI, Paget S. Rheumatoid arthritis. Lancet (London, England). 2009;373(9664):659–72.
3. Firestein GS. The disease formerly known as rheumatoid arthritis. Arthritis Res Ther. 2014;16(3):114.
4. Conigliaro P, Chimenti MS, Triggianese P, Sunzini F, Novelli L, Perricone C, Perricone R. Autoantibodies in inflammatory arthritis. Autoimmun Rev. 2016;15(7):673–83.
5. Moschovakis GL, Bubke A, Friedrichsen M, Falk CS, Feederle R, Forster R. T cell specific Cxcr5 deficiency prevents rheumatoid arthritis. Sci Rep. 2017;7(1):8933.
6. Ueno H. T follicular helper cells in human autoimmunity. Curr Opin Immunol. 2016;43:24–31.
7. Liu X, Nurieva RI, Dong C. Transcriptional regulation of follicular T-helper (Tfh) cells. Immunol Rev. 2013;252(1):139–45.
8. Fazilleau N, Mark L, McHeyzer-Williams LJ, McHeyzer-Williams MG. Follicular helper T cells: lineage and location. Immunity. 2009;30(3):324–35.
9. Le Coz C, Joublin A, Pasquali JL, Korganow AS, Dumortier H, Monneaux F. Circulating TFH subset distribution is strongly affected in lupus patients with an active disease. PLoS One. 2013;8(9):e75319.
10. Xiao F, Zhang HY, Liu YJ, Zhao D, Shan YX, Jiang YF. Higher frequency of peripheral blood interleukin 21 positive follicular helper T cells in patients with ankylosing spondylitis. J Rheumatol. 2013;40(12):2029–37.
11. Wang J, Shan Y, Jiang Z, Feng J, Li C, Ma L, Jiang Y. High frequencies of activated B cells and T follicular helper cells are correlated with disease activity in patients with new-onset rheumatoid arthritis. Clin Exp Immunol. 2013;174(2):212–20.
12. Vinuesa CG, Cook MC. Blood relatives of follicular helper T cells. Immunity. 2011;34(1):10–2.
13. Morita R, Schmitt N, Bentebibel SE, Ranganathan R, Bourdery L, Zurawski G, Foucat E, Dullaers M, Oh S, Sabzghabaei N, et al. Human blood CXCR5(+)CD4(+) T cells are counterparts of T follicular cells and contain specific subsets that differentially support antibody secretion. Immunity. 2011;34(1):108–21.
14. Yu M, Cavero V, Lu Q, Li H. Follicular helper T cells in rheumatoid arthritis. Clin Rheumatol. 2015;34(9):1489–93.
15. Chavele KM, Merry E, Ehrenstein MR. Cutting edge: circulating plasmablasts induce the differentiation of human T follicular helper cells via IL-6 production. J Immunol (Baltimore, Md : 1950). 2015;194(6):2482–5.
16. Aggarwal BB, Kunnumakkara AB, Harikumar KB, Gupta SR, Tharakan ST, Koca C, Dey S, Sung B. Signal transducer and activator of transcription-3, inflammation, and cancer: how intimate is the relationship? Ann N Y Acad Sci. 2009;1171:59–76.
17. Niu Q, Cai B, Huang ZC, Shi YY, Wang LL. Disturbed Th17/Treg balance in patients with rheumatoid arthritis. Rheumatol Int. 2012;32(9):2731–6.
18. Linterman MA, Pierson W, Lee SK, Kallies A, Kawamoto S, Rayner TF, Srivastava M, Divekar DP, Beaton L, Hogan JJ, et al. Foxp3+ follicular regulatory T cells control the germinal center response. Nat Med. 2011;17(8):975–82.
19. Gong Y, Tong J, Wang S. Are follicular regulatory T cells involved in autoimmune diseases? Front Immunol. 2017;8:1790.
20. Sage PT, Sharpe AH. T follicular regulatory cells. Immunol Rev. 2016;271(1):246–59.

21. Sage PT, Sharpe AH. T follicular regulatory cells in the regulation of B cell responses. Trends Immunol. 2015;36(7):410–8.
22. Xu B, Wang S, Zhou M, Huang Y, Fu R, Guo C, Chen J, Zhao J, Gaskin F, Fu SM, et al. The ratio of circulating follicular T helper cell to follicular T regulatory cell is correlated with disease activity in systemic lupus erythematosus. Clin Immunol (Orlando, Fla). 2017;183:46–53.
23. Wen Y, Yang B, Lu J, Zhang J, Yang H, Li J. Imbalance of circulating CD4(+)CXCR5(+)FOXP3(+) Tfr-like cells and CD4(+)CXCR5(+)FOXP3(−) Tfh-like cells in myasthenia gravis. Neurosci Lett. 2016;630:176–82.
24. Dhaeze T, Peelen E, Hombrouck A, Peeters L, Van Wijmeersch B, Lemkens N, Lemkens P, Somers V, Lucas S, Broux B, et al. Circulating follicular regulatory T cells are defective in multiple sclerosis. J Immunol (Baltimore, Md : 1950). 2015;195(3):832–40.
25. Aletaha D, Neogi T, Silman AJ, Funovits J, Felson DT, Bingham CO 3rd, Birnbaum NS, Burmester GR, Bykerk VP, Cohen MD, et al. 2010 Rheumatoid arthritis classification criteria: an American College of Rheumatology/European league against rheumatism collaborative initiative. Arthritis Rheum. 2010;62(9):2569–81.
26. Yao S, Chen L. PD-1 as an immune modulatory receptor. Cancer J (Sudbury, Mass). 2014;20(4):262–4.
27. Bauquet AT, Jin H, Paterson AM, Mitsdoerffer M, Ho IC, Sharpe AH, Kuchroo VK. The costimulatory molecule ICOS regulates the expression of c-Maf and IL-21 in the development of follicular T helper cells and TH-17 cells. Nat Immunol. 2009;10(2):167–75.
28. Riley JL, June CH. The CD28 family: a T-cell rheostat for therapeutic control of T-cell activation. Blood. 2005;105(1):13–21.
29. Raptopoulou AP, Bertsias G, Makrygiannakis D, Verginis P, Kritikos I, Tzardi M, Klareskog L, Catrina AI, Sidiropoulos P, Boumpas DT. The programmed death 1/programmed death ligand 1 inhibitory pathway is up-regulated in rheumatoid synovium and regulates peripheral T cell responses in human and murine arthritis. Arthritis Rheum. 2010;62(7):1870–80.
30. Bryant VL, Ma CS, Avery DT, Li Y, Good KL, Corcoran LM, de Waal MR, Tangye SG. Cytokine-mediated regulation of human B cell differentiation into Ig-secreting cells: predominant role of IL-21 produced by CXCR5+ T follicular helper cells. J Immunol (Baltimore, Md: 1950). 2007;179(12):8180–90.
31. Vogelzang A, McGuire HM, Yu D, Sprent J, Mackay CR, King C. A fundamental role for interleukin-21 in the generation of T follicular helper cells. Immunity. 2008;29(1):127–37.
32. Nurieva RI, Chung Y, Hwang D, Yang XO, Kang HS, Ma L, Wang YH, Watowich SS, Jetten AM, Tian Q, et al. Generation of T follicular helper cells is mediated by interleukin-21 but independent of T helper 1, 2, or 17 cell lineages. Immunity. 2008;29(1):138–49.
33. Yan L, de Leur K, Hendriks RW, van der Laan LJW, Shi Y, Wang L, Baan CC. T follicular helper cells as a new target for immunosuppressive therapies. Front Immunol. 2017;8:1510.
34. Jiang H, Cui N, Yang L, Liu C, Yue L, Guo L, Wang H, Shao Z. Altered follicular helper T cell impaired antibody production in a murine model of myelodysplastic syndromes. Oncotarget. 2017;8(58):98270–9.
35. Xie X, Mu L, Yao X, Li N, Sun B, Li Y, Zhan X, Wang X, Kang X, Wang J, et al. ATRA alters humoral responses associated with amelioration of EAMG symptoms by balancing Tfh/Tfr helper cell profiles. Clin Immunol (Orlando, Fla). 2013;148(2):162–76.
36. Pandya JM, Lundell AC, Hallstrom M, Andersson K, Nordstrom I, Rudin A. Circulating T helper and T regulatory subsets in untreated early rheumatoid arthritis and healthy control subjects. J Leukoc Biol. 2016;100(4):823–33.
37. Ma CS, Avery DT, Chan A, Batten M, Bustamante J, Boisson-Dupuis S, Arkwright PD, Kreins AY, Averbuch D, Engelhard D, et al. Functional STAT3 deficiency compromises the generation of human T follicular helper cells. Blood. 2012;119(17):3997–4008.
38. Eddahri F, Denanglaire S, Bureau F, Spolski R, Leonard WJ, Leo O, Andris F. Interleukin-6/STAT3 signaling regulates the ability of naive T cells to acquire B-cell help capacities. Blood. 2009;113(11):2426–33.
39. Wang M, Wei J, Li H, Ouyang X, Sun X, Tang Y, Chen H, Wang B, Li X. Leptin upregulates peripheral CD4(+)CXCR5(+)ICOS(+) T cells via increased IL-6 in rheumatoid arthritis patients. J Interf Cytokine Res. 2018;38(2):86–92.
40. Deng J, Fan C, Gao X, Zeng Q, Guo R, Wei Y, Chen Z, Chen Y, Gong D, Feng J, et al. Signal transducer and activator of transcription 3 hyperactivation associates with follicular helper T cell differentiation and disease activity in rheumatoid arthritis. Front Immunol. 2018;9:1226.
41. Schmitt N, Bentebibel SE, Ueno H. Phenotype and functions of memory Tfh cells in human blood. Trends Immunol. 2014;35(9):436–42.

3

BATF regulates collagen-induced arthritis by regulating T helper cell differentiation

Sang-Heon Park[1†], Jinseol Rhee[2†], Seul-Ki Kim[1], Jung-Ah Kang[1], Ji-Sun Kwak[1], Young-Ok Son[1], Wan-Su Choi[1], Sung-Gyoo Park[1] and Jang-Soo Chun[1*] (iD)

Abstract

Background: We recently demonstrated that BATF, a member of the activator protein-1 (AP-1) family, regulates osteoarthritic cartilage destruction. Here, we explored the roles and regulatory mechanisms of BATF in collagen-induced arthritis (CIA) in mice.

Methods: CIA and K/BxN serum transfer were used to generate inflammatory arthritis models in wild-type (WT) and *Batf*[−/−] mice. RA manifestations were determined by examining CIA incidence, clinical score, synovitis, synovial hyperplasia, angiogenesis in inflamed synovium, pannus formation, bone erosion, and cartilage destruction. Immune features in RA were analyzed by examining immune cell populations and cytokine production.

Results: BATF was upregulated in the synovial tissues of joints in which inflammatory arthritis had been caused by CIA or K/BxN serum transfer. The increases in CIA incidence, clinical score, and autoantibody production in CIA-induced WT mice were completely abrogated in the corresponding *Batf*[−/−] DBA/1 J mice. Genetic ablation of *Batf* also inhibited CIA-induced synovitis, synovial hyperplasia, angiogenesis in synovial tissues, pannus formation, bone erosion, and cartilage destruction. *Batf* knockout inhibited the differentiation of T helper (Th)17 cells and the conversion of CD4$^+$Foxp3$^+$ cells to CD4$^+$IL-17$^+$ cells. However, BATF did not modulate the functions of fibroblast-like synoviocytes (FLS), including the expressions of chemokines, matrix-degrading enzymes, vascular endothelial growth factor, and receptor activator of NF-κB ligand (RANKL).

Conclusion: Our findings indicate that BATF crucially mediates CIA by regulating Th cell differentiation without directly affecting the functions of FLS.

Keywords: BATF (basic leucine zipper transcription factor, ATF-like), Th cells, Collagen-induced arthritis, Fibroblast-like synoviocytes (FLS), Cartilage, Bone

Background

BATF (basic leucine zipper transcription factor, ATF-like) is a member of the activator protein-1 (AP-1) family whose members regulate various biological functions [1–3]. BATF, which lacks a transactivation domain, heterodimerizes with JUN to bind the AP-1 site for transcriptional regulation [3, 4]. We recently demonstrated that BATF regulates osteoarthritis (OA) in mice by modulating anabolic and catabolic gene expression in chondrocytes [4]. We found that overexpression of BATF upregulated matrix-degrading enzymes and downregulated cartilage

matrix molecules; we also found that BATF expression in mouse joint tissues promoted OA cartilage destruction and that, conversely, knockout of *Batf* in mice (*Batf*[−/−]) suppressed experimental OA [4].

OA and rheumatoid arthritis (RA), which are the most common types of joint arthritis, share certain phenotypic features, such as cartilage destruction [5]. However, these diseases clearly differ in their etiologies, pathogenic mechanisms, and the cell types associated with each pathogenesis. OA is a degenerative joint disease that begins with the destruction of surface articular cartilage [6, 7]. Mechanical stresses (i.e., joint instability) and factors that predispose toward OA (i.e., aging) are important causes of OA pathogenesis [6, 7]. In contrast, RA is an inflammatory autoimmune disease that mainly targets

* Correspondence: jschun@gist.ac.kr
†Sang-Heon Park and Jinseol Rhee contributed equally to this work.
¹School of Life Sciences, Gwangju Institute of Science and Technology, Gwangju 61005, Republic of Korea
Full list of author information is available at the end of the article

the synovium, resulting in destruction of the joint architecture. Various cell types of joint tissues are associated with RA pathogenesis, including T cells, B cells, macrophages, synoviocytes, chondrocytes, and osteoclasts [8–10]. T cell-mediated autoimmune responses play a critical role in the RA pathogenesis, in which interleukin (IL)-17-producing T helper (Th) cells act as crucial effectors [8, 11, 12]. RA is characterized by synovitis with infiltration of immune cells, synovial hyperplasia that arises via proliferation of synovial cells, such as macrophage-like synoviocytes (MLS) and fibroblast-like synoviocytes (FLS), and angiogenesis in the hyperplastic synovium [8–10]. Synovial cells express numerous cytokines that have been implicated in many of the immune processes involved in RA [13]. RA manifestations also include erosion of the bone and cartilage which is caused by the formation of the pannus, which is an aggressive front of hyperplastic synovium. The pannus invades and destroys mineralized cartilage and bone through the action of osteoclasts [8–10].

BATF is known to regulate OA cartilage destruction, and we previously showed that BATF overexpression in joint tissues causes synovial inflammation [4] suggesting that BATF could contribute to inflammatory arthritis. This notion is supported by reports that proinflammatory cytokines, such as IL-1β and IL-6, increase BATF expression in naive CD4$^+$ T cells [14, 15], BATF directly regulates IL-17 expression, and *Batf*-deficient mice show resistance to experimental autoimmune encephalomyelitis [16]. BATF also controls the development of follicular Th cells (Tfh) and class-switch recombination in B cells [17]. Additionally, inhibition of the transcriptional activity of c-Fos/AP-1 suppresses arthritic joint destruction in a mouse RA model [18]. However, while these previous reports suggest that BATF may be involved in RA pathogenesis, the role of BATF and its regulatory mechanisms are not yet well understood.

In this study, we examined whether BATF is required for collagen-induced arthritis (CIA), which is a commonly used experimental model of inflammatory arthritis caused by a T cell-dependent, antibody-mediated autoimmune response directed against cartilage type II collagen [19]. Here, we show that genetic ablation of *Batf* in mice suppresses the manifestations of CIA, including synovitis, synovial hyperplasia, angiogenesis in the inflamed synovium, and cartilage/bone erosion in the joint tissues. We also reveal that BATF regulates CIA by regulating Th cell differentiation without directly affecting the functions of FLS.

Methods
Mice and experimental RA
Male wild-type (WT) and *Batf*$^{-/-}$ DBA/1 J mice were used to generate the CIA models. C57BL/6-background *Batf*$^{-/-}$ mice [4] were backcrossed with DBA/1 J mice to generate *Batf*$^{-/-}$ DBA/1 J mice. All mice were used in accordance

with protocols approved by the Animal Care and Ethics Committees of the Gwangju Institute of Science and Technology. CIA was induced by a standard protocol [19, 20]. Mice were intradermally injected with incomplete Freund's adjuvant alone (nonimmunized; NI) or Freund's adjuvant containing 100 μg collagen type II (CIA). A booster injection was given 21 days later. The incidence and severity of arthritis were evaluated on the indicated days after the first immunization. Severity was evaluated using a clinical score (grade 0–4) of paw swelling [19, 20]. Joint tissues were fixed, decalcified with 0.5 M EDTA, embedded in paraffin, and sectioned at 5-μm thickness. Synovitis was evaluated by hematoxylin and eosin (H&E) staining, and synovial inflammation (grade 0–4) was scored as previously described [19, 20]. The pannus was visualized by H&E staining and quantified by scoring (grade 0–4) [19, 20]. Cartilage destruction was examined by safranin-O staining and scored using the OARSI (Osteoarthritis Research Society International) grading system [4, 20]. Inflammatory arthritis was also induced by K/BxN serum transfer [21] in WT and *Batf*$^{-/-}$ C57BL/6 mice. Arthritic transgenic mice (K/BxN) and nontransgenic littermates (BxN) were generated by crossing KRN T cell receptor (TCR)-transgenic (K/B) mice with nonobese diabetic (NOD) mice. K/BxN and control sera were collected from K/BxN and BxN mice, respectively, and administered intraperitoneally to recipient mice on days 0 and 2. Mice were sacrificed on day 14 after serum transfer.

Immunohistochemistry, immunofluorescence microscopy, and tartrate-resistant acid phosphatase (TRAP) staining
Antigens were retrieved by incubating joint sections at 60 °C overnight with sodium citrate buffer (10 mM sodium citrate, 0.05% Tween 20, pH 6.0). The sections were blocked with 2% bovine serum albumin in phosphate-buffered saline (PBS), and then incubated with primary antibodies, including rabbit anti-BATF (Brookwood Biomedical), rabbit anti-RANKL (receptor activator of NF-κB ligand) (Abcam), goat anti-IL-6 (R&D Systems), rabbit anti-TNF-α (tumor necrosis factor alpha) (Novus Biologicals), and rabbit anti-Ki67 (Abcam). The Dako REAL Envision Detection system was used for chromogenic color development. BATF-expressing cells in synovial tissues were identified by double immunofluorescence labeling of vimentin for FLS, CD11b for macrophages, CD4 for T cells, and B220 for B cells. The following primary antibodies were used: mouse anti-CD4, mouse anti-B220, rat anti-CD11b (Abcam), rabbit anti-BATF (ThermoFisher Scientific), and mouse anti-vimentin (BD Pharmingen). Blood vessels in synovial tissues were detected with mouse anti-CD31 (Dianova). TRAP activity was determined in joint sections as previously described [20, 22], and the numbers of TRAP-positive osteoclasts were counted in

regions containing pannus-cartilage and pannus-bone interfaces.

FLS culture and proliferation assays

FLS were isolated from WT or *Batf* knockout (KO) mice and cultured as described by Zhao et al. [23]. FLS of passages 4–8 were used for further analysis. Pure FLS (> 90% CD90$^+$/< 1% CD14$^+$) were identified by flow cytometry using antibodies against CD90 and CD14 (Abcam). FLS proliferation in culture was quantified by measuring bromodeoxyuridine (BrdU) incorporation [20]. Briefly, FLS cultured in a 96-well plate were treated with or without tumor necrosis factor (TNF)-α (100 ng/ml), and BrdU labeling was detected using the cell proliferation enzyme-linked immunosorbent assay (ELISA) BrdU kit (Roche). Proliferating cells in synovial sections were identified by detecting Ki67 using an antibody obtained from Abcam. The empty adenovirus (Ad-C) and BATF-expressing adenovirus (Ad-*Batf*) were as previously described [4]. FLS were infected with Ad-*Batf* and Ad-C at the indicated multiplicities of infection (MOI) for 2 h, washed, and maintained for 48 h before analysis.

ELISA of autoantibody production

Collagen type II-specific antibodies were measured by ELISA [20]. Sera from NI and CIA mice were loaded to type II collagen-coated 96-well plates, incubated overnight at 4 °C, washed, and incubated for 1 h with alkaline phosphatase-labeled monoclonal antibodies against mouse IgG1, IgG2a, or IgG2b (Immunology Consultants Lab). *p*-Nitrophenyl phosphate was used as a substrate for chromogenic reactions, and the resulting color reaction was quantified using an ELISA plate reader.

RT-PCR, qRT-PCR, and Western blotting

Total RNA was isolated from cultured FLS using the TRI reagent. The isolated RNA was reverse-transcribed, and the resulting cDNA was used for RT-PCR. The PCR primers and experimental conditions were as previously described for BATF, matrix metalloproteinase (MMP)3, and MMP13 [4], as well as CCL2, CCL5, CXCL1, CXCL5, CXCL10, GAPDH, RANKL, and vascular endothelial growth factor (VEGF) [20]. For Western blotting, FLS cells were incubated on ice for 30 min with radioimmune precipitation assay buffer (10 mM sodium phosphate, pH 7.2, 150 mM NaCl, 1% SDS, 1% deoxycholate, 1% Nonidet P-40). Whole-cell lysates were fractionated by polyacrylamide gel electrophoresis and immunoblotted using rabbit anti-BATF (Brookwood Biomedical) and goat anti-Lamin B (Santa Cruz).

Flow cytometric analysis

Thymocytes, splenocytes, and lymphocytes were isolated from 6- to 8-week-old WT and *Batf*$^{-/-}$ mice as previously described [20]. For detection of cell surface antigens, cells (1 × 10^6) were labeled with fluorochrome-conjugated primary antibodies. For detection of intracellular antigens, surface-stained cells were fixed and permeabilized with a permeabilization buffer (eBioscience) or Foxp3/Transcription Factor Staining Buffer (eBioscience). The following antibodies were purchased from eBioscience for cell staining: Alexa Fluor 488®-conjugated anti-mouse CD4 and anti-mouse/rat Foxp3; FITC-conjugated anti-mouse TCRβ and anti-mouse CD8; PerCP Cy5.5-conjugated anti-mouse CD25, anti-mouse CD62L, and anti-mouse interferon (IFN)-γ; APC-conjugated anti-mouse CD4, anti-mouse B220, and anti-mouse IL-17A; PE-conjugated anti-human/mouse CD44, anti-mouse IL-4, anti-mouse CD25, and anti-mouse/rat Foxp3; and eFluor 450®-conjugated anti-mouse CD4, and PE-Cyanine7-conjugated anti-mouse CD4.

In-vitro differentiation of Th cells

CD4$^+$ T cell were isolated from the spleens of WT and *Batf*$^{-/-}$ mice using an EasySep™ Mouse CD4$^+$ T cell Isolation Kit (Stem Cell). The cells (2.5 × 10^5) were cultured for 120 h under Th cell-differentiating conditions [23]. Briefly, for in-vitro differentiation of CD4$^+$ T cells into Th1 cells, isolated cells were cultured with anti-mouse CD3 (5 µg/ml), anti-mouse CD28 (5 µg/ml), IL-12 (20 ng/ml), IL-2 (20 ng/ml), and anti-IL-4 (10 µg/ml). For in-vitro differentiation of CD4$^+$ T cells into Th2 cells, isolated cells were cultured with anti-mouse CD3 (5 µg/ml), anti-mouse CD28 (5 µg/ml), IL-4 (25 ng/ml), IL-2 (20 ng/ml), anti-IFN-γ (10 µg/ml), and anti-IL-12R (10 µg/ml). For in-vitro differentiation of CD4$^+$ T cells into Th17 cells, isolated cells were cultured with anti-mouse CD3 (5 µg/ml), anti-mouse CD28 (5 µg/ml), IL-6 (100 ng/ml), mouse-transforming growth factor (TGF)-β (5 ng/ml), anti-IFN-γ (10 µg/ml), and anti-IL-4 (10 µg/ml). For in-vitro differentiation of CD4$^+$ T cells into Treg cells, isolated cells were cultured with anti-mouse CD3 (5 µg/ml), anti-mouse CD28 (5 µg/ml), mouse-TGF-β (5 ng/ml), and IL-2 (20 ng/ml). After the Th cell differentiation, cytokine production was analyzed by flow cytometry analysis after activation with phorbol-12-myristate 13-acetate (PMA; 50 ng/ml), ionomycin (500 ng/ml), and Brefeldin A solution (eBioscience) for an additional 4 h. To test the plasticity of Treg cells to Th17 cells in vitro, isolated cells were cultured with anti-mouse CD3 (5 µg/ml), anti-mouse CD28 (5 µg/ml), mouse-TGF-β (5 ng/ml), and IL-2 (20 ng/ml) for 2 days. Then, the cells were washed and further incubated with anti-mouse CD3 (5 µg/ml), anti-mouse CD28 (5 µg/ml), IL-6 (100 ng/ml), mouse-TGF-β (5 ng/ml), anti-IFN-γ (10 µg/ml), and anti-IL-4 (10 µg/ml) for 3 days.

Cytokine analysis

For measurement of secreted cytokine levels, lymphocytes were isolated from the lymph nodes of CIA mice. Isolated lymphocytes (1×10^6) were cultured for 4 h with PMA (50 ng/ml) and ionomycin (500 ng/ml) [24]. The LEGEND MAX mouse IL-6 ELISA kit and mouse IL-13 Platinum ELISA kit (Invitrogen) were used to detect IL-6 and IL-10, respectively. The BD Cytometric Bead Array solution (BD Biosciences) and a FACS Canto II flow cytometer (BD Biosciences) were used to measure secreted cytokines such as IL-2, IL-4, IL-10, IL-17A, IFN-γ, and TNF-α.

Statistical analysis

The nonparametric Mann-Whitney U test was used for the analysis of data based on an ordinal grading system, such as the synovitis, pannus, and OARSI grades. For results obtained from ELISA and analyses of joint thickness, TRAP-positive cells, and BrdU incorporation, the data were first tested for conformation to a normal distribution using the Shapiro-Wilk test. The data were analyzed by the Student's t test (pair-wise comparisons) or analysis of variance (ANOVA) with post-hoc tests (multi-comparisons) as appropriate. Significance was accepted at the 0.05 level of probability ($P < 0.05$).

Results

BATF is upregulated in synovial tissues of arthritic joints

To explore the possible functions of BATF in inflammatory arthritis, we first examined the expression patterns of BATF in the arthritic joints of DBA/1 J mice treated with CIA. Immunostaining revealed that BATF expression was markedly increased in the inflamed synovial tissues of CIA (Fig. 1a). In contrast, BATF was not detected (i.e., there was no obvious synovitis or synovial hyperplasia) in the synovial tissues of $Batf^{-/-}$ mice subjected to CIA conditions (Fig. 1a). As expected, TNF-α and IL-6 were also markedly increased in the CIA synovial tissues (Fig. 1b). To identify cell types expressing BATF in synovial tissues, we performed double immunofluorescence staining of BATF with markers of various synovial cell types, including vimentin for FLS, CD4 for T cells, B220 for B cells, and CD11b for macrophages. BATF was detected in subsets of CD4$^+$ T cells (> 80%), CD11b$^+$ macrophages (~ 40%), and vimentin-expressing FLS (< 50%), but not in B220-expressing B cells (Fig. 1c).

Genetic ablation of *Batf* inhibits CIA

We next examined whether BATF regulates CIA. The CIA manifestations observed in WT mice, including CIA incidence, clinical scores, and paw swelling, were completely abrogated in $Batf^{-/-}$ DBA/1 J littermates (Fig. 2a, b). The production of IgG autoantibodies against type II collagen is a key pathological change in RA pathogenesis, and the IgG2a autoantibody is particularly predominant in the CIA model [25]. Consistent with the above results, IgG2a production was markedly increased in the sera of CIA-induced WT mice, but this was completely suppressed in $Batf^{-/-}$ littermates (Fig. 2c). These results collectively indicate that

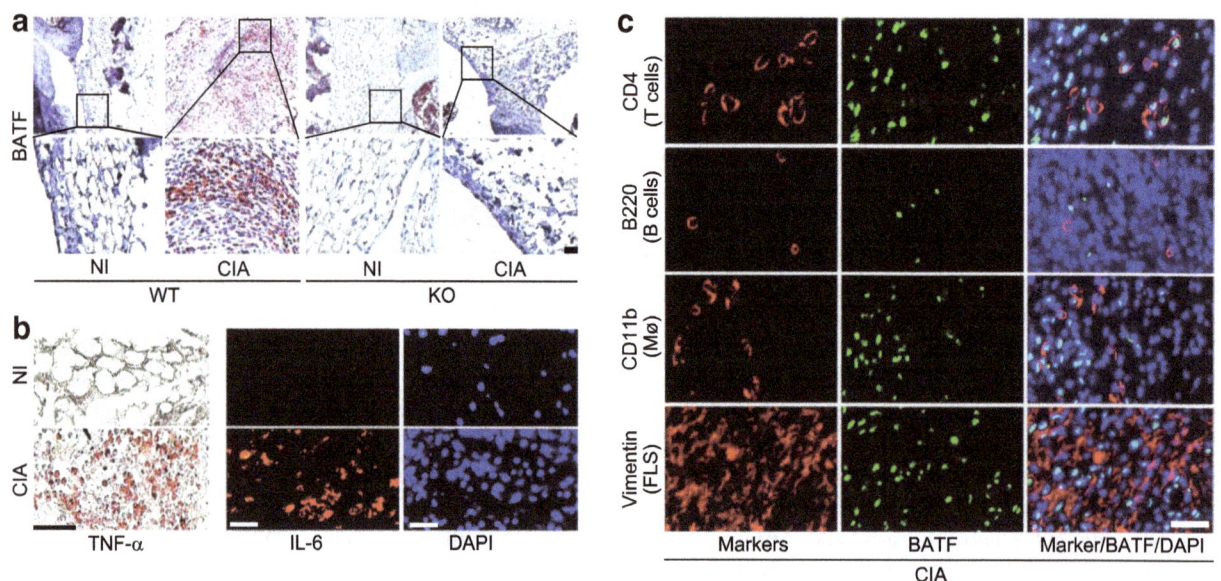

Fig. 1 Upregulation of BATF in arthritic synovial tissues. **a** Representative images (*n* = 10) of BATF immunostaining in synovial tissue sections of nonimmunized (NI) and collagen-induced arthritis (CIA) wild-type (WT) DBA/1 J mice and *Batf*$^{-/-}$ littermates (knockout (KO)). **b** Representative immunostaining images (*n* = 8) of tumor necrosis factor (TNF)-α and interleukin (IL)-6 in CIA synovial tissues determined by immunohistochemical staining and immunofluorescence microscopy, respectively. **c** Representative triple-immunofluorescence microscopic images of mouse CIA synovial sections (*n* = 12) immunostained for BATF, cell type-specific markers, and DAPI. Scale bars = 50 μm

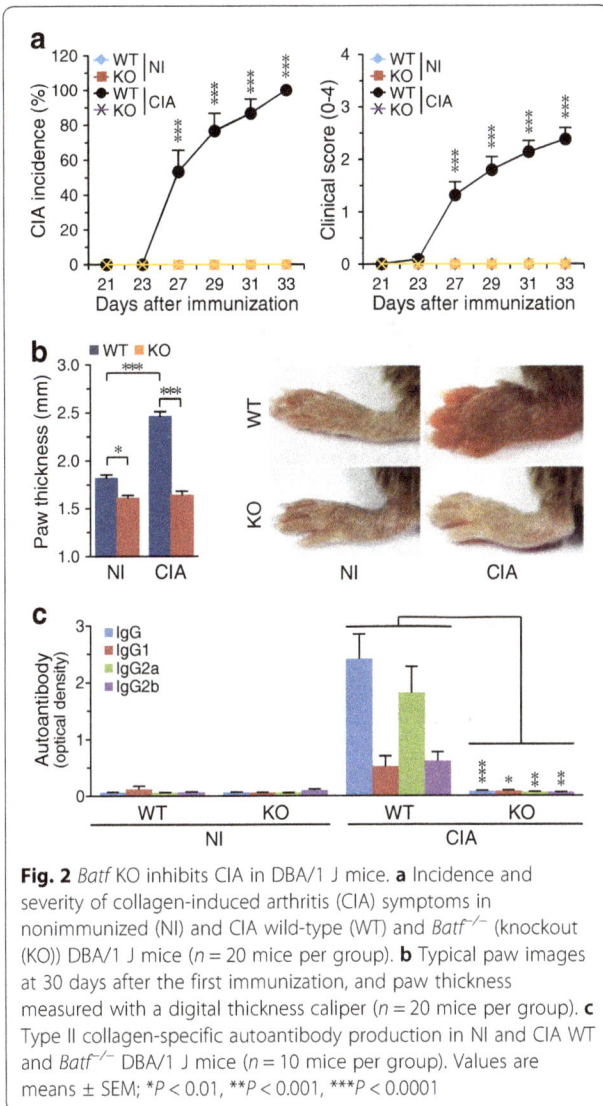

Fig. 2 *Batf* KO inhibits CIA in DBA/1 J mice. **a** Incidence and severity of collagen-induced arthritis (CIA) symptoms in nonimmunized (NI) and CIA wild-type (WT) and *Batf*$^{-/-}$ (knockout (KO)) DBA/1 J mice ($n = 20$ mice per group). **b** Typical paw images at 30 days after the first immunization, and paw thickness measured with a digital thickness caliper ($n = 20$ mice per group). **c** Type II collagen-specific autoantibody production in NI and CIA WT and *Batf*$^{-/-}$ DBA/1 J mice ($n = 10$ mice per group). Values are means ± SEM; *$P < 0.01$, **$P < 0.001$, ***$P < 0.0001$

BATF is required for the pathogenesis of CIA in DBA/1 J mice.

Genetic ablation of *Batf* inhibits CIA-induced synovitis, synovial hyperplasia, and angiogenesis in synovial tissues

CIA is characterized by a synovial hyperplasia that arises through the proliferation of synoviocytes, synovitis with infiltration of immune cells, and angiogenesis in synovial tissues [8–11]. Here, we found that CIA-induced synovitis was significantly blocked in *Batf*$^{-/-}$ mice, as determined by H&E staining and inflammation scoring (Fig. 3a, b). To examine synovial hyperplasia, we determined synovial cell proliferation by Ki67 staining [26]. Ki67 was highly expressed in the synovial tissues of WT mice subjected to CIA-inducing conditions, whereas it was completely absent from those of the corresponding *Batf*$^{-/-}$ mice (Fig. 3c). The inhibition of synovial cell proliferation in *Batf*$^{-/-}$ mice was further confirmed by BrdU incorporation assays

performed using dissociated FLS obtained from WT and *Batf*$^{-/-}$ mice. Compared with WT FLS, *Batf*-deficient FLS showed significantly less proliferation in response to TNF-α (Fig. 3d).

Inflammatory synovial tissues express VEGF, which stimulates angiogenesis to maintain the chronic inflammatory status [27]. Consistent with the above results, neovascularization (as determined by CD31 staining) was observed in CIA-induced WT mice but not in *Batf*$^{-/-}$ mice (Fig. 3e). Previous studies showed that FLS contribute to CIA by producing angiogenic factors associated with blood vessel formation [10, 20, 27, 28], and our group reported that hypoxia-inducible factor (HIF)-2α, which causes RA pathogenesis by modulating FLS functions, stimulates VEGF expression in FLS [20]. Here, we found that overexpression of BATF in FLS did not cause detectable expression of VEGF (Fig. 3f). Additionally, although BATF was upregulated in vimentin-expressing FLS of CIA synovium (Fig. 1c), treatment of FLS with IL-6 or TNF-α, cytokines that critically regulate RA pathogenesis [13], did not induce BATF expression (Fig. 3f). Furthermore, TNF-α- or IL-6-induced upregulation of matrix-degrading enzymes (MMP3 and MMP13), chemokines (CCL2 and CCL5), and chemokine receptors (CXCL1, CXCL5, and CXCL10) in FLS were not affected by *Batf* KO (Fig. 3g).

Genetic ablation of *Batf* inhibits CIA-induced bone and cartilage erosion

As CIA involves the formation of pannus, which invades and destroys mineralized cartilage and bone [8–11], we next examined the possible role of BATF in pannus formation and subsequent bone and cartilage destruction. Indeed, we found that the CIA-induced pannus formation found in WT mice was completely abrogated in *Batf*$^{-/-}$ mice (Fig. 4a). Next, we examined the expression of RANKL, which promotes osteoclast differentiation to stimulate bone erosion [29, 30]. The induction of CIA in WT mice increased the expression of RANKL at the bone/pannus interface, but this was completely abrogated in *Batf*$^{-/-}$ littermates (Fig. 4b). Although FLS are known to produce RANKL [20], BATF overexpression in FLS did not trigger any upregulation of RANKL (Fig. 3f), suggesting that the upregulation of BATF in the FLS of CIA synovium is not directly associated with RANKL expression. In addition, TRAP-positive osteoclasts, which were highly increased at the bone/pannus interface of WT mice, were not observed in *Batf*$^{-/-}$ littermates (Fig. 4c). These results collectively suggest that *Batf* KO inhibits bone erosion under CIA-inducing conditions by blocking RANKL expression and osteoclast differentiation.

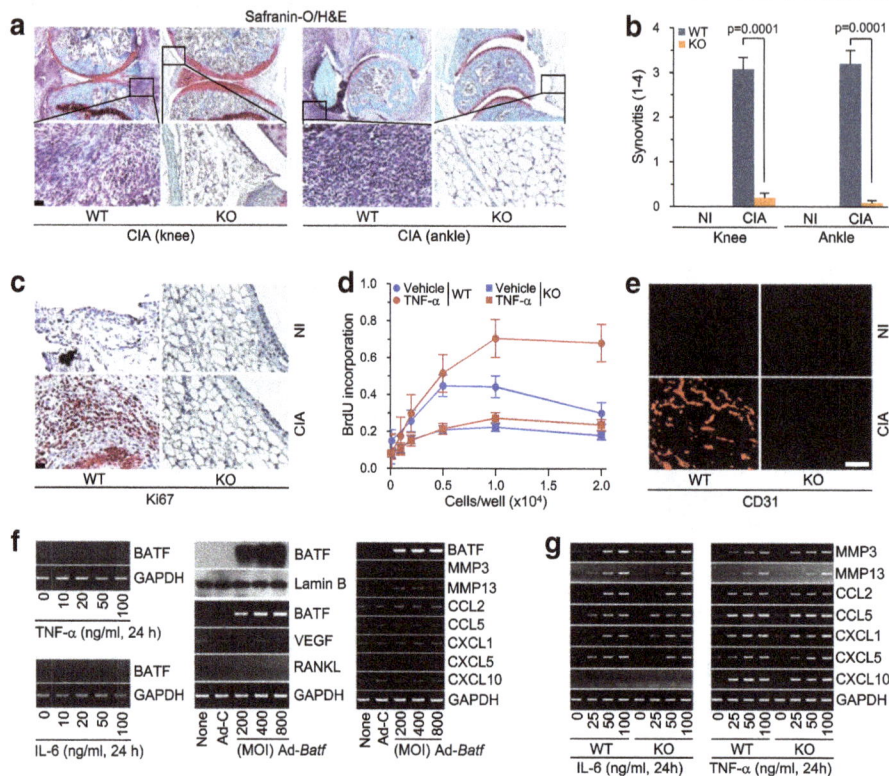

Fig. 3 *Batf* KO inhibits CIA-induced synovitis, synovial hyperplasia, and angiogenesis. H&E staining (**a**) and scoring of synovial inflammation (*n* = 11) (**b**) in knee and ankle joints of nonimmunized (NI) and collagen-induced arthritis (CIA) wild-type (WT) and *Batf*[−/−] (knockout (KO)) DBA/1 J mice. **c** Detection of cell proliferation by Ki67 staining in knee joint sections of NI and CIA WT and *Batf*[−/−] DBA/1 J mice (*n* = 5). **d** Bromodeoxyuridine (BrdU) incorporation assays (*n* = 6) in FLS from WT and *Batf*[−/−] DBA/1 J mice treated with vehicle or tumor necrosis factor (TNF)-α (100 ng/ml for 24 h). **e** Representative images (*n* = 6) of immunofluorescence microscopy of CD31, which was used to detect blood vessels in the ankle joints of NI and CIA WT and *Batf*[−/−] DBA/1 J mice. **f** mRNA levels of the indicated molecules, as detected by RT-PCR in FLS isolated from NI synovium (*n* = 6). FLS were treated with or without the indicated concentrations of TNF-α or IL-6 (left), or with or without 400 MOI (multiplicity of infection) of empty adenovirus (Ad-C) or the indicated MOI of Ad-*Batf* (middle and right). BATF was also detected by Western blotting (middle). Lamin B was detected as a loading control. **g** WT and *Batf* KO FLS were treated with interleukin (IL)-6 or TNF-α. Indicated molecules were detected by RT-PCR (*n* > 5). Values are means ± SEM. Scale bars = 50 μm

CIA in WT mice caused cartilage destruction, as determined by safranin-O staining and OARSI grading (Fig. 4d). Similar to the case of bone erosion, cartilage destruction was completely abrogated in *Batf*[−/−] littermates (Fig. 4d). Cartilage destruction during CIA can be caused by pannus, which invades and destroys mineralized cartilage, or matrix-degrading enzymes produced by synoviocytes and chondrocytes [31, 32]. Although the matrix-degrading enzymes in inflammatory joint tissues are primarily produced by synoviocytes, such as FLS [31, 32], BATF overexpression in FLS did not cause any upregulation of the tested matrix-degrading enzymes (MMP3 and MMP13) or chemokines and chemokine receptors (CCL2, CCL5, CXCL1, CXCL5, and CXCL10) (Fig. 3f). Notably, however, we previously showed that BATF overexpression causes chondrocytes to produce MMP3 and MMP13 [4]. These results collectively suggest that matrix-degrading enzymes produced by chondrocytes, not FLS, may contribute to cartilage destruction during CIA.

Genetic ablation of *Batf* does not affect thymic T cell development

Given that T cells, such as Th17 cells, play crucial roles in inflammatory arthritis [33], we examined whether *Batf* deficiency affected T cell development in DBA/1 J mice. Flow cytometric analysis revealed that thymic T cell development was not affected by *Batf* deletion in DBA/1 J mice (Fig. 5a). However, consistent with a previous report [34], *Batf*[−/−] mice exhibited altered T cell populations in peripheral organs, such as the spleen and lymph nodes (Fig. 5b, c). Compared with WT mice, T cells were slightly reduced in the spleen (Fig. 5b) and lymph nodes (Fig. 5c) of *Batf*[−/−] mice. CD4[+] effector/memory T cells were also slightly reduced in the spleen (Fig. 5b) and lymph nodes (Fig. 5c) of *Batf*[−/−] mice. Overall, although the populations of T cell subsets in the periphery were altered by *Batf* deletion, the degree of alteration was small (i.e., less than 10%) (Fig. 5b, c).

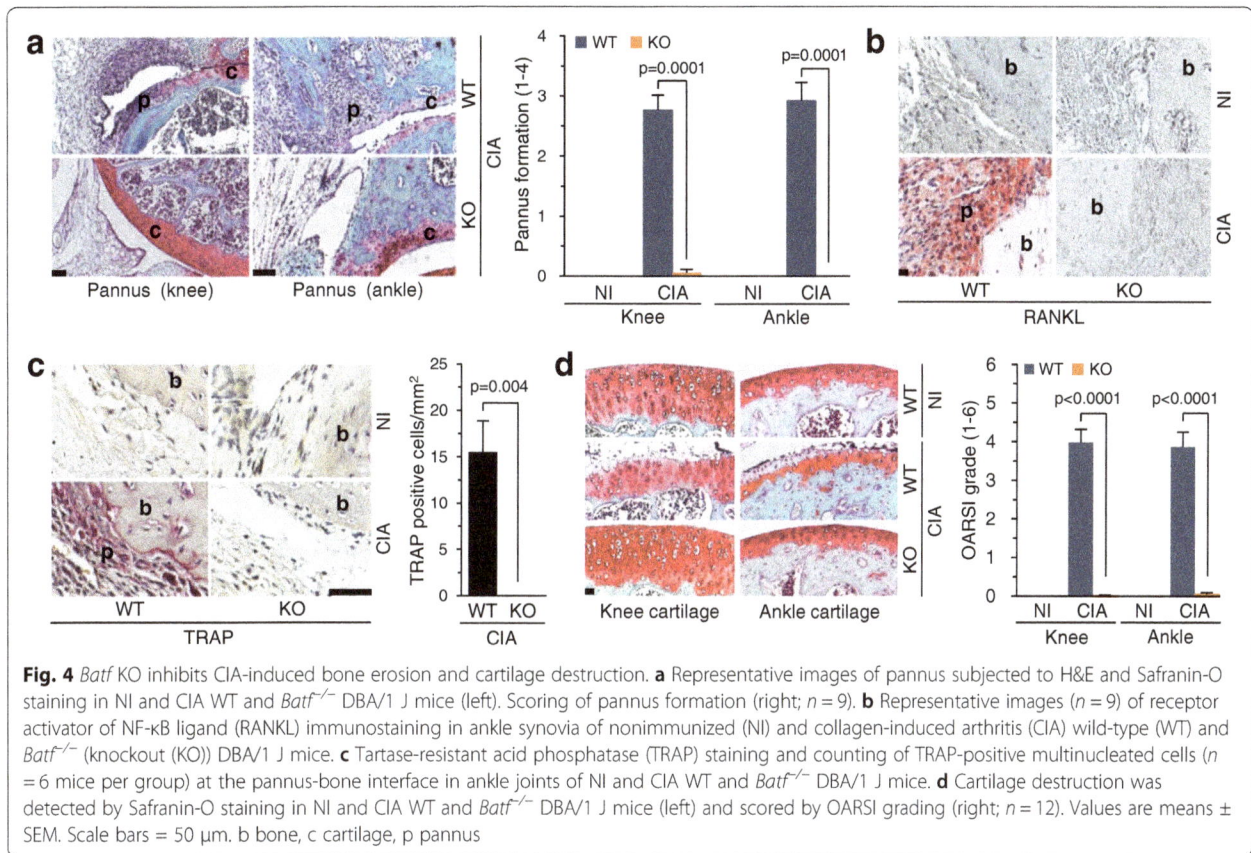

Fig. 4 *Batf* KO inhibits CIA-induced bone erosion and cartilage destruction. **a** Representative images of pannus subjected to H&E and Safranin-O staining in NI and CIA WT and *Batf*−/− DBA/1 J mice (left). Scoring of pannus formation (right; $n = 9$). **b** Representative images ($n = 9$) of receptor activator of NF-κB ligand (RANKL) immunostaining in ankle synovia of nonimmunized (NI) and collagen-induced arthritis (CIA) wild-type (WT) and *Batf*−/− (knockout (KO)) DBA/1 J mice. **c** Tartase-resistant acid phosphatase (TRAP) staining and counting of TRAP-positive multinucleated cells ($n = 6$ mice per group) at the pannus-bone interface in ankle joints of NI and CIA WT and *Batf*−/− DBA/1 J mice. **d** Cartilage destruction was detected by Safranin-O staining in NI and CIA WT and *Batf*−/− DBA/1 J mice (left) and scored by OARSI grading (right; $n = 12$). Values are means ± SEM. Scale bars = 50 μm. b bone, c cartilage, p pannus

Batf KO modulates Th cell differentiation

To further elucidate the functions of BATF, we examined whether *Batf* deficiency affects the in-vitro differentiation of CD4+ T cells into Th cells, including Th1 (CD4+IFNγ+), Th2 (CD4+IL-4+), Th17 (CD4+IL-17A+), and Treg cells (CD4+Foxp3+). Interestingly, *Batf* deletion significantly increased Th2 cell differentiation in *Batf*−/− mice, while in-vitro Th1 and Treg cell differentiations were not affected by *Batf* gene deletion (Fig. 6a). *Batf* gene deletion also significantly reduced Th17 cell differentiation in *Batf*−/− DBA/1 J mice compared with WT control mice (Fig. 6a). Consistent with this finding, the Th17 cell population was significantly reduced in the lymph nodes of *Batf*−/− mice subjected to CIA-inducing conditions (Fig. 6b). Moreover, the CD4+Foxp3+IL-17+ cell population was dramatically reduced in the peripheral lymph nodes of CIA-induced *Batf*−/− mice (Fig. 6c). As the transconversion of Treg cells to Th17 cells can reportedly exacerbate Th17-mediated inflammation [35], we examined whether BATF affects the conversion of Treg cells to Th17 cells in vitro. Indeed, BATF deficiency dramatically abrogated the transconversion of Treg cells to Th17 cells (Fig. 6d), indicating that BATF regulates this conversion. Finally, we analyzed cytokine production in the lymph nodes of *Batf*−/− mice and WT littermates under CIA-inducing conditions. Consistent with the increase in Th2 cell differentiation, the production

of the Th2 cytokines IL-4, IL-10, and IL-13 were increased in CIA-induced *Batf*−/− mice compared with WT littermates (Fig. 6e). Additionally, IL-6 was also increased in CIA-induced *Batf*−/− mice (Fig. 6e). In contrast, the production of the inflammatory cytokines IL-2, IL-17, and TNF-α were reduced in *Batf*−/− mice under CIA-inducing conditions (Fig. 6e).

Genetic ablation of *Batf* does not affect inflammatory arthritis caused by K/BxN serum transfer

Finally, we examined a possible role of BATF in T cell-independent inflammatory arthritis using C57BL/6 mice subjected to K/BxN serum transfer [21]. Immunostaining revealed that BATF expression was markedly increased in the inflamed synovial tissues caused by K/BxN serum transfer (Fig. 7a). However, all examined manifestations of inflammatory arthritis caused by K/BxN serum transfer in WT mice (i.e., paw thickness, synovial inflammation, and cartilage erosion) were not markedly inhibited in *Batf* KO mice (Fig. 7b, c). Our results suggest that BATF is not essential for T cell-independent inflammatory arthritis.

Discussion

We herein show that BATF is required for CIA since *Batf*−/− mice exhibit complete suppression of the manifestations of CIA. We further demonstrate that BATF regulates Th

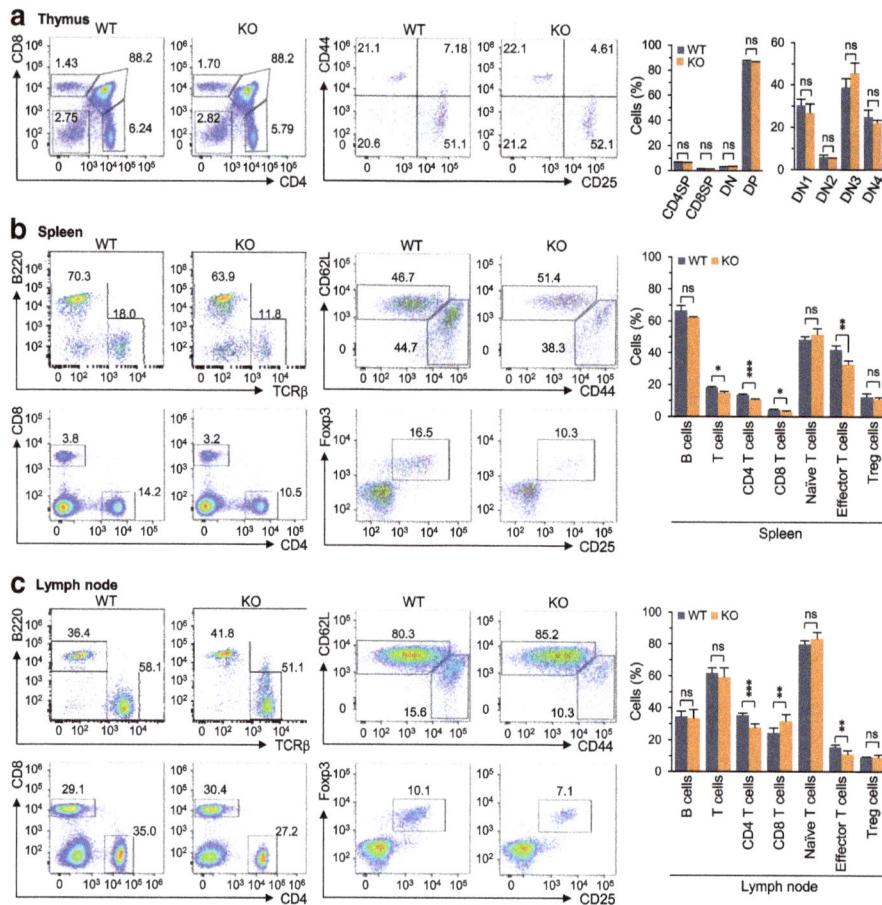

Fig. 5 *Batf* KO does not affect thymic T cell development. **a–c** Representative flow cytometric analysis (*n* = 5 per group) and quantitation of immune cell populations. T cell development in thymus (**a**) and the populations of immune cells in the spleens (**b**) and lymph nodes (**c**) of wild-type (WT) and *Batf⁻/⁻* (knockout (KO)) DBA/1 J mice were analyzed by flow cytometry. Values are presented as means ± SD; *$P < 0.01$, **$P < 0.001$, ***$P < 0.0001$. ns not significant

cell differentiation during CIA. The pathogenesis of RA is associated with enrichment of Th17 cells in the inflamed synovium and enhancement of IL-17 production [8, 9, 36, 37]. A recent report indicated that the conversion of Treg cells to Th17 cells contributes to bone destruction in CIA mice [35], suggesting that an imbalance between these cell populations contributes to CIA. BATF is known to regulate Th17 cell differentiation by modulating the expression of the transcription factor RORγt [16], and to control class-switch recombination in T and B cells [17]. Thus, BATF was previously known to function at multiple hierarchical levels in two cell types to globally regulate switched-antibody responses. Here, we demonstrated that BATF deficiency decreases Th17 cell differentiation both in vivo and in vitro. It was previously reported that a portion of Foxp3-positive cells also expresses IL-17, and that CD4⁺Foxp3⁺IL-17⁺ cells can be found in CIA mice [35]. However, we found here that *Batf* deficiency completely abolished CD4⁺Foxp3⁺IL-17⁺ cell generation under CIA-inducing conditions. An additional interesting finding

of our current study is that BATF regulates Th2 cell differentiation; we demonstrated that IL-4-producing CD4⁺ T cells were increased in CIA-induced *Batf⁻/⁻* mice compared with WT control mice. This is consistent with a previous report that IL-4 negatively regulates the induction and progression of CIA [38]. In addition, BATF is not detected in the infiltrated B cells of CIA synovial tissue. Although this does not rule out expression and the possible role of BATF in B cells of peripheral lymphatic tissues, our results indicate that upregulation of BATF in the infiltrated B cells is not essential for pathogenesis of CIA. Furthermore, we found that T cell-independent inflammatory arthritis caused by K/BxN serum transfer was not affected by *Batf⁻/⁻* mice. Based on these findings, we propose that BATF deficiency alters Th cell differentiation, enabling *Batf⁻/⁻* mice to resist CIA. Thus, BATF inhibition could be a useful strategy for the treatment of RA.

We also report that FLS are not directly associated with the BATF-mediated regulation of CIA, although BATF appears to regulate the proliferation of FLS in

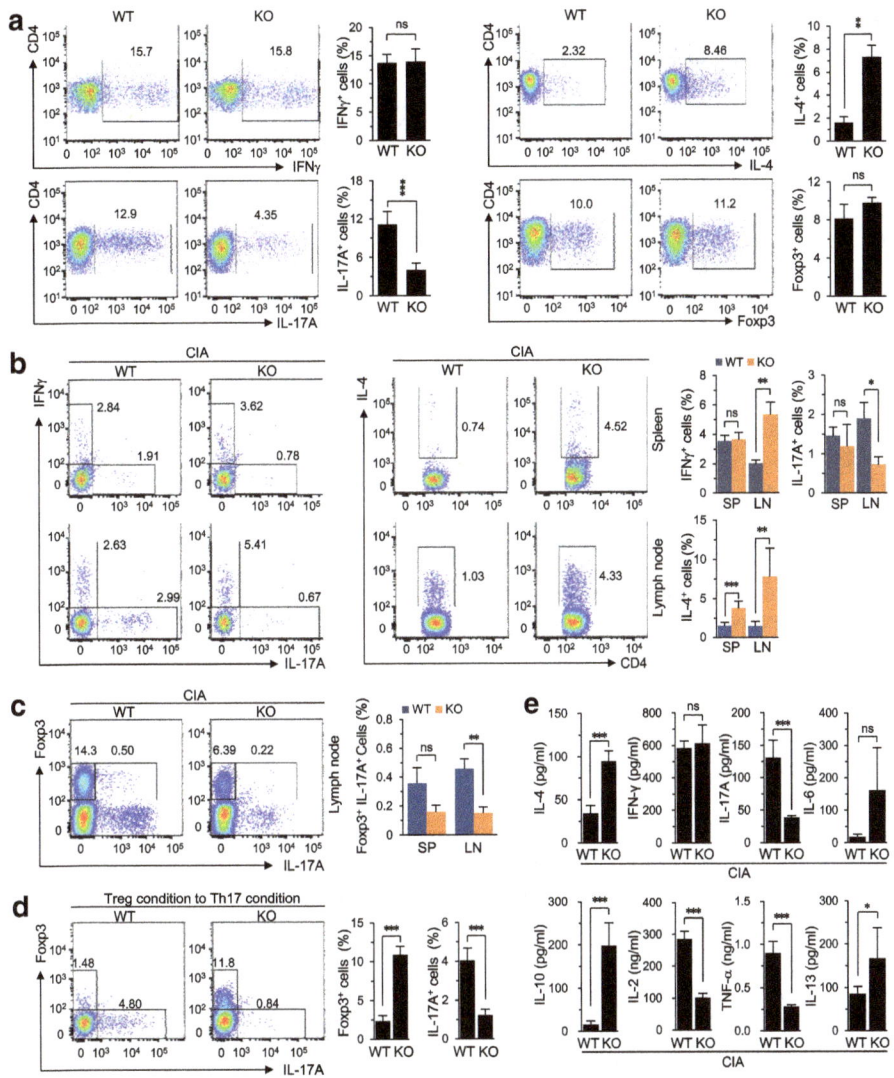

Fig. 6 *Batf* KO reduces Th17 differentiation in CIA. **a** Populations of Th1, Th2, Th17, and Treg cells differentiated from uncommitted CD4+ T cells of wild-type (WT) and *Batf−/−* (knockout (KO)) DBA/1 J mice (*n* = 5). **b** Analysis of interferon (IFN)-γ, interleukin (IL)-17A, and IL-4 producing CD4+ T cells in spleens (SP; top panel) and lymph nodes (LN; bottom panel) of WT and *Batf−/−* DBA/1 J mice 4 to 5 weeks later from CIA induction (*n* = 5 mice per group). **c** Flow cytometric analysis of the productions of Foxp3 and IL-17A in CD4+ T cells from lymph nodes of WT and *Batf−/−* DBA/1 J mice 4 to 5 weeks later from CIA induction (*n* = 5 mice per group) under CIA conditions. **d** Populations of Foxp3+ and IL-17A+ cells in CD4+ T cells cultured under Treg differentiation condition to Th17 differentiation condition (*n* = 5). **e** Cytokine production of total lymph node cells from WT and *Batf−/−* DBA/1 J mice 4 to 5 weeks later from CIA induction (*n* ≥ 5 mice per group). Values are presented as means ± SD; *P < 0.01, **P < 0.001, ***P < 0.0001. ns not significant

response to TNF-α. Accumulating evidence indicates that FLS are key players in RA pathogenesis [10, 28]. Cytokines and chemokines produced by FLS attract T cells to RA synovium, and the interaction of FLS with T cells results in the activation of both cell types. FLS also produce matrix-degrading enzymes involved in cartilage destruction, angiogenic factors associated with neovascularization, and RANKL [10, 28]. The latter factor regulates osteoclastogenesis, which requires physical contact of precursor cells with RANKL-expressing FLS or T cells [29, 30, 39]. We

showed previously that HIF-2α modulates various functions of FLS, including proliferation, the expressions of RANKL and various catabolic factors, and osteoclastogenic potential [20]. Here, we found that, unlike HIF-2α, TNF-α and IL-6 do not cause BATF expression in FLS, and BATF overexpression in FLS does not modulate the expressions of various matrix-degrading enzymes or chemokines. These results collectively support our notion that the ability of BATF to regulate CIA is not due to a direct BATF-mediated modulation of FLS functions.

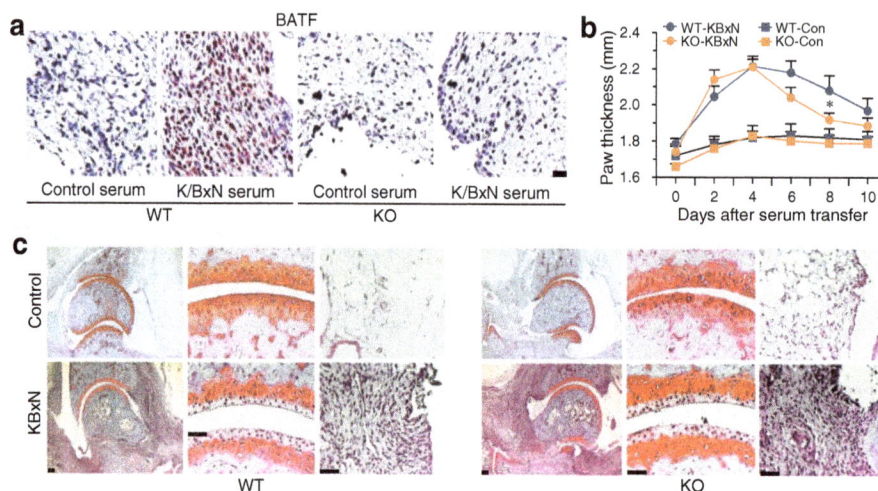

Fig. 7 *Batf* KO does not affect inflammatory arthritis caused by K/BxN serum transfer. **a** Representative immunostaining images (*n* = 6) of BATF immunostaining in synovial tissue sections of C57BL/6 mice transferred with control or K/BxN serum. **b** Paw thickness measured with a digital thickness caliper in wild-type (WT) or *Batf* knockout (KO) mice transferred with control (Con) or K/BxN serum (*n* = 12 mice per group). **c** Typical images of cartilage destruction and synovitis detected by Safranin-O and H&E staining in WT or *Batf* KO mice transferred with control or K/BxN serum (*n* = 12 mice per group). Values are means ± SEM. Scale bars = 50 μm

It has proven difficult to elucidate the role of chondrocytes in cartilage destruction during RA pathogenesis [5]. Such destruction occurs primarily at the interface of the pannus and calcified cartilage [5, 40]. There is evidence that proteoglycans are lost from the superficial zone, where cartilage contacts with synovial fluid, but not with the pannus [5]. Because RA synovium produces various matrix-degrading enzymes [5, 8, 9], cartilage destruction at the superficial zone may be due to synovial cell functions. However, proteoglycans can also be lost from the middle and deep zones of the cartilage [5], suggesting that a chondrocyte may help degrade its own matrix by releasing matrix-degrading enzymes. Indeed, we recently demonstrated that BATF upregulates MMP3 and MMP13 in chondrocytes, leading to cartilage destruction during OA pathogenesis [4]. Therefore, our current and previous [4] results suggest that the BATF-mediated regulation of MMP3 and MMP13 expression in chondrocytes is associated with cartilage destruction during CIA.

The results of the present study collectively indicate that BATF regulates CIA in mice, and our previous work showed that BATF functions as a catabolic regulator of OA cartilage destruction by upregulating catabolic enzymes (e.g., MMP3 and MMP13) in chondrocytes [4]. Thus, despite their different etiologies and pathogeneses, both RA and OA are regulated by BATF. However, different mechanisms are involved; BATF regulates OA pathogenesis by upregulating matrix-degrading enzymes in chondrocytes, whereas it appears to regulate RA pathogenesis by regulating Th cell differentiation. Thus, BATF could be a useful target for the regulation of RA.

Conclusions

In summary, we demonstrated here that BATF regulates CIA, including synovitis, synovial hyperplasia, angiogenesis in the inflamed synovium, cartilage destruction, and bone erosion in the joint tissues. We also reveal that BATF regulates CIA by regulating Th cell differentiation without directly affecting the functions of FLS.

Abbreviations

AP-1: Activator protein-1; BATF: Basic leucine zipper transcription factor, ATF-like; BrdU: Bromodeoxyuridine; CIA: Collagen-induced arthritis; ELISA: Enzyme-linked immunosorbent assay; FLS: Fibroblast-like synoviocytes; H&E: Hematoxylin and eosin; HIF: Hypoxia-inducible factor; IFN: Interferon; IL: Interleukin; KO: Knockout; MLS: Macrophage-like synoviocytes; MMP: Matrix metalloproteinase; NI: Nonimmunized; OA: Osteoarthritis; PMA: Phorbol-12-myristate 13-acetate; RA: Rheumatoid arthritis; RANKL: Receptor activator of NF-κB ligand; TCR: T cell receptor; TGF: Transforming growth factor; Th: T helper; TNF: Tumor necrosis factor; TRAP: Tartase-resistant acid phosphatase; VEGF: Vascular endothelial growth factor; WT: Wild-type

Funding

This work was supported by grants from the National Research Foundation of Korea (2016R1A3B1906090, 2016R1A5A1007318, and 2016R1A2B4008819), the Korea Healthcare Technology R&D project through the Korea Health Industry Development Institute (HI16C0287 and HI14C3484), and the GIST Research Institute (2017).

Authors' contributions

SGP and JSC contributed equally as corresponding authors by conceiving and designing the experiments. SHP, JR, and SKK performed the experiments. JAK, JSK, YS, and WSC analyzed the data. SHP, JR, SGP, and JSC wrote the manuscript. All authors read and approved the final manuscript.

Consent for publication
Not applicable.

Competing interests
The authors declare that they have no competing interests.

Author details
[1]School of Life Sciences, Gwangju Institute of Science and Technology, Gwangju 61005, Republic of Korea. [2]Keimyung University Dongsan Medical Center, Daegu 41931, Republic of Korea.

References
1. Dorsey MJ, Tae HJ, Sollenberger KG, Mascarenhas NT, Johansen LM, Taparowsky EJ. B-ATF: a novel human bZIP protein that associates with members of the AP-1 transcription factor family. Oncogene. 1995;11(11): 2255–65.
2. Li P, Spolski R, Liao W, Wang L, Murphy TL, Murphy KM, Leonard WJ. BATF-JUN is critical for IRF4-mediated transcription in T cells. Nature. 2012; 490(7421):543–6.
3. Murphy TL, Tussiwand R, Murphy KM. Specificity through cooperation: BATF-IRF interactions control immune-regulatory networks. Nat Rev Immunol. 2013;13(7):499–509.
4. Rhee J, Park SH, Kim SK, Kim JH, Ha CW, Chun CH, Chun JS. Inhibition of BATF/JUN transcriptional activity protects against osteoarthritic cartilage destruction. Ann Rheum Dis. 2017;76(2):427–34.
5. Otero M, Goldring MB. Cells of the synovium in rheumatoid arthritis: chondrocytes. Arthritis Res Ther. 2007;9(5):220.
6. Loeser RE, Goldring SR, Scanzello CR, Goldring MB. Osteoarthritis: a disease of the joint as an organ. Arthritis Rheum. 2012;64(6):1697–707.
7. Little CB, Hunter DJ. Post-traumatic osteoarthritis: from mouse models to clinical trials. Nat Rev Rheumatol. 2011;9(8):485–97.
8. McInnes IB, Schett G. The pathogenesis of rheumatoid arthritis. N Engl J Med. 2011;365(23):2205–19.
9. Goronzy JJ, Weyand CM. Developments in the scientific understanding of rheumatoid arthritis. Arthritis Res Ther. 2009;11(5):249–62.
10. Bartok B, Firestein GS. Fibroblast-like synoviocytes: key effector cells in rheumatoid arthritis. Immunol Rev. 2010;233(1):233–55.
11. Bluestone JA, Bour-Jordan H, Cheng M, Anderson M. T cells in the control of organ-specific autoimmunity. J Clin Invest. 2015;125(6):2250–60.
12. Leipe J, Grunke M, Dechant C, Reindl C, Kerzendorf U, Schulze-Koops H, Skapenko A. Role of Th17 cells in human autoimmune arthritis. Arthritis Rheum. 2010;62(10):2876–85.
13. McInnes IB, Schett G. Cytokines in the pathogenesis of rheumatoid arthritis. Nat Rev Immunol. 2007;7(6):429–42.
14. Nurieva RI, Podd A, Chen Y, Alekseev AM, Yu M, Qi S, Huang H, Wen R, Wang J, Hs L, et al. STAT5 protein negatively regulates T follicular helper (Tfh) cell generation and function. J Biol Chem. 2012;287(14):11234–9.
15. Ikeda S, Saijo S, Murayama MA, Shimizu K, Alittsu A, Iwakura Y. Excess IL-1 signaling enhances the development of Th17 cells by downregulating TGF-β-induced Foxp3 expression. J Immunol. 2014;192(4):1449–58.
16. Schraml BU, Hildner K, Ise W, Lee WL, Smith WA, Solomon B, Sahota G, Sim J, Mukasa R, Cemerski S, et al. The AP-1 transcription factor Batf controls T(H)17 differentiation. Nature. 2009;460(7253):405–9.
17. Ise W, Kohyama M, Schraml BU, Zhang T, Schwer B, Basu U, Alt FW, Tang J, Murphy TL, et al. The transcription factor BATF controls the global regulators of class-switch recombination in both B cells and T cells. Nat Immunol. 2011;12(6):536–43.
18. Aikawa Y, Morimoto K, Yamamoto T, Chaki H, Hashiramoto A, Narita H, Hirono S, Shiozawa S. Treatment of arthritis with a selective inhibitor of c-Fos/activator protein-1. Nat Biotechnol. 2008;26(7):817–23.
19. Brand DD, Latham KA, Rosloniec EF. Collagen-induced arthritis. Nat Protoc. 2007;2(5):1269–75.
20. Ryu JH, Chae CS, Kwak JS, Oh H, Shin Y, Huh YH, Lee CG, Park YW, Chun CH, Kim YM, et al. Hypoxia-inducible factor-2α is an essential catabolic regulator of inflammatory rheumatoid arthritis. PLoS Biol. 2014;12(6):e1001881.
21. Matsumoto I, Staub A, Benoist C, Mathis D. Arthritis provoked by linked T and B cell recognition of a glycolytic enzyme. Science. 1999;286(5445):1732–5.
22. Oh H, Ryu JH, Jeon J, Yang S, Chun CH, Park H, Kim HJ, Kim HH, Kwon YG, et al. Misexpression of Dickkopf-1 in endothelial cells, but not in chondrocytes or hypertrophic chondrocytes, causes defects in endochondral ossification. J Bone Miner Res. 2012;27(6):1335–44.
23. Zhao J, Ouyang Q, Hu Z, Huang Q, Wu J, Wang R, Yang M. A protocol for the culture and isolation of murine synovial fibroblasts. Biomed Rep. 2016;5:171–5.
24. Kang JA, Park SH, Jeong SP, Han MH, Lee CR, Lee KM, Kim N, Song MR, Choi M, Ye M, et al. Epigenetic regulation of Kcna3-encoding Kv1.3 potassium channel by cereblon contributes to regulation of CD4[+] T-cell activation. Proc Natl Acad Sci U S A. 2016;113(31):8771–6.
25. Watson WC, Townes AS. Genetic susceptibility to murine collagen II autoimmune arthritis. Proposed relationship to the IgG2 autoantibody subclass response, complement C5, major histocompatibility complex (MHC) and non-MHC loci. J Exp Med. 1985;162(6):1878–91.
26. Scholzen T, Gerdes J. The Ki-67 protein: from the known and the unknown. J Cell Physiol. 2000;182(3):311–22.
27. Fava RA, Olsen NJ, Spencer-Green G, Yeo KT, Berse B, Jackman RW, Sener DR, Dvorak HF, Brown LF. Vascular permeability factor/endothelial growth factor (VPF/VEGF): accumulation and expression in human synovial fluids and rheumatoid synovial tissue. J Exp Med. 1994;180(1):341–6.
28. Bottini N, Firestein GS. Duality of fibroblast-like synoviocytes in RA: passive responders and imprinted aggressors. Nat Rev Rheumatol. 2013;9(1):24–33.
29. Pettit AR, Walsh NC, Manning C, Goldring SR, Gravallese EM. RANKL protein is expressed at the pannus-bone interface at sites of articular bone erosion in rheumatoid arthritis. Rheumatol. 2006;45(9):1068–76.
30. Schett G, Gravallese F. Bone erosion in rheumatoid arthritis: mechanisms, diagnosis and treatment. Nat Rev Rheumatol. 2012;11(11):656–64.
31. Pap T, Shigeyama Y, Kuchen S, Femihough JK, Simmen B, Re G, Billingham M, Gay S. Differential expression pattern of membrane-type matrix metalloproteinases in rheumatoid arthritis. Arthritis Rheum. 2000;43(6):1226–32.
32. Neumann E, Lefevre S, Zimmermann B, Gay S, Muller-Ladner U. Rheumatoid arthritis progression mediated by activated synovial fibroblasts. Trends Mol Med. 2010;16(6):458–68.
33. Lubberts E. The IL-23-IL-17 axis in inflammatory arthritis. Nat Rev Rheumatol. 2015;11(10):562.
34. Betz BC, Jordan-Williams KL, Wang C, Kang SG, Lio J, Logan MR, Kim CH, Taparowsky EJ. Batf coordinates multiple aspects of B and T cell function required for normal antibody responses. J Exp Med. 2010;207(5):933–42.
35. Komatsu N, Okamoto K, Sawa S, Nakashima T, Oh-hora M, Kodama T, Tanaka S, Bluestone JA, Takayanagi H. Pathogenic conversion of Foxp3[+] T cells into TH17 cells in autoimmune arthritis. Nat Med. 2014;20(1):62–8.
36. Nakae S, Nambu A, Sudo K, Iwakura Y. Suppression of immune induction of collagen-induced arthritis in IL-17-deficient mice. J Immunol. 2003;171(11):6173–7.
37. Lubberts E, Joosten LA, Oppers B, van den Bersselaar L, Coenen-de Roo CJ, Kolls JK, Schwarzenberger P, van de Loo FA, van den Berg WB. IL-1-independent role of IL-17 in synovial inflammation and joint destruction during collagen-induced arthritis. J Immunol. 2001;167(2):1004–13.
38. Morita Y, Yang J, Gupta R, Shimizu K, Shelden EA, Endres J, Mule JJ, McDonagh KT, Fox DA. Dendritic cells genetically engineered to express IL-4 inhibit murine collagen-induced arthritis. J Clin Invest. 2001;107(10):1275–84.
39. Maruotti N, Grano M, Colucci S, d'Onofrio F, Cantatore FP. Osteoclastogenesis and arthritis. Clin Exp Med. 2011;11(3):137–45.
40. Edwards JC. Fibroblast biology. Development and differentiation of synovial fibroblasts in arthritis. Arthritis Res. 2000;2(5):344–7.

4

Induction of sustained remission in early inflammatory arthritis with the combination of infliximab plus methotrexate: the DINORA trial

Tanja Alexandra Stamm[1,2], Klaus Peter Machold[2], Daniel Aletaha[2], Farideh Alasti[2], Peter Lipsky[3], David Pisetsky[4], Robert Landewe[5], Desiree van der Heijde[6], Alexandre Sepriano[6], Martin Aringer[7], Dimitri Boumpas[8], Gerd Burmester[9], Maurizio Cutolo[10], Wolfgang Ebner[11], Winfried Graninger[12], Tom Huizinga[6], Georg Schett[13], Hendrik Schulze-Koops[14], Paul-Peter Tak[15,16,17,18], Emilio Martin-Mola[19], Ferdinand Breedveld[20] and Josef Smolen[2,11]*

Abstract

Background: In the present study, we explored the effects of immediate induction therapy with the anti-tumour necrosis factor (TNF)α antibody infliximab (IFX) plus methotrexate (MTX) compared with MTX alone and with placebo (PL) in patients with very early inflammatory arthritis.

Methods: In an investigator-initiated, double-blind, randomised, placebo-controlled, multi-centre trial (ISRCTN21272423, http://www.isrctn.com/ISRCTN21272423), patients with synovitis of 12 weeks duration in at least two joints underwent 1 year of treatment with IFX in combination with MTX, MTX monotherapy, or PL randomised in a 2:2:1 ratio. The primary endpoint was clinical remission after 1 year (sustained for at least two consecutive visits 8 weeks apart) with remission defined as no swollen joints, 0–2 tender joints, and an acute-phase reactant within the normal range.

Results: Ninety patients participated in the present study. At week 54 (primary endpoint), 32% of the patients in the IFX + MTX group achieved sustained remission compared with 14% on MTX alone and 0% on PL. This difference ($p < 0.05$ over all three groups) was statistically significant for IFX + MTX vs PL ($p < 0.05$), but not for IFX + MTX vs MTX ($p = 0.10$), nor for MTX vs PL ($p = 0.31$). Remission was maintained during the second year on no therapy in 75% of the IFX + MTX patients compared with 20% of the MTX-only patients.

Conclusions: These results indicate that patients with early arthritis can benefit from induction therapy with anti-TNF plus MTX compared with MTX alone, suggesting that intensive treatment can alter the disease evolution.

Keywords: Clinical remission, Early arthritis, Rheumatoid arthritis

* Correspondence: josef.smolen@meduniwien.ac.at
[2]Department of Medicine III, Division of Rheumatology, Medical University of Vienna, Waehringer Guertel 18-20, 1090 Vienna, Austria
[11]Department of Internal Medicine, Centre for Rheumatic Diseases, Hietzing Hospital, Wolkersbergenstraße 1, 1130 Vienna, Austria
Full list of author information is available at the end of the article

Background

Rheumatoid arthritis (RA) is a severe chronic inflammatory joint disease that can lead to joint damage and functional impairment. Early therapy with disease-modifying anti-rheumatic drugs (DMARDs) can improve outcomes and limit joint damage and irreversible loss of physical function [1–3]. With the advent of newer therapeutic agents and treatment strategies [4, 5], the goal of remission is achievable in a proportion of patients [6–8]. Importantly, patients in clinical remission usually do not accrue additional joint damage [9, 10]. Despite these benefits of early therapy, drug-free remission is not attainable in the majority of patients [11, 12].

Early in the course of RA, a unique stage called the "window of opportunity" may exist. During this stage, key steps in pathogenesis may be reversible, with DMARD therapy blocking progression to full disease manifestations and potentially leading to sustained remission [13, 14]. Several findings provide support for the window of opportunity hypothesis: an increase in the risk of persistent disease after several months of arthritis symptoms [15, 16]; differences in immunological abnormalities in very early compared with established disease [17, 18]; and the ability of early treatment with a tumour necrosis factor (TNF) inhibitor plus methotrexate (MTX) to allow some patients with RA to achieve a drug-free remission [19, 20]. Information on the existence of the window of opportunity on the basis of current data is limited, however, since some studies did not have a double-blind design, evaluated only a very small number of patients and/or were performed only in a single centre. Furthermore, recent data obtained in patients with early disease suggest that, in those fulfilling the classification criteria of RA, drug-free remission after such induction therapy may be uncommon [12, 21].

Very little is known about the pathogenic processes operative in very early inflammatory arthritis, especially in those subjects who do not meet the classification criteria of RA [17, 18, 22]. Since remission due to MTX therapy alone is rare [23], we reasoned that MTX monotherapy might not be sufficient to induce lasting remission, even at this early stage of disease. Moreover, even though the presence of rheumatoid factor (RF) and anti-citrullinated protein antibodies (ACPA) has been found to identify subjects at increased risk of progressing to RA [24], we elected not to limit entry to subjects that had developed these biomarkers, but rather to examine a broader group of subjects who had developed unexplained inflammatory arthritis within the past 3 months in order to determine whether the presence of these antibodies or even the classification of RA altered the likelihood of progressing to RA despite intense therapy. The goal of this study, therefore, was to determine whether intense therapy with MTX plus infliximab (IFX) compared with MTX alone or placebo had the capacity to induce long-lasting drug-free remission in subjects with a very short period of inflammatory arthritis symptoms who had not received prior DMARD therapy.

Methods

Study design

The Definitive Intervention in New Onset Rheumatoid Arthritis (DINORA) study was a double-blind, randomised, placebo-controlled, multi-centre, investigator-initiated trial of the effects of anti-TNFα chimeric monoclonal antibody IFX in combination with MTX in patients with very early inflammatory arthritis and was conducted at 14 rheumatology centres across Europe (three in Austria, four in the Netherlands, four in Germany, and one each in Greece, Italy, and Spain). The study design is depicted in Additional file 1: Figure SA. The trial was registered at http://www.isrctn.com/ISRCTN21272423. Patient recruitment started in October 2007 and ended in February 2012. The study was conducted in accordance with the Declaration of Helsinki. Ethical committees of each institution approved the study and all patients gave written informed consent.

Patients and randomisation

Patients were eligible for the trial if they had symptom duration of 2 to 12 weeks and had synovial swelling present in at least two joints (66 joint count); at least one joint must have been a metacarpophalangeal, proximal interphalangeal, or metatarsophalangeal (MTP) joint; MTP joints only were considered insufficient for inclusion. Baseline visits were scheduled if clinical joint swelling (arthritis) by history was present for 12 weeks and confirmed at two pre-treatment visits between week 2 and week 12 (Additional file 1: Figure SA). Patients with a positive purified protein derivative (PPD) test or chest radiograph performed at screening suggesting tuberculosis, malignancy, chronic infectious disease, elevated liver enzymes, or patients who were pregnant or planning to become pregnant within 6 months after the last infusion were excluded. Furthermore, patients with a distinct diagnosis made after a routine diagnostic work-up, such as a connective tissue disease, psoriatic arthritis, gout, pseudogout, reactive arthritis, or parvovirus arthritis, were not eligible. Thus, only patients with undifferentiated arthritis or early RA [25] were enrolled in the trial.

Procedures of the study

Patients were randomised into three groups in a 2:2:1 ratio by a computer generated randomisation list to infliximab plus methotrexate (IFX + MTX), MTX monotherapy (MTX), or placebo (PL). For randomisation, patients were stratified for the use of glucocorticoids (users versus non-users, see below) and the presence of ACPA (> 7 units, measured by enzyme-linked immunosorbent assay (ELISA)) or high titre RF (> 50 IU/ml by nephelometry), determined in a central laboratory. Local investigators were blinded to the results of the central RF and ACPA testing and were also discouraged from having these tests performed on site. For reasons of blinding, a "double--dummy-like" administration of study medication was pursued. Every patient was treated with tablets containing MTX or PL and with infusions containing IFX or PL. The study medication code was kept blinded in patients who discontinued prematurely. Patients were followed until week 106. For rescue therapy for patients who discontinued treatment, the protocol recommended leflunomide (20 mg daily without a loading dose) or sulfasalazine (up to 3000 mg/day) with or without low-dose glucocorticoids.

Patients received treatment with IFX + MTX, MTX alone, or PL. In addition, supportive therapy appropriate at this early stage of arthritis was allowed in all three treatment groups. This therapy included non-steroidal anti-inflammatory drugs and, if necessary, glucocorticoids at a dose of no more than 10 mg/day prednisone or equivalent. MTX was dosed orally according to a rapid dose escalation scheme: treatment was started at 10 mg/week and increased to 25 mg/week in three steps with 2-week intervals except in cases of intolerance. IFX was administered by intravenous infusions at a dose of 3 mg/kg at 0, 2, and 6 weeks, and at 5 mg/kg every 8 weeks thereafter (and thus at higher than the minimal dose approved for maintenance therapy).

All core set variables were assessed at every visit. These variables included swollen and tender joint counts (SJC and TJC; using a 66- and 68-joint count, respectively), patient and evaluator global assessments (PGA and EGA, on a 100-mm visual analogue scale (VAS)), patient pain assessment (by VAS), erythrocyte sedimentation rate (ESR; mm/h), C-reactive protein (CRP; mg/dl), American College of Rheumatology (ACR) 20, 50, and 70% response rates [26], and the Health Assessment Questionnaire Disability Index (HAQ) [27]. Furthermore, composite measures of disease activity, such as Clinical and Simplified Disease Activity Index (CDAI and SDAI) [28] and Disease Activity Score 28 (DAS28) using 28-joint counts and ESR [29] were calculated.

Radiographs of hands and feet were taken at baseline, 6 months, 1 year, and 2 years and scored independently using the Sharp-van-der-Heijde (SvdH) method [30] by two readers who were blinded to patient characteristics and group allocation but who were aware of the chronological order of the films. The joint space narrowing (JSN) and erosion scores as well as their sum, representing the total score, were evaluated. The average score of the two readers was used for the analyses. In addition, random-effects models were fitted with and without imputation and by taking into account the scores from

both readers and the interaction between treatment allocation and study visit to assess if the rate of radiological progression between the three treatment groups was significantly different.

Endpoints

Persistent clinical remission at weeks 46 and 54 compared between all three treatment groups was taken as the primary endpoint. Clinical remission was defined as follows: at two consecutive visits, no swollen joint (66-joint count), 0 to at most 2 tender joints (68-joint count but counting unilateral MTPs as one joint), and a CRP level within the normal range (< 0.5 mg/dl) or a normal ESR (< 25 mm/h). At the time of the study design, the ACR/European League Against Rheumatism (EULAR) remission criteria [26] had not yet been developed. The criteria chosen here, however, are consistent with these criteria; similar to the Boolean or index-based remission criteria, they do not allow for more than two affected joints (sum of swollen or tender) and require a normal CRP [10, 28].

In all patients, the last infusion of IFX was planned at week 54 (or earlier, as specified below), whereas MTX was continued at the same dose until week 58 and then tapered in all patients over 4 weeks (weekly reduction by 5 mg/week, last dose at week 62). IFX + MTX, MTX, or PL was discontinued earlier if clinical remission was attained at two consecutive visits after the 14-week visit. Thus, for patients who reached clinical remission at two or more consecutive visits before week 54 (sustained remission), IFX (or PL) was stopped and MTX (or PL) tapered beginning after the second visit in remission (first planned possible IFX withdrawal at week 30; Additional file 1: Figure SA). Since the patients would not know on which regimen they had achieved remission, no blinded infusions were continued from that time-point onward. However, as mentioned above, to qualify for the primary endpoint, patients had to have sustained remission until week 54 irrespective of early withdrawal. The study was continued until week 106 without further study medication to evaluate long-term maintenance of remission; blinding of initial treatment assignment remained intact.

Statistical analysis

The sample size calculation is described in Additional file 2: Supplement S1. Descriptive statistics were used for baseline characteristics and demographic data. We applied a strategy of step-wise hierarchical hypothesis testing [31] to control for type I error of the primary and key secondary (SDAI and DAS28 scores) endpoints. The primary endpoint was analysed at the fixed 46- to 54-week time point (because two visits were needed to define sustained/persistent remission) using Fisher's exact test. Persistent clinical remission at weeks 46 and 54 was evaluated as a categorical variable (in remission or not) and Fisher's exact test was calculated for differences over all three treatment groups. For the primary endpoint analysis, we applied non-responder imputation (NRI) for dichotomous variables from those visits onward at which patients had missing data or for patients who started rescue DMARD therapy, and the last observation carried forward (LOCF) method for continuous variables. In case of a significant result regarding the overall difference between all three groups, the primary endpoint was subsequently assessed comparing each of two groups, respectively: group 1 (IFX + MTX) versus 3 (PL), 1 (IFX + MTX) versus 2 (MTX), and 2 (MTX) versus 3 (PL). Longitudinal data analysis of clinical remission is described in Additional file 2: Supplement S2. Secondary endpoints were tested at years 1 and 2 using either Fisher's exact test for categorical variables or Kruskal-Wallis test for continuous data.

Results

Demographic data and patient flow

Of the 122 screened patients, 90 were randomised and dosed at the baseline visit (Fig. 1). Baseline characteristics and demographic data are described in Table 1. Table 2 depicts the number of patients in clinical remission in the three treatment groups at 6 months, 1 year, and 2 years. Early withdrawal within the first 3 months was seen in three patients in the IFX + MTX group , in two in the MTX group, and in one patient in the PL group.

Clinical remission at 1 year

At week 54 (primary endpoint), more patients in the IFX + MTX group (12/38, 32%) achieved sustained clinical remission compared with 5/36 (14%) on MTX alone and none (0/16, 0%) on PL. The overall difference across all three treatment groups showed statistical significance ($p < 0.05$; Additional file 1: Figure SB). Upon subsequent pairwise comparisons, differences in rates of sustained clinical remission were significant between IFX + MTX and PL (treatment effect: 32%; $p < 0.05$), but not between the IFX + MTX and MTX (treatment effect 18%; $p > 0.05$), nor between MTX and PL (treatment effect 14%; $p > 0.05$). Figure 2 shows sustained remission rates as defined for the primary outcome in a cumulative way over time for each of the treatment groups. By week 30, 10 patients (26%) treated with IFX + MTX had already achieved clinical remission at two consecutive visits and all these patients sustained clinical remission until weeks 46 and 54. It is noteworthy that almost one in three patients receiving IFX + MTX, but only one in seven in the MTX group and none on PL had achieved sustained clinical remission at 1 year. The number needed to treat (NNT) to achieve one additional sustained remission at 52 weeks with IFX + MTX was 3 compared with placebo, while the NNT for MTX alone versus placebo was 7; NNT was 6 when comparing IFX + MTX with MTX

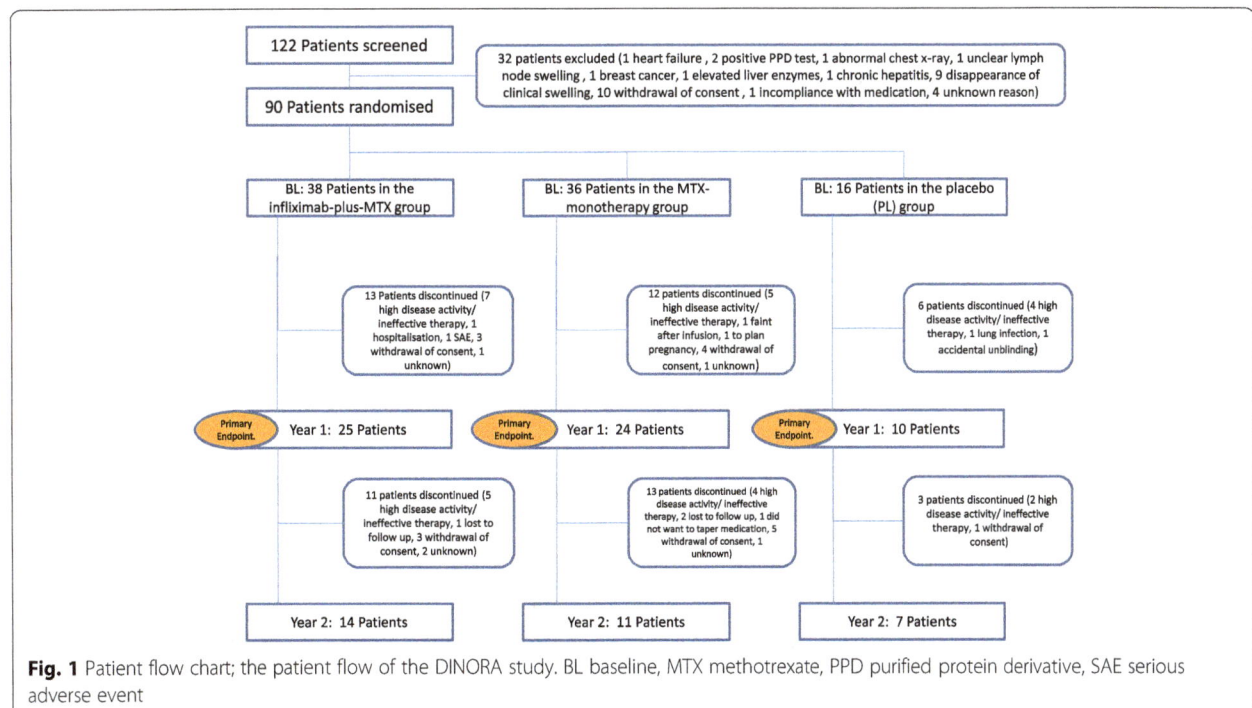

Fig. 1 Patient flow chart; the patient flow of the DINORA study. BL baseline, MTX methotrexate, PPD purified protein derivative, SAE serious adverse event

Table 1 Baseline characteristics of the study sample

	IFX + MTX	MTX	PL	P value
Number of patients (n)	38	36	16	0.4440
Female	26 (68.4%)	28 (77.8%)	9 (56.3%)	0.2833
Age (years), mean ± SD	52.1 ± 14.1	52.9 ± 14.0	54.4 ± 11.2	0.9170
Symptom duration (weeks)[a], mean ± SD	10.3 ± 2.3	9.4 ± 2.3	9.8 ± 1.8	0.0722
Rheumatoid factor positive	13 (34.2%)	13 (36.1%)	7 (43.8%)	0.7988
Patients who used steroids prior to the study	24 (63.2%)	22 (61.1%)	9 (56.3%)	0.8931
Anti-citrullinated protein antibody positive	18 (47.4%)	16 (44.4%)	7 (43.8%)	0.9563
Patients who meet the ACR/EULAR 2010 classification criteria for RA, 2010 [25]	26 (68%)	19 (53%)	12 (75%)	0.2135
Patients who meet the 1987 ARA classification criteria for RA [35]	22 (58%)	19 (53%)	9 (56%)	0.9049
Health Assessment Questionnaire (0–3)	0.9 ± 0.7	0.9 ± 0.6	0.7 ± 0.7	0.2903
Disease Activity Score 28 (DAS28; based on ESR)	5.0 ± 1.4	4.8 ± 1.3	4.7 ± 1.1	0.8464
Simplified Disease Activity Index (SDAI)	34.3 ± 23.8	31.1 ± 14.4	27.5 ± 20.0	0.4771
Clinical Disease Activity Index (CDAI)	25.1 ± 14.7	26.2 ± 13.9	23.5 ± 11.9	0.8951
Swollen joint count (0–28)	7.2 ± 5.7	6.50 ± 5.1	7.4 ± 4.6	0.7048
Tender joint count (0–28)	9.2 ± 7.3	10.3 ± 7.2	7.8 ± 5.6	0.5263
Visual analogue scale pain (mm)	44.0 ± 29.3	44.2 ± 24.3	44.6 ± 22.7	0.9595
Patient global assessment (mm)	48.6 ± 29.0	47.8 ± 24.7	39.6 ± 21.0	0.5274
Evaluator/physician global assessment (mm)	38.6 ± 18.3	46.3 ± 22.3	44.6 ± 20.7	0.3627
C-reactive protein (mg/dl)	1.71 ± 2.40	1.18 ± 1.88	0.98 ± 1.28	0.5567
Erythrocyte sedimentation rate (ESR; mm/h)	23.2 ± 20.3	20.3 ± 21.2	20.4 ± 12.6	0.8129
Total Sharp-van-der-Heide score	2.8 ± 5.4	3 ± 3.8	4.6 ± 8.6	0.4816
Erosion score	1.2 ± 1.8	1.6 ± 2.2	2.2 ± 4.2	0.6019
Joint space narrowing score	1.6 ± 3.8	1.4 ± 2.2	2.4 ± 4.4	0.5658

Data are shown as mean ± standard deviation or n (%) as appropriate
The parameters showed no significant differences between the three groups at baseline
Tables with additional data on baseline characteristics as well as 1-year data for the patients who were in remission at 1 year are provided in Additional file 2 (Tables SC and SD)
ACR American College of Rheumatology, *ARA* American Rheumatism Association, *EULAR* European League Against Rheumatism, *IFX* infliximab, *MTX* methotrexate, *PL* placebo, *RA* rheumatoid arthritis
[a]Symptom duration refers to the first visit when the patients presented themselves at the centres. At the baseline visit, symptom duration of all patients was 12 weeks because baseline visits were scheduled at this time to ensure persistent arthritis for 12 weeks. Patients who had no residual arthritis at the baseline visit were excluded

alone. The results of the longitudinal data analysis are described in Additional file 2: Supplement S3.

Clinical remission at the end of year 2
Maintenance of a remission state until the end of year 2 differed significantly across the three groups ($p = 0.0210$); only 20% of patients in remission on MTX monotherapy at 54 weeks maintained remission, whereas this was the case in 75% of those attaining this state on IFX + MTX despite withdrawal of therapy ($p = 0.0140$ for the comparison between IFX + MTX and MTX groups; Table 2). The NNT to achieve sustained remission at 2 years with IFX + MTX was 2 compared with treatment with MTX alone, and 2 compared with placebo; the NNT for MTX alone versus placebo was 5.

Changes in disease activity and core set variables
At week 54, the proportions of patients with DAS28 < 2.6 and ACR20 responses were significantly different over all three groups ($p < 0.01$ for DAS28 < 2.6 and $p < 0.05$ for ACR20), as well as pain scores measured on a VAS ($p < 0.05$). The stratified differences between treatment groups revealed significance between the IFX + MTX and MTX groups ($p < 0.05$ for DAS28 < 2.6), IFX + MTX and PL ($p < 0.001$ for DAS28 < 2.6; $p < 0.05$ for ACR20; $p < 0.05$ for pain scores), and between MTX and PL ($p < 0.01$ for ACR20; $p < 0.01$ for pain scores).

Patients classified as RA or non-RA at baseline
In the IFX + MTX group, 8/26 (30.8%) of the patients classified as RA [25] achieved clinical remission at the

Table 2 Clinical characteristics of the study sample at 6 months, 1 year, and 2 years

	IFX + MTX n = 38	MTX n = 36	PL n = 16
Clinical remission (primary endpoint), no. of patients in remission (%)			
6 months	10 (26%)	6 (17%)	0
1 year	12 (32%)	5 (14%)	0
2 years	9 (24%)	1 (3%)	3 (19%)
Other definitions of remission, no. of patients in remission (%)			
Disease Activity Score 28 (DAS28)			
6 months	20 (53%)	11 (31%)	1 (6%)
1 year	24 (63%)	13 (36%)	3 (19%)
2 years	23 (61%)	11 (31%)	5 (31%)
Simplified Disease Activity Index (SDAI)			
6 months	16 (42%)	9 (25%)	1 (6%)
1 year	18 (47%)	13 (36%)	1 (6%)
2 years	18 (47%)	13 (36%)	4 (25%)
ACR/EULAR Boolean			
6 months	15 (40%)	8 (22%)	0
1 year	13 (34%)	9 (25%)	1 (6%)
2 years	13 (34%)	10 (28%)	4 (25%)
ACR improvement, responders			
ACR20			
6 months	20 (53%)	18 (50%)	4 (25%)
1 year	22 (58%)	22 (61%)	3 (19%)
2 years	19 (50%)	19 (53%)	3 (19%)
ACR50			
6 months	16 (42%)	13 (36%)	1 (6%)
1 year	17 (45%)	16 (44%)	3 (19%)
2 years	14 (37%)	15 (42%)	3 (19%)
ACR70			
6 months	15 (40%)	6 (17%)	1 (6%)
1 year	14 (37%)	11 (31%)	2 (13%)
2 years	13 (34%)	11 (31%)	3 (19%)
Other secondary outcome parameters (mean ± SD)			
Pain			
6 months	17.3 ± 20.3	22.5 ± 25.2	42.7 ± 31.0
1 year	20.9 ± 23.8	18.3 ± 25.3	45.7 ± 31.8
2 years	23.0 ± 25.1	23.3 ± 29.8	43.5 ± 32.8
Swollen joints (28 joints)			
6 months	2.3 ± 5.2	2.1 ± 4.5	4.9 ± 5.6
1 year	2.3 ± 5.2	2.1 ± 4.3	5.0 ± 5.6
2 years	2.8 ± 5.6	2.4 ± 4.5	5.1 ± 5.6
Tender joints (28 joints)			
6 months	2.9 ± 5.9	4.9 ± 6.2	7.0 ± 6.4
1 year	2.5 ± 5.6	4.2 ± 6.0	7.2 ± 6.8
2 years	3.4 ± 6.5	4.0 ± 6.1	7.1 ± 7.0

Table 2 Clinical characteristics of the study sample at 6 months, 1 year, and 2 years *(Continued)*

	IFX + MTX $n = 38$	MTX $n = 36$	PL $n = 16$
Patient global visual analogue scale (VAS; mm)			
6 months	17.7 ± 6.5	23.1 ± 24.6	35.1 ± 28.2
1 year	21.2 ± 24.0	18.4 ± 24.7	38.0 ± 29.3
2 years	24.3 ± 25.3	24.8 ± 30.0	35.6 ± 29.5
Evaluator global VAS (mm)			
6 months	16.1 ± 22.0	17.2 ± 24.1	34.6 ± 28.0
1 year	14.1 ± 20.8	17.7 ± 24.6	39.3 ± 29.8
2 years	16.6 ± 24.1	18.4 ± 24.7	34.5 ± 31.3
C-reactive protein (mg/dl)			
6 months	0.5 ± 0.9	0.6 ± 1.0	0.8 ± 0.9
1 year	0.5 ± 0.9	0.5 ± 1.0	0.7 ± 0.8
2 years	0.6 ± 1.1	0.6 ± 1.0	0.5 ± 0.8
Erythrocyte sedimentation rate (mm)			
6 months	14.6 ± 12.2	17.8 ± 12.5	14.9 ± 6.9
1 year	14.6 ± 12.3	18.7 ± 13.0	18.3 ± 9.7
2 years	16.5 ± 14.1	17.6 ± 11.2	16.5 ± 10.7
Health Assessment Questionnaire (HAQ)			
6 months	0.30 ± 0.45	0.57 ± 0.64	0.54 ± 0.67
1 year	0.33 ± 0.46	0.52 ± 0.62	0.61 ± 0.66
2 years	0.41 ± 0.52	0.58 ± 0.61	0.62 ± 0.65
X-rays[a]			
6 months	−0.02 ± 0.88	0.07 ± 0.23	0.41 ± 1.53
1 year	0.18 ± 1.06	0.16 ± 0.44	0.0 ± 0.41
2 years	0.36 ± 0.95	0.28 ± 0.67	0.63 ± 1.31

Missing data for continuous variables were imputed using last observation carried forward (LOCF). LOCF was also applied from the time points onwards when patients received other DMARDs as rescue therapy. The denominator for the percentages given is the number of patients initially included in each group and stays consistent for each year

ACR American College of Rheumatology, *EULAR* European League Against Rheumatism, *IFX* infliximab, *MTX* methotrexate, *PL* placebo

[a]Mean change of scores ± SD from baseline of Sharp-van-der-Heijde (SvdH) for patients with complete follow-up data at each time point

primary endpoint (1 year) compared with 4/12 (33.3%) of the patients who did not fulfil RA classification criteria. In the MTX group, 2/19 (10.5%) of the patients classified as RA reached the primary endpoint at 1 year compared with 3/17 (17.6%) of the patients who did not fulfil RA criteria (data not shown). When looking at the 2-year outcome in the IFX + MTX group, 5/26 (19%) of the patients classified as RA [25] achieved clinical remission compared with 4/12 (33.3%) of the patients who did not fulfil RA classification criteria. In the MTX group, 1/19 (5%) patient classified as RA reached the remission at 2 years compared with none who did not fulfil RA criteria (data not shown). Two of the three patients who were in remission after 2 years in the PL group fulfilled the RA classification criteria at baseline, and all three PL patients were ACPA and RF negative. Thus, there was no difference in outcomes whether patients fulfilled the ACR/EULAR classification criteria [25] or not. The

presence of RF made a significant difference in the remission frequency at the 2-year time only point (Chi square test; $p = 0.0399$); the presence of ACPA made no significant difference in the frequency of remission at 6 months, 1 year, or 2 years.

Radiographic changes

Mean change from baseline of the Sharp-van-der-Heide scores [30] did not reveal any noteworthy differences between the three treatment groups (Table 2 and Additional file 2: Figure SC and Table SA).

Adverse events

The occurrences of adverse events (AEs) and serious adverse events (SAEs) are depicted in Table 3. There were no statistically significant differences in the number of patients with AEs between the three treatment groups (Fisher's exact test; data not shown).

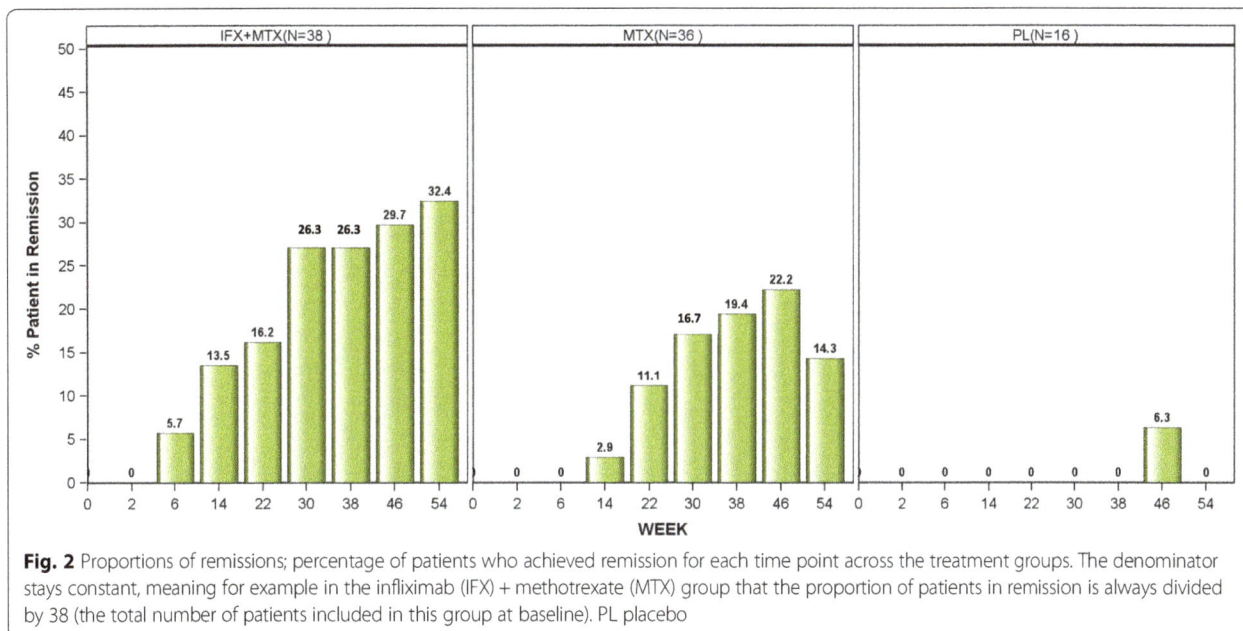

Fig. 2 Proportions of remissions; percentage of patients who achieved remission for each time point across the treatment groups. The denominator stays constant, meaning for example in the infliximab (IFX) + methotrexate (MTX) group that the proportion of patients in remission is always divided by 38 (the total number of patients included in this group at baseline). PL placebo

Discussion

The present trial in patients with very early arthritis yields several important findings on the effects of treatment of early inflammatory arthritis with DMARD therapy. First, as in the SAVE trial [32], our study indicated that spontaneous remission (on placebo and supportive treatment alone) occurred only very rarely in patients with undifferentiated arthritis or very early RA of 12 weeks duration. Secondly, we observed that therapy with anti-TNF plus MTX, while significantly different from PL regarding all outcomes, produced more than twice as many stringently defined remissions when compared with MTX alone (32% and 14%, respectively); while the trend was clear, the difference in response rates did not achieve statistical significance ($p = 0.10$). Thirdly, we found that the majority of those patients who had remission on IFX + MTX therapy maintained remission even after withdrawal of all therapies (overall 24% still had clinical remission at 2 years); in contrast, 80% of those on MTX alone lost their remission state, leaving only 3% of MTX-treated patients in remission at 2 years. Fourthly, the vast majority of patients who achieved sustained drug-free remission had already attained this state within 30 weeks, indicating that the necessity for longer treatment durations to achieve remission does not increase drug-free remission rates. Together, these findings suggest that once joint inflammation is clinically manifest, symptomatic therapy does not impact on the course of disease, that initiation of DMARD therapy is warranted to improve outcomes, and that early intensive treatment with anti-TNF + MTX leads to drug-free remission in 1 of 4 patients. When we assessed other remission definitions, such as SDAI or Boolean remission criteria or DAS28 < 2.6, we saw even higher remission rates in the IFX + MTX group at 1 year (34–63%), but this was also the case for the MTX group and the difference across all three groups was not significant, except for DAS28 < 2.6. These findings might be due to the heterogeneity of the patients in our study; furthermore, our data suggest that aggressive therapy is not always necessary in very early inflammatory arthritis for obtaining sustained drug-free remission, although we did not find any respective predictive markers (data not shown).

In addition to delineating the effects of DMARD therapy on early inflammatory arthritis, this study provides important new information on the validity of the window of opportunity hypothesis. This hypothesis proposes that a short period of intensive therapy early in the disease course may reverse the disease process and produce long-term benefits. Indeed, in this study, almost one-third of the patients receiving IFX + MTX achieved sustained remission, with 9/12 (75%) of those who attained remission in the first year maintaining this state 1 year later without any treatment (or a total of 9/38 (24%) of the randomised patients). This outcome contrasts with that of patients treated with MTX alone since only 1 in 7 achieved remission in the first year, with the majority subsequently losing this state; as a result, only 3% of patients treated with MTX alone had a sustained remission at 2 years. Thus, anti-TNF + MTX induction treatment demonstrated a clear advantage compared with supportive therapy at 1 year and compared with MTX-only therapy at 2 years; in contrast, induction with MTX alone failed to show a significantly better response than placebo. Importantly, the active therapies, in particular anti-TNF plus

Table 3 Patients with adverse events (AEs) and serious adverse events (SAEs)

	Total $n = 90$	IFX + MTX $n = 38$	MTX $n = 36$	PL $n = 16$
Adverse events, n (%)				
Infectious/parasitic disease	31 (35%)	19 (50%)	9 (25%)	3 (19%)
Malignancy	1 (1%)	0	1 (3%)	0
Disease of blood, blood-forming organs, and immune mechanisms (except arthritis)	1 (1%)	1 (3%)	0	0
Endocrine, nutritional, and metabolic diseases	9 (10%)	2 (5%)	5 (14%)	2 (12%)
Disease of the nervous system	17 (19%)	6 (16%)	9 (25%)	2 (13%)
Diseases of the eye	3 (3%)	1 (3%)	2 (6%)	0
Diseases of circulatory system	16 (18%)	6 (16%)	7 (19%)	3 (19%)
Diseases of respiratory system	43 (48%)	23 (61%)	16 (44%)	4 (25%)
Diseases of the digestive system	37 (41%)	15 (39%)	17 (47%)	5 (31%)
Diseases of the skin and subcutaneous tissue	25 (28%)	12 (32%)	8 (22%)	5 (31%)
Diseases of musculoskeletal system and connective tissue	30 (33%)	15 (39%)	9 (25%)	6 (38%)
Diseases of urogenital system (pregnancy, childbirth, and puerperium)	4 (4%)	2 (5%)	2 (6%)	0
Symptoms, signs, and abnormal clinical and laboratory findings not elsewhere classified	27 (30%)	11 (29%)	11 (31%)	5 (31%)
Injury, poisoning and certain other consequences of external causes	9 (10%)	6 (16%)	3 (8%)	0
External causes of morbidity	1 (1%)	1 (3%)	0	0
Total		120	99	35
SAEs (n = 12)				
Hospitalisation due to different reasons[a]		4	1	3
Fainted during blood collection prior to administration of study drug		1	0	0
Significantly raised transaminase levels		1	0	0
Hematuria, followed by a diagnosis of bladder cancer		0	1	0
Hypertensive episode 1 h after the last infusion with study drug		0	1	0

Only 4 (0.9%) of all reported AEs and no SAEs were considered definitely related to the study drug. 155 AEs (37%) and no SAEs were regarded as possibly/probably related to one of the study drugs. No participant died during the 2-year study period. Two SAEs were related to infections (1 gastrointestinal, 1 genitourinary); however, in both cases patients were on PL only. One of these SAEs was related to a malignancy (bladder cancer on MTX monotherapy) and none to tuberculosis

IFX infliximab, *MTX* methotrexate, *PL* placebo

[a]Hyperglycemia (PL), diarrhoea (PL), urinary tract infection (IFX + MTX), urinary tract infection with fever (PL), MTX pneumonitis (opportunistic) infection (IFX + MTX), significant flare of disease activity (IFX + MTX), myocardial infarction more than half a year after last study drug (MTX), and biliary pancreatitis in a time after the study medication (IFX + MTX)

MTX, did not appear to cause major serious adverse events in this early arthritis patient population, with the two observed serious adverse events occurring in patients on supportive care.

While one-third of patients treated with IFX + MTX had a favourable outcome, two-thirds of the patients treated with these agents did not attain remission within the first year. This result is disappointing and could argue against the window of opportunity hypothesis. It is important to note, however, that our results pertain only to the combination of IFX + MTX. As shown in other studies, RA patients can differ in their response to biological agents, perhaps based on their mode of action, and we do not know which patients will respond best to a given targeted therapy [33]. On the other hand, the study outcome is quite promising, since 1 of 4 patients with early arthritis did reach drug-free remission after a short course of an induction therapy with these agents. Importantly, in contrast to other randomised controlled trials in early, although established, RA, we did not observe a gradual decline in responders over the second year [21, 34], suggesting a true abrogation or reversal of the disease process.

Our study has several limitations. First, the study may have been underpowered to show a significant difference between the IFX + MTX and MTX-alone groups. For the purposes of this study, we estimated placebo and spontaneous remission rates on the basis of previous observational studies, and the lack of precise data on remission rates from these trials could have led to difficulties in balancing MTX alone and anti-TNF + MTX responses. Although our results indicate that the majority of patients failed to achieve sustained remission on anti-TNF + MTX, the difference between anti-TNF +

MTX and MTX alone in the first year might have reached statistical significance with a larger sample size. Of note, in this regard, patients treated with MTX alone did not maintain remission until the end of year 2 while IFX + MTX patients did, suggesting relevant differences in the effects of combination therapy compared with monotherapy. The results of our study need to be interpreted with caution; however, they do suggest that early intensive treatment may alter the course of inflammatory arthritis. One notable unexpected finding was the difficulty of recruiting patients into this study which contrasted with our experience from a previous study [32]. We attempted to enrol very early arthritis patients who had to consent to their participation in a long-term (2 years) study at one of their first visits to the rheumatology centre before many of them had the opportunity to recognise and accept the implications of a diagnosis of inflammatory arthritis and possibly RA. Our experiences may be useful in planning future investigator-driven studies with larger sample sizes in this very early arthritis population of patients.

Conclusions

In conclusion, our study provides encouraging evidence that a short-term induction therapy with a TNF inhibitor plus MTX can yield long-term benefit in a considerable proportion of patients with early arthritis, even after cessation of all therapy. In contrast, the data presented indicate that MTX alone will not produce responses that are maintained over time. Placebo or supportive treatment alone neither improves nor reverses disease; these findings represent further evidence that spontaneous remission is rare once the signs and symptoms of RA have emerged. While the current study involves only TNF as a target of biological therapy, the data nevertheless strongly support the possibility that patients with early inflammatory arthritis may have a window of opportunity in which disease reversal is possible.

Abbreviations

ACPA: Anti-citrullinated protein antibodies; ACR: American College of Rheumatology; CRP: C-reactive protein; DAS28: Disease Activity Score 28; DINORA: Definitive Intervention in New Onset Rheumatoid Arthritis; DMARD: Disease-modifying anti-rheumatic drug; EGA: Evaluator global assessment; ESR: Erythrocyte sedimentation rate; EULAR: European League Against Rheumatism; HAQ: Health Assessment Questionnaire Disability Index; IFX: Infliximab; MTP: metatarsophalangeal; MTX: Methotrexate; NNT: Number needed to treat; PGA: Patient global assessment; RA: Rheumatoid arthritis; RF: Rheumatoid factor; SDAI: Simplified Disease Activity Index; SJC: Swollen joint count; TJC: Tender joint count; TNF: Tumour necrosis factor; VAS: Visual analogue scale

Acknowledgements

We are very thankful to all patients who participated in the present study and to the members of the drug safety monitoring board, Hans Bijlsma, Wolfgang Graninger, Hans Hillege, and Frank Wollheim.

Funding

DINORA was designed by the sponsor, the Department of Medicine 3, Medical University of Vienna (MUV), Austria, in collaboration with an international advisory committee. The data were analysed by the sponsor and the Clinical Trial Coordination Center (TCC) in Groningen, The Netherlands. Funds for the planning of the trial were provided by NIH grants AR050880 and AR052465 to DP. The study was funded by a grant from Janssen (previously Centocor). Janssen participated in the design of the protocol and the review of the report. All authors participated in collection and/or interpretation of the data, contributed substantially to the manuscript, and agreed to submit it for publication. All investigators at MUV had full access to the data and vouch for accuracy and completeness of the data and analyses. Individual author disclosures are listed below.

Authors' contributions

KPM, DA, RL, DvdH, MA, DB, GB, MC, WE, WG, TH, GS, HSK, PPT, EMM, and FB were involved in the planning of the study, recruited patients, and participated in writing, reviewing and approval of the analysis and the final manuscript. JS, FA, PL, DP, AS, and TAS were involved in the planning of the study, conducted clinical trial and/or data logistics, performed the data analyses or parts of it and wrote and approved the manuscript. All authors read and approved the final manuscript.

Consent for publication

The present manuscript does not contain any individual person's data, such as individual details, images, or videos.

Competing interests

TAS has received speaker fees from AbbVie, Janssen, MSD, Novartis, and Roche and grant support from AbbVie. MAS has received speaker fees from MSD. KPM has received money from AbbVie (speaker's fees, consulting fees, research grant), Astro (speaker's fees, consulting fees), Baxter (consulting fees), BMS (speaker's fees), Celgene (speaker's fees), Janssen-Cilag (speaker's fees), Lilly (speaker's fees), MSD (speaker's fees), Novartis (speaker's fees, consulting fees), Pfizer (speaker's fees), Roche (speaker's fees), UCB (speaker's fees), Arsanis (consulting fees), and Sandoz (speaker's fees). DA has served as a consultant for and/or received grant/research support from AbbVie, Pfizer, Grünenthal, Merck Medac, UCB, Mitsubishi/Tanabe, Janssen, and Roche. PL received consulting fees from Janssen, EMD Serono, Astra Zeneca, UCB, Roche, Celgene, Sanofi, and Horizon, but none of them relates to the content of this manuscript. RL has received fees for consultation or participation in advisory boards by Abbott/AbbVie, Ablynx, Amgen, Astra-Zeneca, Bristol Myers Squibb, Celgene, Janssen (formerly Centocor), Galapagos, Glaxo-Smith-Kline, Novartis, Novo-Nordisk, Merck, Pfizer, Roche, Schering-Plough, TiGenix, UCB, and Wyeth; research grants from Abbott, Amgen, Centocor, Novartis, Pfizer, Roche, Schering-Plough, UCB and Wyeth and speaker fees from Abbott/AbbVie, Amgen, Bristol Myers Squibb, Janssen (formerly Centocor), Merck, Pfizer, Roche, Schering-Plough, UCB, and Wyeth; furthermore, RL is director of Rheumatology Consultancy BV which is a registered company under Dutch law. DvdH has received consulting fees from AbbVie, Amgen, Astellas, AstraZeneca, BMS, Boeringer Ingelheim, Celgene, Daiichi, Eli-Lilly, Galapagos, Gilead, Janssen, Merck, Novartis, Pfizer, Regeneron, Roche, Sanofi, and UCB and is director of Imaging Rheumatology BV. MA has received advisory Boards and/or speaking fees from AbbVie, Astra Zeneca, BMS, Chugai, GSK, Hexal, Lilly, MSD, Novartis, Pfizer, Roche, Sanofi, and UCB; his institution is clinical trial site for AbbVie, Astra Zeneca, Boehringer Ingelheim, Novartis,

Pfizer, and Roche. GB has received speaker fees from MSD, UCB and Roche and research funds from AbbVie, BMS, UCB, and Roche. MC has received speaker fees from Biogen, Mundipharm, Pfizer and Menarini and research funds from BMS, Horizon, Actelion, Celgene, and MSD. WE has received consulting fees from Novartis and Abbvie. TH has received lecture fees/consultancy fees from Merck, UCB, Bristol Myers Squibb, Biotest AG, Pfizer, GSK, Novartis, Roche, Sanofi-Aventis, Abbott, Crescendo Bioscience, Nycomed, Boeringher, Takeda, Epirus, and Eli Lilly. GS has received speaker fees from BMS, Celgene, Chugai, Lilly, Roche, and UCB. HSK has received speaker fees from AbbVie, Actelion, AstraZeneca, Biogen International, Boehringer Ingelheim, BMS, Celgene, Celltrion, Chugai, Cinfa Biotech, GSK, Hospira, Janssen-Cilag, Lilly, MSD, Medac, Merck, Mundipharma, Novartis, Pfizer, Hexal Sandoz, Roche, and UCB. PPT has become an employee of GlaxoSmithKline. GSK has not been involved in this study. JS has received grants for his institution from Abbvie, Lilly, MSD, Pfizer and Roche and has provided remunerated expert advice to and/or had speaking engagements for Abbvie, Amgen, Astra-Zeneca, Astro, BMS, Boehringer-Ingelheim, Celgene, Celltrion, Chugai, Gilead, Glaxo, ILTOO, Janssen, Lilly, Medimmune, MSD, Novartis-Sandoz, Pfizer, Roche, Samsung, Sanofi, and UCB. The remaining authors declare that they have no competing interests.

Author details

[1]Section for Outcomes Research, Center for Medical Statistics, Informatics, and Intelligent Systems, Medical University of Vienna, Spitalgasse 23, 1090 Vienna, Austria. [2]Department of Medicine III, Division of Rheumatology, Medical University of Vienna, Waehringer Guertel 18-20, 1090 Vienna, Austria. [3]RILITE Research Institute, 250 W Main Street, Charlottesville, Virginia 22902, USA. [4]Medical Research Service Durham VA Medical Center, and Duke University Medical Center, 151G Durham VA Medical Center, 508 Fulton Street, Durham, North Carolina 27705, USA. [5]Department of Medicine, Division of Rheumatology, Academic Medical Center Amsterdam, Amsterdam, The Netherlands. [6]Department of Rheumatology, Leiden University Medical Centre, Albinusdreef 2, PO Box 9600, 2300 RC Leiden, The Netherlands. [7]Division of Rheumatology, Department of Medicine III, University Medical Center and Faculty of Medicine Carl Gustav Carus at the TU Dresden, Fetscherstrasse 74, 01309 Dresden, Germany. [8]Rheumatology Medical School University of Crete, Heraklion and Joint Rheumatology Program, National and Kapodestrian University of Athens, Athens, Greece. [9]Department of Rheumatology and Clinical Immunology, Charité - University Medicine Berlin, Free University and Humboldt University Berlin, Berlin, Germany. [10]Research Laboratory and Division of Rheumatology, Department of Internal Medicine, University of Genova, Viale Benedetto XV, 6, 16132 Genoa, Italy. [11]Department of Internal Medicine, Centre for Rheumatic Diseases, Hietzing Hospital, Wolkersbergenstraße 1, 1130 Vienna, Austria. [12]Department of Rheumatology, Medical University of Graz, Auenbruggerplatz 15, 8036 Graz, Styria, Austria. [13]Department of Internal Medicine 3, Rheumatology and Immunology, Friedrich-Alexander-University Erlangen-Nürnberg (FAU) and Universitätsklinikum Erlangen, Ulmenweg 18, 91054 Erlangen, Germany. [14]Division of Rheumatology and Clinical Immunology, Department of Internal Medicine IV, Ludwig Maximilians University of Munich, Pettenkoferstraße 8a, 80336 Munich, Germany. [15]Amsterdam Rheumatology and Immunology Center, Academic Medical Centre, University of Amsterdam, Amsterdam, the Netherlands. [16]Department of Medicine, Cambridge University, Cambridge, UK. [17]Department of Rheumatology, Ghent University, Ghent, Belgium. [18]GlaxoSmithKline Research & Development, Stevenage, UK. [19]Hospital Universitario La Paz, Paseo de la Castellana 261, 28046 Madrid, Spain. [20]Leiden University Medical Center, Albinusdreef 2, PO Box 9600, 2300 RC Leiden, The Netherlands.

References

1. van der Heide A, Jacobs JW, Bijlsma JW, Heurkens AH, van Booma-Frankfort C, van der Veen MJ, Haanen HC, Hofman DM, van Albada-Kuipers GA, ter Borg EJ, et al. The effectiveness of early treatment with "second-line" antirheumatic drugs. A randomized, controlled trial. Ann Intern Med. 1996; 124(8):699–707.
2. Nell VK, Machold KP, Eberl G, Stamm TA, Uffmann M, Smolen JS. Benefit of very early referral and very early therapy with disease-modifying antirheumatic drugs in patients with early rheumatoid arthritis. Rheumatology (Oxford). 2004; Epub (ahead of print)
3. Lard LR, Visser H, Speyer I, vander Horst-Bruinsma IE, Zwinderman AH, Breedveld FC, Hazes J. Early versus delayed treatment in patients with recent-onset rheumatoid arthritis: comparison of two cohorts who received different treatment strategies. AmJMed. 2001;111(6):446–51.
4. Grigor C, Capell H, Stirling A, McMahon AD, Lock P, Vallance R, Kincaid W, Porter D. Effect of a treatment strategy of tight control for rheumatoid arthritis (the TICORA study): a single-blind randomised controlled trial. Lancet. 2004;364(9430):263–9.
5. Goekoop-Ruiterman YP, de Vries-Bouwstra JK, Kerstens PJ, Nielen MM, Vos K, van Schaardenburg D, Speyer I, Seys PE, Breedveld FC, Allaart CF, et al. DAS-driven therapy versus routine care in patients with recent-onset active rheumatoid arthritis. Ann Rheum Dis. 2010;69(1):65–9.
6. Singh JA, Furst DE, Bharat A, Curtis JR, Kavanaugh AF, Kremer JM, Moreland LW, O'Dell J, Winthrop KL, Beukelman T, et al. 2012 update of the 2008 American College of Rheumatology recommendations for the use of disease-modifying antirheumatic drugs and biologic agents in the treatment of rheumatoid arthritis. Arthritis Care Res. 2012;64(5):625–39.
7. Smolen JS, Landewe R, Breedveld FC, Buch M, Burmester G, Dougados M, Emery P, Gaujoux-Viala C, Gossec L, Nam J, et al. EULAR recommendations for the management of rheumatoid arthritis with synthetic and biological disease-modifying antirheumatic drugs: 2013 update. Ann Rheum Dis. 2014; 73(3):492–509.
8. Mierau M, Schoels M, Gonda G, Fuchs J, Aletaha D, Smolen JS. Assessing remission in clinical practice. Rheumatology(Oxford). 2007;46(6):975–9.
9. Felson DT, Smolen JS, Wells G, Zhang B, van Tuyl LH, Funovits J, Aletaha D, Allaart CF, Bathon J, Bombardieri S, et al. American College of Rheumatology/European league against rheumatism provisional definition of remission in rheumatoid arthritis for clinical trials. Ann Rheum Dis. 2011; 70(3):404–13.
10. Aletaha D, Funovits J, Breedveld FC, Sharp J, Segurado O, Smolen JS. Rheumatoid arthritis joint progression in sustained remission is determined by disease activity levels preceding the period of radiographic assessment. Arthritis Rheum. 2009;60(5):1242–9.
11. Tanaka Y, Takeuchi T, Mimori T, Saito K, Nawata M, Kameda H, Nojima T, Miyasaka N, Koike T, investigators RRRs. Discontinuation of infliximab after attaining low disease activity in patients with rheumatoid arthritis: RRR (remission induction by Remicade in RA) study. Ann Rheum Dis. 2010;69(7): 1286–91.
12. Emery P, Hammoudeh M, FitzGerald O, Combe B, Martin-Mola E, Buch MH, Krogulec M, Williams T, Gaylord S, Pedersen R, et al. Sustained remission with etanercept tapering in early rheumatoid arthritis. N Engl J Med. 2014; 371(19):1781–92.
13. Furst DE. Window of opportunity. J Rheumatol. 2004;31(9):1677–9.
14. Raza K, Saber TP, Kvien TK, Tak PP, Gerlag DM. Timing the therapeutic window of opportunity in early rheumatoid arthritis: proposal for definitions of disease duration in clinical trials. Ann Rheum Dis. 2012;71(12):1921–3.
15. Green M, Marzo-Ortega H, McGonagle D, Wakefield R, Proudman S, Conaghan P, Gooi J, Emery P. Persistence of mild, early inflammatory arthritis: the importance of disease duration, rheumatoid factor, and the shared epitope. Arthritis Rheum. 1999;42(10):2184–8.
16. van der Linden MP, le Cessie S, Raza K, van der Woude D, Knevel R, Huizinga TW, van der Helm-van Mil AH. Long-term impact of delay in assessment of patients with early arthritis. Arthritis Rheum. 2010;62(12): 3537–46.
17. Raza K, Falciani F, Curnow SJ, Ross EJ, Lee CY, Akbar AN, Lord JM, Gordon C, Buckley CD, Salmon M. Early rheumatoid arthritis is characterized by a distinct and transient synovial fluid cytokine profile of T cell and stromal cell origin. Arthritis Res Ther. 2005;7(4):R784–95.
18. de Hair MJ, van de Sande MG, Ramwadhdoebe TH, Hansson M, Landewe R, van der Leij C, Maas M, Serre G, van Schaardenburg D, Klareskog L, et al. Features of the synovium of individuals at risk of developing rheumatoid arthritis: implications for understanding preclinical rheumatoid arthritis. Arthritis Rheumatol. 2014;66(3):513–22.
19. Goekoop-Ruiterman YP, de Vries-Bouwstra JK, Allaart CF, van Zeben D, Kerstens PJ, Hazes JM, Zwinderman AH, Peeters AJ, de Jonge-Bok JM, Mallee

C, et al. Comparison of treatment strategies in early rheumatoid arthritis: a randomized trial. Ann Intern Med. 2007;146(6):406–15.

20. Quinn MA, Conaghan PG, O'Connor PJ, Karim Z, Greenstein A, Brown A, Brown C, Fraser A, Jarret S, Emery P. Very early treatment with infliximab in addition to methotrexate in early, poor-prognosis rheumatoid arthritis reduces magnetic resonance imaging evidence of synovitis and damage, with sustained benefit after infliximab withdrawal: results from a twelve-month randomized, double-blind, placebo-controlled trial. Arthritis Rheum. 2005;52(1):27–35.

21. Emery P, Burmester GR, Bykerk VP, Combe BG, Furst DE, Barre E, Karyekar CS, Wong DA, Huizinga TW. Evaluating drug-free remission with abatacept in early rheumatoid arthritis: results from the phase 3b, multicentre, randomised, active-controlled AVERT study of 24 months, with a 12-month, double-blind treatment period. Ann Rheum Dis. 2015;74(1):19–26.

22. Choi IY, Karpus ON, Turner JD, Hardie D, Marshall JL, de Hair MJ, Maijer KI, Tak PP, Raza K, Hamann J. Stromal cell markers are differentially expressed in the synovial tissue of patients with early arthritis. PLoS One. 2017;12(8): e0182751.

23. Goekoop-Ruiterman YP, Vries-Bouwstra JK, Allaart CF, van Zeben D, Kerstens PJ, Hazes JM, Zwinderman AH, Ronday HK, Han KH, Westedt ML, et al. Clinical and radiographic outcomes of four different treatment strategies in patients with early rheumatoid arthritis (the BeSt study): a randomized, controlled trial. Arthritis Rheum. 2005;52(11):3381–90.

24. Visser H, le Cessie S, Vos K, Breedveld FC, Hazes JM. How to diagnose rheumatoid arthritis early: a prediction model for persistent (erosive) arthritis. Arthritis Rheum. 2002;46(2):357–65.

25. Aletaha D, Neogi T, Silman AJ, Funovits J, Felson DT, Bingham CO III, Birnbaum NS, Burmester GR, Bykerk VP, Cohen MD, et al. 2010 rheumatoid arthritis classification criteria: an American College of Rheumatology/ European League Against Rheumatism collaborative initiative. AnnRheumDis. 2010;69(9):1580–8.

26. Felson DT, Anderson JJ, Boers M, Bombardier C, Furst D, Goldsmith C. American College of Rheumatology preliminary definition of improvement in rheumatoid arthritis. Arthritis Rheum. 1995;38:727–35.

27. Fries JF, Spitz P, Kraines RG, Holman HR. Measurement of patient outcome in arthritis. Arthritis Rheum. 1980;23(2):137–45.

28. Aletaha D, Ward MM, Machold KP, Nell VP, Stamm T, Smolen JS. Remission and active disease in rheumatoid arthritis: defining criteria for disease activity states. Arthritis Rheum. 2005;52(9):2625–36.

29. Prevoo ML, 't Hof MA, Kuper HH, van Leeuwen MA, van de Putte LB, van Riel PL. Modified disease activity scores that include twenty-eight-joint counts. Development and validation in a prospective longitudinal study of patients with rheumatoid arthritis. Arthritis Rheum. 1995;38(1):44–8.

30. van der Heijde D. How to read radiographs according to the sharp/van der Heijde method. J Rheumatol. 2000;27(1):261–3.

31. Genovese MC, Kremer J, Zamani O, Ludivico C, Krogulec M, Xie L, Beattie SD, Koch AE, Cardillo TE, Rooney TP, et al. Baricitinib in patients with refractory rheumatoid arthritis. N Engl J Med. 2016;374(13):1243–52.

32. Machold KP, Landewe R, Smolen JS, Stamm TA, van der Heijde DM, Verpoort KN, Brickmann K, Vazquez-Mellado J, Karateev DE, Breedveld FC, et al. The stop arthritis very early (SAVE) trial, an international multicentre, randomised, double-blind, placebo-controlled trial on glucocorticoids in very early arthritis. AnnRheumDis. 2010;69(3):495–502.

33. Smolen JS, Aletaha D. Rheumatoid arthritis therapy reappraisal: strategies, opportunities and challenges. Nat Rev Rheumatol. 2015;11(5):276–89.

34. Emery P, Breedveld FC, Hall S, Durez P, Chang DJ, Robertson D, Singh A, Pedersen RD, Koenig AS, Freundlich B. Comparison of methotrexate monotherapy with a combination of methotrexate and etanercept in active, early, moderate to severe rheumatoid arthritis (COMET): a randomised, double-blind, parallel treatment trial. Lancet. 2008;372(9636):375–82.

35. Arnett FC, Edworthy SM, Bloch DA, McShane DJ, Fries JF, Cooper NS, Healey LA, Kaplan SR, Liang MH, Luthra HS. The American Rheumatism Association 1987 revised criteria for the classification of rheumatoid arthritis. Arthritis Rheum. 1988;31(3):315–24.

5

Evaluation of ^{99m}Tc-rhAnnexin V-128 SPECT/CT as a diagnostic tool for early stages of interstitial lung disease associated with systemic sclerosis

Janine Schniering[1], Li Guo[1,2], Matthias Brunner[1], Roger Schibli[3,4], Shuang Ye[2], Oliver Distler[1], Martin Béhé[3] and Britta Maurer[1*] ⓘ

Abstract

Background: Given the need for early detection of organ involvement in systemic sclerosis, we evaluated ^{99m}Tc-rhAnnexin V-128 for the detection of early stages of interstitial lung disease (ILD) in respective animal models using single photon emission computed tomography (SPECT/CT).

Methods: In bleomycin (BLM)-challenged mice, fos-related antigen 2 (Fra-2) transgenic (tg) mice and respective controls, lung injury was evaluated by analysis of hematoxylin and eosin (HE) and Sirius red staining, with semi-quantification of fibrosis by the Ashcroft score. Apoptotic cells were identified by TUNEL assay, cleaved caspase 3 staining and double staining with specific cell markers. To detect early stages of lung remodeling by visualization of apoptosis, mice were injected intravenously with ^{99m}Tc-rhAnnexin V-128 and imaged by small animal SPECT/CT. For confirmation, biodistribution and ex vivo autoradiography studies were performed.

Results: In BLM-induced lung fibrosis, inflammatory infiltrates occurred as early as day 3 with peak at day 7, whereas pulmonary fibrosis developed from day 7 and was most pronounced at day 21. In accordance, the number of apoptotic cells was highest at day 3 compared with saline controls and then decreased over time. Epithelial cells (E-cadherin+) and inflammatory cells (CD45+) were the primary cells undergoing apoptosis in the earliest remodeling stages of experimental ILD. This was also true in the pathophysiologically different Fra-2 tg mice, where apoptosis of CD45+ cells occurred in the inflammatory stage. In accordance with the findings on tissue level, at day 3 in the BLM and at week 16 in the Fra-2 tg model, biodistribution and/or ex vivo autoradiography showed increased pulmonary uptake of ^{99m}Tc-rhAnnexin V-128 compared with controls. However, accumulation of the radiotracer and thus the signal intensity in lungs was too low to allow the differentiation of healthy and injured lungs in vivo.

Conclusion: At the tissue level, ^{99m}Tc-rhAnnexin V-128 successfully demonstrated early stages of ILD in two animal models by detection of apoptotic epithelial and/or inflammatory cells. In vivo, however, we did not detect early lung injury. It remains to be investigated whether the same applies to human ILD.

Keywords: Interstitial lung disease, Nuclear imaging, Apoptosis, Systemic sclerosis

* Correspondence: britta.maurer@usz.ch
[1]Center of Experimental Rheumatology, Department of Rheumatology, University Hospital Zurich, Gloriastrasse 25, 8091 Zurich, Switzerland
Full list of author information is available at the end of the article

Background

Systemic sclerosis (SSc) is a devastating multisystem auto-immune connective tissue disease with lung involvement as the primary cause of death [1]. Interstitial lung disease (ILD) occurs early in the disease course and affects 40–70% of patients. Diagnostic tools such as pulmonary function tests (PFTs) or high-resolution computed tomography (HRCT) often only detect irreversibly compromised lung function and structure [2]. Consequently, there is a need for the diagnosis of early, potentially reversible disease stages. This need could be met by nuclear medicine applications such as single photon emission computed tomography (SPECT/CT) and positron emission tomography (PET). These highly sensitive and specific methodologies allow the real-life visualization of pathophysiological processes and have become valuable diagnostic tools in oncology [3].

In SSc-ILD, pulmonary damage at its early stages is characterized by apoptosis of epithelial cells (EPC) (up to 80%) [4] and inflammatory cells caused by, for example, cigarette smoke, infections, environmental exposures or micro-aspiration and/or locally increased oxidative and endoplasmatic reticulum stress [5, 6]. Notably, in experimental animal models of ILD, EPC damage [7] or the delivery of apoptotic cells induce lung fibrosis [8, 9], whereas blocking of apoptotic pathways prevents or attenuates the development [10–12]. Dying cells release cellular contents such as adenosine triphosphate (ATP), uric acid or high-mobility group protein B1 (HMGB-1), some of which being recognized as danger-associated pathogens (DAMPs) [13, 14]. In experimental ILD, signaling via danger receptors, including, for example, toll like receptors (TLRs), initiates innate immune responses, thereby promoting inflammation and fibrosis mainly through the NFkB/inflammasome and IL-1 pathways [15]. In physiologic conditions, the DAMP-mediated influx of inflammatory cells leads to the clearance of apoptotic debris and the resolution of inflammation. In ILD, probably due to a genetic predisposition, exaggerated DAMP signaling occurs with a sustained pro-inflammatory response, part of which is attributed to inefficient phagocytosis of apoptotic cell debris (= efferocytosis) [16, 17]. Among the phagocytosing cells, alternatively activated macrophages, which are predominant in ILD [18, 19], are a major source of transforming growth factor (TGF)β [20]. TGFβ induces apoptosis of EPCs, thereby further enhancing the loss of functional epithelium [21, 22]. Furthermore, TGFβ mediates the differentiation of fibroblasts into myofibroblasts rendering them resistant to apoptosis [23]. This results in massively increased and perpetuated secretion of extracellular matrix proteins. Although less well-investigated, it has been suggested that adaptive immune responses might also be involved in pathogenesis in ILD. Potential mechanisms include cross-presentation of cellular DAMPs from apoptotic epithelial or inflammatory cells by, for example, dendritic cells, which could drive the activity of cytotoxic T cells and thereby increase lung damage [24, 25]. In addition, patient-derived data and data derived from experimental ILD suggest a potential pathogenic involvement of B cells [25–27] and a propensity towards a T helper 2 (Th2) response [28]. Overall, in ILD, there is a vicious cycle of dysregulated pro-apoptotic and anti-apoptotic mechanisms involving different cell types, which identifies apoptosis as an important initiator and driver of lung fibrosis.

One of the first signals of cells undergoing apoptosis is the rapid redistribution of phosphatidylserine (PS) onto the cell surface, where annexin V binds with high affinity. PS constitutes 10–15% of the phospholipids of the inner leaflet of the plasma membrane [29]. Upon the onset of apoptosis, closely following activation of caspase 3, translocation of PS onto the cell surface results in a 100–1000-fold increase of annexin V binding sites per cell [30]. Notably, annexin V may also identify necrotic cells, since the disruption of the membrane of necrotic cells may allow binding of annexin V to PS at the inner leaflet [31]. In human pilot studies, technetium-99 m (^{99m}Tc)-labeled annexin V has been used to detect apoptosis and necrosis in the context of acute myocardial infarction [32] and cardiac allograft rejection [33]. Recent data from animal studies using models of (infectious) endocarditis [34], atherosclerosis [35], myocarditis [36] and rheumatoid arthritis [37] suggest a potential use for the detection of early inflammatory disease stages.

In this study, we aimed to evaluate the potential of ^{99m}Tc-rhAnnexin V-128-based SPECT/CT to visualize early stages of lung remodeling in two representative mouse models of SSc-ILD, the model of bleomycin (BLM)-induced lung fibrosis [38] and the Fos-related antigen 2 (Fra-2) transgenic (tg) mouse model [39, 40].

Methods
Animal experiments

All animal experiments were approved by the cantonal authorities and performed according to the Swiss animal welfare guidelines. For all experiments, mice were randomly assigned into the different study groups.

Model of BLM-induced lung fibrosis

The BLM-induced lung fibrosis model is a commonly used animal model to study pulmonary inflammation and fibrosis mimicking SSc-related ILD. BLM-induced ILD develops in a time-dependent manner with inflammation occurring by day 3 and peaking at day 7, while pulmonary fibrosis develops later starting at day 7 and getting maximal at day 21 after the BLM administration [41]. To induce lung inflammation and fibrosis, female C57Bl6/J mice age 7–8 weeks (Janvier Labs, Le Genest-Saint-Isle, France) were intratracheally instilled with bleomycin sulfate (Baxter, Kantonsapotheke Zurich, Switzerland) at a dosage of 4 U/kg of body weight. Control mice received equivalent volumes of 0.9% saline solution. Mice were sacrificed at days 3, 7, 14 and 21 after the instillation of BLM ($n = 3$–4 receiving saline, $n = 3$–9 receiving BLM).

Fra-2 tg mouse model

Fra-2 tg mice express the transcription factor Fra-2 of the activator protein-1 family under the control of the ubiquitous major histocompatibility complex class I antigen H2Kb promotor [39]. Fra-2 tg mice develop a multi-organ phenotype, most importantly affecting the skin [40, 42] and the lungs [43, 44]. Lung involvement of Fra-2 tg mice is characterized by non-specific interstitial pneumonia with mild interstitial fibrosis and severe proliferative vascular remodeling resembling pulmonary hypertension [43, 44]. Fra-2 tg mice were newly generated and provided by Sanofi Genzyme (Framingham, MA, USA) and back-crossed from a mixed genetic background (C57Bl6/J × CBA) to a pure C57Bl6/J background for more than 10 generations. In this study, 10, 14 and 16 week-old female Fra-2 tg mice ($n = 2$–6) were used. Wild-type littermates ($n = 2$–4) served as controls.

Histological analysis

For histological analysis, lungs were transcardially perfused with sterile phosphate-buffered saline solution (PBS) to remove residual blood, fixed with 10% neutral-buffered formalin and embedded into paraffin. Lung sections (4 μm thick) were stained with hematoxylin and eosin (HE) for the assessment of the overall lung architecture and with Sirius red for the visualization of collagen deposition according to standard protocols. For the analysis of lung fibrosis, the semi-quantitative Ashcroft score was applied as described previously [45]. In brief, successive fields within the lung sections stained with Sirius red to identify fibrotic areas (red) were observed under a microscope at × 100 magnification and allotted a score from 0 (normal) to 8 (total fibrosis) according to the severity (Table 1).

All histological specimens were evaluated by at least two experienced examiners in a blinded fashion. The mean of their individual scores was considered the final fibrotic score. Staining was recorded automatically by the AxioScan.Z1 slidescanner (Carl Zeiss, Feldbach, Switzerland) using a Plan-Apochromat 20×/0.8 M27 objective.

TUNEL assay

To detect apoptotic and necrotic cells in paraffin-embedded lung sections, terminal deoxynucleotidyl transferase (TdT)-mediated dUTP nick end labeling (TUNEL) [46] was performed applying the ApopTag® Fluorescein in Situ Apoptosis Detection Kit (Millipore, USA) according to the manufacturer's instructions. In brief,

Table 1 Fibrotic lung remodeling according to the Ashcroft score [22]

Grade of fibrosis	Histological changes
0	Normal lung
1	Minimal fibrous thickening of alveolar/bronchial walls
2	*Intermediary stage between 1 and 3*
3	Moderate thickening of walls without obvious damage to the lung architecture
4	*Intermediary stage between 3 and 5*
5	Increased fibrosis with definite damage to lung structure and formation of fibrous bands or small fibrous masses
6	*Intermediary stage between 5 and 7*
7	Severe distortion of structure and large fibrous areas; honeycombing lung is placed in this category
8	Total fibrous obliteration of the field

after deparaffinization and rehydration, sections were treated with proteinase K (20 μg/mL) for 15 min at room temperature (RT). Subsequently, equilibration buffer was applied for ~ 10 s, and then the specimens were incubated for 1 h in working strength TdT enzyme solution at 37 °C. Following incubation in stop/wash buffer for 10 min to terminate the reaction, sections were incubated for 30 min in working strength anti-digoxigenin conjugate at RT in the dark to visualize the DNA fragments. Finally, slides were counterstained with 0.5 μg/mL 4′,6-diamidino-2-phenylindole (DAPI) and mounted with fluorescence mounting medium. Sections treated only with reaction buffer, but without TdT enzyme were used as negative controls. To quantify the numbers of apoptotic cells, pictures of six randomly chosen high power fields (HPFs)/slide at × 200 magnification were taken by a blinded examiner using a wide-field fluorescence microscope (Olympus BX53, Volketswil, Switzerland). TUNEL+ nuclei were quantified by automatic counting using Image J (NIH version1.47 t).

Immunohistochemical assessment

To visualize specifically apoptotic cells in paraffin-embedded lung sections, we performed immunohistochemical assessment for cleaved caspase 3. In brief, after deparaffinization and rehydration, antigen was retrieved using 10 mM sodium citrate buffer (pH = 6.0) at 95 °C for 15 min. After blocking endogenous peroxidase activity with 3% hydrogen peroxide for 15 min at RT, sections were treated with 10% normal goat serum (1 h, RT) to prevent unspecific antibody binding and blocked for endogenous biotin using an Avidin/Biotin blocking kit (Vector Laboratories, Burlingame, CA, USA). Afterwards, specimens were incubated with monoclonal rabbit anti-mouse cleaved caspase 3 (1:1000, clone 5A1E, Cell Signaling, USA) overnight at 4 °C. Isotype-matched and concentration-matched IgG was used as a negative control. Afterwards, a biotin-labeled goat anti-rabbit secondary antibody (Vector Laboratories) was applied (1:200, 30 min, RT). This was followed by incubation with the Vectastain ABC Elite HRP kit (Vector Laboratories, 30 min, RT). Finally, staining was visualized using 3,3′-diaminobenzidine (DAB, Vector Laboratories) and counterstained with methyl green.

Staining was recorded automatically by the Zeiss AxioScan.Z1. slidescanner using a Plan-Apochromat 20×/0.8 M27 objective. For cell counting, six randomly selected, non-overlapping HPFs at × 400 magnification were extracted per sample using the Zen 2.0 lite (blue edition) software. All analyses were performed by two blinded examiners.

Immunohistochemical double staining

To identify the cell types undergoing apoptosis, immunohistochemical double staining with cell-type-specific markers were performed. For the double staining, cleaved caspase 3-stained lung sections (without counterstain) were subjected to an additional heat-mediated antigen retrieval step using 10 mM sodium citrate buffer to avoid unspecific staining when using primary antibodies originating from the same species. After repetition of the aforementioned blocking steps, the following primary antibodies were added: monoclonal mouse anti-mouse alpha smooth muscle actin (αSMA, 1:750, clone 1A4, Sigma, Switzerland), monoclonal rat anti-mouse CD45 (1:50, clone 30-F11, BD Pharmingen, San Jose, CA, USA), polyclonal rabbit anti-mouse von Willebrand factor (vWF) (1:100, abcam, Cambridge, UK), and monoclonal mouse anti-mouse E-cadherin (1:400 clone M168, abcam). Isotype-matched and concentration-matched IgGs were used as negative controls. All primary antibodies were incubated overnight at 4 °C except for αSMA with a 1 h incubation time at RT. Next, a direct alkaline phosphatase-labeled goat anti-mouse secondary antibody (Dako, Baar, Switzerland), or biotin-labeled goat anti-rat, anti-mouse, or anti-rabbit secondary antibodies (all from Vector Laboratories) were applied on the sections (30 min, RT). This was followed in the latter case by incubation with the Vectastain ABC Elite HRP kit. Finally, staining was developed using Vector Red (Vector Laboratories) or HistoGreen (Histoprime; Linaris, Wertheim-Bettingen, Germany).

Pictures were recorded at × 400 magnification using the Olympus BX53 microscope in brightfield mode. For semi-quantification of the number of apoptotic leucocytes, epithelial cells, myofibroblasts or endothelial cells, three randomly selected HPFs were taken per sample and double positive cells were manually counted by two blinded examiners.

Biodistribution of ^{99m}Tc-rhAnnexin V-128

After intravenous (i.v.) injection of ~ 10 MBq ^{99m}Tc-rhAnnexin V-128 (kindly provided by Advanced Accelerator Applications, Novartis Company, Saint-Genis Pouilly, France) ex vivo biodistribution studies were performed in BLM-treated mice and saline treated controls at day 3 after the BLM instillation ($n = 3$, each) to assess the radiotracer uptake in the organs and tissues of interest. Mice were killed using carbon dioxide 4 h post injection (p.i.) of the radiotracer and blood was taken, and organs of interest were harvested and weighed. Radioactivity counts were measured in a γ-counter (Packard Cobra II Auto Gamma, Perkin Elmer, Switzerland). The percentage of injected activity per gram tissue (% IA/g) was calculated for each sample.

Ex vivo autoradiography

After i.v. injection of the radiotracer ^{99m}Tc-rhAnnexin V-128 (~ 10 MBq) (1 h p.i. Fra-2 model, 4 h p.i. BLM model), lungs were harvested and embedded in Tissue-Tek O.C.T. compound, and snap frozen at optimal cutting temperature. Fresh frozen sections 8-μm thick were cut using a cryotom and were subsequently exposed on a phosphoimager screen (super resolution type SR, PerkinElmer, Waltham, USA) for 30 min. The phosphoimager screen images were read using a CyclonePlus (PerkinElmer, Waltham, USA).

In vivo imaging using small animal SPECT/CT

BLM-treated, Fra-2 tg mice and respective controls were scanned using a small animal SPECT/CT scanner (NanoSPECT/CT, Mediso, Budapest, Hungary) at 4 h after injection of ~ 10 MBq ^{99m}Tc-rhAnnexin V-128 [36, 47]. Imaging were acquired using the Nucline software (version 1.02, Bioscan). SPECT/CT data were reconstructed iteratively by HiSPECT software (version 1.4.3049, Scivis GmbH, Göttingen, Germany) using ^{99m}Tc γ-energies of 140 keV ± 10%, and visualized with VivoQuant (version 3.0, Invicro, Boston, USA).

Statistical analysis

Statistical analysis was performed using GraphPad Prism (version 7.02, GraphPad Software, La Jolla, CA USA). Non-parametric and non-related data were expressed as median ± min/max values and the Mann-Whitney U test was applied. For parametric, non-related data, expressed as mean ± standard deviation (SD), the unpaired t test was performed. P values less than 0.05 were considered statistically significant.

Results
Apoptosis is an early phenomenon in the development of lung fibrosis in different murine ILD models
Upon BLM challenge, lung remodeling occurred over time with influx of mononuclear cells (days 3–7), loss of

alveoli and thickening of the interstitium (days 7–21) as assessed by HE staining (Fig. 1a). Fibrosis, i.e. the deposition of extracellular matrix proteins as visualized by Sirius Red staining (Fig. 1b) followed the inflammatory stage (days 3–7) and was most pronounced at days 14 and 21, which was also reflected in the semi-quantitative Ashcroft score (median$_{(Q1,Q3)}$ Ashcroft score at day 21 = $5_{(4.4,\ 6.3)}$, $p = 0.0286$; Fig. 1e).To reliably detect apoptosis ex vivo, we performed TUNEL as well as caspase 3 stainings. There was a significant increase in TUNEL+ apoptotic cells as early as day 3 (median$_{(Q1,Q3)}$ = $6.34_{(3.04,10.3)}$ versus $0.75_{(0.42,0.96)}$, $p = 0.0095$; Fig. 1c), which was confirmed by staining for cleaved caspase 3 (Fig. 1d). Semi-quantification showed a rapid decline of apoptotic cells after day 7 (Fig. 1f, g), at which inflammation subsided and fibrosis developed (Fig. 1a, /b). In accordance with the pathophysiology of BLM-induced lung injury, co-staining with specific cell markers identified the

apoptotic cells (cleaved caspase 3+) at days 3, 7, 14 and 21 as EPC (E-cadherin+; Fig. 2a) and leucocytes (CD45+; Fig. 2c) (Additional file 1). At the given time points, apoptosis of endothelial cells (vWF+; Fig. 2b) or fibroblasts (αSMA+; Fig. 2d) did not occur or very rarely occurred (Additional file 1). In summary, in the investigated time period ranging from days 3 to 21, apoptosis peaked at day 3. Then, it decreased rapidly until day 7 and thereafter gradually until day 21, although the numbers of apoptotic cells still remained higher in the lungs of BLM-challenged mice compared to controls (Fig. 1f, g).

In contrast to the model of BLM-induced lung fibrosis, in which - following the route of administration - lung injury started peribronchially and then spread to the interstitium (Fig. 1), in Fra-2 tg mice, and pulmonary vasculopathy was the initial pathophysiologic event starting from week 10 as shown by HE staining (Fig. 3a).

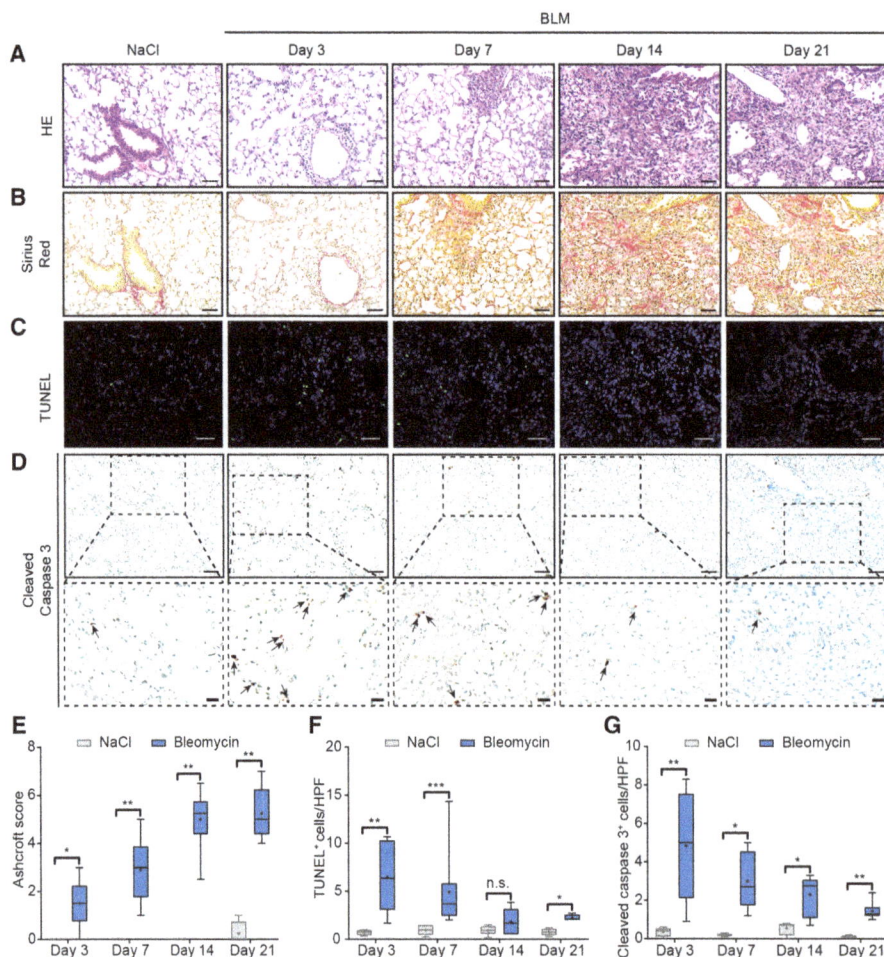

Fig. 1 Time line of apoptosis in the model of bleomycin (BLM)-induced lung fibrosis. Hematoxylin and eosin (HE) staining (× 200) (a); Sirius Red staining (collagen fibers identified by red staining; × 200) (b); TUNEL staining (× 200) (c); cleaved caspase 3 staining (× 200) (d), inlets show higher magnifications (× 400), arrows highlight apoptotic cells; Ashcroft scores (e); semi-quantification of TUNEL+ cells (f) and semi-quantification of cleaved caspase 3+ cells (g): n = 4 (saline) or n = 6–9 (BLM). Data in box plots are expressed as median (line), mean (+) and minimum and maximum values: *p < 0.05, **p < 0.01, ***p < 0.001, Mann-Whitney U test. Scale bars 50 μm and 20 μm for inlets

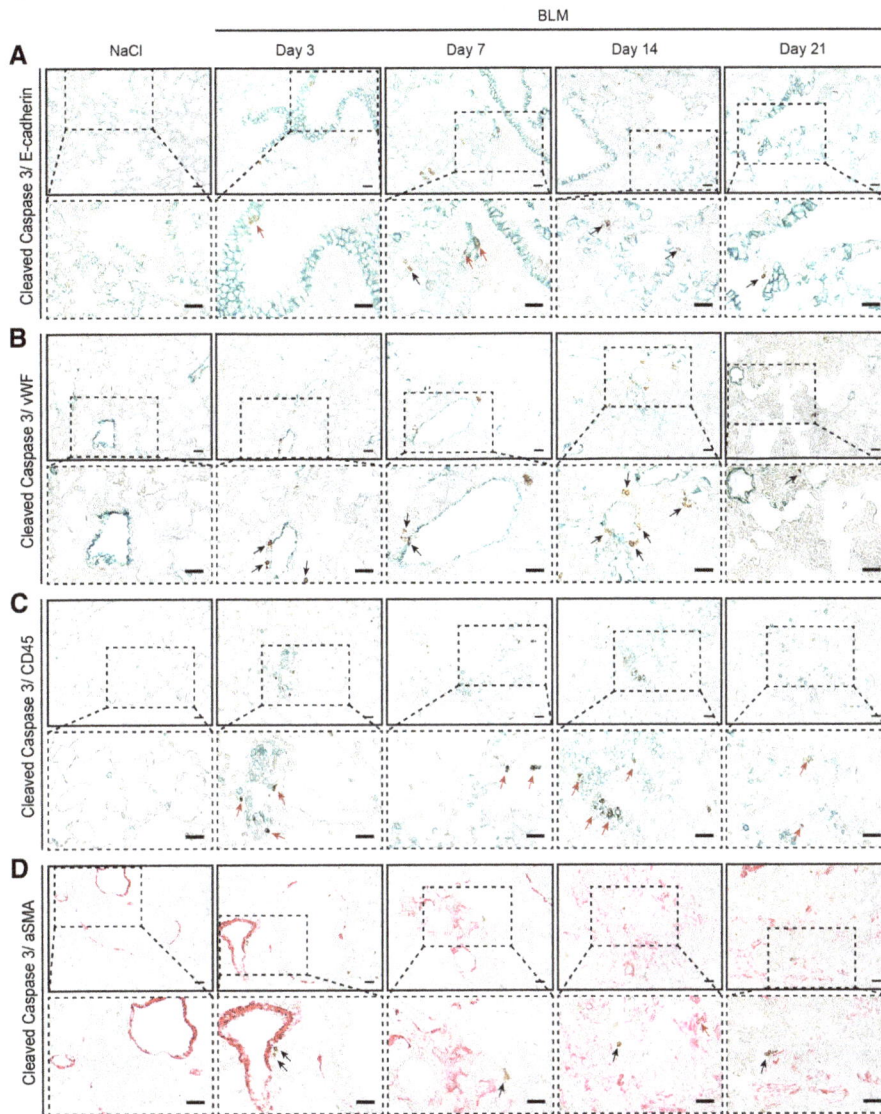

Fig. 2 Identification of cell types undergoing apoptosis in the model of bleomycin (BLM)-induced lung fibrosis. Immunohistochemical co-staining of cleaved caspase 3 (brown) with the epithelial cell marker E-cadherin (green) (**a**), with the endothelial cell marker von Willebrand factor (vWF) (green) (**b**), with the pan-leucocyte marker CD45 (green) (**c**) and with the smooth muscle cell and myofibroblast marker alpha smooth muscle actin (αSMA) (red) (**d**). Magnification is ×400. Inlets represent zoomed images. Representative pictures from three mice each are shown. Scale bars 20 μm. Red arrows highlight double staining with the cell-type-specific markers, black arrows show single stained apoptotic cells

Later, perivascular inflammation (week 14), then interstitial inflammation and to a lesser extent fibrosis (week 16), visualized by Sirius Red staining, occurred (Fig. 3b). With more inflammation in the lungs of Fra-2 tg mice, yet less fibrosis compared to BLM-challenged mice, the semi-quantitative Ashcroft score at the peak of lung remodeling in Fra-2 tg mice (week 16) (median$_{(Q1,Q3)}$ = 4.3 $_{(3.0,\ 4.6)}$, p = 0.0095; Fig. 3e) was not as high as in the respective period of the BLM lung model (day 14) (median$_{(Q1,Q3)}$ = 5.3 $_{(4.4,\ 5.8)}$, p = 0.0048; Fig. 1e). In line with the different pathophysiology, during the period of observation (weeks 10–16) we observed a time-dependent increase in pulmonary apoptotic cells

(TUNEL+, Fig. 3c; cleaved caspase 3+, Fig. 3d) starting from week 10, continuing in week 14 and reaching its peak at week 16 as assessed semi-quantitatively (Figs. 3f, g). Compared with the BLM-challenged mice, co-staining with the respective cell markers (Figs. 4a–d) showed that CD45+ (Fig. 4c) leucocytes accounted for the clear majority of apoptotic cells in the lungs (Additional file 2).

Evaluation of the potential of ^{99m}Tc-rhAnnexin V-128 to visualize apoptosis in different animal models of ILD

Following our observation at the tissue level that apoptosis could serve as a surrogate marker for early lung

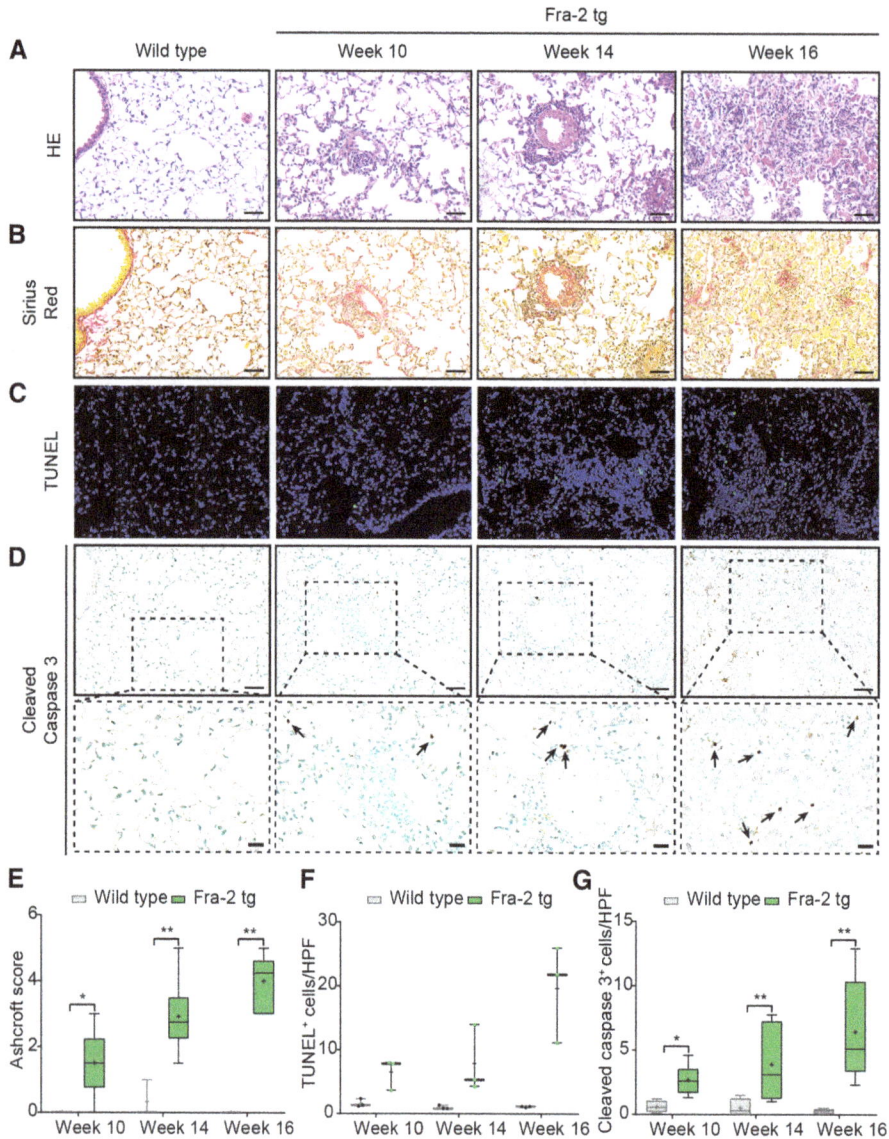

Fig. 3 Time line of apoptosis in the fos-related antigen 2 (Fra-2) transgenic (tg) mouse model. Hematoxylin and eosin (HE) staining (× 20) (**a**); Sirius Red staining (collagen fibers identified by red staining; × 200) (**b**); TUNEL staining (× 200) (**c**); cleaved caspase 3 staining (× 200) (**d**), inlets show higher magnifications (×400), arrows highlight apoptotic cells; Ashcroft scores (**e**), semi-quantification of TUNEL+ cells (**f**) and semi-quantification of cleaved caspase 3+ cells (**g**): $n = 3$–4 (wild type) or $n = 3$–6 (Fra-2 tg). Data in box plots are median (line), mean (+) and minimum and maximum values: $*p < 0.05$, $**p < 0.01$, Mann-Whitney U test. Scale bars 50 μm and 20 μm for inlets

remodeling, we next evaluated the diagnostic potential of the radiotracer ^{99m}Tc-rhAnnexin V-128 in both animal models of experimental ILD. In the BLM lung model, at day 3, biodistribution analysis of ^{99m}Tc-rhAnnexin V-128 revealed a significant difference in the radiotracer uptake (% IA/g) only in the lungs of BLM-treated mice compared to controls (mean ± SD = $0.47 ± 0.09\%$ IA/g versus $0.28 ± 0.05\%$ IA/g; Fig. 5b), yet not in other organs (Fig. 5a). These findings were confirmed by ex vivo autoradiography of frozen lung sections, where a higher accumulation of ^{99m}Tc-rhAnnexin V-128 (4 h p.i.) was observed in BLM-treated mice

compared with controls at day 3 post-instillation (Fig. 5c). In the Fra-2 tg mouse model, ^{99m}Tc-rhAnnexin V-128 clearly demonstrated apoptosis in the inflamed lungs of Fra-2 tg mice using ex vivo autoradiography (1 h p.i.; Fig. 6a).

Despite the encouraging ex vivo results, in vivo imaging of the earliest lung remodeling by visualization of apoptosis with ^{99m}Tc-rhAnnexin V-128 SPECT/CT, in the applied experimental conditions, was not successful (Figs. 5d, 6b). No specific pulmonary accumulation of the radiotracer was observed in either healthy or diseased mice (4 h after injection of the radiotracer).

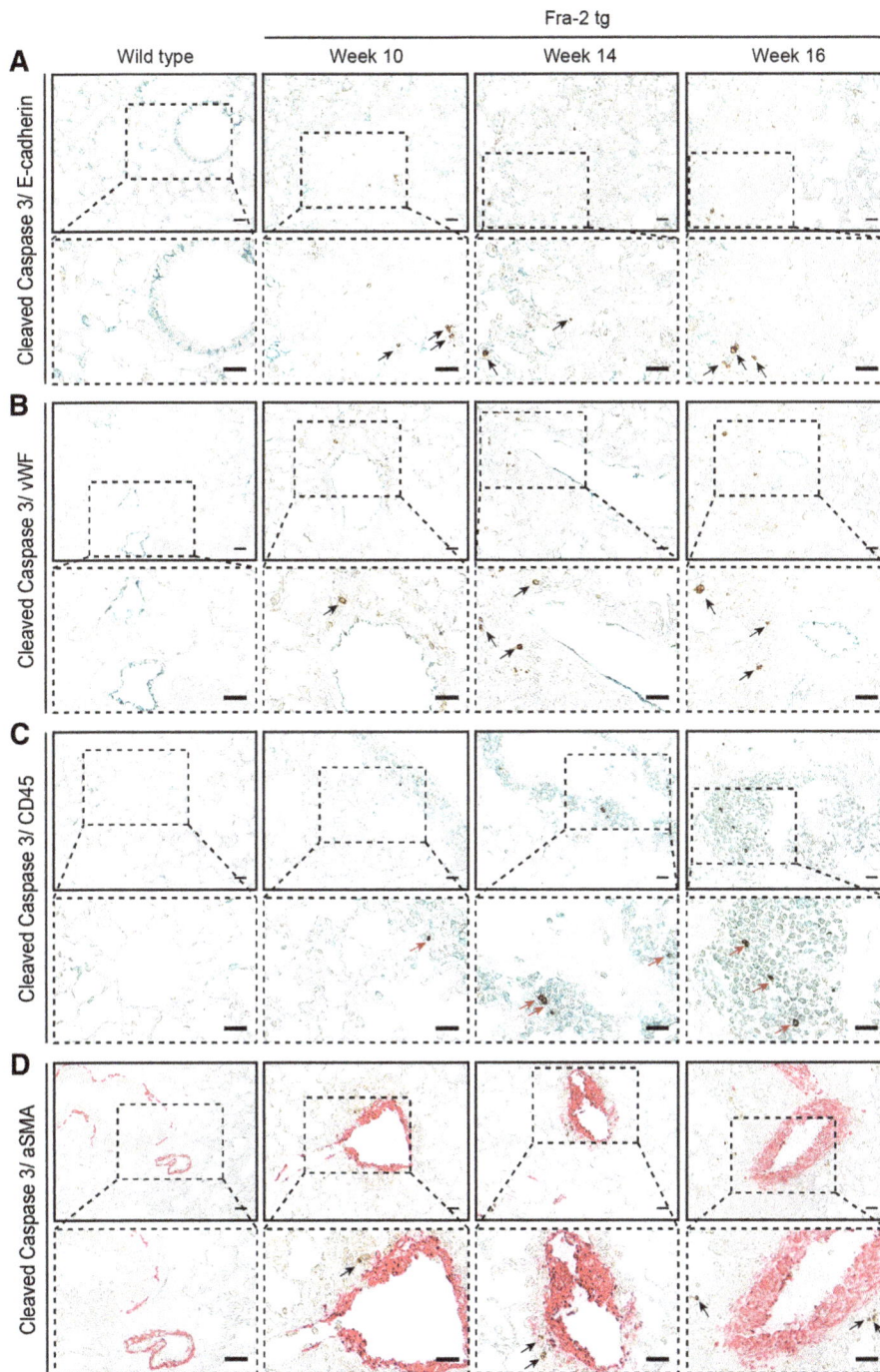

Fig. 4 Identification of cell types undergoing apoptosis in the fos-related antigen 2 (Fra-2) transgenic (tg) mouse model. Immunohistochemical co-staining of cleaved caspase 3 (brown) with the epithelial cell marker E-cadherin (green) (**a**), with the endothelial cell marker von Willebrand factor (vWF) (green) (**b**), with the pan-leucocyte marker CD45 (green) (**c**), and with the smooth muscle cell and myofibroblast marker alpha smooth muscle actin (αSMA) (red) (**d**). Magnification is × 400. Inlets represent zoomed images. Representative pictures from three mice each are shown. Scale bars 20 μm. Red arrows highlight double staining with the cell-type-specific markers, black arrows show single stained apoptotic cells

Discussion

The impending approval of molecular targeted, disease-specific therapies in SSc will provide unique treatment opportunities [48]. However, to improve patient outcome effectively, there is a need for earlier diagnosis of organ involvement to create a real window of opportunity. Sensitive nuclear imaging methodologies allowing the visualization of pathophysiologic processes in real time

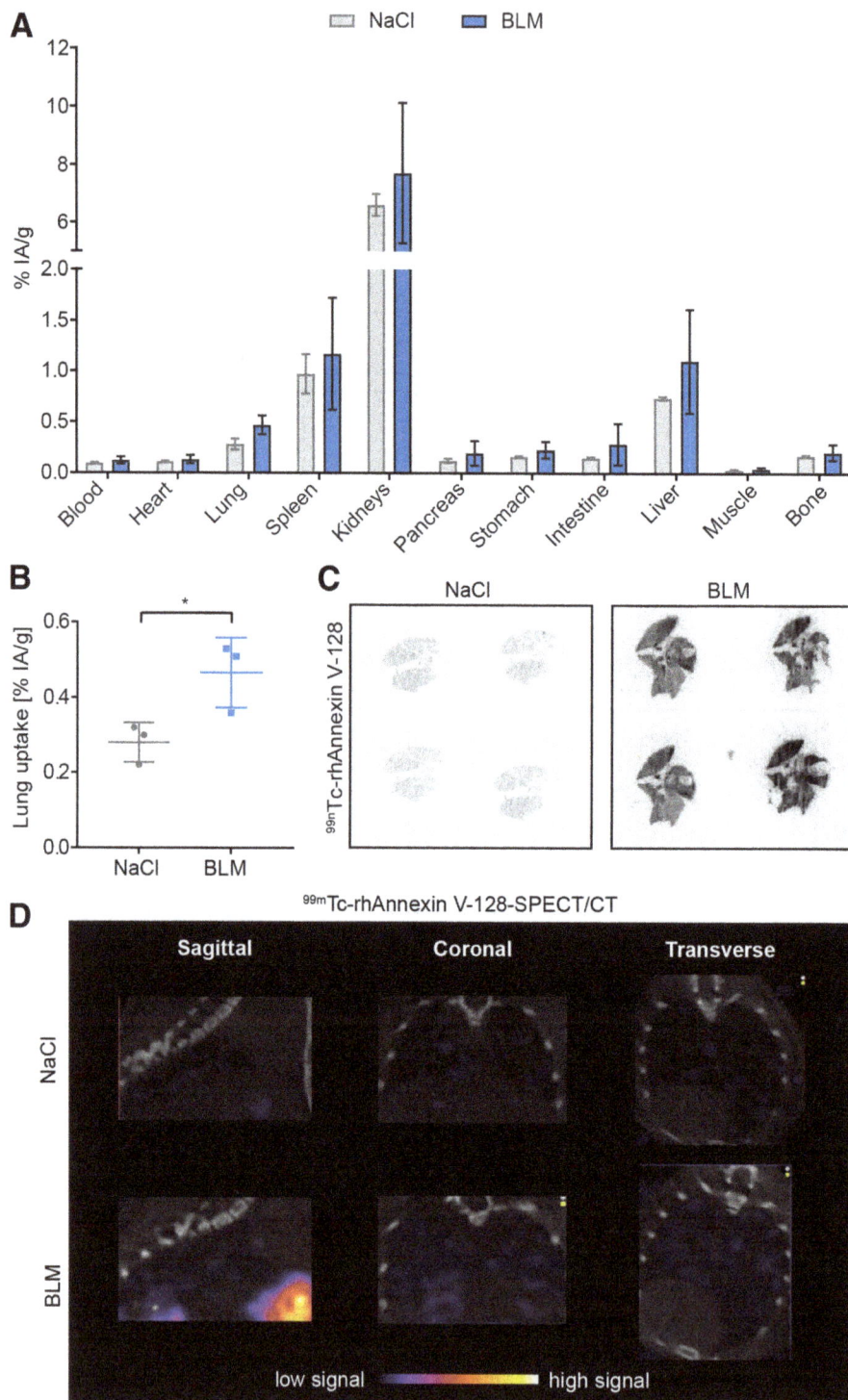

Fig. 5 Imaging of apoptotic cells with ^{99m}Tc-rhAnnexin V-128 in bleomycin (BLM)-treated mice. **a** Biodistribution of ^{99m}Tc-rhAnnexin V-128 in relevant organs of BLM-treated mice and saline controls. **b** Significantly greater lung uptake of the ^{99m}Tc-rhAnnexin V-128 radiotracer (4 h post injection (p.i.)) in the lungs of BLM-treated mice at day 3 after the BLM instillation. **c** Ex vivo autoradiography of frozen lung sections derived from BLM-treated mice and controls showing higher accumulation of ^{99m}Tc-rhAnnexin V-128 (4 h p.i.) in BLM-treated mice versus controls at day 3 post instillation. **d** In vivo single photon emission computed tomography (SPECT/CT) of ^{99m}Tc-rhAnnexin V-128 (4 h p.i.) administrated to BLM-treated mice and saline controls at day 3 post instillation. Herein, the chest cavity including the heart and the lungs is shown. Data are expressed as mean ± SD, $n = 3$, *$p < 0.05$, unpaired parametric Student's t test. % IA/g, percentage of injected activity per gram tissue

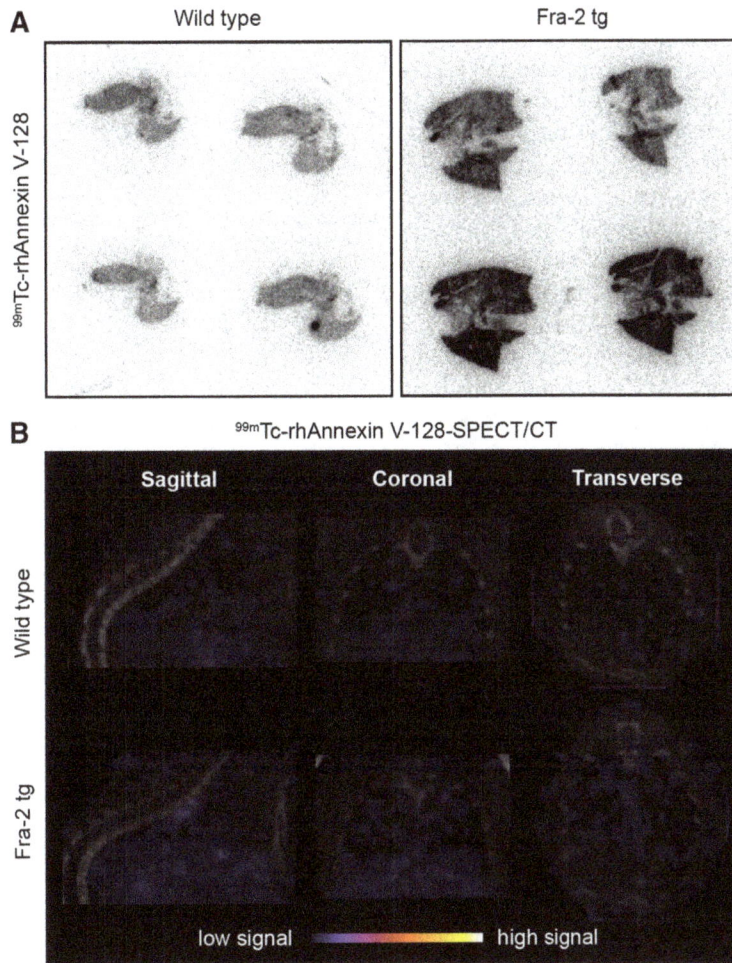

Fig. 6 Imaging of apoptotic cells with ^{99m}Tc-rhAnnexin V-128 in fos-related antigen 2 (Fra-2) transgenic (tg) mice. **a** Ex vivo autoradiography for ^{99m}Tc-rhAnnexin V-128 in the lungs of Fra-2 tg mice versus wild-type mice. Frozen lung sections derived from a Fra-2-tg mouse and a wild-type mouse showed higher accumulation of ^{99m}Tc-rhAnnexin V-128 (1 h post injection (p.i.)) in lungs of transgenic mice. **b** In vivo single photon emission computed tomography (SPECT/CT) of ^{99m}Tc-rhAnnexin V-128 (4 h p.i.) administered to Fra-2 tg mice and wild-type littermates at age 19 weeks. Herein, the chest cavity including the heart and the lungs is shown

have become an integral part of the management of patients with cancer [3]. Although routinely available, the use of ^{18}F-FDG-PET for the diagnosis and monitoring of inflammatory diseases is limited. In inflammatory conditions, increased signal intensity due to metabolic cell activity may reflect both developing and resolving tissue remodeling and is therefore not selective for early inflammatory stages [35, 49]. In (autoimmune) ILD, apoptosis and inflammation represent potentially reversible stages of tissue injury [5, 6].

This led us to investigate the diagnostic potential of ^{99m}Tc-rhAnnexin V-128 SPECT/CT in two pathophysiologically different models of SSc-ILD. In BLM-challenged and Fra-2 tg mice, the radiotracer ^{99m}Tc-rhAnnexin V-128 successfully detected apoptosis in the inflammatory stages as visualized by ex vivo autoradiography and confirmed by biodistribution studies. These results correlated very well with the identification of apoptotic EPC and leukocytes by immunohistochemical fluorescence on tissue level. Most published studies report good correlation between TUNEL-positivity and signal intensity of ^{99m}Tc-rhAnnexin V-128 imaging [36, 50–52]. However, although widely accepted as a surrogate marker for apoptosis, TUNEL staining relies on the detection of DNA strand breaks in the nuclei of dead cells [46], which (a) occur after the up-regulation of annexin V reflecting later stages of apoptosis [53] and (b) are also characteristic of necrotic cells [54]. In the pathogenesis of ILD, apoptosis rather than necrosis plays a key role in the disease initiation and perpetuation [6]. Thus, we additionally performed staining for cleaved caspase 3, which is a marker for early to mediate processes of apoptosis [53]. The fact that we obtained similar results with both staining methodologies indicates that in our models, the majority of cells were apoptotic. At the tissue level, ^{99m}Tc-rhAnnexin V-128 reliably detected apoptosis as assessed by ex vivo autoradiography and biodistribution studies, thereby clearly distinguishing diseased mice from their respective controls. However, in both mouse models, accumulation of the radiotracer and thus the signal intensity in the lungs was too low to allow the diagnosis of ILD in vivo in the tested experimental conditions. Although the most likely explanation is the overall rather low numbers of apoptotic cells in our murine ILD models, we cannot exclude that in our experimental setting the annexin V dose and/or imaging time points were not ideal and might need to be optimized in future trials. However, the number of pulmonary apoptotic cells did not differ from previously published murine ILD studies [39, 43, 55]. In comparison, studies in which ^{99m}Tc-rhAnnexin V-128 SPECT/CT had been used to detect acute myocardial infarction, allograft rejection or infectious/septic states in vivo [32, 33, 36, 47] showed substantially higher percentages or amounts of apoptotic cells per tissue area. In general, nuclear imaging of lung pathology compared with solid organs has inherent challenges, especially in small animals with very rapid breathing rates. Ventilation-triggered, i.e. gated, SPECT/CT imaging [56] has great potential to increase both the quality and quantity of SPECT/CT to such an extent that the detection of apoptosis in lung diseases might become possible, at least in disorders with more severe lung damage (e.g. acute toxic or infectious lung injury). Additional improvement might be achieved by excluding signal interference from the unspecific high uptake of the radiotracer in neighboring metabolic organs (kidneys, liver). This might be realized by, for example, focused imaging of the anatomical region of interest, e.g. the chest instead of the whole body, and/or by the adaptation of computational image reconstruction techniques, e.g. by the analysis of defined regions of interest [34–36]. Additionally, ^{99m}Tc-rhAnnexin V-128 SPECT/CT has also shown some promise for the monitoring of therapeutic responses and overall disease outcome in, for example, infectious or cardiac diseases [32, 47, 50].

Conclusions

In conclusion, ^{99m}Tc-rhAnnexin V-128 allowed successful visualization of early stages of ILD in two animal models by detection of apoptotic epithelial and/or inflammatory cells in ex vivo samples. However, the transfer of ^{99m}Tc-rhAnnexin V-128 SPECT/CT into clinical application to detect early, reversible stages of SSc-ILD remains to be ascertained since in vivo imaging failed to detect lung injury in our two mouse models. Nevertheless, the development of innovative, targeted (nuclear) imaging strategies is currently one of the most challenging prospects in the field of autoimmune diseases to enable the personalized management of these patients.

Abbreviations
% IA/g: Percentage of injected activity per gram tissue; [99m]Tc: Technetium-99 m; ATP: Adenosine triphosphate; BLM: Bleomycin; DAB: 3,3′-Diaminobenzidine; DAMPs: Danger-associated pathogens; EPC: Epithelial cells; Fra-2: Fos-related antigen 2; HE: Hematoxylin and eosin; HMGB-1: High-mobility group protein B1; HPFs: High power fields; HRCT: High-resolution computed tomography; i.v.: Intravenous; ILD: Interstitial lung disease; MBq: MilliBequerel; p.i.: Post injection; PBS: Pphosphate-buffered saline; PET: Positron emission tomography; PFTs: Pulmonary function tests; PS: Phosphatidylserine; RT: Room temperature; SD: Standard deviation; SPECT/CT: Single photon emission computed tomography; SSc: Systemic sclerosis; tg: Transgenic; TGF: Transforming growth factor; TLRs: Toll like-receptors; TUNEL: Terminal deoxynucleotidyl transferase (TdT)-mediated dUTP nick end labeling; vWF: von Willebrand factor; αSMA: Alpha smooth muscle actin

Acknowledgements
We thank Maria Comazzi and Christine de Pasquale for their excellent technical assistance. Furthermore, we thank Advanced Accelerator Applications, a Novartis Company, Saint-Genis Pouilly, France for supplying us with the radiotracer. In addition, we thank Sanofi Genzyme (Framingham, MA, United States) for providing us with the Fra-2 tg mice. Microscopic image recording was performed using equipment maintained by the Center for Microscopy and Image Analysis, University of Zurich.

Funding
This work was supported by supported by the Swiss National Science Foundation (grant CRSII3_154490), Hartmann-Mueller Foundation.

Authors' contributions
JS has made substantial contributions to the conception of the study and the acquisition, analysis and the interpretation of data and was involved in drafting and revising the manuscript. LG and MBr were centrally involved in the acquisition and analysis of data and in revising the manuscript. RS and SY made contributions to the conception and design of the study, the interpretation of the data and the revision of the manuscript. MBe and OD were involved in the experimental design, the acquisition and interpretation of data, in drafting and revising the manuscript. BM made substantial contributions to conception and design of the study and was centrally involved in the acquisition, analysis and interpretation of data and in drafting and revising the manuscript. All authors have given final approval of the version to be published.

Ethics approval
All animal experiments were approved by the cantonal authorities and performed according to the Swiss animal welfare guidelines.

Consent for publication
Not applicable.

Competing interests
JS, MBr, RS, MBe, LG, and SY have no competing interests to declare. OD had a consultancy relationship and/or has received research funding from Actelion, AnaMar, Bayer, Boehringer Ingelheim, ChemomAb, espeRare foundation, Genentech/Roche, GSK, Inventiva, Italfarmaco, Lilly, medac, MedImmune, Mitsubishi Tanabe Pharma, Novartis, Pfizer, Sanofi, Sinoxa and UCB in the area of potential treatments for scleroderma and its complications. In addition, OD has a patent mir-29 licensed for the treatment of systemic sclerosis. The real or perceived potential conflicts listed above are accurately stated.
BM had grant/research support from AbbVie, Protagen, Novartis, congress support from Pfizer, Roche and Actelion. In addition, BM has a patent mir-29 licensed for the treatment of systemic sclerosis. The real or perceived potential conflicts listed above are accurately stated.

Author details
[1]Center of Experimental Rheumatology, Department of Rheumatology, University Hospital Zurich, Gloriastrasse 25, 8091 Zurich, Switzerland. [2]Department of Rheumatology, Renji Hospital, Shanghai Jiao Tong University,

Shanghai, China. ³Center for Radiopharmaceutical Sciences, Villigen-PSI, Switzerland. ⁴Institute of Pharmaceutical Sciences, Department of Chemistry and Applied Biosciences, Zurich, Switzerland.

References

1. Steen VD, Medsger TA. Changes in causes of death in systemic sclerosis, 1972-2002. Ann Rheum Dis. 2007;66(7):940-4.

2. Suliman YA, Dobrota R, Huscher D, Nguyen-Kim TD, Maurer B, Jordan S, Speich R, Frauenfelder T, Distler O. Brief report: pulmonary function tests: high rate of false-negative results in the early detection and screening of scleroderma-related interstitial lung disease. Arthritis Rheumatol. 2015;67(12):3256-61.

3. Kramer-Marek G, Capala J. The role of nuclear medicine in modern therapy of cancer. Tumour Biol. 2012;33(3):629-40.

4. Plataki M, Koutsopoulos AV, Darivianaki K, Delides G, Siafakas NM, Bouros D. Expression of apoptotic and antiapoptotic markers in epithelial cells in idiopathic pulmonary fibrosis. Chest. 2005;127(1):266-74.

5. Wells AU, Denton CP. Interstitial lung disease in connective tissue disease--mechanisms and management. Nat Rev Rheumatol. 2014;10(12):728-39.

6. Ellson CD, Dunmore R, Hogaboam CM, Sleeman MA, Murray LA. Danger-associated molecular patterns and danger signals in idiopathic pulmonary fibrosis. Am J Respir Cell Mol Biol. 2014;51(2):163-8.

7. Sisson TH, Mendez M, Choi K, Subbotina N, Courey A, Cunningham A, Dave A, Engelhardt JF, Liu X, White ES, et al. Targeted injury of type II alveolar epithelial cells induces pulmonary fibrosis. Am J Respir Crit Care Med. 2010;181(3):254-63.

8. Zhao HW, Hu SY, Barger MW, Ma JK, Castranova V, Ma JY. Time-dependent apoptosis of alveolar macrophages from rats exposed to bleomycin: involvement of TNF receptor 2. J Toxicol Environ Health A. 2004;67(17):1391-406.

9. Wang L, Scabilloni JF, Antonini JM, Rojanasakul Y, Castranova V, Mercer RR. Induction of secondary apoptosis, inflammation, and lung fibrosis after intratracheal instillation of apoptotic cells in rats. Am J Physiol Lung Cell Mol Physiol. 2006;290(4):L695-702.

10. Ashley SL, Sisson TH, Wheaton AK, Kim KK, Wilke CA, Ajayi IO, Subbotina N, Wang S, Duckett CS, Moore BB, et al. Targeting inhibitor of apoptosis proteins protects from bleomycin-induced lung fibrosis. Am J Respir Cell Mol Biol. 2016;54(4):482-92.

11. Kuwano K, Kunitake R, Maeyama T, Hagimoto N, Kawasaki M, Matsuba T, Yoshimi M, Inoshima I, Yoshida K, Hara N. Attenuation of bleomycin-induced pneumopathy in mice by a caspase inhibitor. Am J Physiol Lung Cell Mol Physiol. 2001;280(2):L316-25.

12. Wang R, Ibarra-Sunga O, Verlinski L, Pick R, Uhal BD. Abrogation of bleomycin-induced epithelial apoptosis and lung fibrosis by captopril or by a caspase inhibitor. Am J Physiol Lung Cell Mol Physiol. 2000; 279(1):L143-51.

13. Gasse P, Riteau N, Vacher R, Michel ML, Fautrel A, di Padova F, Fick L, Charron S, Lagente V, Eberl G, et al. IL-1 and IL-23 mediate early IL-17A production in pulmonary inflammation leading to late fibrosis. PLoS One. 2011;6(8):e23185.

14. Gasse P, Mary C, Guenon I, Noulin N, Charron S, Schnyder-Candrian S, Schnyder B, Akira S, Quesniaux VF, Lagente V, et al. IL-1R1/MyD88 signaling and the inflammasome are essential in pulmonary inflammation and fibrosis in mice. J Clin Invest. 2007;117(12):3786-99.

15. Artlett CM, Sassi-Gaha S, Rieger JL, Boesteanu AC, Feghali-Bostwick CA, Katsikis PD. The inflammasome activating caspase 1 mediates fibrosis and myofibroblast differentiation in systemic sclerosis. Arthritis Rheum. 2011;63(11):3563-74.

16. Parks BW, Black LL, Zimmerman KA, Metz AE, Steele C, Murphy-Ullrich JE, Kabarowski JH. CD36, but not G2A, modulates efferocytosis, inflammation, and fibrosis following bleomycin-induced lung injury. J Lipid Res. 2013;54(4):1114-23.

17. Morimoto K, Janssen WJ, Terada M. Defective efferocytosis by alveolar macrophages in IPF patients. Respir Med. 2012;106(12):1800-3.

18. Murray LA, Rosada R, Moreira AP, Joshi A, Kramer MS, Hesson DP, Argentieri RL, Mathai S, Gulati M, Herzog EL, et al. Serum amyloid P therapeutically attenuates murine bleomycin-induced pulmonary fibrosis via its effects on macrophages. PLoS One. 2010;5(3):e9683.

19. Prasse A, Pechkovsky DV, Toews GB, Jungraithmayr W, Kollert F, Goldmann T, Vollmer E, Muller-Quernheim J, Zissel G. A vicious circle of alveolar macrophages and fibroblasts perpetuates pulmonary fibrosis via CCL18. Am J Respir Crit Care Med. 2006;173(7):781-92.

20. Voll RE, Herrmann M, Roth EA, Stach C, Kalden JR, Girkontaite I. Immunosuppressive effects of apoptotic cells. Nature. 1997;390(6658): 350-1.

21. Hagimoto N, Kuwano K, Inoshima I, Yoshimi M, Nakamura N, Fujita M, Maeyama T, Hara N. TGF-beta 1 as an enhancer of Fas-mediated apoptosis of lung epithelial cells. J Immunol. 2002;168(12):6470-8.

22. Gregory CD, Devitt A. The macrophage and the apoptotic cell: an innate immune interaction viewed simplistically? Immunology. 2004;113(1):1-14.

23. Horowitz JC, Rogers DS, Sharma V, Vittal R, White ES, Cui Z, Thannickal VJ. Combinatorial activation of FAK and AKT by transforming growth factor-beta1 confers an anoikis-resistant phenotype to myofibroblasts. Cell Signal. 2007;19(4):761-71.

24. Ahrens S, Zelenay S, Sancho D, Hanc P, Kjaer S, Feest C, Fletcher G, Durkin C, Postigo A, Skehel M, et al. F-actin is an evolutionarily conserved damage-associated molecular pattern recognized by DNGR-1, a receptor for dead cells. Immunity. 2012;36(4):635-45.

25. Komura K, Yanaba K, Horikawa M, Ogawa F, Fujimoto M, Tedder TF, Sato S. CD19 regulates the development of bleomycin-induced pulmonary fibrosis in a mouse model. Arthritis Rheum. 2008;58(11):3574-84.

26. Francois A, Gombault A, Villeret B, Alsaleh G, Fanny M, Gasse P, Adam SM, Crestani B, Sibilia J, Schneider P, et al. B cell activating factor is central to bleomycin- and IL-17-mediated experimental pulmonary fibrosis. J Autoimmun. 2015;56:1-11.

27. Lafyatis R, O'Hara C, Feghali-Bostwick CA, Matteson E. B cell infiltration in systemic sclerosis-associated interstitial lung disease. Arthritis Rheum. 2007;56(9):3167-8.

28. Meloni F, Solari N, Cavagna L, Morosini M, Montecucco CM, Fietta AM. Frequency of Th1, Th2 and Th17 producing T lymphocytes in bronchoalveolar lavage of patients with systemic sclerosis. Clin Exp Rheumatol. 2009;27(5):765-72.

29. Zwaal RF, Schroit AJ. Pathophysiologic implications of membrane phospholipid asymmetry in blood cells. Blood. 1997;89(4):1121-32.

30. Tait JF, Smith C, Wood BL. Measurement of phosphatidylserine exposure in leukocytes and platelets by whole-blood flow cytometry with annexin V. Blood Cells Mol Dis. 1999;25(5-6):271-8.

31. Willingham MC. Cytochemical methods for the detection of apoptosis. J Histochem Cytochem. 1999;47(9):1101-10.

32. Hofstra L, Liem IH, Dumont EA, Boersma HH, van Heerde WL, Doevendans PA, De Muinck E, Wellens HJ, Kemerink GJ, Reutelingsperger CP, et al. Visualisation of cell death in vivo in patients with acute myocardial infarction. Lancet. 2000;356(9225):209-12.

33. Narula J, Acio ER, Narula N, Samuels LE, Fyfe B, Wood D, Fitzpatrick JM, Raghunath PN, Tomaszewski JE, Kelly C, et al. Annexin-V imaging for noninvasive detection of cardiac allograft rejection. Nat Med. 2001;7(12): 1347-52.

34. Rouzet F, Dominguez Hernandez M, Hervatin F, Sarda-Mantel L, Lefort A, Duval X, Louedec L, Fantin B, Le Guludec D, Michel JB. Technetium 99m-labeled annexin V scintigraphy of platelet activation in vegetations of experimental endocarditis. Circulation. 2008;117(6):781-9.

35. Kamkar M, Wei L, Gaudet C, Bugden M, Petryk J, Duan Y, Wyatt HM, Wells RG, Marcel YL, Priest ND, et al. Evaluation of apoptosis with 99mTc-rhAnnexin V-128 and inflammation with 18F-FDG in a low-dose irradiation model of atherosclerosis in apolipoprotein E–deficient mice. J Nucl Med. 2016;57(11):1784-91.

36. Peker C, Sarda-Mantel L, Loiseau P, Rouzet F, Nazneen L, Martet G, Vrigneaud JM, Meulemans A, Saumon G, Michel JB, et al. Imaging apoptosis with (99m)Tc-annexin-V in experimental subacute myocarditis. J Nucl Med. 2004;45(6):1081-6.

37. Post AM, Katsikis PD, Tait JF, Geaghan SM, Strauss HW, Blankenberg FG. Imaging cell death with radiolabeled annexin V in an experimental model of rheumatoid arthritis. J Nucl Med. 2002;43(10):1359-65.

38. Germano D, Blyszczuk P, Valaperti A, Kania G, Dirnhofer S, Landmesser U, Luscher TF, Hunziker L, Zulewski H, Eriksson U. Prominin-1/CD133+ lung epithelial progenitors protect from bleomycin-induced pulmonary fibrosis. Am J Respir Crit Care Med. 2009;179(10):939-49.

39. Eferl R, Hasselblatt P, Rath M, Popper H, Zenz R, Komnenovic V, Idarraga MH, Kenner L, Wagner EF. Development of pulmonary fibrosis through a pathway involving the transcription factor Fra-2/AP-1. Proc Natl Acad Sci U S A. 2008;105(30):10525-30.

40. Maurer B, Busch N, Jungel A, Pileckyte M, Gay RE, Michel BA, Schett G, Gay S, Distler J, Distler O. Transcription factor fos-related antigen-2 induces

progressive peripheral vasculopathy in mice closely resembling human systemic sclerosis. Circulation. 2009;120(23):2367–76.

41. Schiller HB, Fernandez IE, Burgstaller G, Schaab C, Scheltema RA, Schwarzmayr T, Strom TM, Eickelberg O, Mann M. Time- and compartment-resolved proteome profiling of the extracellular niche in lung injury and repair. Mol Syst Biol. 2015;11(7):819.

42. Reich N, Maurer B, Akhmetshina A, Venalis P, Dees C, Zerr P, Palumbo K, Zwerina J, Nevskaya T, Gay S, et al. The transcription factor Fra-2 regulates the production of extracellular matrix in systemic sclerosis. Arthritis Rheum. 2010;62(1):280–90.

43. Maurer B, Reich N, Juengel A, Kriegsmann J, Gay RE, Schett G, Michel BA, Gay S, Distler JH, Distler O. Fra-2 transgenic mice as a novel model of pulmonary hypertension associated with systemic sclerosis. Ann Rheum Dis. 2012;71(8):1382–7.

44. Maurer B, Distler JH, Distler O. The Fra-2 transgenic mouse model of systemic sclerosis. Vasc Pharmacol. 2013;58(3):194–201.

45. Ashcroft T, Simpson JM, Timbrell V. Simple method of estimating severity of pulmonary fibrosis on a numerical scale. J Clin Pathol. 1988;41(4):467–70.

46. Gavrieli Y, Sherman Y, Ben-Sasson SA. Identification of programmed cell death in situ via specific labeling of nuclear DNA fragmentation. J Cell Biol. 1992;119(3):493–501.

47. Hardy JW, Levashova Z, Schmidt TL, Contag CH, Blankenberg FG. [99mTc]Annexin V-128 SPECT monitoring of splenic and disseminated Listeriosis in mice: a model of imaging sepsis. Mol Imaging Biol. 2015;17(3):345–54.

48. Dobrota R, Mihai C, Distler O. Personalized medicine in systemic sclerosis: facts and promises. Curr Rheumatol Rep. 2014;16(6):425.

49. Basu S, Zhuang H, Torigian DA, Rosenbaum J, Chen W, Alavi A. Functional imaging of inflammatory diseases using nuclear medicine techniques. Semin Nucl Med. 2009;39(2):124–45.

50. Blankenberg FG, Kalinyak J, Liu L, Koike M, Cheng D, Goris ML, Green A, Vanderheyden JL, Tong DC, Yenari MA. 99mTc-HYNIC-annexin V SPECT imaging of acute stroke and its response to neuroprotective therapy with anti-Fas ligand antibody. Eur J Nucl Med Mol Imaging. 2006;33(5):566–74.

51. Tokita N, Hasegawa S, Maruyama K, Izumi T, Blankenberg FG, Tait JF, Strauss HW, Nishimura T. 99mTc-Hynic-annexin V imaging to evaluate inflammation and apoptosis in rats with autoimmune myocarditis. Eur J Nucl Med Mol Imaging. 2003;30(2):232–8.

52. Bahmani P, Schellenberger E, Klohs J, Steinbrink J, Cordell R, Zille M, Muller J, Harhausen D, Hofstra L, Reutelingsperger C, et al. Visualization of cell death in mice with focal cerebral ischemia using fluorescent annexin A5, propidium iodide, and TUNEL staining. J Cereb Blood Flow Metab. 2011;31(5):1311–20.

53. Naito M, Nagashima K, Mashima T, Tsuruo T. Phosphatidylserine externalization is a downstream event of interleukin-1 beta-converting enzyme family protease activation during apoptosis. Blood. 1997;89(6):2060–6.

54. Grasl-Kraupp B, Ruttkay-Nedecky B, Koudelka H, Bukowska K, Bursch W, Schulte-Hermann R. In situ detection of fragmented DNA (tunel assay) fails to discriminate among apoptosis, necrosis, and autolytic cell death: a cautionary note. Hepatology. 1995;21(5):1465–8.

55. Goto H, Ledford JG, Mukherjee S, Noble PW, Williams KL, Wright JR. The role of surfactant protein a in bleomycin-induced acute lung injury. Am J Respir Crit Care Med. 2010;181(12):1336–44.

56. Guerra L, Ponti E, Morzenti S, Spadavecchia C, Crivellaro C. Respiratory motion management in PET/CT: applications and clinical usefulness. Curr Radiopharm. 2017;10(2):85–92.

6

Sex-based differences in association between circulating T cell subsets and disease activity in untreated early rheumatoid arthritis patients

Jonathan Aldridge[1]*[iD], Jayesh M. Pandya[1], Linda Meurs[1], Kerstin Andersson[1], Inger Nordström[1], Elke Theander[2], Anna-Carin Lundell[1] and Anna Rudin[1]

Abstract

Background: It is not known if sex-based disparities in immunological factors contribute to the disease process in rheumatoid arthritis (RA). Hence, we examined whether circulating T cell subset proportions and their association with disease activity differed in male and female patients with untreated early rheumatoid arthritis (ueRA).

Methods: Proportions of T cell subsets were analyzed in peripheral blood from 72 ueRA DMARD- and corticosteroid-naïve patients (50 females and 22 males) and in 31 healthy age- and sex-matched controls. Broad analysis of helper and regulatory CD4+ T cell subsets was done using flow cytometry. Disease activity in patients was assessed using DAS28, CDAI, swollen joint counts, tender joint counts, CRP, and ESR.

Results: Multivariate factor analyses showed that male and female ueRA patients display distinct profiles of association between disease activity and circulating T cell subset proportions. In male, but not female, ueRA patients Th2 cells showed a positive association with disease activity and correlated significantly with DAS28-ESR, CDAI, and swollen and tender joint counts. Likewise, proportions of non-regulatory CTLA-4+ T cells associated positively with disease activity in male patients only, and correlated with DAS28-ESR. In contrast, there was a negative relation between Th1Th17 subset proportions and disease activity in males only. The proportions of Th17 cells correlated positively with DAS28-ESR in males only, while proportions of Th1 cells showed no relation to disease activity in either sex. There were no significant differences in proportions of T cell subsets between the sexes in patients with ueRA.

Conclusions: Our findings show sex-based differences in the association between T cell subsets and disease activity in ueRA patients, and that Th2 helper T cells may have a role in regulating disease activity in male patients.

Keywords: T cells, Rheumatoid arthritis, Disease activity, Sex

Background

Rheumatoid arthritis (RA) is a chronic and systemic inflammatory disease characterized by synovial inflammation and progressive destruction of joint cartilage and bones [1]. Genetic association studies strongly support the role of CD4+ T cells in promoting RA pathology. So

* Correspondence: Jonathan.aldridge@gu.se
[1]Department of Rheumatology and Inflammation Research, Institute of Medicine, Sahlgrenska Academy of University of Gothenburg, Box 480, S-405 30 Gothenburg, Sweden
Full list of author information is available at the end of the article

far, alleles in the human leukocyte antigen (HLA)-DRB1 region, known as the shared epitope, display the strongest genetic association with RA [2]. Additional genetic loci have also been found to be linked with RA, among them many contain genes linked to T cell activation and function (reviewed in [3]). Still, identification of specific CD4+ T cell phenotypes or functions that are most relevant in this disease, particularly in early and preclinical RA, has been challenging. Traditionally, RA has been thought to be a Th1- and Th17-mediated disorder [1]. However, by combining single-cell analysis and next-generation sequencing in TCR repertoire analysis, it was shown that a majority of the most expanded CD4+ T cell clones from patients with established RA, both in synovial fluid and in peripheral blood, expressed phenotypes other than the Th1 or Th17 subsets [4]. Furthermore, synovial CXCR5^{neg}PD-1^{hi} T peripheral helper (Tph) cells has recently been implicated as contributors in established RA [5]. In a cohort of untreated early RA (ueRA) patients, we also recently demonstrated that the balance of helper T cell subsets in blood of ueRA patients is skewed towards Th2 cells relative to healthy controls [6].

RA has been shown to be a sexually dimorphic condition with current data suggesting that prevalence, disease course, and treatment outcome varies between men and women. The prevalence of RA is approximately threefold higher in females than in males with several observational studies also suggesting that women have a more detrimental disease course than men [7, 8]. For example, in an 8-year prospective follow-up of an early RA study, women had more disability than men despite similar medication [9]. Male RA patients have also shown a higher remission rate than female patients in response to biologic and non-biologic disease-modifying anti-rheumatic drug (DMARD) treatments [7, 8]. However, another study showed that males were only more likely to achieve sustained remission in early RA, not in established RA, when treated with both biologic and non-biologic DMARD [10]. These results indicate that the initial immunological mechanisms responsible for RA may differ in males and females.

There are several disparities between men and women that have been shown to affect both innate and adaptive immune function [11]. Sex hormones are one such contributor, known to affect the immune system via their effects on multiple immune cell subsets as well as on stromal cells [11, 12]. As of yet, results from immunological studies of male and female patients with RA have not been reported separately, except for a recent study where we reported that levels of pro-inflammatory chemokines in blood were higher in ueRA patients than in healthy control (HC) subjects [13]. In this study, there was a positive association between eotaxin levels and disease activity in male patients, while these variables were inversely related among females. When male and female RA patients are reported as a single cohort in studies of immunopathogenesis and biomarkers there is risk that associated data are masked by opposing results by the two sexes. Hence, there is a need to examine both immunological components and their relation to disease activity measures separately in male and female patients with RA. Furthermore, sex-based differences need to be evaluated in a group of DMARD-naïve early RA patients since treatment with biologic and non-biologic DMARD

alter the profile of both immune cells and soluble inflammatory mediators [14, 15].

To address these gaps in knowledge, we here investigated sex-based differences in the association between T cell subset proportions in peripheral blood and disease activity in ueRA patients. Using a broad-scale analysis of T cell subsets based on chemokine receptor expression, and relating these to disease activity measures, we demonstrate differential profiles of association between T cell subsets and disease activity in male and female ueRA patients.

Methods
Patients and healthy controls

The patient group comprised of 72 treatment-naïve subjects who were newly diagnosed with rheumatoid arthritis (RA) according to the American College of Rheumatology (ACR)/European League Against Rheumatism (EULAR) 2010 criteria. The inclusion criteria were as follows: ≥18 years old, ≥ 2 swollen joints and ≥ 2 tender joints (based on 66/68 joint count), rheumatoid factor (RF)-positive or anti-citrullinated protein antibodies (ACPA)-positive or C-reactive protein (CRP) ≥10 mg/L, at least moderate disease activity (> 3.2) by composite index disease activity score in 28 joints (DAS28-CRP), symptom duration < 24 months (retrospective patient-reported symptoms), and no treatment with any DMARD or corticosteroids. Blood samples were drawn from the DMARD- and corticosteroid-naïve patients within 1–2 weeks after RA diagnosis. The patient group was compared to a group of 31 age- and sex-matched HC subjects. Characteristics of female and male ueRA patients and HC are shown in Table 1. The median age of the whole patient cohort (59 years, range 21–80 years) and the HC cohort (55 years, range 20–75 years) was not significantly different ($P = 0.47$). Neither was the median age of ueRA female patients and ueRA male patients significantly different (Table 1). In addition, there were no significant differences between the median age of ueRA female patients and HC female subjects ($P = 0.81$), between the median age of ueRA male patients and HC male subjects ($P = 0.38$), or between the median age of HC female subjects and HC male subjects (Table 1). Furthermore, there was no significant difference between male and female ueRA patients with regard to disease activity measures, or proportions of patients positive for ACPA or RF (Table 1). The patients were recruited at the Rheumatology Clinics at Sahlgrenska University Hospital and at Skåne University Hospital, Sweden. All samples were analyzed at the Clinical Immunology Laboratory at the Sahlgrenska University Hospital in Gothenburg by the same staff to minimize variability. The study was approved by the regional ethics committees of Gothenburg and Lund, Sweden, and all patients signed an informed consent form.

Table 1 Baseline characteristics of female and male early diagnosed untreated RA patients and healthy controls

	ueRA female (n = 50)	ueRA male (n = 22)	P value	HC female (n = 18)	HC male (n = 13)
Age, yr.[a]	60.5 (21–78)	56 (28–80)	0.87[c]	56 (20–72)	55 (27–75)[e]
Symptom duration, months[a,b]	6 (2–23)	3.9 (1–21)	0.07[c]		
CRP, mg/L[a]	9 (0.3–180)	10 (2–113)	0.29[c]		
ESR, mm/hour[a]	28 (5–120)	22.5 (1–85)	0.33[c]		
SJC66[a]	11.5 (3–30)	9 (2–18)	0.08[c]		
TJC68[a]	13 (2–47)	15.5 (3–26)	0.79[c]		
SJC28[a]	9 (2–24)	7 (2–15)	0.15[c]		
TJC28[a]	8.5 (0–27)	9 (1–16)	0.93[c]		
DAS28-CRP[a]	4.9 (2.7–8.3)	5.2 (3.4–6.4)	0.50[c]		
DAS28-ESR[a]	5.3 (2.6–8.7)	5.5 (2.9–6.7)	0.83[c]		
CDAI[a]	28.3 (10.1–68.7)	28.0 (10.5–40.6)	0.40[c]		
ACPA+, n (%)[f]	42 (84)	17 (77)	0.52[d]		
RF+, n (%)[g]	38 (76)	14 (64)	0.40[d]		
ACPA+ and RF+, n (%)[f,g]	35 (70)	13 (59)	0.42[d]		
ACPA- and RF-, n (%)[f,g]	5 (10)	4 (18)	0.44[d]		
Smoker (%)[h]	8 (17)	3 (14)	> 0.99[d]		

ACPA anti-citrullinated protein/peptide antibodies, CDAI clinical disease activity index, CRP C-reactive protein, DAS28 disease activity score in 28 joints, ESR erythrocyte sedimentation rate, HC healthy controls, RF rheumatoid factor, SJC 28/66 swollen joint counts of 28/66, TJC 28/68 tender joint counts of 28/68, ueRA untreated early rheumatoid arthritis

[a]Median and range
[b]Retrospective patient-reported pain in the joints before RA diagnosis
[c]Difference between ueRA female patients and ueRA male patients, Mann-Whitney U test
[d]Difference between ueRA female patients and ueRA male patients, Fisher's exact test
[e]Difference between HC female age and HC male age, P = 0.53, Mann-Whitney U test
[f]Patients with ACPA levels ≥20 IU/ml are considered ACPA+
[g]Patients with RF levels ≥20 IU/ml are considered RF+
[h]Current daily smoker (data available in $n_{female} = 47$, $n_{male} = 22$)

Clinical evaluation

Evaluation of disease activity in patients was done by assessing the following parameters: Swollen Joint Counts of 66 joints (SJC 66), Tender Joint Counts of 68 joints (TJC 68), Swollen Joint Counts in 28 joints status (SJC 28), Tender Joint Counts in 28 joints status (TJC 28), CRP, erythrocyte sedimentation rate (ESR), DAS28 [16], and Clinical Disease Activity Index (CDAI) [17]. ACPA positivity was determined by multiplexed anti-CCP test (BioPlex from BioRad, Hercules, CA, USA) and RF positivity was determined by nephelometry (Beckman Coulter, Brea, CA, USA). Patients with ≥20 IU/ml anti-CCP antibodies or RF in serum were considered ACPA- or RF-positive, respectively.

Definition, analysis and characterization of T cell subsets

Peripheral blood mononuclear cells (PBMCs) were separated from whole blood (sampled from patients within 1–2 weeks after RA diagnosis) using Lymphoprep (Axis-Shield, Oslo, Norway). Small aliquots of fresh blood were used for cell counts (True count, TC) using BD TruCOUNT Absolute Counting Tubes with addition of CD45 PerCP and CD4 APC-H7 antibodies (BD Biosciences, San Jose, CA, USA). In isolated fresh PBMCs, T cell subsets were defined and analyzed using flow cytometry, as previously described in detail [6]. In brief, without any ex vivo stimulations, PBMCs were stained with fluorochrome-conjugated monoclonal antibodies against the following molecules: CD4, CD45RA, CCR4, CCR6, CXCR3, CXCR5, CD127, PD-1, and CD25, and to evaluate FOXP3+ and CTLA-4+ cells, intracellular staining was performed (full list of antibodies available in Additional file 1: Table S1) [6]. Stained samples were acquired by the use of FACSCanto II (BD Biosciences) equipped with FACS Diva software (BD Biosciences). Flow cytometry data was analyzed in FlowJo software (Tree Star, Ashland, OR, USA). T helper subsets were defined by surface chemokine receptor expression. The gating strategy to define different T cell subsets is previously described in [6] and also presented in Fig. 1. The phenotypes of defined T cell subsets were confirmed by lineage specifying transcription factor expression analysis by qPCR and cytokine secretion analysis by Cytometric Bead Array (BD Biosciences) as previously shown [6].

Statistical analysis

Multivariate factor analysis (SIMCA-P+ software; Umetrics, Umeå, Sweden) was used to analyze T cell and disease activity data. Principal component analysis (PCA) was performed in order to evaluate association between

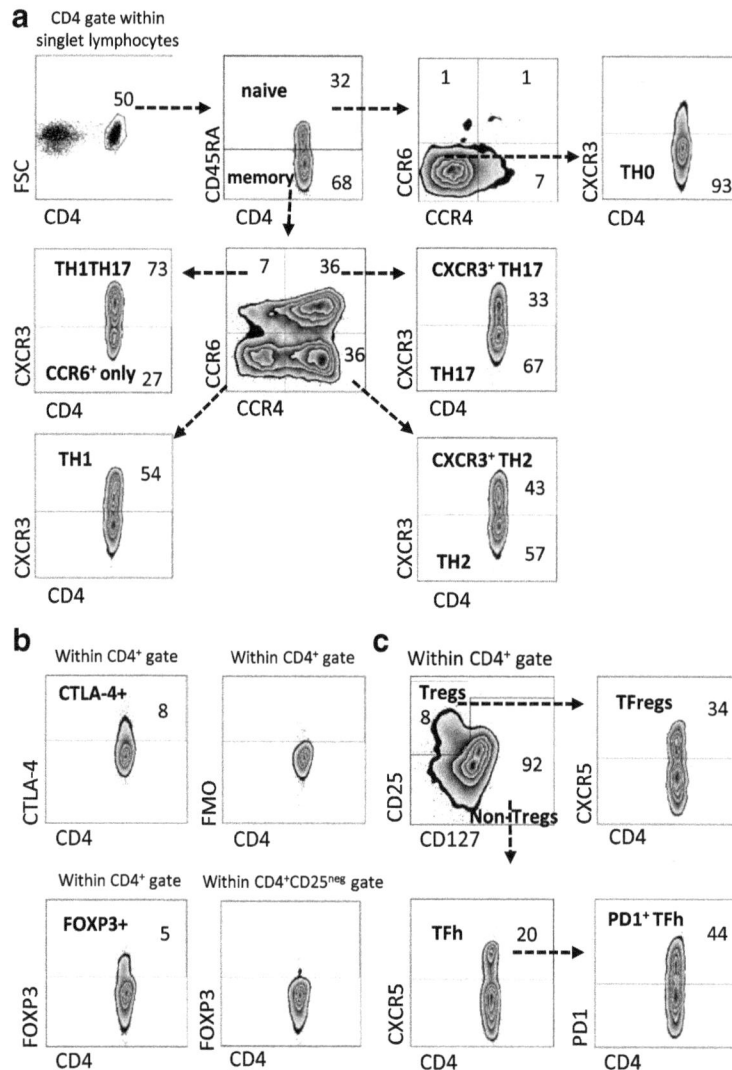

Fig. 1 Gating strategy of CD4+ T cell subsets. The gating strategy (gating result from a representative female RA patient) was as follows: (**a**) singlet PBMCs were gated for lymphocytes and then further gated for CD4+ T cells. CD4+ cells where then divided into naïve (CD45RA+) and memory (CD45RA^{neg}) subsets. From naïve cells, CCR4^{neg}CCR6^{neg}CXCR3^{neg} cells were defined as Th0. Memory cells were divided into four subsets based on CCR4 and CCR6 expression, each of which was the further divided based on CXCR3 expression; Th1 (CCR4^{neg}CCR6^{neg}CXCR3+), Th2 (CCR4+CCR6^{neg}CXCR3^{neg}), CXCR3+Th2 (CCR4+CCR6^{neg}CXCR3+), Th17 (CCR4+CCR6+CXCR3^{neg}), CXCR3+Th17 (CCR4+CCR6+CXCR3+), Th1Th17 (CCR4^{neg}CCR6+CXCR3+), and CCR6+ only (CCR4^{neg}CCR6+CXCR3^{neg}). (**b**) The cutoff for CTLA-4 positivity on CD4+ T cells were determined using fluorescence minus one (FMO) and cutoff for FOXP3 positivity in CD4+ cells was based on FOXP3 expression in CD25^{neg} gated CD4+ cells. (**c**) Regulatory T cells (Tregs) were defined by CD25+CD127^{low} expression, while the remaining cells were defined as non-Tregs. CXCR5+ Tregs were defined as follicular regulatory T cells (TFregs) and CXCR5+ non-Tregs as follicular helper T cells (TFh).

proportions of T cell subsets and disease activity measures. Linear OPLS models were implemented to examine sex-based differences in the associations of T cell subsets with disease activity measures. Orthogonal projection to latent structures discriminant analysis (OPLS-DA) was implemented to investigate sex-based differences in T cell subset proportions in ueRA and HC. The two-class discrimination OPLS-DA model has one predictive component and one orthogonal. Log transformation was used to normalize data and further scaled to unit variance in the SIMCA software by dividing each variable by 1/standard deviation (SD), so that all the variables were given equal weight regardless of their absolute value. The scale presented on the axes of the PCA and OPLS plots is a dimensionless scale, and the loading vector is normalized to length one. The quality of the OPLS models was assessed based on the parameters R2 (i.e. how well the variation of the variables is explained by the model), and Q2, (i.e. how well a variable can be predicted by the model). In order to avoid mass significance, univariate analysis was performed exclusively on the variables that contributed most to the respective OPLS models. Univariate analyses were performed using two-tailed Mann-Whitney U test and two-tailed Spearman's Rank-Order Correlation (GraphPad Prism Software, La Jolla, CA, USA) as described in the figure legends. The strength of correlation was determined based on Spearman's rank correlation coefficient (r) values (r = 0.2–0.39 weak correlation, r = 0.4–0.59 moderate correlation, r = 0.6–0.79 strong correlation, r > 0.8 very strong correlation). A P value ≤0.05 was regarded as being statistically significant (*P ≤ 0.05, **P ≤ 0.01, ***P ≤ 0.001 and ****P ≤ 0.0001).

Results

Male and female untreated early RA patients show different profiles of association between T cell subsets and disease activity

Based on the gating strategy presented in Fig. 1a-c we first examined the proportions of T helper (Th) and regulatory $CD4^+$ T cell subsets in male and female ueRA patients. By the use of cluster analysis, i.e. PCA, we next investigated whether patient sex affects the relationship between proportions of T cell subsets and common disease activity measures used when assessing RA patients (Fig. 2a-b). In both sexes, all disease activity variables were projected in the two right hand quadrants. However, while the Th2, Th17, and $CTLA-4^+$ T cell subset proportions associated positively with several disease activity measures in males (Fig. 2a), none of the T cell subsets were projected in the same quadrant as that of disease activity variables among females (Fig. 2b). Thus, results indicate that the association between T cell subset proportions and disease activity differ in male and female ueRA patients.

Th2 helper T cells correlate with increased disease activity in male but not in female ueRA patients

Having observed sex-based differences in association between T cell subset proportions and disease activity in the PCA analysis, we examined the association of individual helper T cell subsets with multiple disease activity measures, symptom duration, and age using multivariate OPLS analysis. In males, we found that proportions of Th2 cells displayed a positive association with several disease activity measures (Fig. 3a), and correlated significantly with DAS28-ESR, CDAI (Fig. 3b), swollen joint counts (SJC28 $r = 0.45$ $P = 0.05$ and SJC66: $r = 0.48$ $P = 0.03$) and tender joint counts (TJC28 $r = 0.59$ $P = 0.007$ and TJC68: $r = 0.54$ $P = 0.01$). In female ueRA patients, no relation was observed between proportions of Th2 cells and disease activity measures (Fig. 3a-b). In contrast to Th2, proportions of Th1Th17 cells displayed a negative association and inverse correlation with disease

activity measures in male patients, while no relation was observed in females (Fig. 3c-d). The Th17 cells did show patterns of positive association with disease activity in male patients, while females displayed a pattern of negative association (Fig. 3e). However, significant univariate correlation between disease activity measures and proportions of Th17 cells was only observed in male patients (DAS28-ESR, $r = 0.47$ $P = 0.035$). The $CXCR3^+$ Th17 cell proportions in female patients showed significant inverse correlation with swollen joint counts (SJC28, $r = -0.41$ $P = 0.004$ and SJC66, $r = -0.38$ $P = 0.007$).

Although the median level of disease activity was similar in men and women with ueRA, higher disease activity was found in a fraction of the female patients compared to males, which could be a confounding factor for the results. However, exclusion of the female patients with disease activity above the maximum value observed in male patients showed little to no effect to the r and P values in the correlation analyses (relation between Th2 and disease activity before exclusion: $r = 0.022$ and $P = 0.88$ vs after exclusion: $r = 0.097$ and $P = 0.54$). In an attempt to demonstrate that the number of male patients was sufficiently high, additional analyses were performed in which the number of female patients was randomly reduced to 20 (equal to the number of male patients). Univariate analyses were then performed as described previously, investigating the relation between proportions T cell subsets and disease activity. Reduction in the number of females did not have a significant impact on the relation between T cell subset proportions and disease activity (e.g. relation between Th2 and disease activity before reduction: $r = 0.022$ and $P = 0.88$ vs after reduction: $r = -0.082$ and $P = 0.73$). In summary, these findings suggest significant sex-based differences in the contribution of Th2, Th1Th17, and $CXCR3^+$ Th17 cells to disease severity in RA.

$CTLA-4^+$ conventional $CD4^+$ T cell subsets correlate with disease activity in male but not in female ueRA patients

Next, we examined the association between proportions of $CTLA-4^+$, $FOXP3^+$ and regulatory T cell subsets and disease activity in male and female ueRA patients (Fig. 4a-e). We found that the $CTLA-4^+$ T cell fractions displayed a profile of positive association with the majority of disease activity measures in male patients, but not in female patients (Fig. 4a). These results were also corroborated in univariate analysis as the proportions of $CTLA-4^+$ T cells correlated positively with DAS28-ESR in males, while no significant correlations were observed in females (Fig. 4b). CTLA-4 is often used as a marker for regulatory T cells, but CTLA-4 is also expressed by activated conventional T cells. Upon further analyses, we found that both proportions of regulatory and

a Male ueRA patients

R2X=0.44, Q2=0.13

b Female ueRA patients

R2X=0.36, Q2=0.05

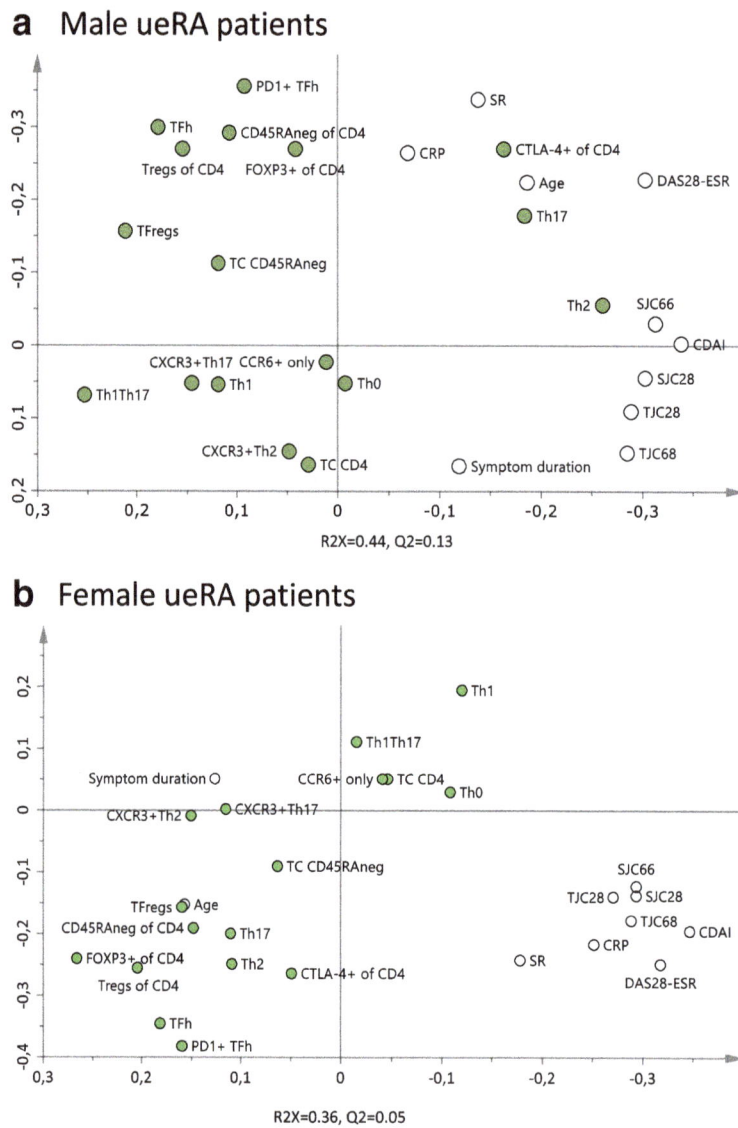

Fig. 2 Relationship between T cell subset proportions and disease activity measures in male and female untreated early RA patients. Principal component analysis (PCA) plots depicting the association between $CD4^+$ T cell subsets proportions and disease activity measures (**a**) in male ($n = 20$–22) and (**b**) in female ($n = 48$–50) ueRA patients. Variables projected close to each other on the same side of the axis associate positively, while variables on opposite sides of an axis associate negatively. *Filled symbols* indicate $CD4^+$ T cell subset variables and *open symbols* indicate disease activity variables

non-regulatory CTLA-4$^+$ T cells showed moderate to strong correlation with DAS28-ESR in males ($r = 0.57$ $P = 0.006$ and $r = 0.62$ $P = 0.002$, respectively). Male regulatory, but not non-regulatory, CTLA-4$^+$ T cells also showed moderate correlation to CDAI, SJC28, SJC66 and TJC28 ($r = 0.54$ $P = 0.01$, $r = 0.44$ $P = 0.04$, r = 0.44 $P = 0.039$ and $r = 0.51$ $P = 0.01$, respectively). In female patients, only regulatory CTLA-4$^+$ T cells showed a weak correlation to DAS28-ESR ($r = 0.29$ $P = 0.05$), whereas no significant correlation between the non-regulatory CTLA-4$^+$ T cell population and disease activity was observed. In contrast to CTLA-4$^+$ T cells, proportions of

FOXP3$^+$ T cells showed no association with disease activity measures in males, but a negative association in females (Fig. 4c). Univariate analysis confirmed a negative correlation between proportions of FOXP3$^+$ T cells and DAS28-ESR (Fig. 4d), SJC66 ($r = -0.34$ $P = 0.02$) and tender joint counts (TJC68: $r = -0.32$ $P = 0.03$) in female patients. The proportions of regulatory T cells (CD25$^+$CD127^{low}CD4$^+$ cells) displayed a weak pattern of negative association with disease activity measures in both sexes, but there were no significant correlations observed in either sex (Fig. 4e). Exclusion of the female patients with disease activity above the maximum value

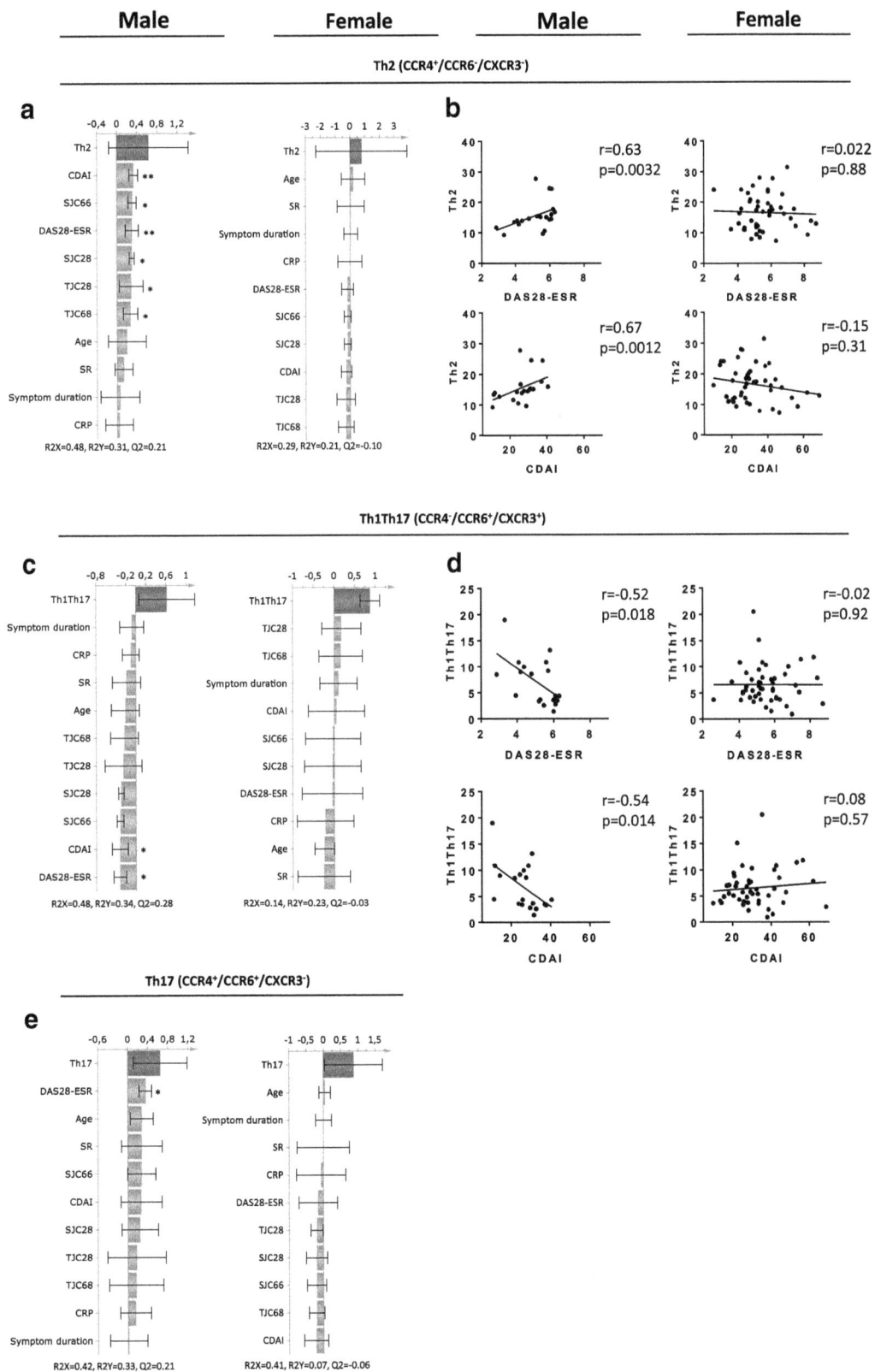

Fig. 3 (See legend on next page.)

observed in male patients showed little to no effect to the r and P values for the correlation analyses (relation between CTLA-4+ and disease activity before exclusion: $r = 0.27$ and $P = 0.060$ vs after exclusion $r = 0.29$ and $P = 0.062$). Thus, although the proportions of CTLA-4$^+$ T cells are elevated in blood of both male and female ueRA patients, this T cell subset correlates with disease activity in males only. Furthermore, non-regulatory CTLA-4$^+$ T cells showed strong correlation to DAS28-ESR in males but not females.

Male and female ueRA patients display a different profile of blood T cell subset proportions compared to their respective healthy controls

Previously, we have shown that ueRA patients display distinct profiles of T cell subset proportions compared to HC [6]. A similar multivariate distinctive pattern was observed in the present study (in a partially overlapping cohort) including a higher number of patients and healthy controls as shown in Additional file 1: Figure S1 [6, 13]. With a larger number of ueRA patients, we here investigated whether sex affects the differential T cell subset profile in ueRA patients in relation to age- and sex-matched HC. T cell subsets that showed the strongest association (positive or negative) with ueRA patients are identified in the OPLS-DA column plots in Fig. 5a and b for males and females respectively. In male patients, the differential profile of T cell subsets between ueRA and HC (Fig. 5a) was less pronounced than in females. Upon univariate analysis, the proportions of CTLA-4$^+$ T cells were significantly higher in male ueRA patients (Fig. 5h), while the fractions of Th1Th17 and CCR6$^+$ only cells were lower in ueRA patients relative to HC (Fig. 5d, g). In contrast, univariate analysis showed that female ueRA patients displayed a strong differential profile of T cell subset proportions compared to HC (Fig. 5b). Female patients had significantly higher proportions of Th2 and Th17 cells as well as elevated fractions of regulatory T cells (CD25$^+$CD127^{low}) and CTLA-4$^+$ T cells compared to HC (Fig. 5c, e, h-i). Both the total count of CD4$^+$ and CD45RA^{neg} T cells (Fig. 5j-k) as well as proportions of Th1Th17 and Th1 T cells were lower in female ueRA patients compared to female HC (Fig. 5d, f). Univariate analysis did not show any

significant differences in T cell subset numbers or proportions between male and female patients with ueRA (Fig. 5c-k). Furthermore, no significant differences in T cell subset proportions between seropositive and seronegative patients was found in either males of females (data not shown).

In conclusion, these results show that there is a differential profile of T cell subset proportions in both male and female ueRA patients compared to their respective HC. Additionally, proportions of the CCR6$^+$ only subset was shown to be higher in male HC than ueRA, which was not observed in females despite 2.3-fold higher number of female participants (Fig. 5g).

Discussion
Sex-based differences in T cell subsets and their clinical relevance have not been explored, neither in early nor established RA. In this study, we found that male and female ueRA patients display distinct profiles of association between disease activity and certain T cell subsets. The proportions of Th2 cells associated positively with disease activity in male but not female ueRA patients, whereas Th1Th17 cells associated negatively with disease activity in male but not in female patients. Moreover, both sexes presented with increased proportions of CTLA-4$^+$ T cells in ueRA, but proportions of these cells associated positively with disease activity in male ueRA patients only. To our knowledge, this is the first study demonstrating sex-based differences in the association between specific T cell subsets and disease activity measures in patients with RA.

The Th1 and Th17 cell subsets have been the target of RA research for many years and patients with established RA have indeed presented elevated frequency of citrulline-specific Th1 cells in circulation [18]. However, previous studies provide inconsistent results regarding the association of circulatory Th1 and Th17 cells with disease activity in RA [19–21]. Furthermore, a recent study showed that Th1 and Th17 cells make up only a small fraction of the most expanded CD4$^+$ T cell clones from patients with established RA, both in peripheral blood and in the synovial fluid [4]. Few studies have explored the role of Th2 cells in RA pathogenesis, but it has been shown that synovial fluid in early arthritis

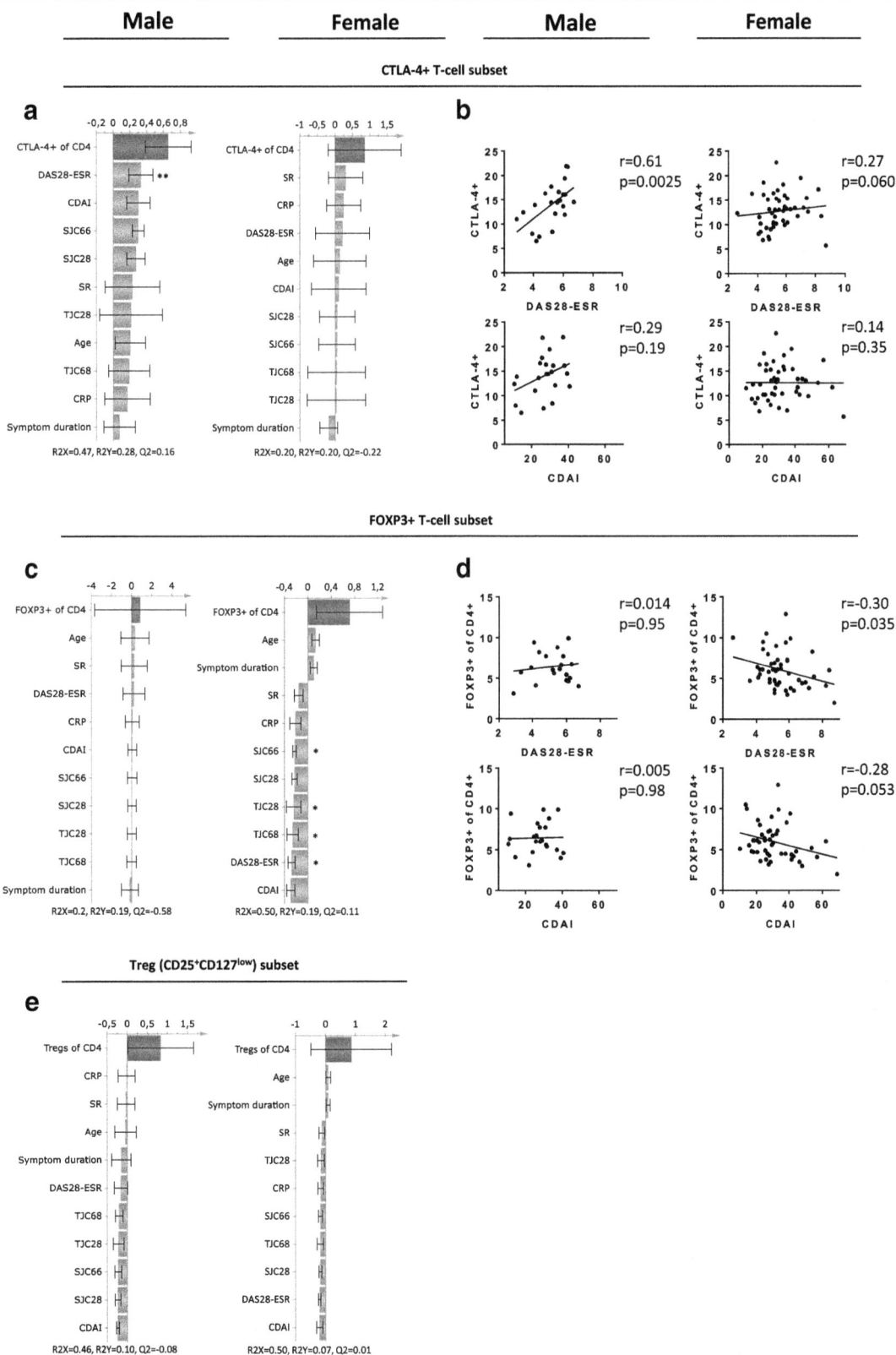

Fig. 4 (See legend on next page.)

Fig. 4 Relationship between CTLA-4+, FOXP3+ and regulatory T cell subset proportions and disease activity measures in untreated early RA patients. Multivariate factor analysis was performed to investigate sex-based differences in the associations of CTLA-4$^+$, FOXP3$^+$, and regulatory T cell subset proportions with multiple disease activity measures in ueRA patients. OPLS column loading plots depicting the association between (**a**) CTLA-4$^+$, (**c**) FOXP3$^+$, and (**e**) regulatory T cell subset proportions (Y-variables) and disease activity measures (X-variables) in male ($n = 22$) and female ($n = 48$–50) ueRA patients. Correlation analyses between the proportion of (**b**) CTLA-4+ or (**d**) FOXP3+ T cell subsets proportions with disease activity measures in male and female ueRA patients, respectively.*$P \leq 0.05$ and **$P \leq 0.01$ (Spearman's rank correlation test). Regression lines are presented in the correlation plots

patients who developed RA had elevated levels of the Th2 cytokine interleukin (IL)-4 [22]. Plasma levels of IL-4 and the Th2-related chemokine eotaxin have also been shown to be elevated in both male and female subjects with no prior symptoms of joint disease who later develop RA [23]. Additionally, we have previously reported that the proportion of Th2 cells in blood are increased in ueRA patients compared to HC in a combined cohort of males and females [6]. In the present study, when analyzing males and females separately, we found that only female ueRA patients displayed significantly elevated proportions of Th2 cells compared to HC. Moreover, we also observed sex-based disparities in the association between Th2 cells and disease activity. Male patients displayed a positive association pattern between Th2 cells and disease activity, while these factors were not related in females. This might explain why no association between Th2 cells and disease activity was previously found when analyzing the group of men and women together [6]. Supporting these sex-based differences, we have recently shown that blood plasma levels of eotaxin associated positively with disease activity in male ueRA patients, whereas it displayed negative association with disease activity in female ueRA patients [13]. Eotaxin, an eosinophil chemoattractant, is associated with Th2 immune response and allergic pulmonary diseases. Thus, our results point towards Th2 cells and eotaxin having a role in regulating the disease activity of male patients with early RA.

As discussed, previous studies provide inconsistent results regarding the association of Th1 and Th17 T cells and disease activity in RA. This may be due to that most such studies were performed on patients with variable disease duration, different treatment protocols, pooled cohorts of males and females, as well as analysis of T cells after ex vivo stimulation and culture. Thus, we here focused our investigation on a more homogenous patient group (untreated early RA) and analyzed fresh isolated PBMC without any intermediary culture or stimulation. We and others have shown that Th1Th17 cells display both Th1 and Th17 characteristics as they express both TBX21 and RORC and produce interferon (IFN)-γ and IL-17 [6, 24]. These cells, which express CXCR3 and CCR6, are also considered important to the disease process of RA [24, 25]. In this study, we show

that proportions of circulating Th1Th17 cells displayed a negative association with clinical disease activity measures in male ueRA patients only. The proportion of circulatory Th17 cells was elevated compared to healthy controls in female patients but showed no significant correlation with disease activity in either sex. In contrast, previous studies have shown negative associations between circulating Th17 cells and disease activity measures in DMARD-naive RA patients with a mean disease duration of 10 and 21 months, respectively [26, 27]. However, the surface markers used to categorize the T cell subsets in these studies were different from ours. The first study defined Th17 cells using the markers CD4 and CD161, while the second study defined Th17 using CD4 combined with intracellular staining of IL-17. Owing to these disparities in defining the cell subsets, the results of the different studies are difficult to compare. Furthermore, sex-related disparities between T cell subsets and disease activity were not investigated in these studies.

We have recently reported that ueRA patients present with increased proportions of circulating CTLA-4 expressing CD4$^+$ T cells compared to HC [6]. In the present study, we demonstrate that this is true for both sexes. However, when we investigated the association between CTLA-4$^+$ T cells and disease activity, we found a positive association between CTLA-4$^+$ T cells and disease activity in male ueRA patients only. Interestingly, RA susceptibility genes involved in T cell regulation (e.g. PTPN22) have also been found to have a stronger association with development of RA in males than in females [28–30]. CTLA-4 is expressed by the majority of regulatory T cells, but also by non-regulatory T cells, and functions as a negative regulator of T cell immune responses by competing with CD28 for binding to the costimulatory molecules CD80/CD86 on APCs [31]. These results suggest that the T cell inhibitory pathways linked to CTLA-4 may be particularly impaired in male ueRA patients, as immunosuppression is not achieved despite increased proportions of T cells expressing CTLA-4. In the present study, the FOXP3$^+$ T cell subset displayed a clear profile of inverse association as well as negative correlations with disease activity measures in female patients. This suggests that at least in female early RA patients, FOXP3$^+$ T cells may be able to regulate disease

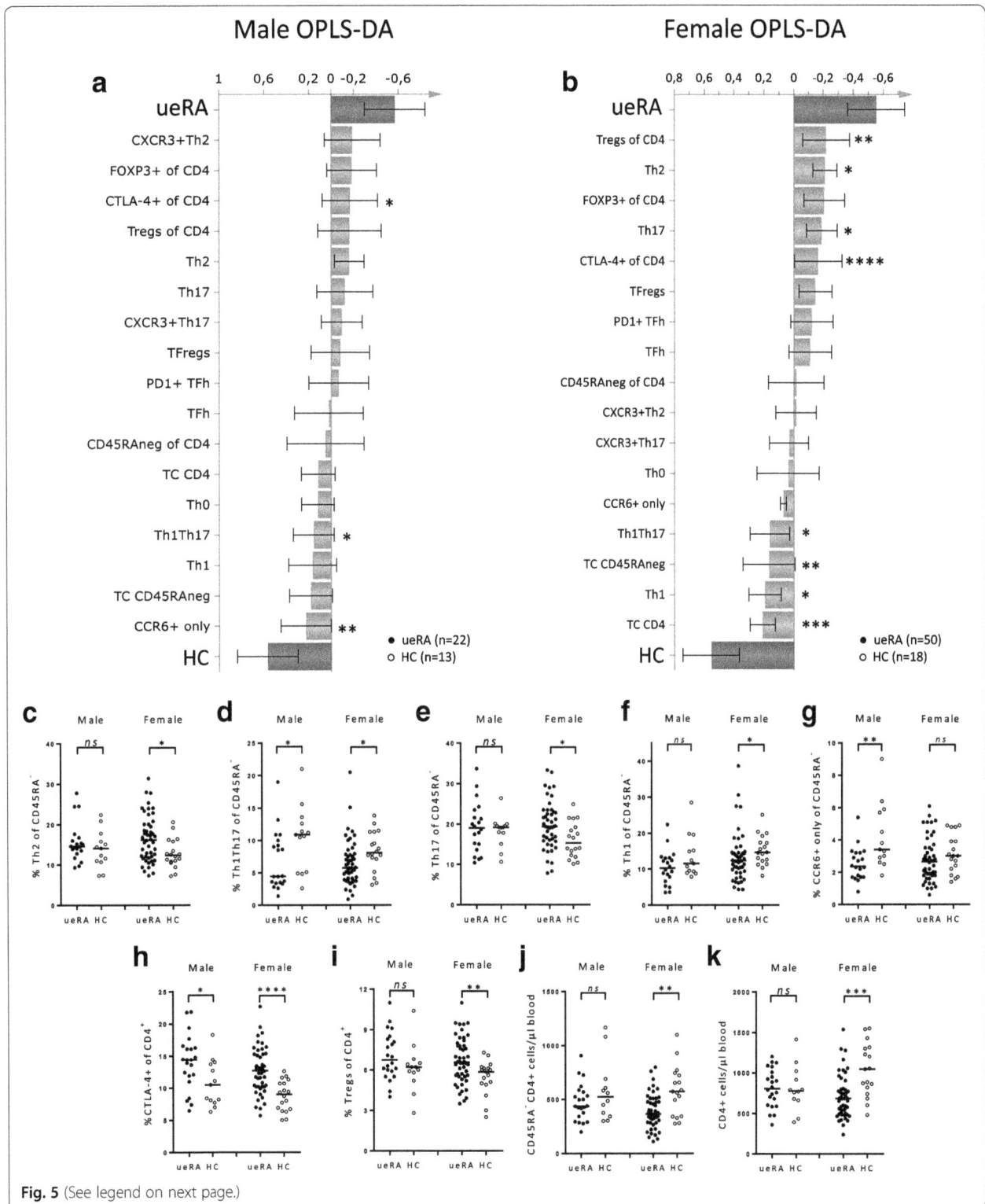

Fig. 5 (See legend on next page.)

(See figure on previous page.)

Fig. 5 Effect of sex on the differential proportions of T cell subsets in untreated early RA patients compared to healthy controls. Multivariate factor analysis was performed to investigate whether the sex affects change in the profile of T cell subsets in ueRA compared to HC. OPLS-DA column loading plots showing the association between ueRA or HC (Y-variables) and T cell subset proportions (X-variables) (**a**) in males (n = 20–22) and (**b**) in females (*n* = 48–50). X-variables (*light grey bars*) pointing in the same direction as ueRA (*top dark grey bar*) are positively associated, whereas X-variables pointing in the opposite direction are positively associated with HC (*bottom dark grey bar*). Comparison of the proportions in CD45RA^{neg}CD4$^+$ cells of (**c**) Th2, (**d**) Th1Th17, (**e**) Th17, (**f**) Th1, (**g**) CCR6$^+$ only, (**h**) CTLA-4$^+$, (**i**) Tregs (CD25$^+$CD127^{low}), and counts of (**j**) CD45RA^{neg}CD4$^+$ (memory cells), and (**k**) all CD4$^+$ cells between ueRA patients and HC are shown for males and females respectively. *Horizontal bars* indicate the median. Two-tailed Mann-Whitney *U* test. *$P \leq 0.05$, **$P \leq 0.01$, ***$P \leq 0.001$ and ****$P \leq 0.0001$

severity to some extent. In male patients, FOXP3$^+$ T cells displayed no association with disease activity measures in multivariate analysis and no statistically significant correlations were found. This could be due to lower number of patients in the male cohort. Alternatively, male ueRA patients might have a higher degree of functional impairment in FOXP3$^+$ regulatory T cells compared to female ueRA patients.

A possible explanation for the lack of positive associations between T cell subset proportions and disease activity in female patients could be that the immunological mechanisms driving early disease may be more heterogeneous in female RA patients compared to males. This could make identifying connections between immunological mechanisms and disease activity in females more difficult. It would also explain the more consistent response to treatment with methotrexate and tumor necrosis factor (TNF) inhibitors observed in males compared to females, even when controlling for baseline disease activity [8].

In our previous study, we observed a distinct profile of circulating T cell subset proportions in ueRA patients compared to HC [6], which was confirmed in the present study including a higher number of patients and healthy controls. When we separated groups into males and females, we found that female ueRA patients displayed a distinct T cell profile compare to HC. The same profile was not observed in male ueRA patients compared to HC, which could in part be due to the lower number of male relative to female patients in the study. However, in the analysis of T cell subsets in relation to disease activity the number of males was clearly sufficient.

Owing to the sexually dimorphic prevalence of RA as well the heterogeneous patient cohorts used in past studies, separation of the male and female patient cohorts and the use of DMARD-naïve early RA patients should be considered the first strength of this study. Secondly, by analyzing fresh PBMC without any ex vivo stimulation before analysis, we avoided the varying methods and duration of stimulation that may have led to inconsistent T cell data in prior studies. Lastly, by the use of multivariate factor analysis we reduced bias and multiplicity problems in the statistical analysis. However, only studying T cells in the circulation and not in the synovial fluid as well as having 2.3 times fewer male than female patients may be considered the major weaknesses.

Conclusion

To the best of our knowledge, this is the first study evaluating sex-based differences in the association between T cell subsets and clinical disease activity measures in RA, more importantly in DMARD-naïve early RA patients. Results from our study point towards differential roles of certain T cell subsets in male and female patients in relation to disease activity in early RA. Specifically, implicating Th2 helper T cells as possible mediators in regulating disease activity of RA in males. Our results also demonstrate that male and female patients with early RA should be clinically evaluated separately and sex-specific differences should be taken into account in the development of immunomodulating therapies targeting RA.

Abbreviations
ACPA: anti-citrullinated protein/peptide antibodies; CDAI: clinical disease activity index; CRP: C-reactive protein; DAS28: disease activity score in 28 joints; DMARD: disease-modifying anti-rheumatic drugs; ESR: erythrocyte sedimentation rate; HC: healthy controls; HLA: human leukocyte antigen; IL: interleukin; OPLS-DA: orthogonal projection to latent structures discriminant analysis; PBMC: peripheral blood mononuclear cells; PCA: principal component analysis; RA: rheumatoid arthritis; RF: rheumatoid factor; SJC 28/66: swollen joint counts of 28/66; TFh: T follicular helper; Th: T helper; TJC 28/68: tender joint counts of 28/68; Tph: T peripheral helper; Tregs: regulatory T cells; ueRA: untreated early rheumatoid arthritis

Acknowledgements
We thank the staff at the Clinical Immunology Laboratory of the Sahlgrenska University Hospital for technical assistance in collecting the flow cytometry data.

Funding
This study was supported by grants from Swedish Research Council (grant 2016–01574); Region Västra Götaland (agreement concerning research and

education of doctors; ALF; grant ALFGBG-143331) and the IngaBritt and Arne Lundberg's foundation. The authors thank Sahlgrenska University Hospital for providing clinical support for the study.

Authors' contributions
JA was involved in analysis and interpretation of the data, designed all figures and wrote the manuscript. JMP and LM produced the patient demography table and were involved in analysis, interpretation of the data, production of figures, and manuscript writing. KA and IN performed experiments and were involved in collecting samples and analysis of the data. ET was involved in collecting samples and clinical data. A-CL was involved in analysis, interpretation of the data and production of figures. AR designed the study, was involved in collecting samples and clinical data, and continuously supervised all aspects of the work. All authors were involved in drafting the manuscript or revising it critically for important intellectual content, and all authors approved the final version to be published. AR has full access to all of the data in the study and takes responsibility for the integrity of the data and the accuracy of the data analysis.

Consent for publication
Not applicable.

Competing interests
None of the authors has any potential conflict of interest related to this manuscript. AR reports that part of her salary for her university full professor position at the Sahlgrenska academy, University of Gothenburg, is covered by grant from AstraZeneca IMed RIA, Gothenburg, Sweden in compensation for an advisory role regarding basic research in inflammation at the company. ET is employed at both Lund University and Janssen Cilag.

Author details
[1]Department of Rheumatology and Inflammation Research, Institute of Medicine, Sahlgrenska Academy of University of Gothenburg, Box 480, S-405 30 Gothenburg, Sweden. [2]Department of Rheumatology, Skåne University Hospital Lund and Malmö, Lund University, Lund, Sweden.

References
1. Firestein GS, McInnes IB. Immunopathogenesis of rheumatoid arthritis. Immunity. 2017;46(2):183–96.
2. Gregersen PK, Silver J, Winchester RJ. The shared epitope hypothesis. An approach to understanding the molecular genetics of susceptibility to rheumatoid arthritis. Arthritis Rheum. 1987;30(11):1205–13.
3. Kim K, Bang SY, Lee HS, Bae SC. Update on the genetic architecture of rheumatoid arthritis. Nat Rev Rheumatol. 2017;13(1):13–24.
4. Ishigaki K, Shoda H, Kochi Y, Yasui T, Kadono Y, Tanaka S, Fujio K, Yamamoto K. Quantitative and qualitative characterization of expanded CD4+ T cell clones in rheumatoid arthritis patients. Sci Rep. 2015;5:12937.
5. Rao DA, Gurish MF, Marshall JL, Slowikowski K, Fonseka CY, Liu Y, Donlin LT, Henderson LA, Wei K, Mizoguchi F, et al. Pathologically expanded peripheral T helper cell subset drives B cells in rheumatoid arthritis. Nature. 2017; 542(7639):110–4.
6. Pandya JM, Lundell AC, Hallstrom M, Andersson K, Nordstrom I, Rudin A. Circulating T helper and T regulatory subsets in untreated early rheumatoid arthritis and healthy control subjects. J Leukoc Biol. 2016;100(4):823–33.
7. Forslind K, Hafstrom I, Ahlmen M, Svensson B, Group BS. Sex: a major predictor of remission in early rheumatoid arthritis? Ann Rheum Dis. 2007; 66(1):46–52.
8. Kvien TK, Uhlig T, Odegard S, Heiberg MS. Epidemiological aspects of rheumatoid arthritis: the sex ratio. Ann N Y Acad Sci. 2006;1069:212–22.
9. Hallert E, Bjork M, Dahlstrom O, Skogh T, Thyberg I. Disease activity and disability in women and men with early rheumatoid arthritis (RA): an 8-year followup of a Swedish early RA project. Arthritis Care Res. 2012;64(8):1101–7.
10. Jawaheer D, Messing S, Reed G, Ranganath VK, Kremer JM, Louie JS, Khanna D, Greenberg JD, Furst DE. Significance of sex in achieving sustained remission in the consortium of rheumatology researchers of North America cohort of rheumatoid arthritis patients. Arthritis Care Res. 2012;64(12):1811–8.
11. Klein SL, Flanagan KL. Sex differences in immune responses. Nat Rev Immunol. 2016;16(10):626–38.
12. Olsen NJ, Gu X, Kovacs WJ. Bone marrow stromal cells mediate androgenic suppression of B lymphocyte development. J Clin Invest. 2001;108(11):1697–704.
13. Pandya JM, Lundell AC, Andersson K, Nordstrom I, Theander E, Rudin A. Blood chemokine profile in untreated early rheumatoid arthritis: CXCL10 as a disease activity marker. Arthritis Res Therapy. 2017;19(1):20.
14. Han BK, Kuzin I, Gaughan JP, Olsen NJ, Bottaro A. Baseline CXCL10 and CXCL13 levels are predictive biomarkers for tumor necrosis factor inhibitor therapy in patients with moderate to severe rheumatoid arthritis: a pilot, prospective study. Arthritis Res Therapy. 2015;18:93.
15. Lina C, Conghua W, Nan L, Ping Z. Combined treatment of etanercept and MTX reverses Th1/Th2, Th17/Treg imbalance in patients with rheumatoid arthritis. J Clin Immunol. 2011;31(4):596–605.
16. Prevoo ML, van 't Hof MA, Kuper HH, van Leeuwen MA, van de Putte LB, van Riel PL. Modified disease activity scores that include twenty-eight-joint counts. Development and validation in a prospective longitudinal study of patients with rheumatoid arthritis. Arthritis Rheum. 1995;38(1):44–8.
17. Anderson J, Caplan L, Yazdany J, Robbins ML, Neogi T, Michaud K, Saag KG, O'Dell JR, Kazi S. Rheumatoid arthritis disease activity measures: American College of Rheumatology recommendations for use in clinical practice. Arthritis Care Res. 2012;64(5):640–7.
18. James EA, Rieck M, Pieper J, Gebe JA, Yue BB, Tatum M, Peda M, Sandin C, Klareskog L, Malmstrom V, et al. Citrulline-specific Th1 cells are increased in rheumatoid arthritis and their frequency is influenced by disease duration and therapy. Arthritis Rheumtol. 2014;66(7):1712–22.
19. Nagafuchi Y, Shoda H, Sumitomo S, Nakachi S, Kato R, Tsuchida Y, Tsuchiya H, Sakurai K, Hanata N, Tateishi S, et al. Immunophenotyping of rheumatoid arthritis reveals a linkage between HLA-DRB1 genotype, CXCR4 expression on memory CD4(+) T cells, and disease activity. Sci Rep. 2016;6:29338.
20. Leipe J, Grunke M, Dechant C, Reindl C, Kerzendorf U, Schulze-Koops H, Skapenko A. Role of Th17 cells in human autoimmune arthritis. Arthritis Rheum. 2010;62(10):2876–85.
21. Miao J, Zhang K, Lv M, Li Q, Zheng Z, Han Q, Guo N, Fan C, Zhu P. Circulating Th17 and Th1 cells expressing CD161 are associated with disease activity in rheumatoid arthritis. Scand J Rheumatol. 2014;43(3):194–201.
22. Raza K, Falciani F, Curnow SJ, Ross EJ, Lee CY, Akbar AN, Lord JM, Gordon C, Buckley CD, Salmon M. Early rheumatoid arthritis is characterized by a distinct and transient synovial fluid cytokine profile of T cell and stromal cell origin. Arthritis Res Therapy. 2005;7(4):R784–95.
23. Kokkonen H, Söderström I, Rocklöv J, Hallmans G, Lejon K, Dahlqvist SR. Up-regulation of cytokines and chemokines predates the onset of rheumatoid arthritis. Arthritis Rheum. 2010;62(2):383–91.
24. Maggi L, Santarlasci V, Capone M, Rossi MC, Querci V, Mazzoni A, Cimaz R, De Palma R, Liotta F, Maggi E, et al. Distinctive features of classic and nonclassic (Th17 derived) human Th1 cells. Eur J Immunol. 2012;42(12):3180–8.
25. Nistala K, Adams S, Cambrook H, Ursu S, Olivito B, De Jager W, Evans JG, Cimaz R, Bajaj-Elliott M, Wedderburn LR. Th17 plasticity in human autoimmune arthritis is driven by the inflammatory environment. Proc Natl Acad Sci U S A. 2010;107(33):14751–6.
26. Chalan P, Kroesen BJ, van der Geest KS, Huitema MG, Abdulahad WH, Bijzet J, Brouwer E, Boots AM. Circulating CD4+CD161+ T lymphocytes are increased in seropositive arthralgia patients but decreased in patients with newly diagnosed rheumatoid arthritis. PLoS One. 2013;8(11):e79370.
27. Edavalath S, Singh A, Soni N, Mohindra N, Kumar S, Misra R. Peripheral blood T helper type 17 frequency shows an inverse correlation with disease activity and magnetic resonance imaging-based osteitis and erosions in disease-modifying anti-rheumatic drug- and steroid-naive established rheumatoid arthritis. Clin Exp Immunol. 2016;186(3):313–20.

28. Plenge RM, Padyukov L, Remmers EF, Purcell S, Lee AT, Karlson EW, Wolfe F, Kastner DL, Alfredsson L, Altshuler D, et al. Replication of putative candidate-gene associations with rheumatoid arthritis in >4,000 samples from North America and Sweden: association of susceptibility with PTPN22, CTLA4, and PADI4. Am J Hum Genet. 2005;77(6):1044–60.

29. Pierer M, Kaltenhauser S, Arnold S, Wahle M, Baerwald C, Hantzschel H, Wagner U. Association of PTPN22 1858 single-nucleotide polymorphism with rheumatoid arthritis in a German cohort: higher frequency of the risk allele in male compared to female patients. Arthritis Res Therapy. 2006;8(3):R75.

30. Stanford SM, Bottini N. PTPN22: the archetypal non-HLA autoimmunity gene. Nat Rev Rheumatol. 2014;10(10):602–11.

31. Romo-Tena J, Gomez-Martin D, Alcocer-Varela J. CTLA-4 and autoimmunity: new insights into the dual regulator of tolerance. Autoimmun Rev. 2013; 12(12):1171–6.

7

Simultaneous quantification of bone erosions and enthesiophytes in the joints of patients with psoriasis or psoriatic arthritis - effects of age and disease duration

David Simon[1], Arnd Kleyer[1], Francesca Faustini[1], Matthias Englbrecht[1], Judith Haschka[1,2], Andreas Berlin[1], Sebastian Kraus[1], Axel J. Hueber[1], Roland Kocijan[1,2], Michael Sticherling[3], Juergen Rech[1*†] and Georg Schett[1*†]

Abstract

Background: Comprehensive simultaneous quantification of bone erosion and enthesiophytes in the joints of patients with psoriatic arthritis (PsA) has not been performed. Herein, we aimed to compare the extent of bone erosion and enthesiophytes in patients with PsA, psoriasis (PSO) and healthy controls, assess the influence of age and disease duration on the development of erosions and enthesiophytes and define their impact on physical function.

Methods: Patients with PsA or with PSO and controls were analysed by high-resolution peripheral quantitative computed tomography (HR-pQCT). The extent of bone erosions and enthesiophytes was assessed and plotted according to different categories of age, duration of PSO and duration of PsA, respectively. In addition, demographic and disease-specific data, including physical function (health assessment questionnaire) were collected.

Results: A total of 203 patients were analysed; 101 had PsA, 55 had PSO and 47 were healthy individuals. Patients with PsA had significantly more and larger erosions ($p = 0.002/p = 0.003$) and enthesiophytes ($p < 0.001$) compared to patients with PSO and healthy controls. Patients with PSO and healthy controls did not differ in erosions, while enthesiophytes were more frequent in patients with PSO than in healthy controls. Bone erosions, but not enthesiophytes, showed strong age-dependency in all three groups. In contrast, enthesiophytes were mostly influenced by the duration of PSO and PsA and, in contrast to bone erosions, were associated with poorer physical function.

Conclusions: Bone erosions are age-dependent, enhanced in PsA and increase with disease duration. Enthesiophytes are less age-dependent, are enhanced in both PSO and PsA and strongly influenced by disease duration. Enthesiophytes impact physical function in PsA suggesting the need for early therapeutic interventions to prevent damage.

Keywords: Psoriatic arthritis, Psoriasis, Bone erosions, Enthesiophytes, Computed tomography, Physical function

Background

Psoriasis (PSO) and psoriatic arthritis (PsA) are common inflammatory disorders, which affect about 3% and 1% of the general population, respectively [1, 2]. Next to inflammation, bone destruction is a hallmark of the disease, especially in PsA. Surprisingly few studies, however, have yet comprehensively addressed bone changes in PsA. It is commonly considered that PsA is not only characterised by catabolic but also by anabolic bone pathologies, which lead to distinct architectural changes of the joints in PsA.

The development of bone erosion in the context of PsA was recognised by Gladman and colleagues 30 years ago, showing that about two thirds of patients with PsA develop radiographically evident erosions (radiographic erosions) and that their extent is related to decline in joint function [3]. Later radiographic studies showed that

* Correspondence: juergen.rech@uk-erlangen.de; georg.schett@uk-erlangen.de
†Jürgen Rech and Georg Schett contributed equally to this work.
[1]Friedrich-Alexander-University Erlangen-Nürnberg (FAU), Department of Internal Medicine 3 – Rheumatology and Immunology, Universitätsklinikum Erlangen, Ulmenweg 18, D-91054 Erlangen, Germany
Full list of author information is available at the end of the article

bone erosion start early in the course of PsA [4–7] and that greater inflammatory activity precipitates more severe erosive damage [8–10]. From the pathophysiological point of view, bone erosions in PsA result from the accumulation of osteoclasts in the joints, which is precipitated by proinflammatory cytokines [11].

Anabolic bone changes in PsA are based on new bone formation. These changes typically occur at insertion sites of tendons to bone. Enthesial inflammation is a key process in PsA and most likely triggered by mechanical stress [12–14]. Skeletal responses at the inflamed enthesial sites then result in the formation of bony spurs, also known as enthesiophytes. As compared to bone erosions, few studies have so far addressed enthesiophytes in PsA. A high-resolution peripheral computed tomography (HR-pQCT)-based study showed that enthesiophytes are key in PsA but are not found as commonly in rheumatoid arthritis [15]. Furthermore, a more recent study revealed that enthesiophytes occur early in patients with PSO without joint involvement, suggesting that they potentially reflect a common process in PSO and PSA [16].

To date, however, no comprehensive analysis of catabolic and anabolic bone damage in patients with PsA has been performed. To better interpret the impact of PsA on catabolic and anabolic bone changes, it is advantageous to investigate appropriate control populations such as healthy individuals and patients with PSO. We therefore simultaneously analysed the extent of catabolic and anabolic bone changes in healthy controls, patients with PSO and patients with PsA, by HR-pQCT and addressed the impact of age, duration of PSO and duration of PsA on respective bone changes.

Methods

Patients

Healthy controls and patients with PsA were part of the Erlangen Imaging Cohort (ERIC), which prospectively assesses articular bone composition in healthy controls and patients with arthritis [17]. Three groups were analysed in a cross-sectional setting: (1) patients with PsA, (2) patients with PSO and (3) healthy controls. Patients with PsA were recruited at the Rheumatology Department of the University of Erlangen-Nuremberg. All patients with PsA had to fulfil the Classification criteria for psoriatic arthritis (CASPAR) criteria [18]. An experienced rheumatologist examined the patients for clinical signs of musculoskeletal involvement (synovitis, enthesitis, dactylitis and/or inflammatory back pain) at the time of imaging. Patients with PSO were recruited at the Dermatology Department of the University of Erlangen-Nuremberg. They were referred to the Rheumatology Department of the same institution for detailed rheumatologic analysis. As with PsA, an experienced

rheumatologist examined the patients for the presence of clinical signs of musculoskeletal involvement. Patients with no current or previous evidence of arthritis, enthesitis or other manifestations of PsA were selected to undergo further evaluation. In addition, healthy controls with comparable age and sex were also investigated. Healthy controls were collected by a field campaign and had no joint pain, swelling or any other sign of inflammatory disease and no personal or family history of such disease. Healthy controls had not to have osteoporosis or any evidence of metabolic diseases such as diabetes mellitus, malabsorption or thyroid dysfunction. Also, renal and hepatic function had to be normal. Subjects receiving glucocorticoids or bisphosphonates (in the present or past) were also excluded.

The study was conducted upon approval of the local ethic committee of the University of Erlangen and with the authorisation of the National Radiation Safety Agency (Bundesamt für Strahlenschutz). Each patient provided informed consent.

Demographic and disease-specific data

Demographic data such as age, sex, body mass index (BMI) and smoking status were collected. As disease-specific parameters, disease severity of psoriasis according to the Psoriasis area severity index (PASI) [19], disease duration of PSO and PsA, involvement of nail and scalp and Health assessment questionnaire (HAQ) data were recorded. In patients with PsA the disease activity 28 score based on erythrocyte sedimentation rate (DAS28-ESR) was collected. C-reactive protein (milligrams per litre) was measured presence of rheumatoid factor and anti-cyclic citrullinated peptides antibodies (ACPA) was assessed. In addition, current medication including disease-modifying anti-rheumatic drugs (DMARDs), glucocorticoids and non-steroidal anti-inflammatory drugs (NSAIDs) was recorded.

High-resolution peripheral quantitative computed tomography (HR-pQCT)

All subjects underwent HR-pQCT scans of the dominant hand using the XtremeCT scanner (SCANCO Medical, Brütisellen, Switzerland). To reduce movement artefacts the hand was immobilised using a custom holder. The region of interest (ROI) was the metacarpal head and the phalangeal base of the metacarpophalangeal (MCP) joints 2 and 3. During the 8.4-min scanning time the MCP region was 80 slices distal to the edge of the third metacarpal head and 242 slices proximal to it were scanned. Resolution was 82 μm isotropic voxels.

Detection of erosions and enthesiophytes on HR-pQCT

Images were analysed using axial slices ($N = 322$). As described before [18], bone was divided into four quadrants representing the palmar (Q1), ulnar (Q2), dorsal

(Q3), and radial (Q4) side, respectively. Thereby exact localization of each erosion or enthesiophyte was possible (Fig. 1). Erosions were defined as breaks in the cortical shell visible in at least two planes [20]. Enthesiophytes were identified as bony proliferations at specific anatomical sites (outside or along the insertion of the capsule). Based on previous studies we have exactly defined these anatomical sites by regions of interest (ROIs) [15–17]. If an erosion or enthesiophyte was found in one (axial) plane, the lesion had to be confirmed in the perpendicular plane (coronal or sagittal).

HR-pQCT scoring

For scoring the number of bone erosions and enthesiophytes per patient, the sum of the respective lesion number in the four aforementioned quadrants in the four assessed regions (metacarpal head 2, metacarpal head 3, phalangeal base 2, phalangeal base 3) was calculated. If in a single quadrant more than one lesion was found, only the largest lesion was scored for its dimension. Enthesiophyte size (millimetres) was defined as the distance between the highest surface of the bone proliferation and the original surface of the cortical bone. Volume of erosions (cubic millimetres) was measured according to a half-ellipsoid formula. Images were

analysed and measured by two independent and blinded readers (DS, SK) using the open source DICOM viewer Osirix V4.1 (Rosslyn, VA, USA): 3D-image software provided by the manufacturer was used for obtaining illustrative 2D and 3D images.

Statistical analysis

Data were collected, organised and analysed through SPSS software for statistics (IBM SPSS 21.0, IBM corporation®, Armonk, NY, USA). Overall, categorical variables are presented as numbers and percentages and continuous variables are provided as mean ± standard deviation (SD) if not stated otherwise. Assumptions of normally distributed continuous variables were tested using quantile-quantile plots and the Kolmogorov-Smirnov and Shapiro-Wilk test. To explore differences in the frequency distributions of categorical variables, the chi-square ($\chi2$) test was applied. We evaluated bivariate relationships between duration of psoriasis, duration of PsA, the HAQ and the occurrence of bone microstructural changes using Spearman correlation analysis. Analysis of the bone microstructure of subgroups (age, PSO duration, PsA duration) was by the Kruskal-Wallis test with subsequent Mann-Whitney U test for pairwise group comparisons in the case of significant Kruskal-Wallis test results. In addition, linear regression

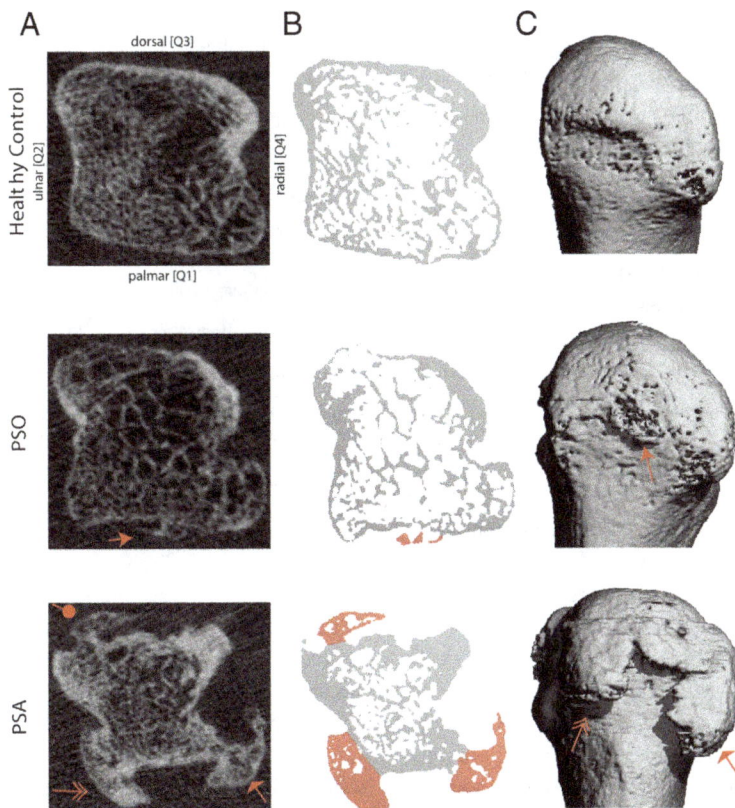

Fig. 1 Examples of bone microstructure in healthy controls, patients with psoriasis (PSO) and patients with psoriatic arthritis (PsA). **a** Axial slices of metacarpal heads. **b** Bi-facially retouched areas of axial slices. **c** Palmar reconstruction of the associated metacarpal head. Arrows mark bone proliferation

was modelled, with the total number of enthesiophytes/erosions, size of enthesiophytes and volume of erosions, respectively, as the dependent variable, while age, sex, BMI, PASI and skin disease duration were entered as independent variables. P values < 0.05 were regarded as significant.

Results

Demographic and clinical features of the patients with psoriatic disease

In total, 203 individuals were analysed for catabolic and anabolic bone changes in their joints. Among these, 101 individuals (51 women/50 men) had a diagnosis of PsA, 55 (20 women/35 men) had PSO without clinical musculoskeletal involvement and 47 individuals were healthy controls (23 women/24 men). Mean age and sex distribution were comparable among the three groups. Body mass index was significantly higher in patients with PsA or PSO compared to healthy controls, representing the well-recognised association between the disease and obesity. Smoking habits were comparable among the three groups. Patients with PsA had a mean duration of 18.9 ± 14.8 years of skin disease and 6.4 ± 7.3 years of joint disease. Patients with PSO had comparable disease duration of 15.2 ± 15.4 years: 21% of patients with PsA and 51% of patients with PSO reported of nail disease, while the prevalence of scalp involvement was 29% in patients with PSO and 20% in patients with PsA. Skin and musculoskeletal disease activity in patients with PsA, as evaluated by the PASI (3.4 ± 5.5), DAS28-ESR (2.98 ± 1.48) and HAQ (0.8 ± 0.8) was low, most likely due to effective treatment of PsA. Further disease-specific characteristics of the patient groups are shown in Table 1.

Inter-observer agreement for catabolic and anabolic bone changes

Inter-observer agreement for the detection of bone lesions was very high. The intraclass correlation coefficient (ICC) was 0.96 for detection of erosions and 0.95 for detection of enthesiophytes, respectively. Regarding the extent of the lesions, the ICC for measuring the size of enthesiophytes was 0.94 and for measuring the volume of erosions it was 0.90.

Comparison of enthesiophytes in patients with psoriasis and patients with psoriatic arthritis

In the PsA group 963 enthesiophytes were identified, while in the PSO group only 306 enthesiophytes were observed. The average number of enthesiophytes per patient was significantly higher in patients with PsA. In PsA, we detected 9.5 ± 6.7 enthesiophytes per patient, while 5.6 ± 3.3 enthesiophytes per patient were detected in PSO (p < 0.001) (Table 2). In both groups the majority of enthesiophytes were found at the metacarpal heads and the most affected sides were the dorsal and palmar side of the metacarpal heads, where functional entheses can be found. A significant (p < 0.001)

Table 1 Demographic and disease-specific characteristics of patients with psoriatic arthritis (PsA), patients with psoriasis (PSO) and healthy controls (HC)

	PsA	PSO	HC	P values
Demographic characteristics				
Number of subjects	101	55	47	–
Sex (male/female)	50/51	35/20	24/23	0.220
Age (years)	50.8 ± 13.2	49.0 ± 11.4	45.7 ± 12.9	0.056
Body mass index	28.1 ± 5.7	27.9 ± 5.6	25.0 ± 4.7	0.011
Smokers, N (%)	28 (27.7)	16 (29.1)	11 (23.4)	0.875
Disease specific characteristics				
Duration of PSO (years)	18.9 ± 14.8	15.2 ± 15.4	–	0.071
Duration of PsA (years)	6.4 ± 7.3	–	–	–
PASI (units)	3.4 ± 5.5	6.2 ± 8.0	–	0.007
HAQ	0.8 ± 0.8	0.4 ± 0.5	–	0.003
DAS28-ESR (units)	2.98 ± 1.48	–	–	–
Phenotypic characteristics				
Nail involvement, N (%)	21 (20.8)	28 (50.9)	–	0.004
Scalp involvement, N (%)	20 (19.8)	16 (29.1)	–	0.659
Other clinical characteristics				
Positive ACPA, N (%)	1 (1.0)	0	–	0.452
Positive low-titre RF, N (%)[a]	9 (8.9)	4 (7.3)	–	0.681
C-reactive protein (mg/L)[b]	4.9 ± 6.5	3.8 ± 4.6	–	0.228
Treatment modalities				
Current csDMARDs, N (%)	52 (51.5)	9 (16.4)	–	< 0.001
Current bDMARDs, N (%)	49 (48.5)	4 (7.3)	–	< 0.001
Current Glucocorticoids, N (%)	19 (18.8)	0 (0)	–	0.001
Current NSAIDs, N (%)	31 (30.7)	6 (10.9)	–	0.005
No systemic treatment, N (%)	13 (12.9)	41 (74.5)	–	< 0.001

ACPA anti-citrullinated protein antibody, *bDMARDs* biologic disease-modifying anti-rheumatic drugs, *csDMARDs* conventional synthetic disease-modifying anti-rheumatic drugs, *DAS28-ESR* disease activity score 28 based on erythrocyte sedimentation rate, *N* number, *NSAIDs* non-steroidal anti-inflammatory drugs, *PASI* Psoriasis area and severity index, *HAQ* health assessment questionnaire, *RF* rheumatoid factor
[a] < 50 IE/mL
[b] Normal value < 5 mg/mL

difference between the PsA and PSO subgroup was detected in the extent of the enthesiophytes, with an increased enthesiophyte size of 6.8 ± 5.6 mm in the PsA group and 4.0 ± 2.2 mm in the PSO group.

Comparison of erosions in patients with psoriasis and patients with psoriatic arthritis

In the PsA group 140 erosions were detected, while in the PSO group 27 erosions were detected. With respect to the

Table 2 Anabolic and catabolic bone changes in healthy controls (HC), patients with psoriasis (PSO) and patients with psoriatic arthritis (PsA)

A. Effects of age

N	HC	PSO	PsA
	(18/22/7)	(11/36/8)	(20/55/26)
Number of enthesiophytes			
20–40 years	2.41 ± 1.94	5.00 ± 2.49	7.50 ± 5.65
41–60 years	3.29 ± 1.77	6.00 ± 3.50	9.09 ± 6.20
> 60 years	3.86 ± 1.22	3.71 ± 1.98	11.96 ± 7.71
Number of erosions			
20–40 years	0.12 ± 0.33	0.27 ± 0.90	1.05 ± 1.82
41–60 years	0.33 ± 0.48	0.50 ± 0.94	1.26 ± 1.87
> 60 years	1.29 ± 0.95	0.86 ± 1.07	2.00 ± 2.95
Size of enthesiophytes (mm)			
20–40 years	1.44 ± 1.10	3.37 ± 1.61	5.26 ± 5.56
41–60 years	2.24 ± 1.15	4.40 ± 2.37	6.33 ± 4.96
> 60 years	2.69 ± 0.74	3.01 ± 1.56	8.82 ± 6.70
Volume of erosions (mm^3)			
20–40 years	0.06 ± 0.20	0.28 ± 0.91	1.92 ± 3.61
41–60 years	0.53 ± 1.08	0.99 ± 2.25	2.95 ± 5.71
> 60 years	4.84 ± 6.31	1.99 ± 3.33	5.27 ± 12.58

B. Effects of disease duration

N	PSO in PSO	PSO in PsA	PSA in PsA
	(27/21/7)	(40/40/21)	(78/17/6)
Number of enthesiophytes			
0–10 years	5.50 ± 2.49	7.91 ± 3.82	8.72 ± 5.33
11–20 years	4.80 ± 2.14	10.72 ± 7.88	10.13 ± 8.36
> 20 years	6.60 ± 4.56	11.00 ± 8.26	18.17 ± 10.93
Number of erosions			
0–10 years	0.67 ± 1.11	0.71 ± 1.45	1.31 ± 2.17
11–20 years	0.53 ± 0.92	1.33 ± 2.17	1.06 ± 1.81
> 20 years	0.20 ± 0.45	2.65 ± 2.82	3.50 ± 2.67
Size of enthesiophytes (mm)			
0–10 years	4.07 ± 1.67	5.33 ± 3.20	6.05 ± 4.59
11–20 years	3.21 ± 1.49	7.65 ± 6.60	7.61 ± 6.96
> 20 years	5.09 ± 3.19	8.38 ± 7.24	13.59 ± 9.71
Volume of erosions (mm^3)			
0–10 years	1.21 ± 2.61	1.57 ± 3.16	2.71 ± 5.01
11–20 years	1.03 ± 2.29	3.08 ± 9.75	4.87 ± 14.36
> 20 years	0.18 ± 0.39	6.72 ± 9.24	7.44 ± 11.41

N numbers of subjects in the three different age categories

number of erosions there was a significant difference between the PsA and PSO subgroup ($p = 0.002$) with patients with PsA having more erosions (1.4 ± 2.2) than patients with PSO (0.5 ± 0.9). The sides most affected by erosions were the radial sides of the metacarpal heads. There was a

significant difference in the volume of erosions between patients with PsA and patients with PSO ($p = 0.003$), with higher erosion volumes in PsA (6.3 ± 9.7 mm^3) than in PSO (3.3 ± 3.1 mm^3).

Comparison of erosions and enthesiophytes in patients with psoriasis or psoriatic arthritis and healthy controls

We then compared catabolic and anabolic bone damage in patients with PsA with the ones identified in healthy controls. The number ($p = 0.002$) and size ($p = 0.004$) of bone erosions was significantly greater in patients with PsA compared to healthy controls. Furthermore, analysis of enthesiophytes showed a similar picture: again the number and size of enthesiophytes (both $p < 0.001$) was significantly greater in patients with PsA than in healthy controls. As already described [16], patients with PSO did not differ in the number of erosions compared to healthy controls, but in PSO the number of enthesiophytes was significantly greater ($p < 0.001$).

Influence of age on bone erosions in psoriasis and psoriatic arthritis

The analysis of number and extent of bone erosions in three age groups (20–40 years, 41–60 years and more than 60 years) revealed a continuous increase in erosive bone changes with age in healthy controls and in patients with PSO or PsA (Table 2, Fig. 2), suggesting that age is a key determinant of erosive damage in the joints. Nonetheless, patients with PsA were most affected by erosive bone damage among all age groups. Hence, the amount of erosive bone changes in a 20 to 40-year old patient with PsA was as high as in healthy individuals aged over 60 years. Healthy individuals and patients with PSO did not substantially differ in erosive changes. While erosions were absent in young healthy individuals and patients with PSO, they significantly increased with age over 60 years.

Influence of age on enthesiophytes in psoriasis and psoriatic arthritis

Age did not influence the burden of enthesiophytes in healthy controls and patients with PSO. In patients with PsA, the number of enthesiophytes moderately increased with age (20–40 years, 7.50 ± 5.65; 41–60 years, 9.09 ± 6.20, $p = 0.015$; > 60 years, 11.96 ± 7.71, $p = 0.001$). Similarly, the size of enthesiophytes increased with age in patients with PsA (20–40 years, 5.26 ± 5.56 mm; 41–60 years, 6.33 ± 4.96 mm, $p = 0.006$; 20–40 years, 5.26 ± 5.56 mm; > 60 years, 8.82 ± 6.70 mm, $p = 0.001$).

Influence of disease duration on bone erosions in psoriasis and psoriatic arthritis

We next analysed to which extent the duration of PSO and PsA influence the burden of erosive damage in PsA. Bone erosions significantly increased with the duration

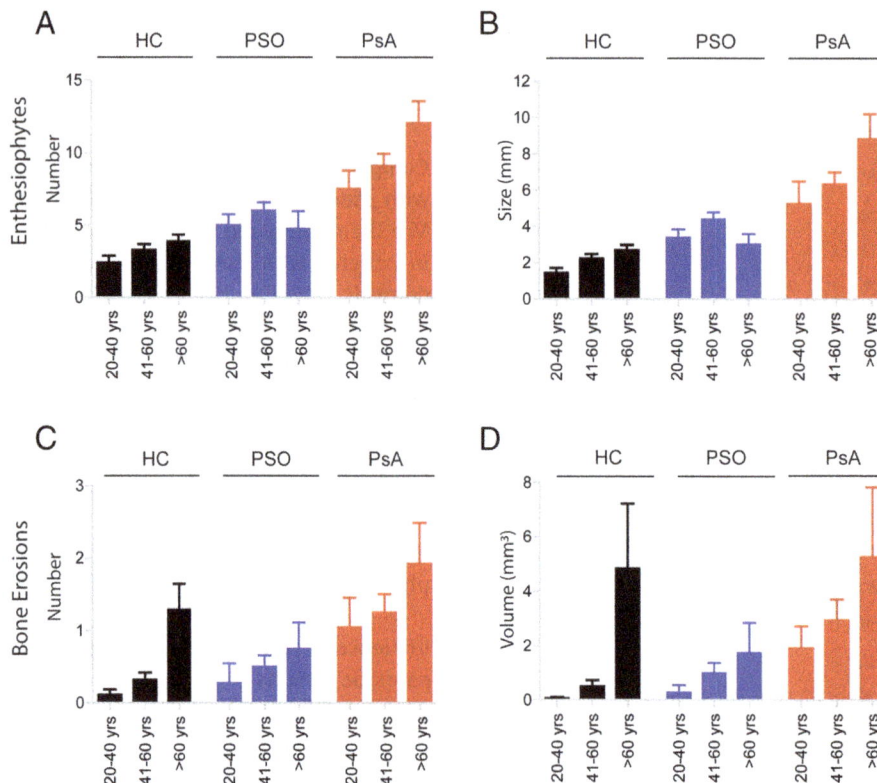

Fig. 2 Effect of age on anabolic and catabolic bone changes in healthy controls (HC), patients with psoriasis (PSO) and psoriatic patients with arthritis (PsA). Mean (SE) values of enthesiophyte number (**a**), enthesiophyte size (**b**), erosion number (**c**) and erosion volume (**d**) in healthy controls (black), patients with PSO (blue) and patients with PsA (red) in the different age categories: (i) 20–40 years, (ii) 41–60 years and (iii) over 60 years

of psoriatic skin disease (Fig. 3, Table 2). Hence, their numbers (2.65 ± 2.82) and volumes $(6.72 \pm 9.24$ mm^3) were significantly greater in patients with PsA with psoriasis of more than 20 years duration compared those with 11–20 years $(p = 0.015$ and $p = 0.003$, respectively) and less than 10 years disease duration (both $p < 0.001$). Not surprisingly, the duration of PsA also affected erosive damage (Fig. 3, Table 2): Patients with long disease duration $(> 20$ years) had significantly more erosions (3.50 ± 2.67), compared to those with disease duration between 11 and 20 years $(p = 0.019)$ or less than 10 years $(p = 0.015)$. In patients with PSO, overall erosive changes were very mild and not related to duration of psoriasis.

Influence of disease duration on enthesiophytes in psoriasis and psoriatic arthritis

With respect to anabolic bone changes, we found that duration of skin disease influenced enthesiophyte burden both in patients with PSO and patients with PsA. While patients with PSO had mild increases in enthesiophytes with duration of psoriasis, this effect was more pronounced in PsA (Table 2). Furthermore, duration of PsA influenced the burden of enthesiophytes as well. Number (18.17 ± 10.93) and size (13.59 ± 9.71) of enthesiophytes were more than twofold greater in patients with PsA with disease duration of

more than 20 years compared to those with shorter disease duration (11–20 years, $p = 0.048$; < 10 years, $p = 0.009$) (Table 2).

Association between specific clinical variables and catabolic and anabolic microstructural changes

Duration of PSO significantly correlated with the number of enthesiophytes $(p = 0.005)$, the size of enthesiophytes $(p = 0.011)$, the number of erosions $(p = 0.002)$ and the volume of erosions $(p = 0.010)$. Duration of PsA significantly correlated with the number and size of enthesiophytes (both $p < 0.001$) and the number and volume of erosions (both $p < 0.001$). Most importantly the number and size of enthesiophytes but not number and volume of erosions correlated with physical function as measured by the HAQ score $(p = 0.001$, $p = 0.002)$. Furthermore, the burden of erosions and enthesiophytes was higher $(p = 0.028$ and $p < 0.001$, respectively) in patients taking biological DMARDs compared to patients not taking biological DMARDs, reflecting the more severe disease course in patients starting biological DMARDs.

Testing the influence of certain demographic and clinical parameters on the bone microstructure

Using a regression model including sex, age, PASI, BMI and duration of skin disease to determine the factors

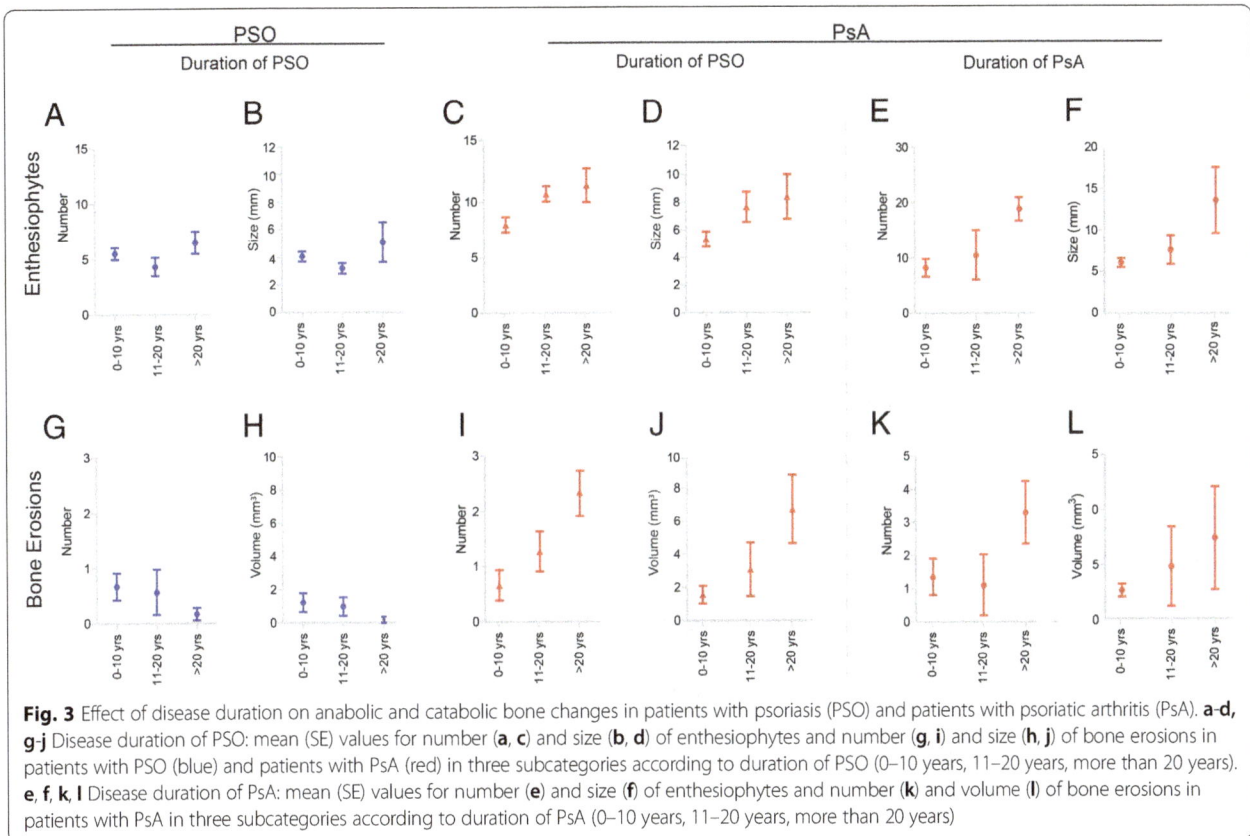

Fig. 3 Effect of disease duration on anabolic and catabolic bone changes in patients with psoriasis (PSO) and patients with psoriatic arthritis (PsA). **a–d, g–j** Disease duration of PSO: mean (SE) values for number (**a**, **c**) and size (**b**, **d**) of enthesiophytes and number (**g**, **i**) and size (**h**, **j**) of bone erosions in patients with PSO (blue) and patients with PsA (red) in three subcategories according to duration of PSO (0–10 years, 11–20 years, more than 20 years). **e, f, k, l** Disease duration of PsA: mean (SE) values for number (**e**) and size (**f**) of enthesiophytes and number (**k**) and volume (**l**) of bone erosions in patients with PsA in three subcategories according to duration of PsA (0–10 years, 11–20 years, more than 20 years)

that independently influence erosion and enthesiophytes numbers, respectively, the only variable that remained significant was the duration of skin disease ($p = 0.031$; $p = 0.023$). Using the same model and determining the extent of erosions and enthesiophytes underlined once more the importance of the duration of skin disease, as it was the only variable influencing the size of enthesiophytes and the volume of bone erosions ($p = 0.005$ $p = 0.034$).

Discussion

This cross-sectional study simultaneously analysed erosions and enthesiophytes in patients with PsA and compared data with findings obtained in two control populations - healthy controls and patients with PSO. The analyses revealed significantly increased catabolic and anabolic bone changes in the hand joints of patients with PsA, not only confirming the bone-destructive nature of the disease but also the co-occurrence of enthesiophytes as a typical feature of PsA. While it has already been described that erosive damage accumulates with longer disease duration, no data on enthesiophytes were available that showed their relationship with disease duration.

HR-pQCT is a highly sensitive technique for picking up bone erosions and enthesiophytes in the peripheral joints [15, 16, 20]. On the other hand, previous HR-pQCT

studies have shown that healthy individuals also have a certain degree of intra-articular bone changes [16, 20]. Therefore, bone damage observed in PsA has to be validated against data obtained in healthy individuals. Furthermore, recent data has also revealed specific bone changes in PSO in the absence of clinical joint disease, particularly enthesiophytes [16]. To consider these findings we also included a group of patients with psoriasis in this analysis. Compared to healthy controls and patients with PSO the burden of structural damage was significantly higher in PsA, showing more bone erosions and more enthesiophytes.

Bone erosions were dependent on age and disease duration of PsA. Erosions reflect accumulating mechanical and inflammatory damage in the joints. In accordance, erosive damage was greatest in patients with PsA. No difference was found between healthy controls and patients with PSO. A remarkable finding was that with increase in age, bone erosions did not only increase in patients with PsA, but also in patients with PSO and healthy controls. While individuals without inflammatory joint disease (healthy controls and patients with psoriasis) most likely accrue damage due to mechanical triggers, in patients with PsA the additional inflammatory trigger appears to speed up erosions. Hence, the average 20 to 40-year old patient with PsA already exhibits a burden of bone erosions, which equals that of an individual who is over 60 years old and does not have inflammatory joint disease. These findings also indicate that judgement on the burden of erosive bone damage in an individual with PsA has to consider age as an important influencing factor. The influence of inflammation as an enhancer of progression of bone erosions is also supported by the notion that the duration of PsA is associated with the burden of bone erosions. This clinical observation is substantiated by earlier mechanistic data showing that key cytokines involved in the pathogenesis of psoriatic disease, like IL-17 and TNF-alpha, potently affect bone homeostasis by enhancing bone resorption while suppressing bone formation [21–24]. Hence the longer the bone is exposed to the inflammatory micro-environment in PsA, the more likely bone erosion occurs.

In contrast to bone erosions, enthesiophytes were not only increased in PsA but also in PSO. This finding supported previous findings showing that enthesiophytes are also present in PSO [16]. Furthermore, age dependency of enthesiophytes is less pronounced. These anabolic bone changes appear to be specifically induced by the disease itself, highlighting the role of enthesial inflammation in PsA and providing an opportunity to detect musculoskeletal involvement very early in the process of psoriatic disease. Longitudinal studies will be needed to clarify whether such lesions predict the onset of PsA. Enthesiophytes are formed at sites of functional entheses substantiating the concept of the "synovio-entheseal complex", which is based on biomechanical stress- induced inflammation [12–14]. Given that enthesiophytes likely represent irreversible lesions, these findings particularly stress the importance of early therapeutic interventions in PsA. This consideration is even more important since our analyses showed that primarily enthesiophytes, but not bone erosions, impact the physical function of Patients with PsA.

Our data show that PsA, at present, is still associated with significant bone destructive changes, most likely because of late recognition of the disease and consequently late start of anti-inflammatory treatment [25]. These findings thereby foster the importance of implementation of early and tightly controlled treatment regimen in PsA in order to prevent the development of bone damage. In this context it is noteworthy that several different biological DMARD treatments have already shown structural benefits in the treatment of PsA, hence providing the possibility to interfere at least with the catabolic aspect of bone damage in PsA [26–28].

Conclusions

In summary, PsA acts as a strong enhancer of age-related catabolic bone damage. In contrast, enthesiophytes, as signs of anabolic bone damage, are less age-dependent but primarily depend on the duration of PsA. Small enthesiophytes occur before clinical joint involvement and increase in size with progressive disease. Taken together, these findings highlight the destructive nature of PsA and the necessity for an early intervention to limit the burden of bone damage in PsA.

Abbreviations
ACPA: Anti-cyclic citrullinated peptides antibodies; BMI: Body mass index; CASPAR: Classification criteria for psoriatic arthritis; DAS28-ESR: Disease activity 28 score based on erythrocyte sedimentation rate; DMARDs: Disease-modifying anti-rheumatic drugs; HAQ: Health assessment questionnaire; HR-pQCT: High-resolution peripheral quantitative computed tomography; IL-17: Interleukin-17; MCP: Metacarpophalangeal; NSAIDs: Non-steroidal anti-inflammatory drugs; PASI: Psoriasis Area Severity Index; PsA: Psoriatic arthritis; PSO: Psoriasis; ROI: Region of interest; TNF: Tumour necrosis factor

Funding
This study was supported by the Deutsche Forschungsgemeinschaft (CRC1181), the Marie Curie project OSTEOIMMUNE, the IMI-funded project RTCure and the Pfizer Competitive Grant Award Germany.

Authors' contributions
DS, AK, FF, JH, AB and RK collected the data. DS, ME, AJH, MS, JR and GS analysed and interpreted the data. DS, AK, FF and GS prepared and revised the manuscript. DS, AK and GS designed the study. All authors read and approved the final manuscript.

Consent for publication
Not applicable.

Competing interests
The authors declare that they have no competing interests.

Author details
[1]Friedrich-Alexander-University Erlangen-Nürnberg (FAU), Department of Internal Medicine 3 – Rheumatology and Immunology, Universitätsklinikum Erlangen, Ulmenweg 18, D-91054 Erlangen, Germany. [2]St. Vincent Hospital, Medical Department II, the VINFORCE Study Group, Academic Teaching Hospital of Medical University of Vienna, Vienna, Austria. [3]Department of Dermatology, University of Erlangen-Nuremberg, Erlangen, Germany.

References
1. Gelfand JM, Gladman DD, Mease PJ, Smith N, Margolis DJ, Nijsten T, et al. Epidemiology of psoriatic arthritis in the population of the United States. J Am Acad Dermatol. 2005;53(4):573.
2. Catanoso M, Pipitone N, Salvarani C. Epidemiology of psoriatic arthritis. Reumatismo. 2012;64(2):66–70.
3. Gladman DD, Shuckett R, Russell ML, Thorne JC, Schachter RK. Psoriatic arthritis (PSA)--an analysis of 220 patients. Q J Med. 1987;62(238):127–41.
4. Torre Alonso JC, Rodriguez Perez A, Arribas Castrillo JM, Ballina Garcia J, Riestra Noriega JL, Lopez LC. Psoriatic arthritis (PA): a clinical, immunological and radiological study of 180 patients. Br J Rheumatol. 1991;30(4):245–50.

5. Gladman DD, Stafford-Brady F, Chang CH, Lewandowski K, Russell ML. Longitudinal study of clinical and radiological progression in psoriatic arthritis. J Rheumatol. 1990;17(6):809–12.

6. Scarpa R, Cuocolo A, Peluso R, Atteno M, Gisonni P, Iervolino S, et al. Early psoriatic arthritis: the clinical spectrum. J Rheumatol. 2008;35(1):137–41.

7. Palazzi C, D'Agostino L, D'Amico E, Pennese E, Petricca A. Asymptomatic erosive peripheral psoriatic arthritis: a frequent finding in Italian patients. Rheumatology (Oxford). 2003;42(7):909–11.

8. Gladman DD, Farewell VT, Nadeau C. Clinical indicators of progression in psoriatic arthritis: multivariate relative risk model. J Rheumatol. 1995; 22(4):675–9.

9. Queiro-Silva R, Torre-Alonso JC, Tinture-Eguren T, Lopez-Lagunas I. A polyarticular onset predicts erosive and deforming disease in psoriatic arthritis. Ann Rheum Dis. 2003;62(1):68–70.

10. Gladman DD, Farewell VT. Progression in psoriatic arthritis: role of time varying clinical indicators. J Rheumatol. 1999;26(11):2409–13.

11. Ritchlin CT, Haas-Smith SA, Li P, Hicks DG, Schwarz EM. Mechanisms of TNF-alpha- and RANKL-mediated osteoclastogenesis and bone resorption in psoriatic arthritis. J Clin Invest. 2003;111(6):821–31.

12. McGonagle D, Lories RJ, Tan AL, Benjamin M. The concept of a "synovio-entheseal complex" and its implications for understanding joint inflammation and damage in psoriatic arthritis and beyond. Arthritis Rheum. 2007;56(8):2482–91.

13. Jacques P, Lambrecht S, Verheugen E, Pauwels E, Kollias G, Armaka M, et al. Proof of concept: enthesitis and new bone formation in spondyloarthritis are driven by mechanical strain and stromal cells. Ann Rheum Dis. 2014; 73(2):437–45.

14. Benjamin M, McGonagle D. The anatomical basis for disease localisation in seronegative spondyloarthropathy at entheses and related sites. J Anat. 2001;199(Pt 5):503–26.

15. Finzel S, Englbrecht M, Engelke K, Stach C, Schett G. A comparative study of periarticular bone lesions in rheumatoid arthritis and psoriatic arthritis. Ann Rheum Dis. 2011;70(1):122–7.

16. Simon D, Faustini F, Kleyer A, Haschka J, Englbrecht M, Kraus S, et al. Analysis of periarticular bone changes in patients with cutaneous psoriasis without associated psoriatic arthritis. Ann Rheum Dis. 2016;75(4):660–6.

17. Simon D, Kleyer A, Stemmler F, Simon C, Berlin A, Hueber AJ, et al. Age- and sex-dependent changes of intra-articular cortical and trabecular bone structure and the effects of rheumatoid arthritis. J Bone Miner Res. 2017; 32(4):722–30.

18. Taylor W, Gladman D, Helliwell P, Marchesoni A, Mease P, Mielants H. Classification criteria for psoriatic arthritis: development of new criteria from a large international study. Arthritis Rheum. 2006;54(8):2665–73.

19. Fredriksson T, Pettersson U. Severe psoriasis–oral therapy with a new retinoid. Dermatologica. 1978;157(4):238–44.

20. Stach CM, Bauerle M, Englbrecht M, Kronke G, Engelke K, Manger B, et al. Periarticular bone structure in rheumatoid arthritis patients and healthy individuals assessed by high-resolution computed tomography. Arthritis Rheum. 2010;62(2):330–9.

21. Lam J, Takeshita S, Barker JE, Kanagawa O, Ross FP, Teitelbaum SL. TNF-alpha induces osteoclastogenesis by direct stimulation of macrophages exposed to permissive levels of RANK ligand. J Clin Invest. 2000;106(12): 1481–8.

22. Bertolini DR, Nedwin GE, Bringman TS, Smith DD, Mundy GR. Stimulation of bone resorption and inhibition of bone formation in vitro by human tumour necrosis factors. Nature. 1986;319(6053):516–8.

23. Sato K, Suematsu A, Okamoto K, Yamaguchi A, Morishita Y, Kadono Y, et al. Th17 functions as an osteoclastogenic helper T cell subset that links T cell activation and bone destruction. J Exp Med. 2006;203(12):2673–82.

24. Uluckan O, Jimenez M, Karbach S, Jeschke A, Grana O, Keller J, et al. Chronic skin inflammation leads to bone loss by IL-17-mediated inhibition of Wnt signaling in osteoblasts. Sci Transl Med. 2016;8(330):330ra337.

25. Coates LC, Moverley AR, McParland L, Brown S, Navarro-Coy N, O'Dwyer JL, et al. Effect of tight control of inflammation in early psoriatic arthritis (TICOPA): a UK multicentre, open-label, randomised controlled trial. Lancet. 2015;386(10012):2489–98.

26. van der Heijde D, Kavanaugh A, Gladman DD, Antoni C, Krueger GG, Guzzo C, et al. Infliximab inhibits progression of radiographic damage in patients with active psoriatic arthritis through one year of treatment: results from the induction and maintenance psoriatic arthritis clinical trial 2. Arthritis Rheum. 2007;56(8):2698–707.

27. Kavanaugh A, Ritchlin C, Rahman P, Puig L, Gottlieb AB, Li S, et al. Ustekinumab, an anti-IL-12/23 p40 monoclonal antibody, inhibits radiographic progression in patients with active psoriatic arthritis: results of an integrated analysis of radiographic data from the phase 3, multicentre, randomised, double-blind, placebo-controlled PSUMMIT-1 and PSUMMIT-2 trials. Ann Rheum Dis. 2014;73(6):1000–6.

28. van der Heijde D, Landewe RB, Mease PJ, McInnes IB, Conaghan PG, Pricop L, et al. Brief report: Secukinumab provides significant and sustained inhibition of joint structural damage in a phase III study of active psoriatic arthritis. Arthritis Rheumatol. 2016;68(8):1914–21.

8

Investigation of myositis and scleroderma specific autoantibodies in patients with lung cancer

Zoe E. Betteridge[1], Lynsey Priest[2], Robert G. Cooper[3], Neil J. McHugh[1,4], Fiona Blackhall[2,5] and Janine A. Lamb[6]* ⓘ

Abstract

Background: The close temporal association between onset of some connective tissue diseases and cancer suggests a paraneoplastic association. Adult patients with scleroderma with anti-RNA polymerase III autoantibodies and adult patients with dermatomyositis with anti-transcriptional intermediary factor 1 (anti-TIF1) or anti-nuclear matrix protein 2 (anti-NXP2) autoantibodies have a significantly increased risk of developing cancer. Autoantibodies may serve as biomarkers for early detection of cancer and also could be relevant for prediction of responses to immune therapies. We aimed to test whether myositis and scleroderma specific or associated autoantibodies are detectable in individuals with lung cancer.

Methods: Serum from 60 Caucasian patients with lung cancer (30 with small cell lung cancer, 30 with non-small cell lung cancer) was screened for myositis and scleroderma specific and associated autoantibodies by radiolabelled immunoprecipitation.

Results: Anti-TIF1, anti-NXP2 or anti-RNA polymerase III autoantibodies were not detected in any of the 60 patients with lung cancer. Anti-glycyl-transfer RNA (tRNA) synthetase (anti-EJ) autoantibodies were detected in one patient with non-small cell lung cancer. No other known myositis or scleroderma autoantibodies were identified.

Conclusions: Myositis and scleroderma specific autoantibodies, including anti-TIF1, anti-NXP2 and anti-RNA polymerase III, are rare in patients with lung cancer without an autoimmune disease. We report here the first case of anti-EJ autoantibodies being detected in a patient with lung cancer without clinical or radiographic evidence of the anti-synthetase syndrome.

Keywords: Idiopathic inflammatory myopathies, Myositis, Scleroderma, Cancer, Autoantibodies, Anti-glycyl-tRNA synthetase

Background

A close temporal association has been observed between the onset of some autoimmune connective tissue diseases (CTD) and various cancers, suggesting that the appearance of a CTD may sometimes represent a paraneoplastic phenomenon. For example, adult patients with dermatomyositis (DM) with anti-transcription intermediary factor 1 (anti-TIF1) autoantibodies have a dramatically increased risk of developing cancer compared to the general population [1]. Presence of anti-nuclear matrix protein 2 (anti-NXP2) autoantibodies similarly is associated with an

increased cancer risk in adult DM [2]. A meta-analysis of five studies [3] showed that the pooled standardized incidence ratio for lung cancer among patients with DM is 19.74 (95% confidence interval 18.91–20.58), second only to lymphatic and haematopoietic cancers.

DM comprises a subgroup of the idiopathic inflammatory myopathies (IIM), a rare CTD spectrum characterized by inflammation of skeletal muscle (myositis) causing weakness and associated disability. Extra-muscular manifestations occur in the lungs and skin, and temporally associated cancers are common. In addition to clinical classification, IIM can be accurately classified according to the presence of approximately 20 myositis-specific and associated autoantibodies (MSA/MAA), identified in 60–70% of adult patients with IIM. MSA are almost mutually

---
* Correspondence: Janine.Lamb@manchester.ac.uk
[6]Centre for Epidemiology, Faculty of Biology, Medicine and Health, Manchester Academic Health Science Centre, University of Manchester, Manchester, UK
Full list of author information is available at the end of the article

exclusive, and predictive of an individual patient's clinical phenotype, including disease progression and treatment response characteristics [4]. "Cancer associated myositis" has been defined as myositis occurring in association with an incident cancer diagnosed 3 years either side of myositis onset, and a treatment-induced cancer cure can be associated with a simultaneous regression of the myositis. Recent evidence suggests that scleroderma also represents a paraneoplastic phenomenon, being similarly temporally associated with cancers in some anti-RNA polymerase III-positive patients [5]. The mechanism underlying this close temporal association between cancer onset and certain serologically defined subgroups of myositis and scleroderma is unknown.

In patients with cancer, a large number of autoantibodies directed against intracellular tumour-associated antigens have been identified. These autoantibodies may be detected in patients' serum prior to the initial presentation of clinical cancer signs. Current theories suggest that autoantibody production in patients with cancer may result from changes in tissue protein expression, altered protein structure, defects in tolerance and inflammation and aberrant tissue degradation mechanisms [6]. Inflammation in the tumour microenvironment may facilitate the release of certain intracellular antigens to create reactive neo-epitopes via aberrant protein expression and/or altered protein structure through somatic mutation or conformational change. These changes facilitate the generation of autoantibodies against these altered proteins.

For paraneoplastic rheumatic diseases, a model has been proposed whereby a mutation in an incident cancer causes an increase in neo-antigen expression, triggering an autoimmune anti-tumour cytolytic response. This leads to successful autoimmune-mediated elimination of the responsible cancer in some patients [7]. Although the malignancy may be the antigen source initiating the autoimmune anti-tumour cytolytic response, a cross-reaction against regenerating cells in other target tissues (e.g. muscle and skin cells in patients with dermatomyositis) may initiate a self-propagating "feed-forward" loop of tissue damage and induced autoimmunity in genetically susceptible individuals. These observations support the "immunosurveillance" hypothesis; the continual eradication of nascent tumour cells via immunoediting and triggering of cellular and humoral immune responses.

In view of the possible association between incident cancers and induced secondary autoimmunity, we undertook a pilot study to ascertain whether serotyping by the gold standard of radiolabelled immunoprecipitation (IP) would uncover evidence of clinically covert CTD-associated autoantibody generation in patients with primary lung cancer and without clinically overt connective tissue disease.

Methods

Patient cohort

Caucasian patients with lung cancer had already been recruited via the ChemoRes EU Framework 6 integrated project (https://www.cruk.manchester.ac.uk/Our-Research/CEP/Areas-of-Interaction-with-Other-Teams), designed to improve the outcome of cancer chemotherapy. These patients were recruited into a prospective, single-centre study being conducted at the Christie Hospital, Manchester, UK. To be eligible for ChemoRes study inclusion, small cell lung cancer (SCLC) had to be histologically or cytopathologically confirmed, and disease had to naïve to chemotherapy and staged and managed using standard treatment protocols. Non-small cell lung cancer (NSCLC) had to histologically proven and radiologically confirmed as stage IIIA, IIIB or IV disease, and also had to be naïve to chemotherapy [8]. For our pilot serological study we opportunistically recruited 30 each of these patients with SCLC and NSCLC from ChemoRes. All patients gave their written, informed consent to the ethically approved study protocols. Peripheral blood samples for IP testing were collected in the 7 days prior to commencing their planned ChemoRes treatment, and serum was separated according to standard operating procedures and good clinical laboratory practice. Clinical data including age, gender, ethnicity, diagnosis and smoking status were collected.

Autoantibody testing

Autoantibody testing for myositis and scleroderma specific and associated autoantibodies: Jo-1, PMScl, snRNP, Mi-2, Ku, PL12, PL7, EJ, KS, OJ, Zo, Ha, Topo, U3, SRP, TIF1, SAE, MDA5, Ro60, La, RNA Polymerase I-III, AMA, Th/To, NXP2, EIF3 and EIF2B, was carried out by IP using radiolabelled ^{35}S-methionine on patient serum, as described previously [9]. Serum from patients positive for known myositis and scleroderma autoantibodies were included as controls. Antibody positivity by IP was confirmed using the EUROLINE Autoimmune Inflammatory myopathies (IgG) recombinant line-blot technology (Euroimmun, Lübeck, Germany).

When patients immunoprecipitated bands at 140 kDa/155 kDa, their samples were screened also by TIF1γ ELISA using rTIF1γ (Origene, USA), according to standard protocols. All samples were tested in duplicate with a positive cutoff defined as > 3 SD above the mean of 40 healthy controls.

Results

Demographic data for the two patient cohorts are shown in Table 1. Myositis specific autoantibodies against glycyl-transfer RNA (tRNA) synthetase (anti-EJ) were identified by IP in one patient with NSCLC (Additional file 1: Figure S1). This antibody specificity was also positive by line-blot testing, with a semi-quantitative value of +++.

Table 1 Patient demographics

Characteristic	SCLC (n = 30)	NSCLC (n = 30)
Age at onset, years		
Median	68	67
Range	48–82	53–78
Sex		
Female	18	15
Male	12	15
Diagnosis		
Limited	13	
Extensive	17	
Adenocarcinoma		12
Squamous cell carcinoma		8
Other		2
Not documented		8
Smoking status		
Current smoker	14	6
Former smoker	14	14
Never-smoker	0	3
Not documented	2	7

SCLC small cell lung cancer, NSCLC non-small cell lung cancer

Although TIF1γ autoantibodies have been strongly associated with malignancy in dermatomyositis, none of the 60 patients with lung cancer tested positive for anti-TIF1, anti-NXP2 or anti-RNAP III autoantibodies (by either IP or TIF1γ ELISA), indicating that these autoantibodies are rare in patients with lung cancer without an autoimmune disease. No other known myositis or scleroderma autoantibodies were identified.

A total of 55 patients (including the patient with anti-EJ) had one or more unknown bands on IP, which did not correspond to any known CTD autoantigen. Although these were generally moderate or strong bands, indicating the possible presence of an autoantibody, 10 patients (5 with SCLC and 5 with NSCLC) had only weak bands thought to represent non-specific binding: the remaining 5 patients were completely negative by IP; all had SCLC.

Anti-glycl-tRNA synthetase (anti-EJ)-positive patient

The anti-EJ-positive patient was female, and aged 67 years. She was a former smoker, starting at age 17 years, but stopped 2 years prior to her lung cancer diagnosis. The patient originally presented with right arm and shoulder discomfort with reduced shoulder movements, initially diagnosed as arthritis. She had normal exercise tolerance at presentation. A computerized tomography (CT) scan revealed a large spiculated mass in the posterior segment of the right upper lobe. Significantly enlarged lymph nodes were seen in the supraclavicular, right paratracheal, prevascular, subcarinal and right hilar regions. The CT scan showed no evidence of interstitial lung disease. Histological analysis confirmed poorly differentiated adenocarcinoma. Immunohistochemical analysis demonstrated positivity for cytokeratin 7, thyroid transcription factor-1 and carcinoembryonic antigen 125. Tumour cells were negative for cytokeratin 20, gross cystic disease fluid protein 15 and oestrogen receptor, in keeping with metastatic adenocarcinoma, primary non-small cell lung cancer. Somatic mutation in the epidermal growth factor receptor (*EGFR*) gene or presence of anaplastic lymphoma receptor tyrosine kinase (*ALK*) gene fusion was not present. Following four cycles of carboplatin and gemcitabine, follow-up CT demonstrated progressive disease with increase in the size of the lung mass plus satellite lesions plus a new right pleural effusion, even though the patient had improved symptomatically. The patient survived 155 days (5.1 months) from the date of her consent to participate in the ChemoRes study.

Discussion

In this pilot study, we used IP to interrogate for the presence of myositis and scleroderma specific and associated autoantibodies in individuals with primary lung cancer. We identified one patient with NSCLC with autoantibodies against glycyl-tRNA synthetase (anti-EJ), subsequently confirmed by line-blot testing. No other CTD autoantibodies were identified, including antibodies against TIF1γ, NXP2 or RNAP III. We conclude that known myositis and scleroderma specific and associated autoantibodies are rare in patients with lung cancer without a known CTD. These results are in keeping with those from a recent study that similarly tested for anti-TIF1γ, anti-NXP2, and anti-RNAP III autoantibodies in patients with breast cancer without rheumatic disease [10]. Taken together, these findings suggest that immune-mediated anti-tumor cytolytic responses in patients with cancer rarely induce paraneoplastic CTDs, or that patients with cancer without an associated CTD fail to mount an immune response sufficiently strong to induce paraneoplastic consequences. Although five patients in our study were autoantibody negative by IP, the remaining patients had unidentified bands, potentially indicating the presence of autoantibodies targeting unknown antigens. This is consistent with the large number of autoantibodies that have been reported in cancer, and the role of immune homeostasis and a humoral immune response in cancer pathogenesis [6].

To our knowledge, this is the first report of anti-glycyl-tRNA synthetase autoantibodies in a patient without a known anti-synthetase syndrome. Anti-EJ autoantibodies are identified in only ~1% of adult Caucasian patients with IIM [4].

A limitation of this pilot study is the lack of follow-up clinical data relating to complete ascertainment of CTD or anti-synthetase syndrome development; the patient seropositive for anti-EJ lived only 155 days following consent to participate in the ChemoRes study. Patients were recruited as part of a project to improve the outcome of cancer chemotherapy, and so were referred to oncologists rather than rheumatologists. Subtle CTD clinical features therefore could have been overlooked. Alternatively, anti-EJ autoantibodies may have been detectable in this patient's serum prior to the development of overt CTD clinical signs, as reported in patients seropositive for rheumatoid factor before they develop overt rheumatoid arthritis. The median age of lung cancer onset in this pilot study was 68 years and 67 years in SCLC and NSCLC, respectively. In a large international study of IIM, the mean age of IIM onset was ~ 50 years, and was 57 years in those with malignancy, with a median interval between IIM onset and associated cancer diagnoses of only 1 month [11], suggesting possible selection against patients with cancer-associated myositis in the present study.

There is currently an unmet clinical need for biomarkers to facilitate early detection of lung and other cancers. Recent progress in the treatment of lung cancer with immune therapies reinforces the need to better understand host immune responses in the context of lung cancer. Although the presence of a cancer-associated autoantibody or paraneoplastic syndrome could potentially signify a tumuor more likely to respond to an immunomodulatory approach, the low prevalence of CTD autoantibodies identified in this series counters their potential utility in an unselected population. Notably, however, the relatively small number of patients with cancer included in this study limits our ability to detect rare or low-frequency autoantibodies; utility in screening should be addressed using larger cohorts with longitudinal follow-up data.

Conclusions

In patients with lung cancer without an associated CTD, myositis and scleroderma specific and associated autoantibodies, including anti-TIF1, anti-NXP2 and anti-RNAP III, are rare. We identified one patient with NSCLC with anti-EJ autoantibodies, the first time that this anti-synthetase autoantibody has been reported in a patient without anti-synthetase syndrome clinical features.

Abbreviations

CT: Computerized tomography; CTD: Connective tissue disease; DM: Dermatomyositis; ELISA: Enzyme-linked immunosorbent assay; IIM: Idiopathic inflammatory myopathies; IP: Immunoprecipitation; MSA/MAA: Myositis specific/myositis associated autoantibodies; NSCLC: Non-small cell lung cancer; NXP2: Nuclear matrix protein 2; SCLC: Small cell lung cancer; TIF1: Transcriptional intermediary factor 1; tRNA: Transfer RNA

Acknowledgements

This work was supported by the National Institute for Health Research (NIHR) Christie Clinical Research Facility. The views expressed are those of the author(s) and not necessarily those of the National Health Service (NHS), the NIHR or the Department of Health.

Authors' contributions

ZEB and LP performed, analysed and interpreted the patient data and autoantibody data. ZEB, RGC, NJMcH, FB and JAL wrote the manuscript. All authors read and approved the final manuscript.

Consent for publication

Not applicable.

Competing interests

The authors declare that they have no competing interests.

Author details

[1]Department of Pharmacy and Pharmacology, University of Bath, Bath, UK. [2]Division of Molecular and Clinical Cancer Sciences, University of Manchester, Manchester, UK. [3]MRC/ARUK Centre for Integrated Research into Musculoskeletal Ageing, University of Liverpool, Liverpool, UK. [4]Royal National Hospital for Rheumatic Diseases, Royal United Hospitals Foundation Trust, Bath, UK. [5]CRUK Lung Cancer Centre of Excellence, The Christie NHS Foundation Trust, Wilmslow Road, Manchester, UK. [6]Centre for Epidemiology, Faculty of Biology, Medicine and Health, Manchester Academic Health Science Centre, University of Manchester, Manchester, UK.

References

1. Trallero-Araguas E, Rodrigo-Pendas JA, Selva-O'Callaghan A, Martinez-Gomez X, Bosch X, Labrador-Horrillo M, Grau-Junyent JM, Vilardell-Tarres M. Usefulness of anti-p155 autoantibody for diagnosing cancer-associated dermatomyositis: a systematic review and meta-analysis. Arthritis Rheum. 2012;64(2):523–32.
2. Fiorentino DF, Chung LS, Christopher-Stine L, Zaba L, Li S, Mammen AL, Rosen A, Casciola-Rosen L. Most patients with cancer-associated dermatomyositis have antibodies to nuclear matrix protein NXP-2 or transcription intermediary factor 1gamma. Arthritis Rheum. 2013;65(11): 2954–62.
3. Olazagasti JM, Baez PJ, Wetter DA, Ernste FC. Cancer risk in dermatomyositis: a meta-analysis of cohort studies. Am J Clin Dermatol. 2015;16(2):89–98.
4. Betteridge Z, McHugh N. Myositis-specific autoantibodies: an important tool to support diagnosis of myositis. J Intern Med. 2016;280(1):8–23.
5. Shah AA, Xu G, Rosen A, Hummers LK, Wigley FM, Elledge SJ, Casciola-Rosen L. Brief report: anti-RNPC-3 antibodies as a marker of cancer-associated scleroderma. Arthritis Rheumatol. 2017;69(6):1306–12.
6. Zaenker P, Gray ES, Ziman MR. Autoantibody production in cancer–the humoral immune response toward autologous antigens in cancer patients. Autoimmun Rev. 2016;15(5):477–83.
7. Shah AA, Casciola-Rosen L, Rosen A. Review: cancer-induced autoimmunity in the rheumatic diseases. Arthritis Rheumatol. 2015;67(2):317–26.
8. Krebs MG, Sloane R, Priest L, Lancashire L, Hou JM, Greystoke A, Ward TH, Ferraldeschi R, Hughes A, Clack G, et al. Evaluation and prognostic significance of circulating tumor cells in patients with non-small-cell lung cancer. J Clin Oncol. 2011;29(12):1556–63.
9. Betteridge Z, Gunawardena H, North J, Slinn J, McHugh N. Identification of a novel autoantibody directed against small ubiquitin-like modifier activating enzyme in dermatomyositis. Arthritis Rheum. 2007;56(9):3132–7.
10. Shah AA, Rosen A, Hummers LK, May BJ, Kaushiva A, Roden RBS, Armstrong DK, Wigley FM, Casciola-Rosen L, Visvanathan K. Evaluation of cancer-associated myositis and scleroderma autoantibodies in breast cancer patients without rheumatic disease. Clin Exp Rheumatol. 2017;35(Suppl 106(4)):71–4.
11. Lilleker JB, Vencovsky J, Wang G, Wedderburn LR, Diederichsen LP, Schmidt J, Oakley P, Benveniste O, Danieli MG, Danko K, et al. The EuroMyositis registry: an international collaborative tool to facilitate myositis research. Ann Rheum Dis. 2018;77(1):30–9.

9

An explorative study on deep profiling of peripheral leukocytes to identify predictors for responsiveness to anti-tumour necrosis factor alpha therapies in ankylosing spondylitis: natural killer cells in focus

Ursula Schulte-Wrede[1], Till Sörensen[2], Joachim R. Grün[1,4], Thomas Häupl[2], Heike Hirseland[1], Marta Steinbrich-Zöllner[3], Peihua Wu[3], Andreas Radbruch[1,5], Denis Poddubnyy[3,6], Joachim Sieper[3], Uta Syrbe[3] and Andreas Grützkau[1*] [ID]

Abstract

Background: Therapeutic targeting of tumour necrosis factor (TNF)-α is highly effective in ankylosing spondylitis (AS) patients. However, since one-third of anti-TNF-treated AS patients do not show an adequate clinical response there is an urgent need for new biomarkers that would aid clinicians in their decision-making to select appropriate therapeutic options. Thus, the aim of this explorative study was to identify cell-based biomarkers in peripheral blood that could be used for a pre-treatment stratification of AS patients.

Methods: A high-dimensional, multi-parametric flow cytometric approach was applied to identify baseline predictors in 31 AS patients before treatment with the TNF blockers adalimumab (TNF-neutralisation) and etanercept (soluble TNF receptor).

Results: As the major result, the frequencies of natural killer (NK) cells, and in particular CD8-positive (CD8+) NK cell subsets, were most predictive for therapeutic outcome in AS patients. While an inverse correlation between classical CD56+/CD16+ NK cells and reduction of disease activity was observed, the CD8+ NK cell subset behaved in the opposite direction. At baseline, responders showed significantly increased frequencies of CD8+ NK cells compared with non-responders.

Conclusions: This is the first study demonstrating that the composition of the NK cell compartment has predictive power for prediction of therapeutic outcome for anti-TNF-α blockers, and we identified CD8+ NK cells as a potential new player in the TNF-α-driven chronic inflammatory immune response of AS.

Keywords: Ankylosing spondylitis, Etanercept, CD8+ NK cells, TNF-alpha blocker, Predictive biomarker

* Correspondence: gruetzkau@drfz.de
[1]German Rheumatism Research Center Berlin (DRFZ), an Institute of the Leibniz-Association, Immune Monitoring Core Facility, Charitéplatz 1, 10117 Berlin, Germany
Full list of author information is available at the end of the article

Background

Ankylosing spondylitis (AS) is a multifactorial chronic inflammatory rheumatic disease belonging to the group of rheumatic diseases known as spondyloarthritis (SpA) which primarily affects the axial skeleton [1]. AS has a prevalence of about 1.43 million in the European population [2] with an onset in adolescence [3] and a two-times higher occurrence in men than women [4]. The pathogenesis of AS is still obscure; it is assumed that AS is mainly caused by both genetic factors, which implies the expression of the major histocompatibility complex (MHC) I antigen human leukocyte antigen B27 (HLA-B27) [5], and also by environmental factors such as enterobacterial antigens [6]. To alleviate the axial symptoms of AS patients, non-steroidal anti-inflammatory drugs (NSAIDs) are delivered as first-line therapy. Anti-tumour necrosis factor (TNF) blocking therapy is applied only in patients with constantly high disease activity who are non-responsive to conventional NSAID treatment [7, 8]. At present, there are five anti-TNF-α agents approved for the treatment of AS: infliximab [9], a monoclonal chimeric antibody; etanercept, a soluble human TNF receptor (sTNFR)2 fusion protein [10]; adalimumab, a humanised monoclonal antibody [11]; golimumab, a fully human monoclonal antibody [12]; and certoluzimab, a Fab fragment of a humanised monoclonal antibody [13]. Most of these biologics are also successfully administered in rheumatoid arthritis (RA), psoriasis (Pso), juvenile inflammatory arthritis (JIA), and inflammatory bowel disease (IBD). The biological functions of TNF-α are mediated by binding to the membrane receptors TNFR1 (p55) or TNFR2 (p75). While TNFR1 is ubiquitously expressed in all lymphoid and myeloid immune cells and body cells [14], the expression of TNFR2 is mainly restricted to T cells [15] and natural killer (NK) cells [16]. In addition, TNFR2 can be found to be expressed in endothelial and mesenchymal cells, cells of the central nervous system (CNS), oligodendrocytes and cardiac myocytes [17], and a few other cell types [18]. According to their functions, TNFR1 is primarily associated with pro-apoptotic processes, while TNFR2 is responsible for processes ensuring survival of cells [19].

Although targeting of TNF-α is very effective in AS, around one-third of treated patients show only a poor response that can be partly attributed to the development of anti-drug antibodies (ADAb) resulting in reduced bioavailability [20]. The most likely precondition for swapping to another anti-TNF agent is partial or entire failure of effectiveness along with side effects [21]. With respect to these adverse reactions and the high costs of anti-TNF agents leading to high economic burden for the health care systems, it is desirable to stratify patients according to treatment predictors prior to biological therapy. Various demographic and clinical parameters such as high baseline disease activity, short disease duration, young age, male sex, and presence of HLA-B27 have been shown to correlate with adequate clinical short- and long-term response [22–26]. In addition, modern imaging techniques, such as magnetic resonance imaging (MRI), are used to correlate bone and tissue destruction with treatment response [27]. However, these techniques are time consuming and expensive when used as a standard pre-treatment assessment. Another level of therapy response prediction was investigated when responsiveness to anti-TNF agents was related to the presence of different TNF-α genotypes. It was reported that patients with TNF-α–308 G/G, –857 C/C, or –1031 T/T genotypes showed a better response to anti-TNF agents than patients without these polymorphisms [28, 29]. Apart from these observations, there are no reliable predictive biomarkers for anti-TNF responsiveness in AS. Using a multi-parametric flow cytometric approach, we aimed to identify cell-based biomarkers in the peripheral blood of AS patients that are able to predict a successful therapeutic response to TNF inhibitors before starting therapy. As a result, we found that a low pre-treatment frequency of a CD8-expressing subpopulation of NK cells is associated with a lack of therapeutic response.

Methods

Subjects

Ethics statement

The study was performed in accordance with the 1964 Declaration of Helsinki and approved by the Charité University Medicine ethics committee I of Charité Campus Mitte. All patients provided written informed consent to participate in the study. Furthermore, we declare that this manuscript contains no information or images that could lead to identification of a study participant.

A total of 31 AS patients (22 male, 9 female) of whom 81% were positive for HLA-B27, recruited from the rheumatology outpatient clinics of the Charité, and 10 healthy controls (HC; 7 male, 3 female) participated in the study. The patients had an average age of 38 ± 10.2 years and the HC averaged 34 ± 10.7 years. All patients fulfilling the modified New York criteria [30] and who were eligible for anti-TNF inhibitor treatment because of persistently high disease activity (Bath Ankylosing Spondylitis Disease Activity Index (BASDAI) > 4) despite treatment with NSAIDs or who were unable to take NSAIDs due to contraindications were included in the study (Table 1). Disease activity was assessed according to the BASDAI index consisting of a score range from 0 (no symptoms) to 10 (high disease activity). The mean baseline BASDAI prior to TNF inhibitor therapy was 6.2 ± 1.3 (Table 1).

Table 1 Demographic and disease characteristics of AS patients treated with ETN and ADA, respectively

	ADA- and ETN-treated AS patients (n = 31)	ETN-treated AS patients (n = 15)	ADA-treated AS patients (n = 16)
Demographics			
Sex (M:F)	22:9	11:4	11:5
Age (years)	38 ± 10.2	37.7 ± 11.5	38.3 ± 9.2
Disease status			
DD (months)	140.8 ± 117.9	145.1 ± 135.4	136.8 ± 103.8
BASDAI at baseline	6.2 ± 1.3	6.2 ± 1.5	6.2 ± 1.2
BASDAI red. (%)	47.6 ± 31.3	51.1 ± 31.7	44.3 ± 31.6
BASDAI assessment (months)	3.1 ± 1.4	3 ± 1	3.2 ± 1.6
BASDAI50 (R:NR)	19:12	10:5	9:7
CRP (mg/dl)	1.5 ± 1.7	1.3 ± 1.1	1.6 ± 2.2
HLA-B27-positive (%)	81	87	75
ESR (mm/h)	33.2 ± 21.9	31.7 ± 22.3	34.6 ± 22.3

Results are displayed as mean ± SD unless otherwise indicated

ADA adalimumab, *AS* ankylosing spondylitis, *BASDAI* Bath Ankylosing Disease Activity Index, *BASDAI red.* percental BASDAI reduction after 1–6 month of therapy, *BASDAI50* percental BASDAI reduction according to an improvement of 50%, *CRP* C-reactive protein, *DD* disease duration, *ESR* erythrocyte sedimentation rate, *ETN* etanercept, *F* female, *HLA* human leukocyte antigen, *M* male, *NR* non-responder, *R* responder

Prior to the start of TNF inhibitor therapy, 10 ml heparinised blood was taken to perform flow cytometric analysis. Fifteen patients were treated with etanercept (Enbrel; Amgen, and Pfizer) and 16 patients with adalimumab (Humira; AbbVie Inc.). The BASDAI score was obtained at baseline and at follow-up visits [31]. The response to treatment was assessed between 1 and 6 months after the start of therapy and defined as a 50% BASDAI reduction (BASDAI50 response) relative to baseline BASDAI (Additional file 1: Table S1).

Blood sample preparation, antibody staining, and flow cytometry measurement

Blood sample preparation and antibody staining procedures were as described previously [32]. Cells obtained from the blood of patients prior to treatment were stained for 50 different surface antigens in a seven-colour staining combined to 10 tubes (Table 2). After staining, cells were fixed with 1% paraformaldehyde and analysed within 24 h. We did not include a live/dead cell staining, but cell debris, erythrocytes, and thrombocytes were excluded according to their SSC/FSC characteristics.

Data acquisition was accomplished with a FACS-Canto™ II Flow Cytometer (BD Biosciences, USA) with an average cell count of one million cells per sample. To warrant reproducibility and to survey the instruments' performance, a BD™ Cytometer Setup and Tracking Beads were regularly used before each measurement. In addition, we have always monitored the quality of antibody staining directly after data acquisition by monitoring each individual fluorescence channel used for each particular staining tube. For this 20,000 randomly selected events were plotted. Samples which did not pass this quality check were excluded from further analysis.

Data analysis and statistical analysis

Two different software tools were applied to analyse the complex datasets generated by this unsupervised flow cytometry approach, which is based on both manual and automatic bioinformatic strategies identify potential candidate phenotypes. In the first approach, the relevant

Table 2 Staining matrix showing antibodies and their corresponding fluorochrome conjugates measured in ten separate staining tubes

Fluorochrome	T1	T2	T3	T4	T5	T6	T7	T8	T9	T10
Pacific Blue	CD3	CD3	CD3	CD3	CD3	CD3	CD3	CD3	CD3	CD3
FITC	CD27	CD64	CD244	CD35	CD46	CD45RA	BDCA2	CD138	CD134	CD28
PE	IgD/ CD14/ CD56	CD33/ NKG2D	CD163/ CRTH-2	CD119	CD88	CXCR4	CD1c	CD38	ICOS	CD31
PE-Cy5	CD45RA	HLA-DR	CD128b	CD107a	CD21	CD62L	HLA-DR	HLA-DR	CD154	CD45RA
PE-Cy7	CD8	CD56/ CD14	CD14	CD14	CD14	CCR7	CD14	CD69	CD69	CD69
APC	CD19	CD32	CCR2	CD120b	CD55	CXCR3	CD11c	CD20	CD25	CD152
APC-Cy7	CD4/ CD16	CD4/ CD16	CD4/ CD16	CD4/ CD16	CD4/ CD16	CD4/ CD16	CD19	CD19	CD4/ CD16	CD4/ CD16

T1–T10 represents the respective staining tubes

statistics such as mean fluorescence intensities (MFIs) and absolute cell numbers of manually analysed data were transferred as a comma-separated value (CSV) file format to an Access database as shown previously [32]. This primary data analysis including colour compensation and gate setting was performed by FACSDIVA v6.0 software (BD Biosciences, USA). The second approach utilised the automated classification algorithm immunoClust, which processes uncompensated raw data and therefore excludes any operator-dependent gating or compensation artefacts [33]. Population clustering and comparative meta-clustering of immunoClust assume finite mixture models and use Expectation Maximisation (EM)-iterations with an integrated classification likelihood (ICL) criterion to stabilise the number of reasonable clusters. For meta-clustering, a probability measure on Gaussian distributions was invented, which is based on the Bhattacharyya Coefficients. Meta-clusters were manually annotated and classified.

Linear regression and receiver operating characteristic (ROC) analysis performed with Prism 5 (GraphPad Software, Inc.) was used to elucidate associations between candidate markers and clinical parameters. For statistical data analysis, the Welch corrected t test was used where p values < 0.05 were determined as statistically significant.

Results

Patient baseline characteristics and their clinical responses

The study design encompassed 31 AS patients with high disease activity indicated by a baseline BASDAI of 6.2 ± 1.3 before treatment with adalimumab (ADA; $n = 16$) or etanercept (ETN; $n = 15$). The patient demographic and baseline clinical characteristics are summarised in Table 1 and showed no significant differences between the ADA- and ETN-treated patients.

The average BASDAI assessment date was 3.1 ± 1.4 month after the start of treatment. After 1 to 6 months of treatment, the relative reduction of disease activity assessed by BASDAI was 51.1 ± 31.7% for ETN-treated patients and 44.3 ± 31.6% for patients who received ADA. According to the BASDAI response criteria, five patients in the ETN group and seven patients in the ADA group failed to respond (Additional file 1: Table S1).

Clinical parameters available at baseline, such as disease duration, baseline BASDAI, C-reactive peptide (CRP) levels, and erythrocyte sedimentation rate (ESR), as well as the expression of HLA-B27, allowed no discrimination between patients who would respond to TNF-α blockers and those who would fail.

For data analysis, we have applied an unsupervised, automated cell clustering approach, immunoClust [33], to identify potential immunophenotypic parameters that

enable classification of AS patients into responders (R) and non-responders (NR) prior to anti-TNF treatment. Since the freshly obtained patient blood was immediately processed we have not performed dead cell staining, but we gated for live cells according to cell size and granularity defined by forward scatter (FSC) and sideward scatter (SSC) characteristics, respectively.

The presented two-dimensional clustering approach with patients clustered in the vertical direction and immunophenotypic parameters clustered in the horizontal direction gives an overview of all leukocyte subsets including certain activation markers that are differentially expressed in R and NR. For the identification of significant parameters by the immunoClust algorithm, FCS files (Flow Cytometry Standard file format) of uncompensated raw data were used and finally disclosed 36 parameters when all patient samples were considered. Analysing ETN- and ADA-treated patients separately revealed 21 and 27 parameters, respectively (Fig. 1).

Although using all these parameters did not allow an error-free classification of R and NR, all samples were grouped into two main clusters which were enriched for R and NR, respectively (Fig. 1a). Surprisingly, more than 50% of the discriminating parameters could be clearly assigned to NK cell subsets if all patients were analysed together (Fig. 1a). For further analysis of NK cell-related subsets, and knowing that ETN and ADA have different modes of action to neutralise the effect of TNF-α, we continued to investigate both treatment groups separately to identify therapy-specific response signatures. Using this approach, the majority of parameters that significantly discriminate between NR and R in the ETN group (Fig. 1b) and ADA group (Fig. 1c) were related to the NK cell compartment. The best classification of R and NR was achieved in the group of ETN-treated patients. Here, only two of 10 R were grouped as NR and one single of five NR was grouped as R.

Validation of classical NK cells and CD8-positive NK cells as potential immunological biomarkers for an anti-TNF-α therapy prediction

Since both the percentage distribution of classical NK cells in general and the ratio of CD8-positive and CD8-negative NK cells in particular appeared to be the most promising predictors for an anti-TNF therapy response, we looked at the CD8 receptor expression on NK cells in more detail. In Fig. 2 the general gating strategy to define classical $CD56^{dim}CD16^+$ NK cells is shown. In Additional file 2 (Figure S1), backgating for monocytes and NK cells demonstrates that, despite labelling multiple antigens by the same fluorochrome (CD14/CD56/IgD labelled to PE), unravelling of these complex stainings with respect to NK cells, monocytes, T cells, and B cells is possible.

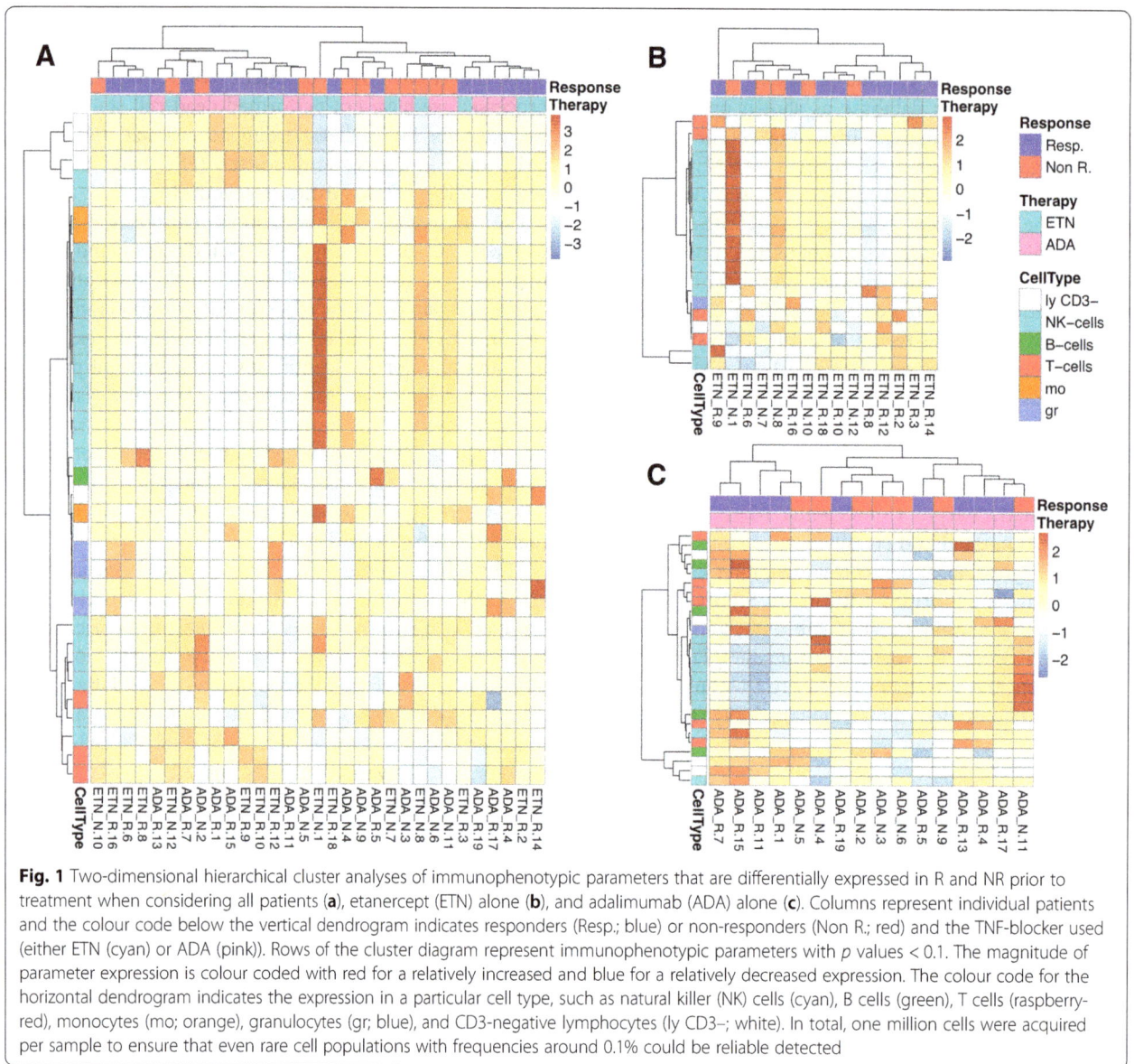

Fig. 1 Two-dimensional hierarchical cluster analyses of immunophenotypic parameters that are differentially expressed in R and NR prior to treatment when considering all patients (**a**), etanercept (ETN) alone (**b**), and adalimumab (ADA) alone (**c**). Columns represent individual patients and the colour code below the vertical dendrogram indicates responders (Resp.; blue) or non-responders (Non R.; red) and the TNF-blocker used (either ETN (cyan) or ADA (pink)). Rows of the cluster diagram represent immunophenotypic parameters with p values < 0.1. The magnitude of parameter expression is colour coded with red for a relatively increased and blue for a relatively decreased expression. The colour code for the horizontal dendrogram indicates the expression in a particular cell type, such as natural killer (NK) cells (cyan), B cells (green), T cells (raspberry-red), monocytes (mo; orange), granulocytes (gr; blue), and CD3-negative lymphocytes (ly CD3-; white). In total, one million cells were acquired per sample to ensure that even rare cell populations with frequencies around 0.1% could be reliable detected

At first, a lymphocyte scatter gate (G1) was set (Fig. 2a). Next T and B cells were excluded out of the lymphocyte population (G2) to determine the percentage of $CD56^{dim}CD16^+$ NK cells (G3). Subsequently, the CD8-positive NK cells were quantified by sub-gating as shown exemplarily for five responders (R2, R9, R16, R12, and R18) and five non-responders (NR1, NR7, NR8, NR10, and NR12) (Fig. 2b).

Figure 3 shows the frequencies of CD8-positive NK cells for healthy controls ($n = 10$), anti-TNF R ($n = 19$), and anti-TNF NR ($n = 12$). A significantly higher frequency of CD8 receptor-bearing NK cells was observed in the R group compared with NR (Fig. 3). Comparing the percentage of CD8-positive NK cells to HC, AS patients who will not respond showed significantly lower frequencies of

CD8-expressing NK cells (Fig. 3). Individual values for frequencies and absolute counts of NK cells and CD8-positive subsets are given in Additional file 1 (Table S1).

Next, we performed Spearman's rank correlation and linear regression analyses which showed a significant inverse correlation of frequencies of classical NK cells and an improved therapy outcome if all 31 patients were included (Fig. 4a; $p = 0.01$, $r^2 = 0.19$).

Surprisingly, a positive, linear correlation was found when we focused on the analysis of CD8- expressing NK cells (Fig. 4b). Here, the frequency of CD8-positive cells related to the cells of the total NK cells (G3) clearly correlated with a successful therapy response. This correlation was statistically significant when all patients were considered ($p = 0.002$, $r^2 = 0.29$).

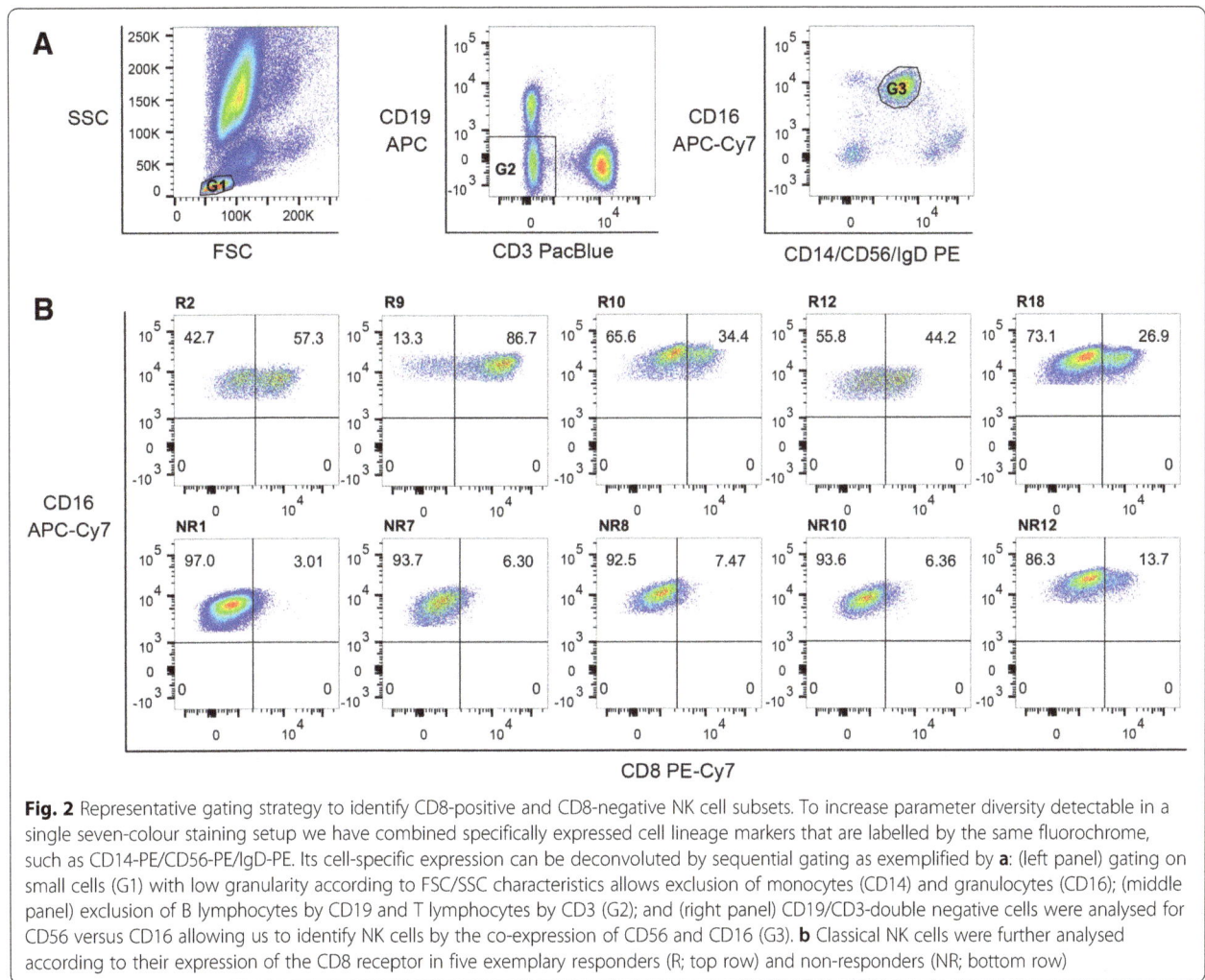

Fig. 2 Representative gating strategy to identify CD8-positive and CD8-negative NK cell subsets. To increase parameter diversity detectable in a single seven-colour staining setup we have combined specifically expressed cell lineage markers that are labelled by the same fluorochrome, such as CD14-PE/CD56-PE/IgD-PE. Its cell-specific expression can be deconvoluted by sequential gating as exemplified by **a**: (left panel) gating on small cells (G1) with low granularity according to FSC/SSC characteristics allows exclusion of monocytes (CD14) and granulocytes (CD16); (middle panel) exclusion of B lymphocytes by CD19 and T lymphocytes by CD3 (G2); and (right panel) CD19/CD3-double negative cells were analysed for CD56 versus CD16 allowing us to identify NK cells by the co-expression of CD56 and CD16 (G3). **b** Classical NK cells were further analysed according to their expression of the CD8 receptor in five exemplary responders (R; top row) and non-responders (NR; bottom row)

Furthermore, reverse regression analyses, displayed by ROC curves, were performed to verify the quality of classical and especially CD8-positive NK cells as suitable cellular biomarkers for predicting an anti-TNF therapy outcome (Fig. 4c, d). If all samples were included for this analysis, the frequency of classical NK cells was the most promising parameter as a baseline predictor (Fig. 4c; $p = 0.008$, area under the curve (AUC) = 0.79). Slightly improved values were obtained if the frequency of CD8-positive NK cells was used (Fig. 4d; $p = 0.007$, AUC = 0.79). Therefore, our data implicate that the appearance of CD8-positive NK cells is a robust biomarker for the prediction of an anti-TNF-α response at baseline.

Discussion

To our knowledge, this is the first study aiming to identify cellular biomarkers in peripheral blood to stratify AS patients upfront with regard to subsequent responsiveness to anti-TNF-α therapy. To date, there are no quantifiable laboratory parameters available that can be used for a personalised response prediction [34]. Although higher values of CRP, ESR, and serum amyloid A (SAA), together with the presence of HLA-B27, have been reported to be useful baseline predictors for a successful anti-TNF-α therapy response in AS, the robustness, sensitivity, and specificity fail if applied to individual patients [35, 36]. Even our data, such as the age of patients, disease duration, CRP levels, or blood sedimentation, did not allow any prediction of future responsiveness.

Other potential new biomarkers described, such as single nucleotide polymorphisms (SNPs) and activity of endoplasmic reticulum aminopeptidase (ERAP)-1 [37], serum levels of matrix metalloproteinase (MMP)-3 [38], or vascular endothelial growth factor (VEGF) [39], have not yet reached a standard in the clinical diagnostic routine of AS. Generally, it is challenging to correlate quantifiable parameters to the disease activity BASDAI score, which is calculated on the basis of a patient's subjective assessment of well-being and therefore is only of limited value when used as an absolute variable.

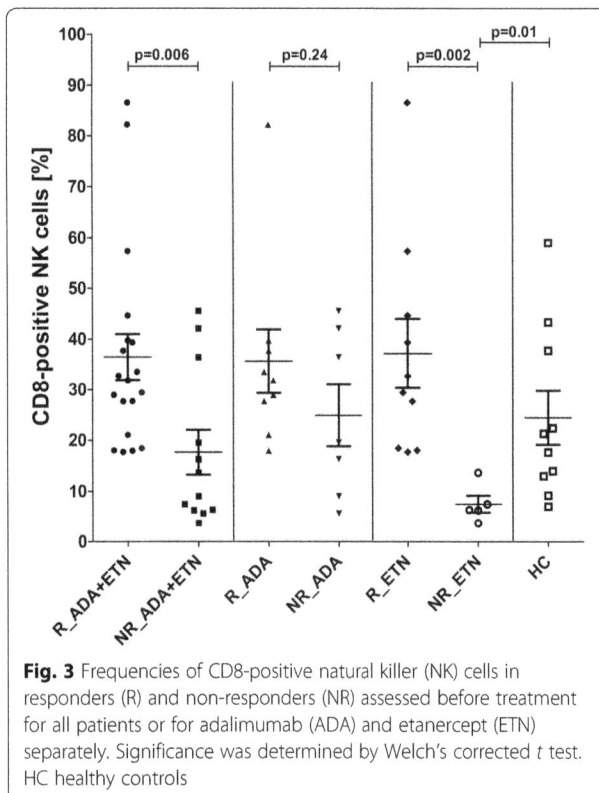

Fig. 3 Frequencies of CD8-positive natural killer (NK) cells in responders (R) and non-responders (NR) assessed before treatment for all patients or for adalimumab (ADA) and etanercept (ETN) separately. Significance was determined by Welch's corrected *t* test. HC healthy controls

In our explorative study presented here we used an integrated multi-parametric flow cytometry and a new unsupervised data clustering approach to identify possible cellular biomarkers that are qualitatively or quantitatively different in responders and non-responders. A similar approach has been successfully used to classify active AS patients from healthy donors according to specific phenotypical changes in blood [32]. A comprehensive overview about immunophenotypical changes described so far in different autoimmune diseases is given by Alegria et al. [40].

Principally, at first view, an increased frequency of the major $CD56^{dim}CD16^{+}$ NK cell subset was indicative for a weak therapeutic anti-TNF response. This finding is in line with other reports showing that innate immunity and particularly NK cells may play a central role in the pathogenesis of various autoimmune diseases both in a protective and pathogenic manner. Their frequency and functionality were investigated in chronic inflammation, such as rheumatoid arthritis [41], multiple sclerosis [42], psoriasis [43], and systemic lupus erythematosus [44]. Despite some conflicting results, an overall decrease and a cytolytic impairment of circulating NK cells could be observed. In AS, the functionality of NK cells is described to be likewise impaired [45] but, in contrast to other autoimmune diseases, an increased NK cell number is reported [46, 47]. We could confirm this observation if comparing the non-responder group with normal donors (Fig. 3a); however, the NK cell frequency in the responder cohort was similar to the

number of healthy individuals. The strong association between NK cells and the aetiology of AS is underlined by the capability of the disease-dependent elevated killer cell immunoglobulin-like receptors (KIRs) to recognise the HLA-B27 antigen, which is expressed in 80–90% of AS patients [48, 49]. Concomitant with a pathogenetic upregulated frequency of $KIR3DL1^{+}$ NK cells in AS, interferon (IFN)γ production is correspondingly diminished [50]. Moreover, activated $KIR3DL2^{+}$ NK cells are increased in SpA and may play a pathogenic role.

An in-depth analysis of the NK cell compartment revealed that the frequency of classical NK cells expressing the CD8 antigen showed a significant and positive correlation with anti-TNF responsiveness. It is known that about 40% of NK cells variably express CD8 in an α/α homodimeric form whereas the CD8-positive subset is described to exhibit enhanced cytotoxic features as compared with its CD8-negative counterpart [51, 52]. We could not detect significant age- or sex-related differences with respect to the frequency of CD8-positive NK cells either in the group of healthy controls or in that of AS patients. Thus, our data imply that NK cells expressing the CD8αα homodimer are directly or indirectly involved in the immunosuppressive effect exerted by anti-TNF-α blockers.

If CD8αα-expressing NK cells are directly involved it can be assumed that their increased cytotoxic activity and/or their diminished behaviour regarding cytotoxicity-induced apoptosis are responsible for the improved responsiveness of TNF blockers. Alternatively, it can be hypothesised that an engagement of CD8αα receptors on NK cells to molecules of the HLA-I family can cause an increased secretion of the pro-inflammatory cytokines TNF-α and IFNγ [53], which in turn promote both TNF receptor (TNFR) synthesis and its proteolysis to a soluble form [54]. By this mechanism, endogenously synthesised sTNFRs [55, 56] can co-operatively support the action of therapeutic TNF inhibitors [57, 58]. These non-signalling 'decoy' receptors are still competent for binding TNF and thus may function as a natural TNF antagonist comparable to ETN [59]. Since we have included adalimumab- and etanercept-treated patients in our study, it was interesting to know if differences in the prediction of responsiveness were detectable when either TNF-α was neutralised by ADA or scavenged by the sTNFR2 fusion protein (ETN). Although group size reduction was responsible for a less statistical power of prediction analysis, we could ascertain a better correlation with respect to ETN-treated patients compared with ADA-treated patients. Therefore, these findings are encouraging for validation in new independent cohorts of appropriate group sizes. If this result could be validated it would indicate diverse and more complex modes of action going beyond the mere neutralising effect of TNF-α blockers.

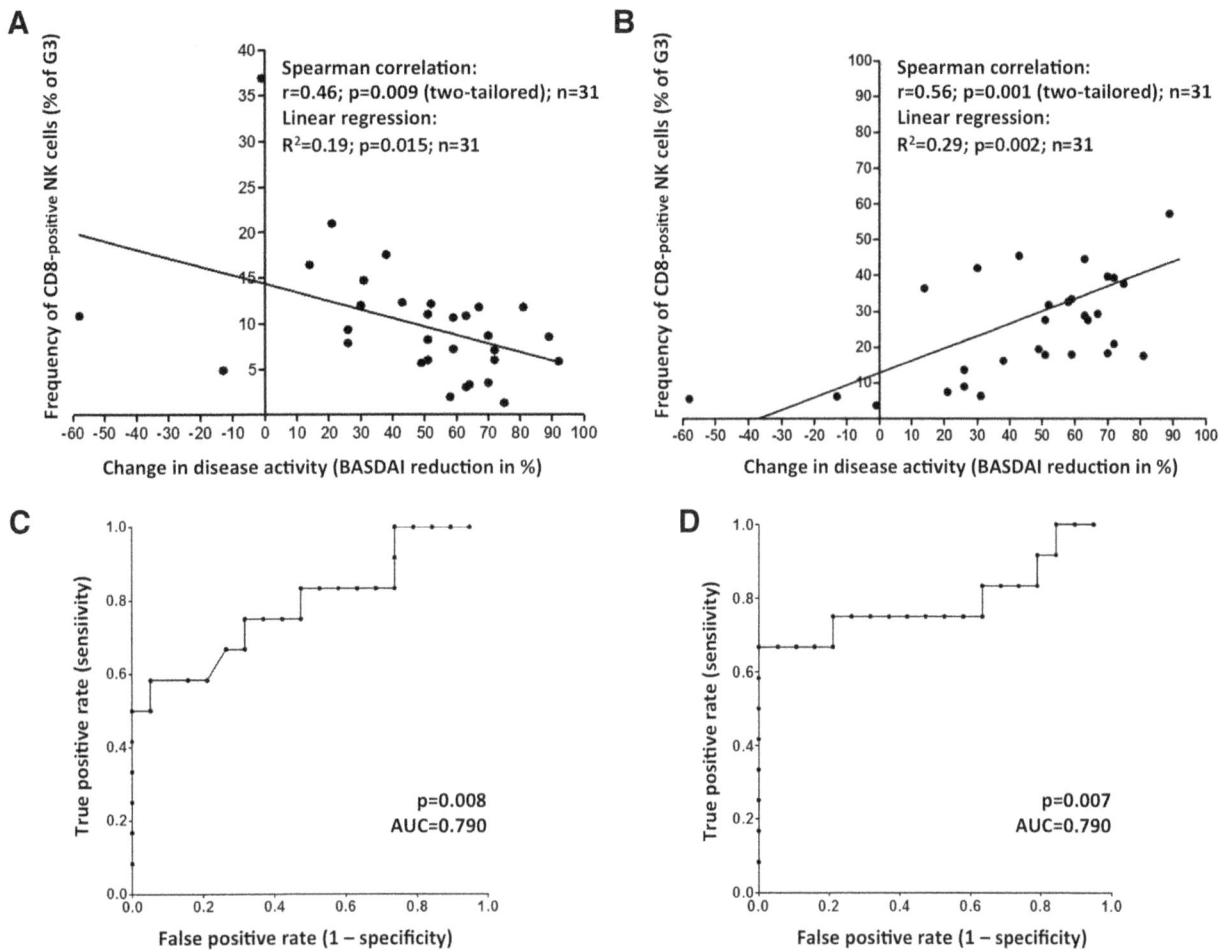

Fig. 4 Linear regression and Spearman's rank correlation analyses showing relative reduction of Bath Ankylosing Spondylitis Disease Activity Index (BASDAI) values within 1 to 6 months after treatment with ADA and ETN (*n* = 31), associated with changes in frequencies of classical natural killer (NK) cells (**a**) and CD8-positive NK cells (**b**). ROC curves for all patients demonstrating the value of classical (**c**) and CD8-expressing NK cells (**d**) as prognostic markers according to increasing area under the curve (AUC) values

To elucidate possible differences in the TNFR expression in CD8-positive and CD8-negative NK cell subsets isolated from healthy individuals, we performed global gene expression analyses but could not detect any differential expression of TNFR1, TNFR2, or TNF-α (data not shown). Comparing the expression of TNFR1 and TNFR2 in healthy individuals, it was obvious that higher expression levels were detectable for TNFR2 (data not shown). Unfortunately, thus far we have had no opportunity for analysing cells isolated from AS patients to test if TNFRs or TNF-α were differentially expressed under chronic inflammatory conditions. Thus, according to our data, it can be postulated that CD8-positive NK cells are obviously capable of amplifying the neutralising effect of TNF-blockers, but it remains unclear why this amplification is preferentially observed in ETN- and not in ADA-treated patients.

Conclusions

Although our findings are promising, a further validation of CD8-positive NK cells as a potential biomarker for TNF responsiveness is necessary in an independent cohort of AS and other rheumatic and gastrointestinal diseases where anti-TNF blockers are successfully administered. Nevertheless, our study is a first proof of the concept that cellular response signatures can be identified in peripheral blood by an extensive immunophenotyping approach. Even though the exact mechanism of how CD8-positive NK cells and the therapeutic effect of TNF-α blockers are interrelated in AS is only poorly understood thus far, monitoring these cells by flow cytometry offers an interesting new diagnostic option with respect to the challenges of an individualised therapy concept, at least in the field of chronic inflammatory rheumatic diseases.

Abbreviations

ADA: Adalimumab; AS: Ankylosing spondylitis; BASDAI: Bath Ankylosing Spondylitis Disease Activity Index; CRP: C-reactive protein; ERAP: Endoplasmic reticulum aminopeptidase; ESR: Erythrocyte sedimentation rate; ETN: Etanercept; HC: Healthy controls; IBD: Inflammatory bowel disease; JIA: Juvenile inflammatory arthritis; KIR: Killer cell immunoglobulin-like receptor; MFI: Mean fluorescence intensity; MMP: Matrix metalloproteinase; NK: Natural killer; NR: Non-responders; NSAID: Non-steroidal anti-inflammatory drug; Pso: Psoriasis; R: Responders; RA: Rheumatoid arthritis; SAA: Serum amyloid A; SNP: Single nucleotide polymorphism; SpA: Spondyloarthritis; sTNFR: Soluble human tumour necrosis factor receptor; TNF: Tumour necrosis factor; VEGF: Vascular endothelial growth factor

Funding

This study was funded by the following grants: IMI JU-funded Project BeTheCure (grant no. 115142–2), the German Research Foundation (DFG) (grant no. SFB 650 TPZ06), the German Federal Ministry of Education and Research (BMBF) within the framework of the e:Med research and funding concept sysINFLAME (grant no. 01ZX1306B), and Leibniz ScienceCampus Chronic Inflammation (http://www.chronische-entzuendung.org). These funders had no involvement in the study design, in the collection, analysis, and interpretation of the data, in the writing of the report, or in the decision to submit the paper for publication.

Authors' contributions

US-W performed experiments, analysed data, and wrote the manuscript. TS, JRG, and TH analysed data. MS-Z, HH, and PW performed experiments. AR and JS designed the experimental strategy. US and DP characterised the patients and determined clinical inclusion criteria. AG designed the experimental strategy, analysed data, and wrote the manuscript. All authors read and approved the final manuscript.

Consent for publication

Not applicable.

Competing interests

The authors declare that they have no competing interests.

Author details

[1]German Rheumatism Research Center Berlin (DRFZ), an Institute of the Leibniz-Association, Immune Monitoring Core Facility, Charitéplatz 1, 10117 Berlin, Germany. [2]Department of Rheumatology and Clinical Immunology, Charité - Universitätsmedizin Berlin, Berlin, Germany. [3]Department of Gastroenterology, Infectiology and Rheumatology, Charité - Universitätsmedizin Berlin, Berlin, Germany. [4]German Rheumatism Research Center Berlin (DRFZ), an Institute of the Leibniz-Association, Bioinformatics Group, Berlin, Germany. [5]German Rheumatism Research Center Berlin (DRFZ), an Institute of the Leibniz-Association, Cell Biology Group, Berlin, Germany. [6]German Rheumatism Research Center Berlin (DRFZ), an Institute of the Leibniz-Association, Epidemiology Unit, Berlin, Germany.

References

1. Braun J, Sieper J. Ankylosing spondylitis. Lancet. 2007;369:1379–90.
2. Dean LE, et al. Global prevalence of ankylosing spondylitis. Rheumatology (Oxford). 2014;53:650–7. https://doi.org/10.1093/rheumatology/ket387.
3. Feldtkeller E, Khan M, van der Heijde D, van der Linden S, Braun J. Age at disease onset and diagnosis delay in HLA-B27 negative vs. positive patients with ankylosing spondylitis. Rheumatol Int. 2003;23:61–6.
4. Hill HF, Hill AG, Bodmer JG. Clinical diagnosis of ankylosing spondylitis in women and relation to presence of HLA-B27. Ann Rheum Dis. 1976; 35:267–70.
5. Brewerton DA, et al. Ankylosing spondylitis and HL-A 27. Lancet. 1973;1:904–7.
6. Trull A, Ebringer A, Panayi G, Ebringer R, James DC. HLA-B27 and the immune response to enterobacterial antigens in ankylosing spondylitis. Clin Exp Immunol. 1984;55:74–80.

7. Coates LC, Marzo-Ortega H, Bennett AN, Emery P. Anti-TNF therapy in ankylosing spondylitis: insights for the clinician. Ther Adv Musculoskelet Dis. 2010;2:37–43.
8. Sieper J, Braun J, Rudwaleit M, Boonen A, Zink A. Ankylosing spondylitis: an overview. Ann Rheum Dis. 2002;61(Suppl 3):iii8–18.
9. Braun J, et al. Efficacy and safety of infliximab in patients with ankylosing spondylitis over a two-year period. Arthritis Rheum. 2008;59:1270–8.
10. Dijkmans B, et al. Etanercept in the long-term treatment of patients with ankylosing spondylitis. J Rheumatol. 2009;36:1256–64. https://doi.org/10.3899/jrheum.081033.
11. van der Heijde D, et al. Adalimumab effectiveness for the treatment of ankylosing spondylitis is maintained for up to 2 years: long-term results from the ATLAS trial. Ann Rheum Dis. 2009;68:922–9.
12. Deodhar A, et al. Golimumab administered subcutaneously every 4 weeks in ankylosing spondylitis: 5-year results of the GO-RAISE study. Ann Rheum Dis. 2015;74:757–61.
13. Landewe R, et al. Efficacy of certolizumab pegol on signs and symptoms of axial spondyloarthritis including ankylosing spondylitis: 24-week results of a double-blind randomised placebo-controlled phase 3 study. Ann Rheum Dis. 2014;73:39–47.
14. Aggarwal BB, Gupta SC, Kim JH. Historical perspectives on tumor necrosis factor and its superfamily: 25 years later, a golden journey. Blood. 2012; 119:651–65.
15. Ware C, et al. Tumor necrosis factor (TNF) receptor expression in T lymphocytes. Differential regulation of the type I TNF receptor during activation of resting and effector T cells. J Immunol. 1991;147:4229–38.
16. Mason A, et al. Regulation of NK cells through the 80-kDa TNFR (CD120b). J Leukoc Biol. 1995;58:249–55.
17. Yang L, Lindholm K, Konishi Y, Li R, Shen Y. Target depletion of distinct tumor necrosis factor receptor subtypes reveals hippocampal neuron death and survival through different signal transduction pathways. J Neurosci. 2002;22:3025–32.
18. Faustman DL, Davis M. TNF receptor 2 and disease: autoimmunity and regenerative medicine. Front Immunol. 2013;4(478):1–8.
19. Naude PJ, den Boer JA, Luiten PG, Eisel UL. Tumor necrosis factor receptor cross-talk. FEBS J. 2011;278:888–98.
20. Vincent FB, et al. Antidrug antibodies (ADAb) to tumour necrosis factor (TNF)-specific neutralising agents in chronic inflammatory diseases: a real issue, a clinical perspective. Ann Rheum Dis. 2013;72:165–78.
21. Haberhauer G, Strehblow C, Fasching P. Observational study of switching anti-TNF agents in ankylosing spondylitis and psoriatic arthritis versus rheumatoid arthritis. Wien Med Wochenschr. 2010;160:220–4.
22. Arends S, et al. Baseline predictors of response and discontinuation of tumor necrosis factor-alpha blocking therapy in ankylosing spondylitis: a prospective longitudinal observational cohort study. Arthritis Res Ther. 2011;13:R94.
23. Arends S, van der Veer E, Kallenberg CG, Brouwer E, Spoorenberg A. Baseline predictors of response to TNF-alpha blocking therapy in ankylosing spondylitis. Curr Opin Rheumatol. 2012;24:290–8.
24. Lord PA, et al. Predictors of response to anti-TNF therapy in ankylosing spondylitis: results from the British Society for Rheumatology biologics register. Rheumatology (Oxford). 2010;49:563–70.
25. Maneiro JR, Souto A, Salgado E, Mera A, Gomez-Reino JJ. Predictors of response to TNF antagonists in patients with ankylosing spondylitis and psoriatic arthritis: systematic review and meta-analysis. RMD Open. 2015;1: e000017.
26. Rudwaleit M, Listing J, Brandt J, Braun J, Sieper J. Prediction of a major clinical response (BASDAI 50) to tumour necrosis factor alpha blockers in ankylosing spondylitis. Ann Rheum Dis. 2004;63:665–70.
27. Rudwaleit M, et al. MRI in predicting a major clinical response to anti-tumour necrosis factor treatment in ankylosing spondylitis. Ann Rheum Dis. 2008;67:1276–81.
28. Seitz M, Wirthmuller U, Moller B, Villiger PM. The −308 tumour necrosis factor-alpha gene polymorphism predicts therapeutic response to TNFalpha-blockers in rheumatoid arthritis and spondyloarthritis patients. Rheumatology (Oxford). 2007;46:93–6.
29. Tong Q, et al. TNF-alpha −857 and −1031 polymorphisms predict good therapeutic response to TNF-alpha blockers in Chinese Han patients with ankylosing spondylitis. Pharmacogenomics. 2012;13:1459–67.
30. van der Linden S, Valkenburg HA, Cats A. Evaluation of diagnostic criteria for ankylosing spondylitis. A proposal for modification of the New York criteria. Arthritis Rheum. 1984;27:361–8.

31. Garrett S, et al. A new approach to defining disease status in ankylosing spondylitis: the Bath Ankylosing Spondylitis Disease Activity Index. J Rheumatol. 1994;21:2286–91.

32. Steinbrich-Zollner M, et al. From transcriptome to cytome: integrating cytometric profiling, multivariate cluster, and prediction analyses for a phenotypical classification of inflammatory diseases. Cytometry A. 2008;73: 333–40.

33. Sörensen T, Baumgart S, Durek P, Grützkau A, Häupl T. ImmunoClust—an automated analysis pipeline for the identification of immunophenotypic signatures in high-dimensional cytometric datasets. Cytometry A. 2015;87: 603–15.

34. Reveille J. Biomarkers for diagnosis, monitoring of progression, and treatment responses in ankylosing spondylitis and axial spondyloarthritis. Clin Rheumatol. 2015;34:1009–18.

35. de Vries MK, et al. Erythrocyte sedimentation rate, C-reactive protein level, and serum amyloid a protein for patient selection and monitoring of anti-tumor necrosis factor treatment in ankylosing spondylitis. Arthritis Rheum. 2009;61:1484–90.

36. Luc M, et al. C-reactive protein predicts tumor necrosis factor-alpha blocker retention rate in axial ankylosing spondylitis. J Rheumatol. 2007;34:2078–81.

37. Evans D, et al. Interaction between ERAP1 and HLA-B27 in ankylosing spondylitis implicates peptide handling in the mechanism for HLA-B27 in disease susceptibility. Nat Genet. 2011;43:761–7.

38. Arends S, et al. Serum MMP-3 level as a biomarker for monitoring and predicting response to etanercept treatment in ankylosing spondylitis. J Rheumatol. 2011;38:1644–50.

39. Poddubnyy D, et al. Elevated serum level of the vascular endothelial growth factor predicts radiographic spinal progression in patients with axial spondyloarthritis. Ann Rheum Dis. 2014;73:2137–43.

40. Carvajal Alegria G, Gazeau P, Hillion S, Daien CI, Cornec DYK. Could lymphocyte profiling be useful to diagnose systemic autoimmune diseases? Clinic Rev Allerg Immunol. 2017;53:219–36.

41. Aramaki T, et al. A significantly impaired natural killer cell activity due to a low activity on a per-cell basis in rheumatoid arthritis. Mod Rheumatol. 2009;19:245–52.

42. Vranes Z, Poljakovic Z, Marusic M. Natural killer cell number and activity in multiple sclerosis. J Neurol Sci. 1989;94:115–23.

43. Cameron AL, Kirby B, Griffiths CE. Circulating natural killer cells in psoriasis. Br J Dermatol. 2003;149:160–4.

44. Ewan PW, Barrett HM, Pusey CD. Defective natural killer (NK) and killer (K) cell function in systemic lupus erythematosus. J Clin Lab Immunol. 1983; 10:71–6.

45. Conigliaro P, Scrivo R, Valesini G, Perricone R. Emerging role for NK cells in the pathogenesis of inflammatory arthropathies. Autoimmun Rev. 2011;10: 577–81.

46. Lopez-Botet M, Moretta L, Strominger J. NK-cell receptors and recognition of MHC class I molecules. Immunol Today. 1996;17:212–4.

47. Mousavi T, et al. Phenotypic study of natural killer cell subsets in ankylosing spondylitis patients. Iran J Allergy Asthma Immunol. 2009;8:193–8.

48. Azuz-Lieberman N, et al. The involvement of NK cells in ankylosing spondylitis. Int Immunol. 2005;17:837–45.

49. Chan AT, Kollnberger SD, Wedderburn LR, Bowness P. Expansion and enhanced survival of natural killer cells expressing the killer immunoglobulin-like receptor KIR3DL2 in spondylarthritis. Arthritis Rheum. 2005;52:3586–95.

50. Scrivo R, Morrone S, Spadaro A, Santoni A, Valesini G. Evaluation of degranulation and cytokine production in natural killer cells from spondyloarthritis patients at single-cell level. Cytometry B Clin Cytom. 2011;80:22–7.

51. Addison EG, et al. Ligation of CD8alpha on human natural killer cells prevents activation-induced apoptosis and enhances cytolytic activity. Immunology. 2005;116:354–61.

52. Srour EF, Leemhuis T, Jenski L, Redmond R, Jansen J. Cytolytic activity of human natural killer cell subpopulations isolated by four-color immunofluorescence flow cytometric cell sorting. Cytometry. 1990;11:442–6.

53. Gibbings D, Befus AD. CD4 and CD8: an inside-out coreceptor model for innate immune cells. J Leukoc Biol. 2009;86:251–9.

54. Fischer R, Kontermann RE, Maier O. Targeting sTNF/TNFR1 signaling as a new therapeutic strategy. Antibodies. 2015;4:48–70.

55. Solomaon KA, Pesti N, Wu G, Newton RC. Cutting edge: a dominant negative form of TNF-alpha converting enzyme inhibits proTNF and TNFRII secretion. J Immunol. 1999;163:4105–8.

56. Wallach D, et al. Soluble and cell surface receptors for tumor necrosis factor. Agents Actions Suppl. 1991;35:51–7.

57. Meusch U, et al. In vitro response pattern of monocytes after tmTNF reverse signaling predicts response to anti-TNF therapy in rheumatoid arthritis. J Transl Med. 2015;13:256. https://doi.org/10.1186/s12967-015-0620-z.

58. Pinckard JK, Sheehan KC, Arthur CD, Schreiber RD. Constitutive shedding of both p55 and p75 murine TNF receptors in vivo. J Immunol. 1997;158:3869–73.

59. Higuchi M, Aggarwal BB. TNF induces internalization of the p60 receptor and shedding of the p80 receptor. J Immunol. 1994;152:3550–8.

10

GPR120 is an important inflammatory regulator in the development of osteoarthritis

Yuanfeng Chen[1,3,4†], Dan Zhang[2†], Ki Wai Ho[3†], Sien Lin[3,4], Wade Chun-Wai Suen[3,5], Huantian Zhang[1], Zhengang Zha[1], Gang Li[3,4*] and Po Sing Leung[2*]

Abstract

Background: The aim of this study was to investigate the regulatory role of G-protein coupled receptor 120 (GPR120) in the development and progression of osteoarthritis (OA).

Methods: GPR120 knockout (KO) and wild-type (WT) mice were used to create an animal model of OA by means of anterior cruciate ligament transection (ACLT) surgery. The severity of OA was staged and evaluated by histological examination, microcomputed tomography scan and enzyme-linked immunosorbent assay (ELISA). The anti-inflammatory effects of the GPR120 agonist docosahexaenoic acid (DHA) on human chondrocytes were further evaluated by specific inflammatory markers. In addition, the healing progression of a skin defect model was determined with histological assays.

Results: The GPR120-KO mice displayed an accelerated development of OA after ACLT. The secondary inflammation, cartilage degeneration, and subchondral bone aberrant changes were significantly elevated in the early phase of OA in KO mice relative to those in WT mice. In addition, we found that GPR120 levels were downregulated in OA patients compared with control subjects, whereas GPR120 activation with DHA exhibited anti-inflammatory effects in primary human chondrocytes in vitro. Moreover, results from the skin defect model showed that GPR120 agonism with DHA enhanced wound repair in mice, as shown by the downregulation of the number of CD68[+] cells.

Conclusions: Our study suggests that GPR120 is an important inflammatory mediator during the development of OA, and that it is a potential marker for the diagnosis of high-risk patients with OA.

Keywords: G-protein coupled receptors, Polyunsaturated fatty acids, Proinflammatory mediators, Cartilage, Subchondral bone, Skin defect, Diagnostic markers

Background

Osteoarthritis (OA) is one of the leading causes of physical disability and affects nearly 80% of individuals older than 75 years in the US [1]. Current pharmacological therapies are mainly targeted at the level of symptomatic control, which is less effective for disease progression. Better understanding of the pathogenesis of OA is crucial for the design and development of novel therapeutic agents. Obesity is one of the primary risk factors for OA, but the underlying mechanisms involved have yet to be determined [2]. It is believed that an increased loading by weight gain on the joints is attributable to the obesity-accelerated OA; however, the mechanical factors alone do not account for the higher incidence of OA in nonweight-bearing joints, such as the hands [3]. Interestingly, previous studies have shown that morbidly obese mice do not develop OA when fed with standard or low-fat diet [4]. These findings suggest that other factors rather than adiposity or body weight contribute to OA in obesity, such as lipid metabolism homeostasis or the circulating levels of adipokines.

* Correspondence: gangli@cuhk.edu.hk; psleung@cuhk.edu.hk
†Yuanfeng Chen, Dan Zhang and Ki Wai Ho contributed equally to this work.
³Department of Orthopaedics & Traumatology, Li Ka Shing Institute of Health Sciences and Lui Che Woo Institute of Innovative Medicine, Faculty of Medicine, The Chinese University of Hong Kong, Prince of Wales Hospital, Shatin, Hong Kong SAR, People's Republic of China
²School of Biomedical Sciences, Faculty of Medicine, The Chinese University of Hong Kong, Hong Kong, Hong Kong SAR, People's Republic of China
Full list of author information is available at the end of the article

It was reported that obesity-associated oxidative stress induces lipolysis of adipocytes and thus increases the circulating levels of free fatty acids (FAs) [5] . The circulating FAs can serve as either proinflammatory or anti-inflammatory molecules for metabolic signaling; for example, the saturated FAs can activate macrophages to secrete tumor necrosis factor (TNF)-α and interleukin (IL)-1, thereby activating the proinflammatory pathways [5]. In this regard, the derivatives of ω-6 polyunsaturated FAs (PUFA) are involved in joint pain [6, 7], while ω-3 FAs are reported to reduce spontaneous OA in animals on a low-fat diet [8]. Generally, by binding its receptor, ω-3 PUFA gives rise to anti-inflammatory oxylipins such as protectins and resolvins, whereas ω-6 PUFA produce proinflammatory oxylipins including numerous prostaglandins and leukotrienes [9]. Furthermore, it has been reported that the surface of cartilage is covered with a layer of phospholipids that serves as a boundary lubricant during joint loading [10]. Therefore, changes in the composition of this lubrication layer due to either injury or abnormal lipid metabolism may impact the function of the articular joint and potentially lead to the onset of OA [11]. These findings imply that free FAs or metabolic factors play a relatively direct role in the process of joint degeneration, but the regulatory roles of the ω-3 FAs and their receptors in the development of OA still need to be further investigated.

G-protein coupled receptor 120 (GPR120), or free fatty acid receptor 4 (FFA4), is known to bind with ω-3 and stabilize the metabolic homeostasis via cascades of physiological activities [12, 13]. Activation of GPR120 with its agonists such as docosahexaenoic acid (DHA) has an insulinotropic effect on pancreatic beta-cell secretion and survival, with therapeutic potential for obesity-associated type 2 diabetes [14]. In fact, GPR120 stimulation confers protection from obesity and diabetes by inhibiting inflammatory responses, modulating hormone secretions from the gastrointestinal tract and pancreas, and regulating lipid and/or glucose metabolism in adipose, liver, and muscle tissues [15]. However, whether GPR120 plays a role in OA is still largely unknown. The objective of this study was to investigate the role of GPR120 in the development of OA and whether it can be a potential marker for the diagnosis of high-risk patients with OA.

Methods
GPR120 knockout mice
GPR120 global knockout (KO) mice (Ffar4[tm1(KOMP)Vlcg], http://velocigene.com/komp/detail/15078) were produced by the Knockout Mice Project (KOMP) Repository (UCSD, CA, USA) as has been reported previously [16]. Briefly, the targeting vector was constructed by ligating the fragments of 5' and 3' homology recombination arms and the fragment for the *lacZ*-ployA-loxP-hUbCpro-*neo*[r]-ployA-loxP cassette. The targeting vector was

introduced into C57BL/6 embryonic stem cells, where the original DNA was replaced by homologous recombination. The coding region of mouse GPR120 consists of three exons, exons 1–3. The major parts of exon 1 and 3 and the whole of exon 2 were replaced with the aforementioned cassette. Using heterozygous GPR120 KO mouse sperm provided by KOMP, we established GPR120 KO mice by performing in-vitro fertilization. Our experimental procedures were approved by the Animal Experimental Ethics Committee of the Chinese University of Hong Kong (ref. 13/044/GRF-5).

Genotyping
The last 3–5 mm of mouse tails were digested with 100 μl 50 mM NaOH for approximately 25 min in a water bath at 95 °C, and then centrifuged to remove cell debris. Real-time polymerase chain reaction (RT-PCR) analysis was performed using 1 μl genomic DNA to determine the expression of the tag gene Neomycinresistance (Neo[r]) and GPR120. Primers for the genotyping are listed in Additional file 1.

Clinical sample collection
The study was approved by the Joint Chinese University of Hong Kong-New Territories East Cluster Clinical Research Ethics Committee (ethical approval code CRE-2013.248) or the First Affiliated Hospital of Guangzhou University of Chinese Medicine Clinical Research Ethics Committee (ethical approval code YJ-2015.034) and informed consent was obtained from each donor. The clinical specimens (cartilage or fat tissues) were obtained from patients with OA during total knee arthroplasty surgery ($n = 10$; seven women and three men; age 62.3 ± 4.5 years, range 45–72 years) in the Prince of Wales Hospital, Chinese University of Hong Kong. The clinical samples for the control group were collected from bone fracture patients with no previous history of OA during fracture surgery in the First Affiliated Hospital of Guangzhou University of Chinese Medicine ($n = 9$; five women and four men; age 58.8 ± 3.6 years, range 32–77 years).

Animal models
Male GPR120-KO mice or wild-type (WT) mice, 12 weeks old and weighing 20–25 g, were used in this study (ref. 13/044/GRF-5). Animals were acclimatized to local vivarium conditions at a temperature of 24–26 °C and humidity of 70% with free access to water and a pelleted commercial diet in the mouse house under specific pathogen-free (SPF) conditions. For the OA model, WT or KO mice were used for the OA and control groups ($n = 10$). In the OA group, the right knee joint of the mice received anterior cruciate ligament and medial collateral ligament transection (ACLT) surgery as previously described [17]. In the sham-operated group

(n = 10), only the skin of the right knee joint was resected. Samples were collected at 6 weeks after the operations. At 4 and 6 weeks postoperation, WT and KO mice from each group were randomly selected and killed for the collection of blood serum and right knee joint samples.

For the skin defect model (ref. 17–145-ITF), WT or KO mice were used in each group (n = 5). The dorsolateral skin of the mice was first punched using a 4-mm skin biopsy punch and the mice were then divided into docosahexaenoic acid (DHA; Cayman Chemical, USA) and control groups. In the DHA group, the mice were treated daily with 180 µl DHA (7 mg/ml) by gavage administration; in the control group, the mice were given phosphate-buffered saline (PBS) by gavage. Photos of the wound were taken for 8 consecutive days and wound sizes were estimated using ImageJ software (National Institutes of Health, Bethesda, MD.). All mice were sacrificed at day 8 and skin samples were collected.

Cell experiments

Nonfibrillated cartilage samples (OARSI scores of 0–3) collected from patients during total knee arthroplasty surgery were analyzed in this study. The cartilage tissues were washed and minced into pieces before being sequentially digested with 0.25% trypsin (Life, USA) for 20 min and 0.2% (2 mg/ml) type II collagenase (Sigma, USA) for 24 h at 37 °C. After centrifugation, the supernatants were removed and the chondrocytes were cultured in alpha minimum essential medium (α-MEM) + 10% fetal bovine serum (FBS) (both from Invitrogen Corp., Carlsbad, CA, USA). The cell type was identified by collagen II immunostaining.

For the inflammatory induction study in the TNF-α + DHA group, chondrocyte cells at passages 2 to 3 were seeded on 24-well plates (5×10^4 cells/well) in serum-free Dulbecco's modified Eagle's medium (DMEM) and treated with 50 ng/ml TNF-α (Sigma, USA) and 10 µg/ml DHA (Cayman Chemical, USA). For the TNF-α group, cells were treated with 50 ng/ml TNF-α; neither TNF-α nor DHA were applied to the cells in the control group. Cells were harvested after 24 h of incubation.

The gene expression levels of chemokine (C-C motif) ligand 2 (Ccl2), cyclooxygenase 2 (Cox2), IL-1β, matrix metallopeptidase (MMP)-13, and glyceraldehyde 3-phosphate dehydrogenase (GAPDH) for chondrocytes induced by TNF-α were determined using RT-PCR. Primer sequences are listed in Additional file 2.

Enzyme-linked immunosorbent assay (ELISA) measurements

For the human clinical samples, fat tissues were collected (1×1 cm^3) from the OA patient group and the non-OA patient control group. Samples were weighed, mechanically homogenized and ground into powder with liquid nitrogen, and then were treated with ice-cold tissue protein extraction reagents (Life Technologies, Pleasanton, CA, USA). Samples were then centrifuged and tested using a GPR120 ELISA examination kit according to the protocol suggested by the manufacturer (Fine Test, China).

For the animal samples from the OA model, a 1-ml blood sample was collected by cardiac puncture immediately after the mice were sacrificed. The blood sample was then centrifuged and the TNF-α level tested using a TNF-α ELISA kit according to the protocol suggested by the manufacturer (Dakewe, China).

Microcomputed tomography (µCT) assessment

The right knee joints of mice from the OA model were fixed overnight in 10% formalin. Samples were then analyzed using high-resolution µCT scan (µCT40, Scanco Medical, Basserdorf, Switzerland). Three dimensional (3D) reconstructions of the mineralized tissues were performed using a global threshold (216 mg hydroxyapatite/cm^3) and a Gaussian filter (sigma = 0.8, support = 2) was used for noise suppression. One hundred sagittal images of the tibial subchondral bone were used to perform the 3D histomorphometric analysis. The bone mineral density (BMD), bone volume/total tissue volume (BV/TV), trabecular thickness (Tb.Th) and structure model index (SMI) were analyzed as the 3D structural parameters.

Histological and immunochemical examinations

Mouse tissue samples including colon tissues from GPR120 KO mice, right knee joints collected from the OA model, the skin of the back from the skin defect model, and the human chondrocytes were fixed in 10% formalin, while the knee joint was additionally treated with 10% ethylenediaminetetraacetic acid (EDTA) for decalcification for 14 days before paraffin embedding. Frozen samples were embedded in the optimum cutting temperature (OCT) compound (Sakura Finetek, Zoeterwoude, The Netherlands) and then sectioned at 5 µm thick for skin and right knee joint samples and 6 µm thick for colon samples at the sagittal-oriented position for Safranin-O/fast green, hematoxylin and eosin (H&E), and immunofluorescent staining.

For immunofluorescent staining, the colon tissues and human chondrocyte were incubated with primary antibodies to chicken anti-beta galactosidase (Abcam, 1:100, ab9361) and rabbit anti-Collagen II (Abcam, 1:300, ab34712), respectively, overnight at 4 °C. Secondary antibodies conjugated with fluorescence goat anti-chicken or goat anti-rabbit CY3 (Life Technologies, Pleasanton, CA, USA; 1:800) were added, and slides were incubated at room temperature in the dark for 1 h. Photographs of the selected areas were taken under a microscope.

Immunostaining was performed using a standard protocol as previously reported [18, 19]. We incubated the sections with primary antibodies to rabbit MMP13

(Abcam, 1:50, ab3208) and collagen X (Abcam, 1:80, ab58632), Osterix (Abcam, 1:600, ab22552), and CD68 (Boster, 1:100, BA2966) overnight at 4 °C. For immuno-histochemical staining, a horseradish peroxidase–strep-tavidin in the detection system (Dako, Carpinteria, CA, USA) was subsequently used, followed by counterstain-ing with hematoxylin. Photographs of the selected areas were taken under a light microscope. We counted the number of positively stained cells and repeated in tripli-cate in three randomly selected sections in the area of interest per specimen, and the numbers of cells were sta-tistically analyzed.

Statistical analysis

In accordance with the ARRIVE guidelines [20], we have reported measures of precision and n to provide an indi-cation of significance. All statistical analyses were per-formed using the statistical software SPSS 15.0. The data were analyzed by one-way analysis of variance (ANOVA), except for data on wound healing analysis which were tested by two-way ANOVA. Data are reported as mean and 95% confidence interval (CI). The graphs were gener-ated using GraphPad Prism 6 (GraphPad Software, San Diego, CA, USA).

Results

Validation of GPR120-KO mice

Genotyping result showed that only WT mice showed ex-pression of GPR120 at the genomic DNA (Fig. 1a) or mRNA level (Fig. 1b, c), while such expression was not de-tected in GPR120-KO mice. β-galactosidase activity is a surrogate of GPR120, and immunofluorescent staining also showed that β-galactosidase-positive cells (red) could be found in colon tissue of the KO mice while it was ab-sent in WT mice (Fig. 1d). These results indicated that knockout of the GPR120 gene was successfully generated. In addition, changes in body weight of the KO and the WT mice were also found to be not statistically different (mean 33.97, 95% CI 28.97–38.98 g, versus 30.99, 95% CI 29.41–32.56 g, respectively; $n = 10$; $p > 0.05$) (Fig. 1e). Taken together, these results provide evidence of the suc-cessful establishment of the GPR120 KO mice.

Acceleration of cartilage degeneration in GPR120-KO mice with surgically induced OA

Safranin-O/fast green staining showed that there were significantly more degenerative features in the knee joint samples of KO mice compared with those of WT mice at 4 weeks postoperation, while the cartilage dam-age is obvious in both groups 6 weeks after the OA sur-gery. No abnormal cartilages were observed in the sham group (Fig. 2a). Based on the OARSI histologic grading system, the scores indicated that KO mice showed more severe cartilage degeneration (16.5, 95%

CI 15.02–17.98; $n = 10$) than WT mice (6.9, 95% CI 5.441–8.358; $n = 10$; $p = 0.0034$) at 4 weeks postopera-tion, and the cartilage damage was significantly worse in both KO and WT mice at 6 weeks postoperation (19.52, 95% CI 16.32–22.72, and 19.38, 95% CI 17.49–21.27, respectively; $n = 10$; $p > 0.05$). For the sham group, both KO and WT mice showed minimum carti-lage damage (0.6, 95% CI 0.2306–0.9694, versus 0.6, 95% CI 0.23–0.97, respectively; $n = 10$; $p > 0.05$) (Fig. 2a and Additional file 3). Moreover, the percentage of type X collagen (ColX)-positive chondrocytes and MMP13+ chondrocytes in cartilage were both higher in the KO mice (46.2, 95% CI 39.35–53.04, and 50.19, 95% CI 46.11–54.28, respectively; $n = 5$; $p < 0.01$) than in WT mice (32.70, 95% CI 27.66–37.74, and 32.92, 95% CI 26.73–39.11, respectively; $n = 5$) at 4 weeks after sur-gery (Fig. 2b, c and Additional file 4A, B). In the sham control group, both KO and WT mice showed the low-est percentage of ColX+ chondrocytes (KO: 25.96, 95% CI 19.22–32.70; WT: 27.51, 95% CI 23.19–31.82; $n = 5$) and MMP13+ chondrocytes (KO: 23.88, 95% CI 16.66–31.09; WT: 25.95, 95% CI 17.34–34.56; $n = 5$). The highest percentage of ColX+ (KO: 57.46, 95% CI 51.75–63.17; WT: 52.86, 95% CI 46.93–58.79; $n = 5$) and MMP13+ chondrocytes (KO: 56.82, 95% CI 52.23–61.41; WT: 52.14, 95% CI 46.86–57.41; $n = 5$) were found in both KO and WT mice at 6 weeks postopera-tion (Fig. 2b, c and Additional file 4A, B).

Aggravation of abnormal bone remodeling in subchondral bone in GPR120-KO mice with surgically induced OA

The 3D reconstructed images from μCT showed the microarchitecture of the mouse subchondral bone in all groups (Fig. 3a). The results showed that, at 4 weeks after OA surgery, the abnormal bone formation in sub-chondral bone was significantly more severe in KO mice (BMD: 481.5, 95% CI 464.5–498.6 mg/cm³, $n = 10$; BV/TV: 0.5515, 95% CI 0.5130–0.5901, $n = 10$) than in WT mice (BMD: 429.5, 95% CI 406.9–452.1 mg/cm³, $n = 10$, $p = 0.0256$; BV/TV: 0.4630, 95% CI 0.4162–0.5097, $n = 10$, $p = 0.0359$) (Fig. 3b, c). At 6 weeks after operation, the abnormal bone formation was severe in both KO (BMD: 496.3, 95% CI 461.9–532.1 mg/cm³, $n = 10$; BV/TV: 0.5619, 95% CI 0.5225–0.6014, $n = 10$) and WT mice (BMD: 498.4, 95% CI 472.1–524.7 mg/cm³, $n = 10$, $p = 0.7446$; BV/TV: 0.5913, 95% CI 0.5441–0.6385, $n = 10$, $p = 0.736$) (Fig. 3b, c). In the sham control group, ab-normal bone formation was mild in both KO (BMD: 447.9, 95% CI 429.0–466.8 mg/cm³, $n = 10$; BV/TV: 0.4935, 95% CI 0.4543–0.5326, $n = 10$) and WT mice (BMD: 424.2, 95% CI 407.2–441.1 mg/cm³, $n = 10$, $p = 0.22$; BV/TV: 0.4482, 95% CI 0.3971–0.4992, $n = 10$, $p = 0.3957$) (Fig. 3b, c).

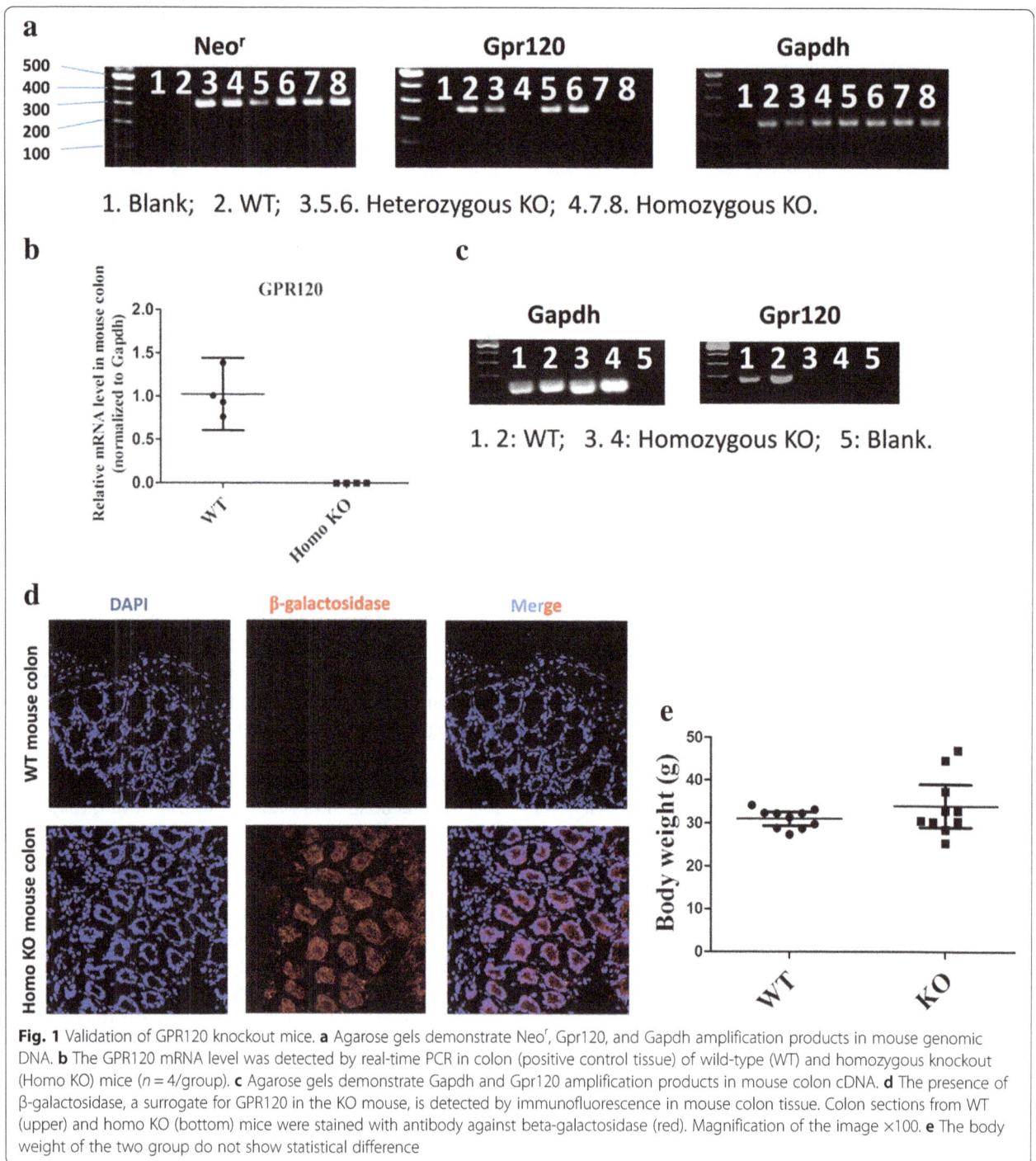

Fig. 1 Validation of GPR120 knockout mice. **a** Agarose gels demonstrate Neo^r, Gpr120, and Gapdh amplification products in mouse genomic DNA. **b** The GPR120 mRNA level was detected by real-time PCR in colon (positive control tissue) of wild-type (WT) and homozygous knockout (Homo KO) mice ($n = 4$/group). **c** Agarose gels demonstrate Gapdh and Gpr120 amplification products in mouse colon cDNA. **d** The presence of β-galactosidase, a surrogate for GPR120 in the KO mouse, is detected by immunofluorescence in mouse colon tissue. Colon sections from WT (upper) and homo KO (bottom) mice were stained with antibody against beta-galactosidase (red). Magnification of the image ×100. **e** The body weight of the two group do not show statistical difference

Trabecular bone thickness (Tb.Th.) in KO mice (0.1505, 95% CI 0.1436–0.1575 mm; $n = 10$) was higher than that in WT mice (0.1292, 95% CI 0.1219–0.1364 mm; $n = 10$; $p = 0.0217$) at 4 weeks postoperation, and at 6 weeks after surgery Tb.Th was at the highest level for both WT and KO mice (0.155, 95% CI 0.1438–0.1662 mm, and 0.1676, 95% CI 0.1616–0.1736 mm, respectively; $n = 10$; $p > 0.05$) (Additional file 4D). Tb.Th. was lowest in KO and WT mice from the sham group (0.1208, 95% CI 0.1145–

0.1272 mm, and 0.1108, 95% CI 0.1016–0.1201 mm, respectively; $n = 10$) (Additional file 4D). Furthermore, KO mice had a significantly more decreased SMI (−1.167, 95% CI −1.846 to −0.4884; $n = 10$) than WT mice (0.0036, 95% CI−0.6356 to 0.6283; $n = 10$; $p > 0.05$) at 4 weeks after the OA surgery, though no statistically significant differences were found (Additional file 4E). SMI was at the lowest level for both WT and KO mice (−1.985, 95% CI −3.073 to −0.8975, and −0.6783, 95% CI −1.351 to −0.005,

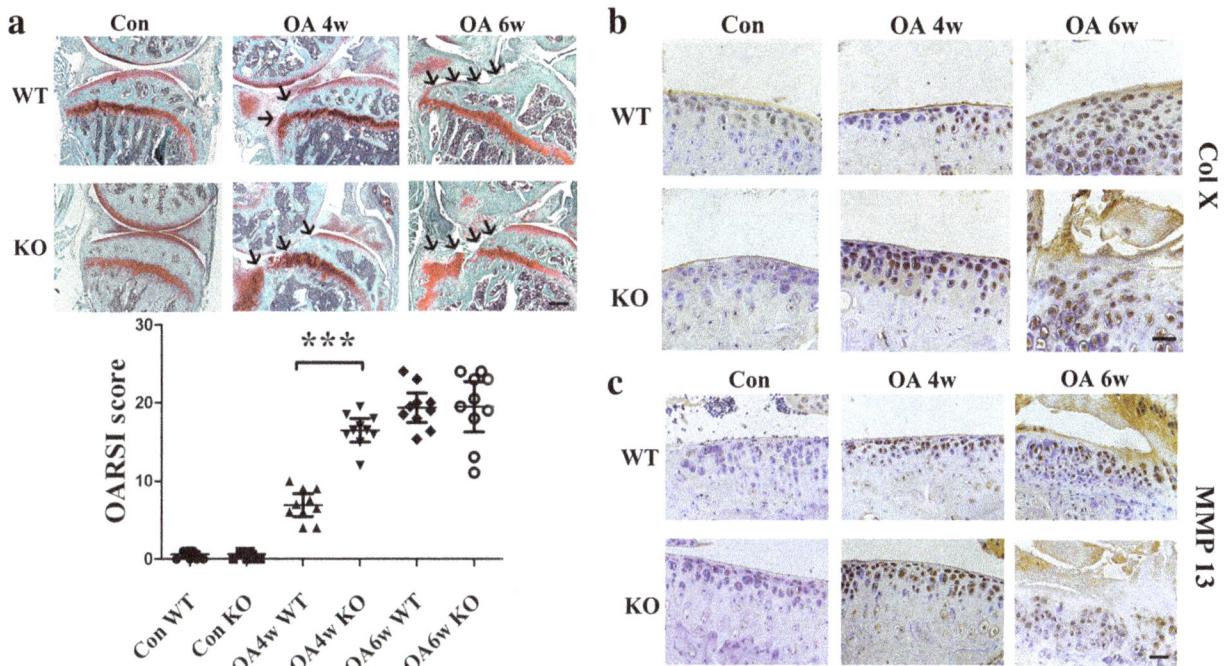

Fig. 2 a Safranin-O/fast green staining and quantification of the histologic results using the Osteoarthritis Research Society International Cartilage Histopathology Assessment System (OARSI score) indicated articular cartilage damage in all groups. Black arrows show the damaged region of the cartilage. *******p* < 0.01, compared with the wild-type (WT) osteoarthritis (OA) mice at 4 weeks (4w). Scale bar = 400 μm. Immunohistochemical analysis of **b** type X collagen (COL X)- and **c** matrix metalloproteinase 13 (MMP13)-positive chondrocytes (brown) in articular cartilage showed that GPR120 knockout (KO) mice significantly increased the numbers of COL X- and MMP13-positive chondrocytes compared with the WT mice 4 weeks after the OA surgery. The fewest numbers of positive cells could be found in the sham control (Con) in both KO and WT mice, and the highest numbers of COL X- and MMP13-positive cells can be found in OA at 6 weeks (6w) for both KO and WT mice. Scale bar = 50 μm

respectively; $n = 10$; $p > 0.05$) at 6 weeks postoperation; in the controls, SMI in WT mice was 0.2041 (95% CI −0.1689 to 0.5772) and in KO mice it was −0.054 (95% CI −0.4845 to 0.375). There were no statistically significant differences (Additional file 4E).

Furthermore, the results of immunohistochemistry staining with Osterix, an osteoprogenitor, revealed that KO mice had a significantly higher increase in numbers of Osterix-positive cells in the subchondral bone marrow than WT mice 4 weeks after OA surgery (KO: 277.8, 95% CI 250.9–304.7; WT: 151.2, 95% CI 130.8–171.6; $n = 5$, $p < 0.001$) (Fig. 3d and Additional file 4C), while at 6 weeks postoperation an upregulated number of Osterix-positive cells could be observed in both KO and WT mice (KO: 335.2, 95% CI 293.3–377.1; WT: 323.6, 95% CI 285.3–361.9; $n = 5$). Only a few Osterix-positive cells could be found in the sham control groups for both KO and WT mice (KO: 112.6, 95% CI 87.83–137.4; WT: 115.4, 95% CI 78.30–152.5; $n = 5$) (Fig. 3d and Additional file 4C).

Upregulation of plasma levels of TNF-α in GPR120-KO mice with surgically induced OA

ELISA showed that the level of TNF-α was significantly higher in KO mice (18.04, 95% CI 5.08–30.56 pg/ml; $n = 5$) when compared with that of WT mice (5.54, 95% CI

3.436–7.645 pg/ml; $n = 5$; $p = 0.022$) at 4 weeks after the OA surgery (Fig. 4a). At 6 weeks after the operation, TNF-α was at a high level in both KO (15.15, 95% CI −1.347 to 31.65 pg/ml; $n = 5$) and WT mice (12.62, 95% CI 4.442–20.81 pg/ml; $n = 5$). The sham control group showed the lowest TNF-α level in both KO (6.3, 95% CI −1.820 to 14.42 pg/ml; $n = 5$) and WT mice (9.234, 95% CI −1.162 to 19.63 pg/ml; $n = 5$) (Fig. 4a).

Downregulation of GPR120 expression in OA patients

ELISA was used to analyze the human clinical samples collected from the OA or non-OA patients during surgery. The result indicated that the GPR120 level was significantly more downregulated in OA patients (470.5, 95% CI 368.9–572.1 pg/ml; $n = 10$) than non-OA patients (803.6, 95% CI 700.2–907 pg/ml; $n = 9$; $p = 0.0349$) (Fig. 4b).

GPR120 activation-induced inhibition of inflammatory factor expression in human chondrocytes

The result of immunofluorescent staining showed that the primary human chondrocytes expressed Collagen II (a chondrocyte marker) (Additional file 5). It has been reported that the chondrocytes express GPR120 [21] and, in this study, the RT-PCR result showed that DHA, a GPR120 agonist, could induce anti-inflammatory

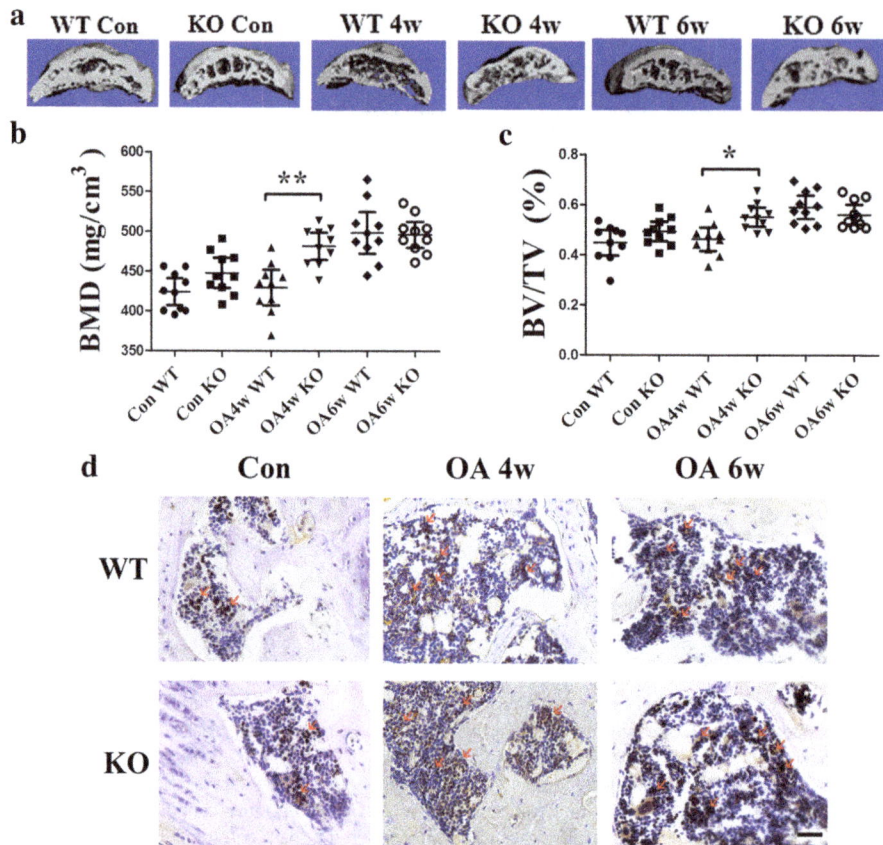

Fig. 3 a 3D μCT images of the tibia subchondral bone medial compartment (sagittal view) of mice in all groups. Quantitative analysis of structural parameters of subchondral bone by μCT. **b** Bone mineral density (BMD) and **c** bone volume/total tissue volume (BV/TV), $n = 10$ per group. *$p < 0.05$, compared with the wild-type (WT) osteoarthritis (OA) mice at 4 weeks (4w). **d** Immunohistochemical analysis of Osterix-positive cells (brown, red arrow) in the tibial subchondral region. The result showed that GPR120 knockout (KO) mice significantly increased the numbers of Osterix-positive cells in subchondral bone compared with the WT mice 4 week after OA surgery. Scale bar = 50 μm. 6w 6 weeks, Con sham control

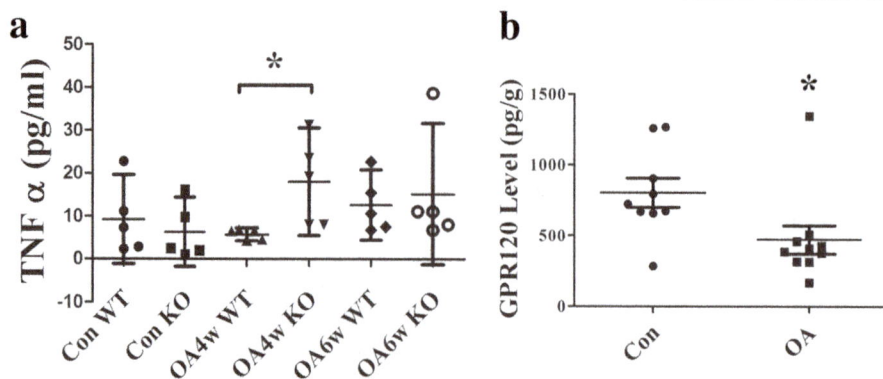

Fig. 4 ELISA showing **a** the tumor necrosis factor alpha (TNFα) level in serum in all groups ($n = 5$ for each group; *$p < 0.05$, compared with the wild-type (WT) osteoarthritis (OA) mice at 4 weeks (4w)) and **b** the GPR120 level in OA ($n = 10$) and non-OA patients ($n = 9$). *$p < 0.05$, compared with sham control (Con). 6w 6 weeks

effects in primary human chondrocytes. The mRNA expression levels of the proinflammatory genes Ccl2, Cox2, and IL-1β in the TNF-α + DHA group (3.05, 95% CI 1.305–4.79; 1.58, 95% CI 0.8351–2.334; 72.93, 95% CI −32.57 to 176.7; respectively; $n = 6$) were significantly more reduced than those in the TNF-α group (15.26, 95% CI 8.374–22.14; 3.1, 95% CI 1.821–4.378; 277.01, 95% CI 83.63–470.4; respectively; $n = 6$; $p < 0.05$) (Fig. 5). Consistent with this, the TNF-α + DHA group (0.75, 95% CI 0.415–1.087; $n = 6$) had more dramatically down-regulated MMP13 mRNA levels than the TNF-α group (4.05, 95% CI 0.9548–7.153; $n = 6$; $p < 0.05$) (Fig. 5).

GPR120 activation-induced protective effect on wound repair in mice

The DHA-treated GPR120 mice showed significantly improved tissue regeneration with thickened epithelium (Additional file 6A). All mice demonstrated a certain degree of regeneration, including re-epithelialization and new formation of sebaceous glands or hair follicles, while only the DHA-treated mice showed accelerated wound repair (Additional file 6B). The infiltration of inflammatory cells to the wound margins was evaluated using the macrophage marker CD68, and the number of CD68-positive cells significantly decreased in the DHA-treated mice (146.5, 95% CI 119.1–174; $n = 5$) compare with the control mice (63.47, 95% CI 38.84–88.09; $n = 5$; $p < 0.001$) (Additional file 6C, D).

Discussion

This study demonstrated that GPR120 is an important inflammatory regulator in the development of OA and wound healing. Several studies have shown that ω-3 PUFA bind to its receptor GPR120 to give rise to

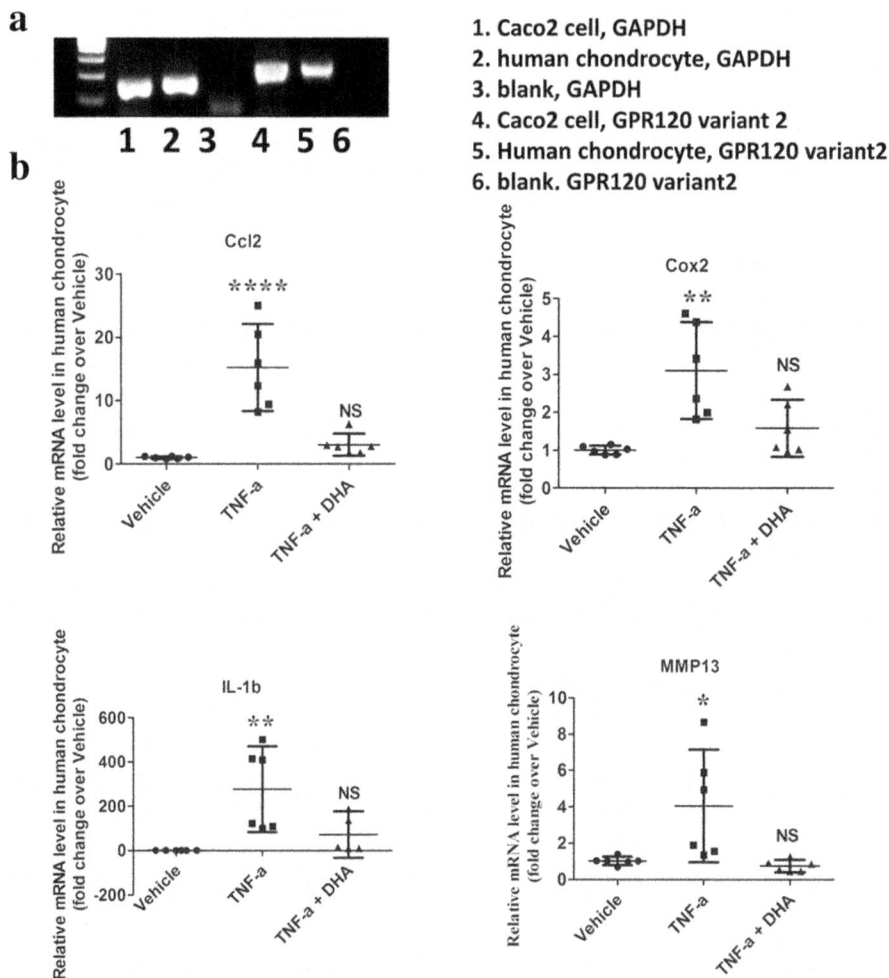

1. Caco2 cell, GAPDH
2. human chondrocyte, GAPDH
3. blank, GAPDH
4. Caco2 cell, GPR120 variant 2
5. Human chondrocyte, GPR120 variant2
6. blank. GPR120 variant2

Fig. 5 The GPR120 agonist DHA exhibits anti-inflammatory effects on primary human chondrocytes. **a** Agarose gels demonstrate Gapdh and Gpr120 amplification products in human colorectal tumor cell Caco2 (positive control) and human chondrocyte cell cDNA. **b** Human chondrocytes were exposed to 50 ng/ml human tumor necrosis factor alpha (TNFα) with or without 25 μM docosahexaenoic acid (DHA) for 48 h. The mRNA expression levels of the proinflammatory genes Ccl2, Cox2, IL-1β, and MMP13 were assessed ($n = 6$/group). *$p < 0.05$, **$p < 0.01$, ****$p < 0.0001$ compared with corresponding vehicle group. NS not significant

anti-inflammatory oxylipins such as protectins and resolvins, whereas ω-6 PUFA produce proinflammatory oxylipins including numerous prostaglandins and leukotrienes [9]. Additionally, it has been reported that the surface of cartilage is covered by a layer of phospholipids [10]. Any compositional changes in this lubrication layer due to either injury or abnormal lipid metabolism may have an impact on the function of the articular joint and potentially lead to the onset of OA [11]. Recently, several studies have demonstrated that lipid metabolic homeostasis plays an important role in cartilage degeneration during the development of OA [22, 23]. In our study, the results were consistent with the previous studies, showing that cartilage degeneration was significantly increased in the early phase of OA (i.e., 4 weeks postoperation) under the GPR120-KO condition; these observations were shown by the increases in the OARSI score and the expression of MMP13 and COLX (Fig. 2 and Additional files 3 and 4), as demonstrated by Safranin O/fast green and immunohistochemical staining, relative to the changes in WT mice.

Changes in subchondral bone play a key role in the regulation of OA progression [24]. In addition, bone marrow lesions are closely associated with pain, which has been implicated to predict the severity of cartilage damage in OA [25]. In-vitro studies have previously reported that GPR120 signaling negatively regulates osteoclast differentiation, survival, and function [26]. Moreover, it has also been shown that GPR120 activation-mediated cellular signaling determines the bi-potential of osteogenic and adipogenic differentiation of bone marrow-derived mesenchymal stem cells (BMSCs) in a dose-dependent manner [27]. Given that BMSCs and osteoclasts play a pivotal role in bone remodeling of the subchondral bone, these prior study findings point to the activation of GPR120 signaling as being of physiological importance for bone homeostasis. In fact, several in-vivo studies have shown that downregulation of the ω-3-GPR120 signaling leads to abnormalities in bone remodeling or osteophyte formation of subchondral bone in animal model of OA [22, 23]. Interestingly, we also found that subchondral bone aberrant changes in GPR120-KO mice were specifically increased in the early phase of OA (at 4 weeks postoperation) when compared with WT mice in the present study (Fig. 3 and Additional file 4).

It is known that inflammatory cytokines are the key regulators of OA [19, 28–30], while the activation of FA signaling has a critical role in the regulation of anti-inflammation during OA and wound healing. For example, activation of GPR120 with ω-3 PUFA is negatively correlated with the severity of OA and the area of wound healing, whereas it is positively correlated with adiponectin, an adipokine capable of promoting insulin sensitization and priming macrophages toward the M2 anti-inflammatory phenotype [23, 31, 32]. More

interestingly, it has been shown that infiltration of macrophages within human adipose tissue significantly inhibits GPR120 expression [33]. In light of these findings, it is plausible to postulate that the downregulation of GPR120 expression can disrupt the lipid metabolic homeostasis, thus aggravating the level of inflammatory responses and ultimately leading to the vicious cycle in the process of OA and would healing. In corroboration with previous findings, our in-vitro studies firstly demonstrated that activation of GPR120 signaling inhibits the expression of inflammatory factors in human chondrocytes (Fig. 5). Secondly, our in-vivo studies further demonstrated that the level of secondary inflammation in GPR120-KO mice was dramatically increased in the early phase of OA (at 4 weeks postoperation) when compared with WT mice (Fig. 4a). In addition, our skin defect model indicated that GPR120 agonism with DHA could accelerate the wound repair and downregulate the inflammation level at the wound, as evidenced by the lowered number of CD68$^+$ macrophages (Additional file 6). Our study findings are in agreement with a recent study reporting that the defected wound closure and cartilage regeneration may share a common, heritable, and OA-associated genetic trait [34].

One of the major obstacles to developing a new treatment option for OA is the lack of an effective and minimally invasive method to predict, diagnose, and monitor its disease progression. To address this issue, considerable efforts have been recently made for the identification of biomarkers in a clinical setting. In this regard, a lot of research for biomarkers has been focused on the release of cartilage matrix proteins, such as the collagens, proteoglycans, or cartilage oligomeric matrix protein, in the serum and synovial fluid [35–37]. Accumulated evidence has emerged that the development of OA is not only due to cartilage damage, but also to both systemic and local intra-articular metabolic factors, notably inflammation, which appear to play a pivotal role in joint degeneration [38, 39]. In additional to matrix degradation products, inflammatory cytokines and lipid metabolic factors may therefore be potential biomarkers of OA that are associated with disease mechanisms [40, 41]. Towards this end, one of the novel findings in the present study is that the expression level of GPR120 was found to be downregulated significantly more in patients with OA than in non-OA patients (Fig. 4b).

A limitation of this study is the relatively low number of mice in each group. More time points are also needed for this OA model to further evaluate the effect of GPR120 on OA progression. Also, we collected the OA and non-OA groups for the clinical specimen test without applying Kellgren grading in the assessment which might help us to understand the level of GPR120 in OA patients at different stages. Future research should consider using a larger sample size, design multiple time points in the animal study, and use Kellgren grading in the assessment to further dissect the effects of GPR120 on OA progression.

Conclusions

In conclusion, our data indicate that GPR120 plays an important role in metabolic homeostasis by showing that GPR120 downregulation is able to interrupt the metabolic homeostasis. The dysregulated metabolism may subsequently lower the capability of immunoregulation and elicit more severe immunological reactions upon injury. In addition, the assessment of the GPR120 level may potentially be applied as a diagnostic marker for high-risk OA patients. This is the first study to report that downregulation of GPR120 is a high-risk factor for the pathogenesis of OA, and these data provide a scientific basis for the development of new minimally invasive methods (such as fat tissue biopsy) to identify the high-risk OA patients who could receive supplementation with GPR120 agonists as a potential preventative and therapeutic approach to OA.

Abbreviations
3D: Three-dimensional; ACLT: Anterior cruciate ligament transection; ANOVA: Analysis of variance; BMD: Bone mineral density; BMSC: Bone marrow-derived mesenchymal stem cell; BV/TV: Bone volume/total tissue volume; Ccl2: Chemokine C-C motif ligand 2; CI: Confidence interval; Col X: Type X collagen; Cox2: Cyclooxygenase 2; DHA: Docosahexaenoic acid; ELISA: Enzyme-linked immunosorbent assay; FA: Fatty acid; GAPDH: Glyceraldehyde 3-phosphate dehydrogenase; GPR120: G-protein coupled receptor 120; KO: Knockout; IL: Interleukin; MMP: Matrix metallopeptidase; μCT: Microcomputed tomography; OA: Osteoarthritis; PUFA: Polyunsaturated fatty acids; RT-PCR: Real-time polymerase chain reaction; SMI: Structure model index; Tb.Th: Trabecular thickness; TNF: Tumor necrosis factor; WT: Wild-type

Funding
This work was partially supported by grants from the Hong Kong Government Research Grant Council, General Research Fund (14119115, 14160917, 9054014 N_CityU102/15, and T13–402/17-N), the National Natural Science Foundation of China (8143004981772322, 81602360, 81672224, and 81741045), the Hong Kong Innovation Technology Commission Funds (ITS/UIM-305), the Guangzhou Provincial Science and Technology Project of China (2014Y2–00084), and the China Postdoctoral Science Foundation (No. 61 fund). This study was also supported in part by SMART program, Lui Che Woo Institute of Innovative Medicine, The Chinese University of Hong Kong, and the research was made possible by resources donated by Lui Che Woo Foundation Limited.

Authors' contributions
YC, DZ, and KWH carried out the study design, animal experiments, data collection, analysis, and manuscript preparation. SL and HZ carried out the animal experiments. WCWS carried out manuscript preparation and review; ZZ provided materials and manuscript review. GL and PSL have contributed to the funding for supporting this research project and supervised all the experiments. All authors read and approved the final manuscript.

Consent for publication
Not applicable.

Competing interests
The authors declare that they have no competing interests.

Author details
[1]Institute of Orthopedic Diseases and Center for Joint Surgery and Sports Medicine, the First Affiliated Hospital, Jinan University, Guangzhou, People's Republic of China. [2]School of Biomedical Sciences, Faculty of Medicine, The Chinese University of Hong Kong, Hong Kong, Hong Kong SAR, People's Republic of China. [3]Department of Orthopaedics & Traumatology, Li Ka Shing Institute of Health Sciences and Lui Che Woo Institute of Innovative Medicine, Faculty of Medicine, The Chinese University of Hong Kong, Prince of Wales Hospital, Shatin, Hong Kong SAR, People's Republic of China. [4]The CUHK-ACC Space Medicine Centre on Health Maintenance of Musculoskeletal System, The Chinese University of Hong Kong Shenzhen Research Institute, Shenzhen, People's Republic of China. [5]Department of Haematology, University of Cambridge, Cambridge CB2 0PT, UK.

References
1. Lawrence RC, Felson DT, Helmick CG, Arnold LM, Choi H, Deyo RA, Gabriel S, Hirsch R, Hochberg MC, Hunder GG, et al. Estimates of the prevalence of arthritis and other rheumatic conditions in the United States. Part II. Arthritis Rheum. 2008;58(1):26–35.
2. Aspden RM. Obesity punches above its weight in osteoarthritis. Nat Rev Rheumatol. 2011;7(1):65–8.
3. Felson DT, Chaisson CE. Understanding the relationship between body weight and osteoarthritis. Baillieres Clin Rheumatol. 1997;11(4):671–81.
4. Griffin TM, Huebner JL, Kraus VB, Guilak F. Extreme obesity due to impaired leptin signaling in mice does not cause knee osteoarthritis. Arthritis Rheum. 2009;60(10):2935–44.
5. Nguyen MT, Favelyukis S, Nguyen AK, Reichart D, Scott PA, Jenn A, Liu-Bryan R, Glass CK, Neels JG, Olefsky JM. A subpopulation of macrophages infiltrates hypertrophic adipose tissue and is activated by free fatty acids via toll-like receptors 2 and 4 and JNK-dependent pathways. J Biol Chem. 2007; 282(48):35279–92.
6. Bagga D, Wang L, Farias-Eisner R, Glaspy JA, Reddy ST. Differential effects of prostaglandin derived from omega-6 and omega-3 polyunsaturated fatty acids on COX-2 expression and IL-6 secretion. Proc Natl Acad Sci U S A. 2003;100(4):1751–6.
7. Pincus T, Koch G, Lei H, Mangal B, Sokka T, Moskowitz R, Wolfe F, Gibofsky A, Simon L, Zlotnick S, et al. Patient Preference for Placebo, Acetaminophen (paracetamol) or Celecoxib Efficacy Studies (PACES): two randomised, double blind, placebo controlled, crossover clinical trials in patients with knee or hip osteoarthritis. Ann Rheum Dis. 2004;63(8):931–9.
8. Knott L, Avery NC, Hollander AP, Tarlton JF. Regulation of osteoarthritis by omega-3 (n-3) polyunsaturated fatty acids in a naturally occurring model of disease. Osteoarthritis Cartilage. 2011;19(9):1150–7.
9. Norling LV, Perretti M. The role of omega-3 derived resolvins in arthritis. Curr Opin Pharmacol. 2013;13(3):476–81.
10. Sarma AV, Powell GL, LaBerge M. Phospholipid composition of articular cartilage boundary lubricant. J Orthop Res. 2001;19(4):671–6.
11. Kosinska MK, Ludwig TE, Liebisch G, Zhang R, Siebert HC, Wilhelm J, Kaesser U, Dettmeyer RB, Klein H, Ishaque B, et al. Articular joint lubricants during osteoarthritis and rheumatoid arthritis display altered levels and molecular species. PLoS One. 2015;10(5):e0125192.
12. Oh DY, Talukdar S, Bae EJ, Imamura T, Morinaga H, Fan W, Li P, Lu WJ, Watkins SM, Olefsky JM. GPR120 is an omega-3 fatty acid receptor mediating potent anti-inflammatory and insulin-sensitizing effects. Cell. 2010;142(5):687–98.
13. Ichimura A, Hirasawa A, Poulain-Godefroy O, Bonnefond A, Hara T, Yengo L, Kimura I, Leloire A, Liu N, Iida K, et al. Dysfunction of lipid sensor GPR120 leads to obesity in both mouse and human. Nature. 2012;483(7389):350–4.
14. Zhang D, So WY, Wang Y, Wu SY, Cheng Q, Leung PS. Insulinotropic effects of GPR120 agonists are altered in obese diabetic and obese non-diabetic states. Clin Sci. 2017;131(3):247–60.
15. Zhang D, Leung PS. Potential roles of GPR120 and its agonists in the management of diabetes. Drug Des Devel Ther. 2014;8:1013–27.
16. Quesada-Lopez T, Cereijo R, Turatsinze JV, Planavila A, Cairo M, Gavalda-Navarro A, Peyrou M, Moure R, Iglesias R, Giralt M, et al. The lipid sensor GPR120 promotes brown fat activation and FGF21 release from adipocytes. Nat Commun. 2016;7:13479.

17. Hayami T, Pickarski M, Zhuo Y, Wesolowski GA, Rodan GA, Duong LT. Characterization of articular cartilage and subchondral bone changes in the rat anterior cruciate ligament transection and meniscectomized models of osteoarthritis. Bone. 2006;38(2):234–43.

18. Chen Y, Sun Y, Pan X, Ho K, Li G. Joint distraction attenuates osteoarthritis by reducing secondary inflammation, cartilage degeneration and subchondral bone aberrant change. Osteoarthritis Cartilage. 2015;23(10): 1728–35.

19. Chen Y, Lin S, Sun Y, Pan X, Xiao L, Zou L, Ho KW, Li G. Translational potential of ginsenoside Rb1 in managing progression of osteoarthritis. J Orthop Translat. 2016;6:27–33.

20. Kilkenny C, Browne WJ, Cuthill IC, Emerson M, Altman DG. Improving bioscience research reporting: the ARRIVE guidelines for reporting animal research. Osteoarthritis Cartilage. 2012;20(4):256–60.

21. Koren N, Simsa-Maziel S, Shahar R, Schwartz B, Monsonego-Ornan E. Exposure to omega-3 fatty acids at early age accelerate bone growth and improve bone quality. J Nutr Biochem. 2014;25(6):623–33.

22. Huang MJ, Wang L, Jin DD, Zhang ZM, Chen TY, Jia CH, Wang Y, Zhen XC, Huang B, Yan B, et al. Enhancement of the synthesis of n-3 PUFAs in fat-1 transgenic mice inhibits mTORC1 signalling and delays surgically induced osteoarthritis in comparison with wild-type mice. Ann Rheum Dis. 2014; 73(9):1719–27.

23. Wu CL, Jain D, McNeill JN, Little D, Anderson JA, Huebner JL, Kraus VB, Rodriguiz RM, Wetsel WC, Guilak F. Dietary fatty acid content regulates wound repair and the pathogenesis of osteoarthritis following joint injury. Ann Rheum Dis. 2015;74(11):2076–83.

24. Suri S, Walsh DA. Osteochondral alterations in osteoarthritis. Bone. 2012; 51(2):204–11.

25. Hunter DJ, Zhang Y, Niu J, Goggins J, Amin S, LaValley MP, Guermazi A, Genant H, Gale D, Felson DT. Increase in bone marrow lesions associated with cartilage loss: a longitudinal magnetic resonance imaging study of knee osteoarthritis. Arthritis Rheum. 2006;54(5):1529–35.

26. Kim HJ, Yoon HJ, Kim BK, Kang WY, Seong SJ, Lim MS, Kim SY, Yoon YR. G protein-coupled receptor 120 signaling negatively regulates osteoclast differentiation, survival, and function. J Cell Physiol. 2016;231(4):844–51.

27. Gao B, Huang Q, Jie Q, Lu WG, Wang L, Li XJ, Sun Z, Hu YQ, Chen L, Liu BH, et al. GPR120: a bi-potential mediator to modulate the osteogenic and adipogenic differentiation of BMMSCs. Sci Rep. 2015;5:14080.

28. Wei L, Fleming BC, Sun X, Teeple E, Wu W, Jay GD, Elsaid KA, Luo J, Machan JT, Chen Q. Comparison of differential biomarkers of osteoarthritis with and without posttraumatic injury in the Hartley guinea pig model. J Orthop Res. 2010;28(7):900–6.

29. Elsaid KA, Jay GD, Chichester CO. Reduced expression and proteolytic susceptibility of lubricin/superficial zone protein may explain early elevation in the coefficient of friction in the joints of rats with antigen-induced arthritis. Arthritis Rheum. 2007;56(1):108–16.

30. Kanbe K, Takagishi K, Chen Q. Stimulation of matrix metalloprotease 3 release from human chondrocytes by the interaction of stromal cell-derived factor 1 and CXC chemokine receptor 4. Arthritis Rheum. 2002;46(1):130–7.

31. Ohashi K, Parker JL, Ouchi N, Higuchi A, Vita JA, Gokce N, Pedersen AA, Kalthoff C, Tullin S, Sams A, et al. Adiponectin promotes macrophage polarization toward an anti-inflammatory phenotype. J Biol Chem. 2010; 285(9):6153–60.

32. Wu CL, Kimmerling KA, Little D, Guilak F. Serum and synovial fluid lipidomic profiles predict obesity-associated osteoarthritis, synovitis, and wound repair. Sci Rep. 2017;7:44315.

33. Trayhurn P, Denyer G. Mining microarray datasets in nutrition: expression of the GPR120 (n-3 fatty acid receptor/sensor) gene is down-regulated in human adipocytes by macrophage secretions. J Nutr Sci. 2012;1:e3.

34. Rai MF, Hashimoto S, Johnson EE, Janiszak KL, Fitzgerald J, Heber-Katz E, Cheverud JM, Sandell LJ. Heritability of articular cartilage regeneration and its association with ear wound healing in mice. Arthritis Rheum. 2012;64(7):2300–10.

35. Bay-Jensen AC, Reker D, Kjelgaard-Petersen CF, Mobasheri A, Karsdal MA, Ladel C, Henrotin Y, Thudium CS. Osteoarthritis year in review 2015: soluble biomarkers and the BIPED criteria. Osteoarthritis Cartilage. 2016;24(1):9–20.

36. Bauer DC, Hunter DJ, Abramson SB, Attur M, Corr M, Felson D, Heinegard D, Jordan JM, Kepler TB, Lane NE, et al. Classification of osteoarthritis biomarkers: a proposed approach. Osteoarthritis Cartilage. 2006;14(8):723–7.

37. Kraus VB, Burnett B, Coindreau J, Cottrell S, Eyre D, Gendreau M, Gardiner J, Garnero P, Hardin J, Henrotin Y, et al. Application of biomarkers in the development of drugs intended for the treatment of osteoarthritis. Osteoarthritis Cartilage. 2011;19(5):515–42.

38. Thijssen E, van Caam A, van der Kraan PM. Obesity and osteoarthritis, more than just wear and tear: pivotal roles for inflamed adipose tissue and dyslipidaemia in obesity-induced osteoarthritis. Rheumatology. 2015;54(4):588–600.

39. Berenbaum F. Osteoarthritis as an inflammatory disease (osteoarthritis is not osteoarthrosis!). Osteoarthritis Cartilage. 2013;21(1):16–21.

40. Daghestani HN, Kraus VB. Inflammatory biomarkers in osteoarthritis. Osteoarthritis Cartilage. 2015;23(11):1890–6.

41. King LK, Henneicke H, Seibel MJ, March L, Anandacoomarsmy A. Association of adipokines and joint biomarkers with cartilage-modifying effects of weight loss in obese subjects. Osteoarthritis Cartilage. 2015;23(3):397–404.

11

Effect of subcutaneous tocilizumab treatment on work/housework status in biologic-naïve rheumatoid arthritis patients using inverse probability of treatment weighting: FIRST ACT-SC study

Yoshiya Tanaka[1*], Hideto Kameda[2], Kazuyoshi Saito[1,3], Yuko Kaneko[4], Eiichi Tanaka[5], Shinsuke Yasuda[6], Naoto Tamura[7], Keishi Fujio[8], Takao Fujii[9], Toshihisa Kojima[10], Tatsuhiko Anzai[11], Chikuma Hamada[12^], Yoshihisa Fujino[1], Shinya Matsuda[1] and Hitoshi Kohsaka[13]

Abstract

Background: Following the onset of rheumatoid arthritis (RA), patients experience a functional decline caused by various joint symptoms which affects their activities of daily living and can lead to reduced work productivity. We evaluated the effect of a 52-week treatment with tocilizumab by subcutaneous injection (TCZ-SC) among biologic-naive Japanese house workers (HWs) and paid workers (PWs) with RA in a real-world clinical practice.

Methods: This multicenter, observational, prospective study enrolled 377 and 347 RA patients into TCZ-SC and conventional synthetic disease-modifying antirheumatic drugs (csDMARDs)-alone groups, respectively. The primary endpoint was the change in percentage of overall work impairment (OWI) among PWs at week 52 assessed using the Work Productivity and Activity Impairment Questionnaire (WPAI). Inverse probability of treatment weighting analyses were used to compare treatments. The Work Functioning Impairment Scale, disease activity, quality of life (QOL) measures, and safety were also assessed.

Results: The weighted change in OWI from baseline for PWs was −18.9% (TCZ-SC group) and −19.0% (csDMARDs group) at week 52, without a significant between-group difference (adjusted treatment difference 0.1, 95% confidence interval (CI) −6.3 to 6.5; $P = 0.978$). Changes in WPAI activity impairment in the overall group (between-group difference −6.4, 95% CI −10.7 to −2.2; $P = 0.003$) and HWs (−9.5, 95% CI − 16.0 to −2.9; $P = 0.005$) were significantly better with TCZ-SC than with csDMARDs at week 52. TCZ-SC-treated HWs showed significant improvement in all QOL assessments (Frenchay Activities Index, EuroQol 5 Dimension (EQ-5D), Japanese Health Assessment Questionnaire Disability Index (HAQ-DI), and 6-item Kessler scale (K6)) at week 52; PWs did not show any between-group differences for these QOL measures. Disease activity (Disease Activity Score 28-erythrocyte sedimentation rate, Clinical Disease Activity Index, and Simplified Disease Activity Index) and QOL measures (EQ-5D, HAQ-DI, and K6) improved over time in the overall group. No new safety concerns were raised with TCZ-SC.

(Continued on next page)

* Correspondence: tanaka@med.uoeh-u.ac.jp
^Deceased
[1]University of Occupational and Environmental Health, 1-1 Iseigaoka, Yahatanishi-ku, Kitakyushu, Fukuoka 807-0804, Japan
Full list of author information is available at the end of the article

(Continued from previous page)

Conclusions: Despite the lack of differences in OWI between groups at week 52, the overall group (particularly HWs) receiving TCZ-SC in addition to csDMARDs showed significant improvements in activity impairment, disease activity, and QOL versus those receiving csDMARDs alone. This study may promote the evaluation of work productivity improvements in HWs and PWs by RA treatment.

Keywords: Disease activity, Work disability, Quality of life, Rheumatoid arthritis, Tocilizumab,

Background

The decrease in work productivity caused by rheumatoid arthritis (RA), whether it be for paid work or housework, has been gaining increasing attention [1–3]. Participation in work-related activities was added as one of the overarching principles of the primary goals of RA treatment [4]. It is estimated that, 6 months after the onset of RA, patients experience functional decline secondary to joint symptoms caused by joint inflammation and cartilage destruction. This not only affects activities of daily living, such as home activities, recreation, and social relations, but also results in reduced work productivity among house workers (HWs) and paid workers (PWs) [5–10]. Furthermore, it has been reported that, in Japanese patients with RA, work productivity and activity impairment are strongly correlated with the extent of physical disability and quality of life (QOL) [11].

The assessment methods for work productivity status are absenteeism (the decrease in number of actual working days by disease), presenteeism (the loss in the demonstration of the subject's original working ability by disease activity), and overall work impairment (OWI; the sum of absenteeism and presenteeism). The Work Productivity and Activity Impairment Questionnaire (WPAI) is one of the recommended assessment methods for work productivity in RA patients [12, 13].

Recent advancements in the understanding of the molecular and cellular mechanisms of RA have led to the identification of novel targets and the development of effective biologic agents, such as tumor necrosis factor inhibitors [14] and anti-interleukin (IL)-6 receptor antibodies [15]. Tocilizumab (TCZ) is an anti-IL-6 receptor antibody that blocks the IL-6 receptor and inhibits the binding between IL-6 and its receptor. TCZ (in solution for intravenous administration) was approved for the treatment of RA in Japan in April 2008, in Europe in 2009, and in the US in 2010. Additionally, TCZ by subcutaneous injection (TCZ-SC) was approved in Japan in March 2013; thus, there are now two formulations available for RA patients.

No clinical studies have reported on the efficacy of TCZ in improving work productivity, either for paid work or housework, among RA patients. Therefore, in this study, we evaluated the effect of TCZ-SC based on improvements in work productivity and activity impairment among biologic-naive Japanese HWs and PWs with RA in a real-world clinical practice.

Methods

Study design

This was a multicenter, observational, prospective study in which patients were enrolled by central registration from 82 participating centers in Japan. The planned study period spanned from October 2013 to September 2015. The planned observation period was from October 2013 to December 2017.

The treatment period was 104 weeks for the TCZ-SC ± conventional synthetic disease-modifying antirheumatic drugs (csDMARDs) group, and 52 weeks for the csDMARD-alone group. As the main report of this research, we focus on reporting the comparison between treatment groups at 52 weeks.

Patients

The inclusion criteria were: diagnosis of RA according to the 2010 American College of Rheumatology (ACR)/European League Against Rheumatism (EULAR) 2010 Classification Criteria; previous treatment with more than one csDMARD; performing remunerated work as an employee of a given company or family business (i.e., PW), or performing a central role in the housework within a household (i.e., HW); Disease Activity Score in 28 joints using the erythrocyte sedimentation rate (DAS28-ESR) ≥ 3.2; biologic-naive; prescribed TCZ-SC for the first time; receiving a csDMARD (except for tofacitinib) dose increase; receiving a csDMARD (except for tofacitinib) as add-on therapy; switching to a csDMARD (except for tofacitinib) treatment from other csDMARD(s); and written informed consent. Patients with any contraindication for use of the drugs evaluated in this study and those judged as ineligible for participation in this study by the investigators were excluded.

Study oversight and conduct

Ethical approval was obtained from the institutional review board of each institution. The study was conducted in accordance with the Declaration of Helsinki and "Ethical Guidelines for Clinical Research" of the Ministry of Health, Labour and Welfare. Urgent events, such as adverse events (AEs), were reported to the research steering committee.

Accordingly, the institutional review board and research steering committee determined the continuity of the patients in the study as well as that of the study itself. All patients provided written informed consent to participate in this study before being registered in the electronic data capturing system.

Study treatment

In the TCZ-SC ± csDMARDs group, the dose was prescribed by the treating physician according to the prescribing information in the package insert [16]. In the csDMARDs-alone group, the dose of each csDMARD was prescribed according to the prescribing information in the corresponding package insert. Starting a csDMARD alone or in combination, as well as dose changes, switching to other csDMARDs, or adding other csDMARDs was permitted in the TCZ-SC ± csDMARDs group. Dose changes, switching, or addition of another csDMARD was also permitted in the csDMARDs-alone group.

Assessments

The registration questionnaire was obtained at study registration. Patient demographic and disease characteristics were evaluated at baseline. The WPAI, Work Functioning Impairment Scale (WFun) [17], Frenchay Activities Index (FAI) [18], EuroQol 5 Dimension (EQ-5D) [19], Japanese Health Assessment Questionnaire Disability Index (HAQ-DI) [20, 21], and 6-item Kessler psychological distress scale (K6) [22] were assessed at baseline and at weeks 12, 24, and 52. DAS28-ESR, Clinical Disease Activity Index (CDAI) [23], and the Simplified Disease Activity Index (SDAI) [23] were assessed at baseline and at weeks 12, 24, 36, and 52. AEs were assessed continuously. The duration of assessments was approximately 52 weeks plus an additional 28 days (allowance).

Discontinuation criteria were as follows: 1) patient withdrawal; 2) physician's decision because of AEs; 3) patients in the TCZ-SC ± csDMARDs group who switched from TCZ-SC to other biological agents; 4) patients in the csDMARDs-alone group who started treatment with biological agents, including TCZ and/or tofacitinib; and 5) other cases judged to require discontinuation by treating physicians.

Endpoints

The primary endpoint was the change in the percentage of OWI among PWs at week 52 as assessed using the WPAI. The secondary endpoints for efficacy were as follows: change in the percentage of presenteeism (in PWs), absenteeism (in PWs), and activity impairment of daily work by WPAI (PWs and HWs); change in employment rate by WPAI (PWs); changes in WFun (PWs); and changes in disease activity by DAS28-ESR, CDAI, and remission rate. WPAI parameters were scored in the following way:

absenteeism = (hours absent from work due to RA) / (hours absent from work due to RA + hours actually worked); and percentage of OWI = absenteeism + [(1 − absenteeism) × presenteeism].

The secondary endpoints for QOL were as follows: changes in FAI among HWs; changes in EQ-5D; changes in HAQ-DI (some questions were replaced to accommodate Japanese lifestyle differences and have been validated/confirmed) [20]; and changes in K6 improvement factor.

Additional exploratory analyses were conducted to assess the relationship between characteristics and each assessment outcome. Safety was assessed based on all AEs reported.

Sample size calculation

Based on previous studies in Japan and the US reporting WPAI of PWs with RA as the main endpoint [5, 24], we assumed that the mean percentage of OWI (primary endpoint) was 30% to 40% at baseline. We also assumed that the percent change in OWI from baseline in the TCZ-SC and csDMARDs-alone groups at week 52 would be 40% and 15% (i.e., − 12% and −4.5% change from baseline considering a value of 30% at baseline), respectively. We used the Monte Carlo Simulation, repeated 10,000 times, to investigate the target population. Using the Wilcoxon rank sum test, we calculated the sample size to achieve a 5% two-sided significance level of 5% and 80% power. As a result, we estimated the need for a total of 160 PWs in both groups. Considering a possible drop out/discontinuation rate of 50% among PWs, we set the target population at 800 patients: 400 patients in the TCZ-SC ± csDMARDs group and 400 patients in the csDMARDs-alone group. Patient enrollment was continued until the number of PWs (excluding HWs) reached at least 200 in the TCZ-SC ± csDMARDs group.

Study population

Efficacy analysis sets were the intention-to-treat set (patients whose treatment plan was determined among registered patients, except for any patient who did not provide written informed consent, or duplicated patients) and the modified intention-to-treat (mITT) set (patients in the TCZ-SC or csDMARDs-alone groups who received TCZ-SC or corresponding csDMARDs one or more times, except for patients with significant protocol deviations such as erroneous registration, lacking data for efficacy evaluations, or lacking baseline data for propensity score estimation). The safety analysis set included all patients in the TCZ-SC or csDMARDs-alone groups who received TCZ-SC or the corresponding csDMARDs one or more times, respectively, among the registered patients in this study. All analyses were conducted using the mITT population.

Statistical analysis

In contrast to randomized controlled trials, it is difficult to compare the efficacy in an observational study because of the treatment selection bias. Therefore, we adjusted patient characteristics between groups using propensity scores. Propensity scores were estimated using a multivariate logistic regression model predicting treatment with TCZ-SC based on the following key variables: background (age, weight, disease duration, salary, education, and occupation); concomitant use of glucocorticoids and/or methotrexate, rheumatoid factor, anti-cyclic citrullinated peptide antibody; disease activity and severity (class, stage, DAS28-ESR, CDAI, and SDAI); and questionnaires (percentage of OWI, absenteeism, presenteeism, activity impairment, EQ-5D, HAQ-DI, and K6).

The mean change from baseline and differences between treatment groups were estimated by linear regression with a robust variance estimator adjusted by the inverse probability of treatment weighting (IPTW) method. The last observation carried forward (LOCF) method was used for missing data. The primary adjustment method for confounding was changed from propensity score matching to IPTW by the research steering committee based only on baseline information, excluding post-treatment measurement values, as prespecified in the protocol.

Sensitivity analysis for estimating propensity scores confirmed the robustness of the present analyses by the model selection method (backward selection) using the clinically significant factors and selected variables. Additionally, we performed the Wilcoxon rank sum test after propensity score matching, a stratified analysis with five strata based on propensity score and regression analyses adjusting for clinically significant factors. Data insufficiently adjusted by IPTW (i.e., methotrexate yes/no) were separately and additionally adjusted by using sensitivity analysis to avoid any effects on the primary statistics.

An exploratory, linear regression analysis was conducted to investigate background factors possibly related to activity impairment and OWI improvement in PWs. The absolute standard partial regression coefficient for each baseline factor was calculated to assess the treatment response to TCZ-SC and csDMARDs. All statistical analyses were performed using SAS 9.3 version (SAS Institute Inc., Cary, NC, USA).

Results

Patients

A total of 377 and 347 patients were enrolled in the TCZ-SC and csDMARDs-alone groups, respectively (Fig. 1). At 52 weeks, 256 and 241 patients, respectively, remained under study treatment in the TCZ-SC and csDMARDs-alone groups.

The main reasons for discontinuation in the TCZ-SC group were investigator's decision (9.3%), insufficient efficacy (6.1%), patient request (4.5%), AEs (4.2%), and patient withdrawal (1.9%). In the csDMARDs-alone group, most patients discontinued because they began treatment with a biological drug (12.4%), followed by investigator decision (11.5%), and patient request (3.7%).

At baseline (unadjusted data) in the mITT population, over 75% of patients among PWs and HWs in the TCZ-SC and csDMARDs-alone groups were women (PWs 75.4% and 78.1%, HWs 88.3% and 93.9%, respectively), had a mean (± standard deviation (SD)) age of over 51 years (PWs 51.5 ± 12.1 and 55.0 ± 11.5 years, HWs 64.5 ± 12.6 and 65.5 ± 12.0 years, respectively), and a mean (± SD) disease duration of over 4 years (PWs 5.77 ± 8.23 and 4.36 ± 5.83 years, HWs 8.09 ±10.58 and 5.99 ± 7.76 years, respectively). Regarding the Steinbrocker Stage and Class and DAS28-ESR score, disease activity was higher in both PWs and HWs in the TCZ-SC group compared with PWs and HWs in the csDMARDs-alone group. The OWI of the PWs also indicated a higher impairment in the TCZ-SC group at baseline compared with the csDMARDs-alone group (Table 1). Additional file 1 shows the baseline and clinical characteristics of the mITT population after adjustment using IPTW. Most characteristics were sufficiently adjusted for by using IPTW since the absolute value of the standardized difference was lower than 0.1. In the TCZ-SC and csDMARDs-alone groups, 74.5% and 72.1% of PWs and 94.6% and 77.0% of HWs, respectively, were women. In the TCZ-SC and csDMARDs-alone groups, the mean (± SD) age of PWs was 52.2 ± 12.1 and 53.0 ± 10.9 years, respectively, and that of HWs was 64.6 ± 11.8 and 64.8 ± 11.5 years, respectively. Results for mean disease duration were also similar after adjusting for these variables (PWs 5.27 ± 7.18 and 5.28 ± 7.08 years, HWs 6.57 ± 9.87 and 6.44 ± 8.10 years). Similar results were obtained for the overall population when comparing the adjusted and unadjusted results of TCZ-SC and csDMARDs-alone groups (Additional file 2).

Efficacy

Primary endpoint

Table 2 summarizes the results related to the mean change in the percentage of OWI using WPAI at week 52 and adjusted using IPTW. The weighted change in OWI from baseline for PWs was −18.9% in the TCZ-SC group and −19.0% in the csDMARDs-alone group at week 52, without a significant difference between groups (adjusted treatment difference 0.1%, 95% confidence interval (CI) −6.3% to 6.5%; $P = 0.978$).

Secondary endpoints for efficacy and QOL

After adjustment using IPTW, differences among PWs between the TCZ-SC and csDMARDs-alone groups in

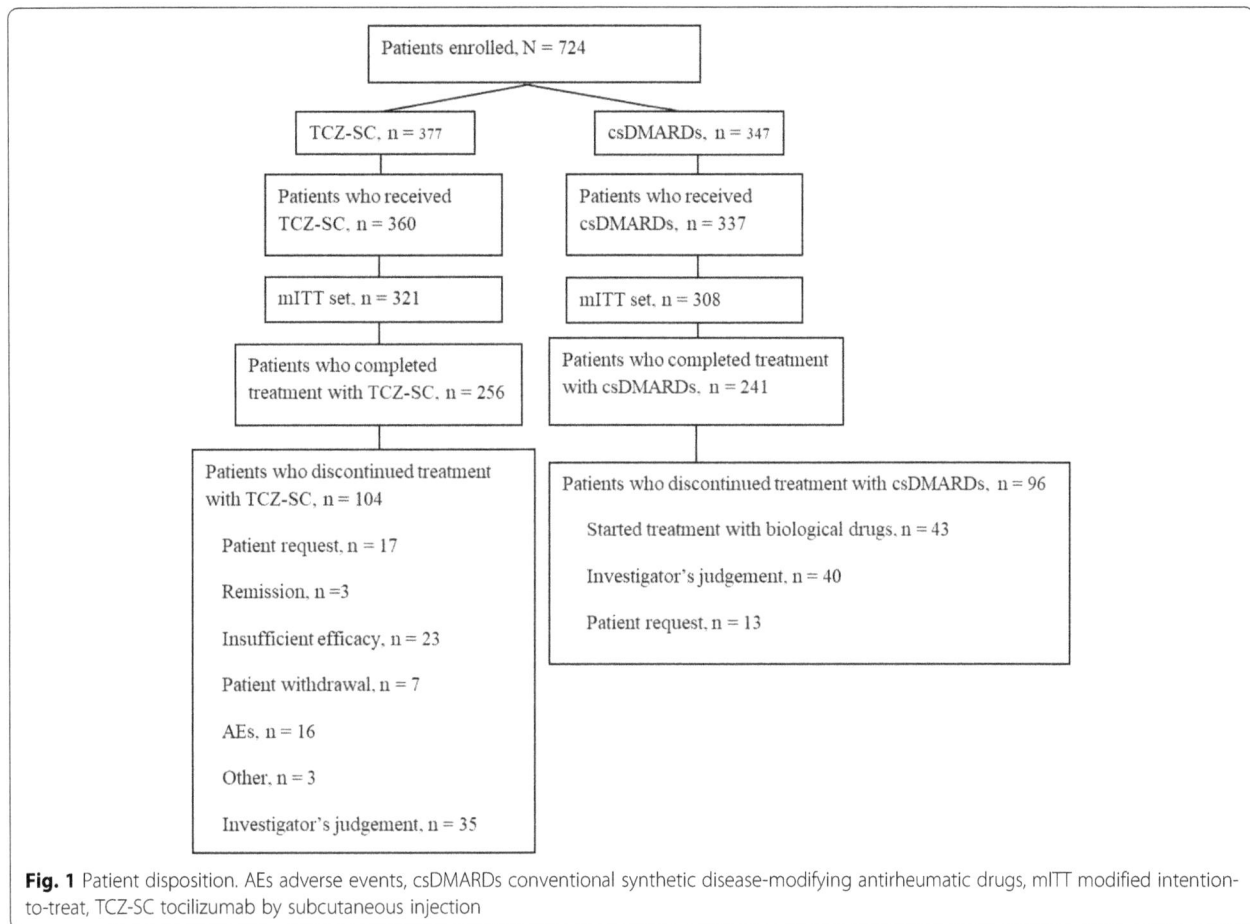

Fig. 1 Patient disposition. AEs adverse events, csDMARDs conventional synthetic disease-modifying antirheumatic drugs, mITT modified intention-to-treat, TCZ-SC tocilizumab by subcutaneous injection

the percentage of presenteeism (−0.5%, 95% CI −6.7% to 5.6%) and absenteeism (−1.1%, 95% CI −4.8% to 2.7%) at week 52 were not significantly different ($P = 0.868$ and 0.580, respectively). The changes in WPAI activity impairment in the overall group (between-group difference −6.4%, 95% CI −10.7% to −2.2%) and in HWs (−9.0%, 95% CI −16.0% to −2.9%) were significantly better in the TCZ-SC group compared with the csDMARDs-alone group at week 52 ($P = 0.003$ and 0.005, respectively).

The weighted changes by IPTW method over time in WPAI, DAS28-ESR, CDAI, and SDAI in the overall population are shown in Fig. 2a–d. For these secondary endpoints, significant differences were observed in all assessments in the overall population. Improvements were observed for WPAI and disease activity (DAS28-ESR, CDAI, and SDAI), indicating improvements in treatment efficacy from baseline to 12 weeks.

Regarding the changes in disease activity according to DAS28-ESR at week 52 (Table 2), improvements in disease activity in the overall group (between-group difference −1.344, 95% CI −1.601 to −1.087; $P < 0.001$), in PWs (−0.999, 95% CI −1.386 to −0.612; $P < 0.001$), and HWs (−1.674, 95% CI −2.050 to −1.298; $P < 0.001$) were significantly greater in the TCZ-SC group compared with the csDMARDs-alone group. Changes in disease activity according to CDAI and SDAI were only significantly different for the overall population and HWs ($P < 0.001$ for all).

The unadjusted changes in DAS28-ESR and CDAI in PWs over time indicated that disease activity decreased in both treatment groups (Fig. 3a, b). Regarding the changes in QOL measures at week 52 (Table 2), TCZ-SC-treated HWs showed significant improvement in overall QOL, as well as in FAI, EQ-5D, HAQ-DI, and K6, at week 52. PWs did not show any between-group differences for these QOL measures. There were no significant between-group differences in the changes in WFun at week 52 (0.0, 95% CI −1.3 to 1.3; $P = 0.983$).

Regarding the remission rates at week 52 (Table 3), after adjustment using IPTW and according to DAS28-ESR, significantly more patients in the overall population (67.9%), PWs (66.3%), and HWs (70.3%) treated with TCZ-SC achieved remission at week 52 ($P < 0.0001$ for all), compared with those receiving csDMARDs alone. According to CDAI and SDAI, significantly more patients in the overall population and HWs treated with TCZ-SC achieved remission at week 52 ($P < 0.0001$), compared with those receiving csDMARDs alone.

Table 1 Baseline characteristics of paid workers and house workers (unadjusted data) (modified intention-to-treat set)

	Paid worker			House worker		
	TCZ-SC group (n = 167)	csDMARDs-alone group (n = 160)	Standardized difference csDMARDs vs TCZ-SC	TCZ-SC group (n = 154)	csDMARDs-alone group (n = 148)	Standardized difference csDMARDs vs TCZ-SC
Sex, female, n (%)	126 (75.4)	125 (78.1)	0.063	136 (88.3)	139 (93.9)	0.198
Age (years), mean (SD)	51.5 (12.1)	55.0 (11.5)	0.299	64.5 (12.6)	65.5 (12.0)	0.085
Weight (kg), mean (SD)	57.01 (11.65)	56.02 (11.35)	−0.086	52.43 (9.22)	51.87 (10.16)	−0.058
Disease duration (years), mean (SD)	5.77 (8.23)	4.36 (5.83)	−0.197	8.09 (10.58)	5.99 (7.76)	−0.226
Income[a], n (%)						
< 1,000,000 yen	5 (3.0)	8 (5.0)	0.103	15 (9.7)	13 (8.8)	−0.033
1,000,000−< 2,000,000 yen	12 (7.2)	17 (10.6)	0.121	24 (15.6)	20 (13.5)	−0.059
2,000,000−< 3,000,000 yen	18 (10.8)	23 (14.4)	0.109	35 (22.7)	24 (16.2)	−0.165
3,000,000−< 5,000,000 yen	50 (29.9)	49 (30.6)	0.015	49 (31.8)	40 (27.0)	−0.105
5,000,000−< 7,000,000 yen	37 (22.2)	25 (15.6)	−0.167	17 (11.0)	19 (12.8)	0.056
≥ 7,000,000 yen	42 (25.1)	36 (22.5)	−0.062	14 (9.1)	24 (16.2)	0.216
Unknown	3 (1.8)	2 (1.3)	−0.045	0 (0.0)	8 (5.4)	0.338
Job, n (%)						
Full-time/unknown	81 (48.5)	72 (45.0)	−0.070	–	–	–
Part-time	51 (30.5)	58 (36.3)	0.121	–	–	–
Private business	35 (21.0)	30 (18.8)	−0.055	–	–	–
Housework	–	–	–	154 (100.0)	148 (100.0)	–
Methotrexate, n (%)	130 (77.8)	153 (95.6)	0.543	98 (63.6)	133 (89.9)	0.653
Steinbrocker stage, n (%)						
Stage I	69 (41.3)	71 (44.4)	0.062	33 (21.4)	55 (37.2)	0.351
Stage II	54 (32.3)	60 (37.5)	0.108	66 (42.9)	46 (31.1)	−0.246
Stage III	22 (13.2)	17 (10.6)	−0.079	30 (19.5)	21 (14.2)	−0.142
Stage IV	22 (13.2)	12 (7.5)	−0.187	25 (16.2)	26 (17.6)	0.036
Steinbrocker class, n (%)						
Class 1	43 (25.7)	59 (36.9)	0.242	24 (15.6)	40 (27.0)	0.282
Class 2	114 (68.3)	95 (59.4)	−0.186	107 (69.5)	97 (65.5)	−0.084
Class 3/4	10 (6.0)	6 (3.8)	−0.104	23 (14.9)	11 (7.4)	−0.240
DAS28-ESR, mean (SD)	5.110 (1.261)	4.527 (0.991)	−0.514	5.546 (1.183)	4.882 (1.008)	−0.605

Table 1 Baseline characteristics of paid workers and house workers (unadjusted data) (modified intention-to-treat set) (Continued)

	Paid worker			House worker		
	TCZ-SC group (n = 167)	csDMARDs-alone group (n = 160)	Standardized difference csDMARDs vs TCZ-SC	TCZ-SC group (n = 154)	csDMARDs-alone group (n = 148)	Standardized difference csDMARDs vs TCZ-SC
CDAI, mean (SD)	23.995 (11.588)	17.823 (8.713)	−0.602	26.773 (13.514)	19.053 (10.120)	−0.647
SDAI, mean (SD)	25.902 (2.852)	19.086 (9.284)	−0.608	31.075 (26.411)	20.868 (10.805)	−0.506
Rheumatoid factor, n (%)						
Positive	112 (67.1)	100 (62.5)	−0.020	99 (64.3)	95 (64.2)	−0.150
Negative	32 (19.2)	30 (18.8)	0.020	24 (15.6)	33 (22.3)	0.150
ACPA, n (%)						
Positive	100 (59.9)	78 (48.8)	−0.104	90 (64.3)	95 (64.2)	−0.123
Negative	26 (15.6)	26 (16.3)	0.104	18 (11.7)	20 (13.5)	0.123
WPAI						
Absenteeism = 0, n (%)	117 (70.1)	118 (73.8)	0.082	–	–	–
Absenteeism > 0, n (%)	44 (26.3)	37 (23.1)	−0.075	–	–	–
Presenteeism (%), mean (SD)	45.9 (32.2)	34.8 (26.9)	−0.373	–	–	–
OWI (%), mean (SD)	48.7 (32.9)	37.0 (29.2)	−0.346	–	–	–
AI (%), mean (SD)	53.6 (31.6)	40.8 (26.7)	−0.440	58.8 (27.5)	45.2 (27.9)	−0.492
WFun, mean (SD)	16.4 (8.7)	14.0 (7.5)	−0.290	–	–	–
EQ-5D, mean (SD)	0.596 (0.140)	0.656 (0.137)	0.434	0.564 (0.152)	0.654 (0.163)	0.569
HAQ-DI, mean (SD)	0.917 (0.709)	0.643 (0.585)	−0.421	1.255 (0.759)	0.959 (0.647)	−0.419

[a]100 yen = 0.9 US$

ACPA antibodies to citrullinated peptide antigens, CDAI clinical disease activity index, csDMARD conventional synthetic disease-modifying antirheumatic drug, DAS28-ESR disease activity score in 28 joints using the erythrocyte sedimentation rate, EQ-5D EuroQol 5 dimension, HAQ-DI health assessment questionnaire disability index, SD standard deviation, SDAI simplified disease activity index, TCZ-SC tocilizumab by subcutaneous injection, WFun work functioning impairment scale, WPAI work productivity and activity impairment questionnaire

Table 2 Adjusted mean change in WPAI, Work Functioning Impairment Scale, DAS28-ESR, and QOL measures at week 52

	PWs or HWs	TCZ-SC group	csDMARDs-alone group	Difference between TCZ-SC group − csDMARDs-alone group (95% confidence interval)	P value (TCZ-SC group vs csDMARDs-alone group)
WPAI					
OWI (%)	PWs	−18.9	−19.0	0.1 (−6.3, 6.5)	0.978
Presenteeism (%)	PWs	−17.7	−17.2	−0.5 (−6.7, 5.6)	0.868
Absenteeism (%)	PWs	−7.1	−6.0	−1.1 (−4.8, 2.7)	0.580
Activity impairment (%)	Overall	−22.3	−15.8	−6.4 (−10.7, −2.2)	0.003
	PWs	−22.5	−19.4	−3.1 (−8.8, 2.7)	0.293
	HWs	−24.0	−14.5	−9.5 (−16.0, −2.9)	0.005
Work Functioning Impairment Scale					
WFun	PWs	−3.2	−3.2	0.0 (−1.3, 1.3)	0.983
Disease activity					
DAS28-ESR	Overall	−2.732	−1.388	−1.344 (−1.601, −1.087)	< 0.001
	PWs	−2.576	−1.577	−0.999 (−1.386, −0.612)	< 0.001
	HWs	−2.953	−1.279	−1.674 (−2.050, −1.298)	< 0.001
CDAI	Overall	−13.932	−10.340	−3.591 (−5.440, −1.742)	< 0.001
	PWs	−12.951	−11.679	−1.272 (−3.484, 0.939)	0.259
	HWs	−15.399	−9.427	−5.972 (−8.964, −2.980)	< 0.001
SDAI	Overall	−16.014	−11.521	−4.494 (−6.528, −2.459)	< 0.001
	PWs	−14.117	−12.338	−1.778 (−4.163, 0.607)	0.143
	HWs	−18.391	−11.388	−7.003 (−10.507, −3.499)	< 0.001
QOL					
FAI	HWs	1.8	0.7	1.0 (0.0, 2.1)	0.054
EQ-5D	Overall	0.147	0.092	0.055 (0.023, 0.086)	< 0.001
	PWs	0.154	0.123	0.031 (−0.015, 0.077)	0.182
	HWs	0.162	0.075	0.087 (0.036, 0.137)	< 0.001
HAQ-DI	Overall	−0.355	−0.238	−0.117 (−0.207, −0.027)	0.011
	PWs	−0.349	−0.286	−0.063 (−0.176, 0.050)	0.274
	HWs	−0.381	−0.226	−0.155 (−0.305, −0.005)	0.042
K6	Overall	−2.2	−1.1	−1.2 (−1.8, −0.6)	< 0.001
	PWs	−1.9	−1.2	−0.6 (− 1.3, 0.0)	0.065
	HWs	−3.0	−1.1	−1.8 (−2.9, −0.8)	< 0.001

Adjusted-weight analysis by inverse probability treatment weighting method
Last observation carried forward method was applied for missing data due to patient discontinuation
CDAI clinical disease activity index, *csDMARD* conventional synthetic disease-modifying antirheumatic drug, *DAS28-ESR* disease activity score in 28 joints using the erythrocyte sedimentation rate, *EQ-5D* EuroQol 5 dimension, *FAI* Frenchay activities index, *HAQ-DI* health assessment questionnaire disability index, *HW* house worker, *K6* 6-item Kessler psychological distress scale, *OWI* overall work impairment, *PW* paid worker, *QOL* quality of life, *SDAI* simplified disease activity index, *TCZ-SC* tocilizumab by subcutaneous injection, *WFun* work functioning impairment scale, *WPAI* work productivity and activity impairment questionnaire

Figure 2e–g shows the weighted mean changes in EQ-5D, HAQ-DI, and K6 over time in the overall population. There were improvements in QOL assessments in both treatment groups. Figure 3c shows the unadjusted changes of HAQ-DI in PWs over time. Body function, as measured by HAQ-DI, improved from baseline in both groups as well.

Additionally, we conducted exploratory analyses to identify factors possibly related to the differences in efficacy results of activity impairment (Table 4) and OWI (Table 5) and the treatment received. Regarding overall activity impairment outcomes, all parameters analyzed were significantly related to TCZ-SC treatment. However, HAQ-DI, CDAI, SDAI, and K6 did not show a significant relationship with csDMARDs alone treatment. Regarding overall work impairment outcomes, all parameters analyzed, except for K6 and CDAI, were significantly related to TCZ-SC treatment;

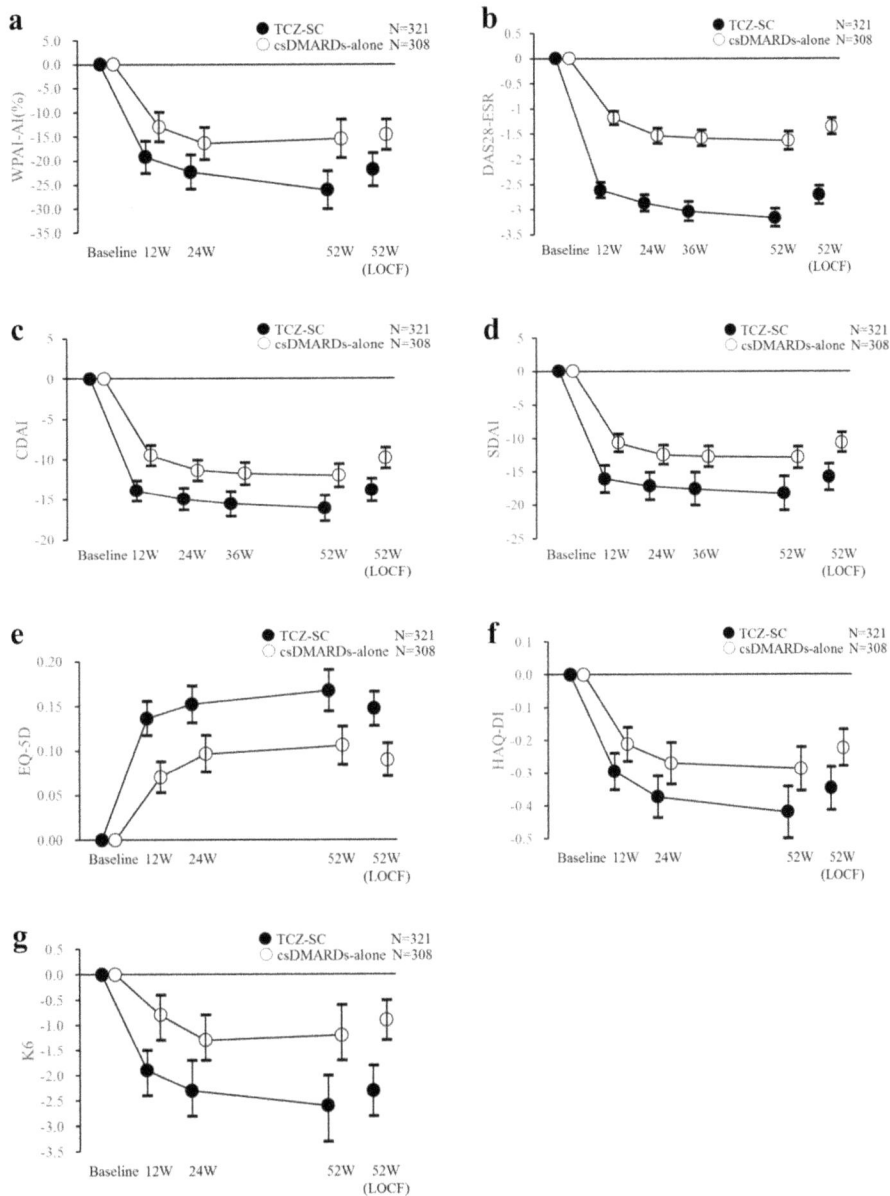

Fig. 2 Mean change in WPAI-AI, DAS28-ESR, CDAI, SDAI, EQ-5D, HAQ-DI, and K6 over time. Mean change from baseline and 95% confidence interval in (**a**) WPAI-AI, (**b**) DAS28-ESR, (**c**) CDAI, (**d**) SDAI, (**e**) EQ-5D, (**f**) HAQ-DI, and (**g**) K6 over time (overall population) adjusted using the inverse probability of treatment weighting (IPTW) method. AI activity impairment, CDAI clinical disease activity index, csDMARDs conventional synthetic disease-modifying antirheumatic drugs, DAS28-ESR disease activity score in 28 joints using the erythrocyte sedimentation rate, EQ-5D EuroQol 5 dimension, HAQ-DI health assessment questionnaire, K6 6-item Kessler psychological distress scale, LOCF last observation carried forward, SDAI simplified disease activity index, TCZ-SC tocilizumab by subcutaneous injection, W weeks, WPAI Work Productivity and Activity Impairment

furthermore, all parameters analyzed, except for CDAI and SDAI, were significantly related to csDMARD treatment.

Safety and adverse events

The results for AEs are summarized in Table 6. The most frequent AEs in the TCZ-SC group ($n = 358$) were nasopharyngitis (15 (4.2%)), stomatitis (11 (3.1%)), liver dysfunction (8 (2.2%)), and leukopenia (11 (3.1%)). In the csDMARDs group ($n = 336$), the most frequent AEs were nasopharyngitis (13 (3.9%)) and liver dysfunction (11 (3.3%)).

Discussion

The present study is the first to assess the effect of TCZ-SC and/or csDMARDs on WPAI in PWs and HWs among Japanese patients with RA. We did not identify any significant difference between PWs treated with TCZ-SC and/or

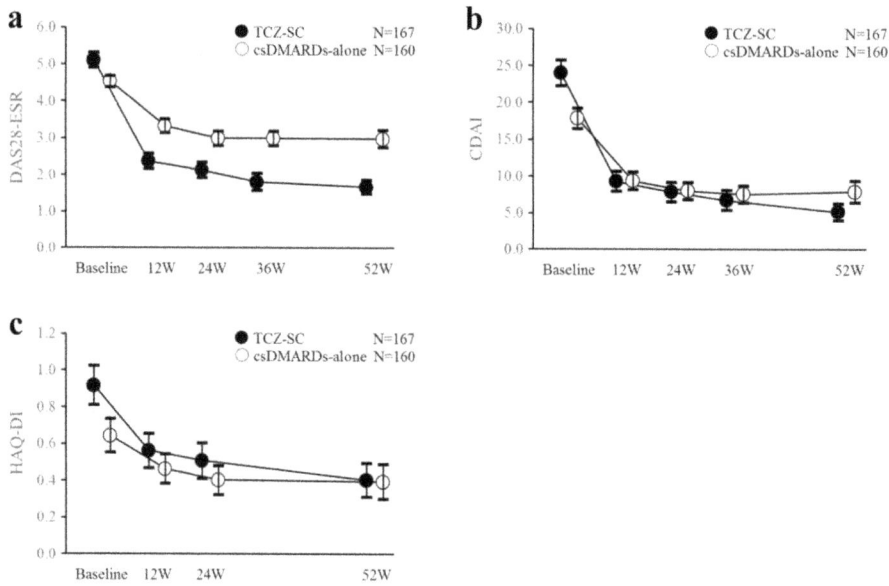

Fig. 3 Mean change (unadjusted) in DAS28-ESR, CDAI, and HAQ-DI among paid workers. Unadjusted mean change from baseline and 95% confidence interval in (**a**) DAS28-ESR, (**b**) CDAI, and (**c**) HAQ-DI. CDAI clinical disease activity index, csDMARDs conventional synthetic disease-modifying antirheumatic drugs, DAS28-ESR disease activity score in 28 joints using the erythrocyte sedimentation rate, HAQ-DI Health Assessment Questionnaire Disability Index, TCZ-SC tocilizumab by subcutaneous injection, W weeks

csDMARDs in terms of the change in OWI according to the WPAI at 52 weeks. However, we did observe an improvement in OWI from baseline in both treatment groups, meaning that RA treatment intervention was effective in decreasing disease activity, improving function, and improving overall QOL. These findings are consistent with a previous, large-scale study that evaluated the effects of adalimumab on WPAI in Japanese RA patients [5]. Previous studies of etanercept plus methotrexate in Latin America [25] and Asia [26]

showed similar improvements in patient-reported outcomes, including WPAI. A previous study comparing baricitinib with placebo and adalimumab reported statistically significant improvements in absenteeism ($P \leq$ 0.05), presenteeism ($P \leq 0.001$), and work productivity loss ($P \leq 0.001$) with baricitinib compared with placebo; however, improvements compared with adalimumab were not statistically significant at week 52 [27].

Despite the result in OWI in the present study, improvement in the percentage of activity impairment in

Table 3 Remission rate in each group by DAS28-ESR, CDAI, and SDAI

Remission rate	PWs or HWs	TCZ-SC group, n (%)	csDMARDs-alone group, n (%)	Odds ratio for TCZ-SC group/csDMARDs-alone group (95% confidence interval)	P value (TCZ-SC group vs csDMARDs-alone group)
DAS28-ESR	Overall	205.0 (67.9)	64.6 (21.7)	6.778 (4.508, 10.189)	< 0.0001
	PWs	104.1 (66.3)	39.7 (25.5)	5.689 (3.146, 10.287)	< 0.0001
	HWs	102.0 (70.3)	22.8 (16.1)	9.153 (4.814, 17.403)	< 0.0001
CDAI	Overall	125.5 (39.2)	58.5 (19.2)	2.549 (1.631, 3.982)	< 0.0001
	PWs	62.4 (37.3)	43.0 (27.1)	1.564 (0.860, 2.845)	0.1427
	HWs	70.2 (45.9)	16.1 (11.1)	5.635 (2.757, 11.516)	< 0.0001
SDAI	Overall	132.1 (41.8)	57.4 (19.1)	2.855 (1.828, 4.458)	< 0.0001
	PWs	65.8 (40.1)	41.6 (26.5)	1.811 (0.991, 3.309)	0.0535
	HWs	73.0 (48.1)	16.1 (11.3)	6.052 (2.981, 12.288)	< 0.0001

Adjusted odds ratio by the logistic regression model using last observation carried forward; adjusted-weight analysis by inverse probability treatment weighting method
Remission was defined as DAS28-ESR < 2.6, CDAI ≤2.8, and SDAI ≤3.3
CDAI clinical disease activity index, csDMARD conventional synthetic disease-modifying antirheumatic drug, DAS28-ESR disease activity score in 28 joints using the erythrocyte sedimentation rate, HW house worker, PW paid worker, SDAI simplified disease activity index, TCZ-SC tocilizumab by subcutaneous injection

Table 4 Exploratory analysis of relationships between overall activity impairment outcomes and type of drug received

Activity impairment measures	TCZ-SC group				csDMARDs-alone group			
	n	Standardized regression coefficient	95% CI	P value	n	Standardized regression coefficient	95% CI	P value
Presenteeism (%)	143	−0.4861	−0.6470, −0.3252	< 0.0001	148	−0.4328	−0.5887, −0.2769	< 0.0001
Overall work impairment (%)	143	−0.4819	−0.6437, −0.3202	< 0.0001	148	−0.3913	−0.5491, −0.2336	< 0.0001
Activity impairment (%)	143	−0.6345	−0.7747, −0.4943	< 0.0001	148	−0.6486	−0.7876, −0.5096	< 0.0001
HAQ-DI	143	−0.4828	−0.6415, −0.3241	< 0.0001	148	−0.1584	−0.3360, 0.0201	0.0815
EQ-5D	143	0.3635	0.1960, 0.5311	< 0.0001	148	0.3181	0.1446, 0.4916	0.0004
DAS28-ESR	143	−0.3305	−0.4950, −0.1661	0.0001	148	−0.1802	−0.3533, −0.0072	0.0414
CDAI	143	−0.1950	−0.3674, −0.0226	0.0270	148	−0.1127	−0.2819, 0.0564	0.1897
SDAI	143	−0.2289	−0.4003, −0.0576	0.0092	148	−0.1113	−0.2810, 0.0585	0.1971
WFun	143	−0.3549	−0.5266, −0.1832	< 0.0001	148	−0.1680	−0.3353, −0.0007	0.0491
K6	143	−0.1895	−0.3661, −0.0130	0.0355	148	−0.1497	−0.3216, 0.0222	0.0873

CDAI clinical disease activity index, *CI* confidence interval, *csDMARD* conventional synthetic disease-modifying antirheumatic drug, *DAS28-ESR* disease activity score in 28 joints using the erythrocyte sedimentation rate, *EQ-5D* EuroQol 5 dimension, *HAQ-DI* health assessment questionnaire disability index, *K6* 6-item Kessler psychological distress scale, *SDAI* simplified disease activity index, *TCZ-SC* tocilizumab by subcutaneous injection, *WFun* work functioning impairment scale

the overall population and among HWs was significantly better in the TCZ-SC group compared with the csDMARDs-alone group at week 52. This difference between treatment groups remained significant after adjusting for baseline characteristics using the IPTW method. This finding shows that, compared with the csDMARDs-alone treatment, TCZ-SC treatment resulted in improvement in disease activity (CDAI, SDAI, and DAS28) and significant improvement in QOL (EQ-5D, HAQ-DI, and K6). A recent, 48-week, observational study on adalimumab in Japan, focusing on work-related outcomes, showed that, compared with baseline, adalimumab treatment significantly improved measures of productivity loss due to absenteeism, presenteeism, OWI, and activity impairment in RA patients in all

employment types, including PWs and HWs ($P < 0.01$) [28]. A fairly recent observational study in the US focused on work and activity impairment in employed moderate to severe RA patients and showed that etanercept led to significant reductions in overall work and activity impairment ($P \leq 0.0001$) [1]. Furthermore, results of past studies have shown that total body inflammation and fatigue can be suppressed by inhibiting IL-6 [29]. In the present study, both clinical indexes and daily life (activity impairment) tended to improve in HWs and even in PWs. Although these changes did not reach statistical significance, these tendencies aligned with the results reported in previous studies. We consider that improvement in fatigue affected the improvement in activity impairment (daily life).

Table 5 Exploratory analysis of the relationships between overall work impairment outcomes and type of drug received

Work impairment measures	TCZ-SC group				csDMARDs-alone group			
	n	Standardized regression coefficient	95% CI	P value	n	Standardized regression coefficient	95% CI	P value
Presenteeism (%)	143	−0.5751	−0.7214, −0.4289	< 0.0001	147	−0.6999	−0.8240, −0.5758	< 0.0001
Overall work impairment (%)	143	−0.5950	−0.7393, −0.4507	< 0.0001	147	−0.6845	−0.8094, −0.5595	< 0.0001
Activity impairment (%)	143	−0.4754	−0.6287, −0.3221	< 0.0001	147	−0.5008	−0.6562, −0.3453	< 0.0001
HAQ-DI	143	−0.4107	−0.5707, −0.2508	< 0.0001	147	−0.1920	−0.3696, −0.0145	0.0343
EQ-5D	143	0.2840	0.1164, 0.4516	0.0011	147	0.2872	0.1126, 0.4618	0.0014
DAS28-ESR	143	−0.2961	−0.4581, −0.1342	0.0004	147	−0.2434	−0.4140, −0.0729	0.0055
CDAI	143	−0.1629	−0.3320, 0.0061	0.0587	147	−0.1608	−0.3287, 0.0070	0.0602
SDAI	143	−0.2030	−0.3709, −0.0351	0.0182	147	−0.1639	−0.3321, 0.0043	0.0560
WFun	143	−0.3748	−0.5403, −0.2092	< 0.0001	147	−0.1875	−0.3544, −0.0206	0.0280
K6	143	−0.1408	−0.3142, 0.0327	0.1108	147	−0.2002	−0.3704, − 0.0300	0.0215

Adjusted for sex, age, disease duration, job type, use of methotrexate, Steinbrocker stage, and Steinbrocker class
CDAI clinical disease activity index, *CI* confidence interval, *csDMARD* conventional synthetic disease-modifying antirheumatic drug, *DAS28-ESR* disease activity score in 28 joints using the erythrocyte sedimentation rate, *EQ-5D* EuroQol 5 dimension, *HAQ-DI* health assessment questionnaire disability index, *K6* 6-item Kessler psychological distress scale, *SDAI* simplified disease activity index, *TCZ-SC* tocilizumab by subcutaneous injection, *WFun* work functioning impairment scale

Table 6 Summary of adverse events in the safety analysis set

	TCZ-SC group, n (%)	csDMARDs-alone group, n (%)
n	358	336
AEs	127 (35.5)	99 (29.5)
Drug-related AEs	85 (23.7)	–
Serious AEs	32 (8.9)	11 (3.3)
Serious drug-related AEs	21 (5.9)	–
AEs leading to discontinuation of study treatment	33 (9.2)	28 (8.3)
Drug-related AEs leading to discontinuation of study treatment	29 (8.1)	–

AE adverse event, *csDMARD* conventional synthetic disease-modifying antirheumatic drug, *TCZ-SC* tocilizumab by subcutaneous injection

In the present study, according to DAS28-ESR, significantly more patients in the overall population, as well as PWs and HWs, treated with TCZ-SC achieved remission at week 52 ($P < 0.0001$ for all) compared with those receiving csDMARDs alone. However, by CDAI and SDAI, only those in the overall population and HWs treated with TCZ-SC achieved remission at week 52 ($P < 0.0001$). A study by Radner et al. that assessed the benefit of remission over low disease activity in RA showed that patients who achieved remission achieved better function, health-related QOL, and productivity [30].

Regarding the main differences in baseline characteristics between groups by type of work performed, HWs had greater disease severity at baseline than PWs. Similar findings were reported previously [5]. Although a tendency for improvement was observed in terms of other work productivity indices and QOL measures, no differences within the groups were observed for PWs, and a remarkable improvement in QOL measures was observed among HWs. The greater disease severity among HWs may be the reason this population experienced significantly greater improvements in overall QOL measures at week 52 compared with PWs.

An improvement in work productivity/activity impairment could be determined by differences in the treatment received as shown by the results of the presented analysis. Additionally, differences in disease severity, duration, treatment, and working conditions between PWs and HWs at baseline might have also contributed to this result. Similar conclusions were drawn in the study by Takeuchi et al. [5]. Furthermore, differences in the mechanical load on the affected joints between PWs and HWs could also be attributable to the differences in work productivity/activity impairment between PWs and HWs receiving TCZ-SC in addition to csDMARDs compared with those receiving csDMARDs alone.

Regarding the exploratory results, among PWs factors related to symptom improvement differed by study drug according to the results for HAQ-DI. These results indicated that TCZ-SC administration to patients with high HAQ-DI at baseline might result in greater improvement in work productivity and activity impairment.

The planned method for the primary analysis was changed from propensity score matching to IPTW to include all applicable patients in the analysis set because the planned sample size with a balanced number of patients was insufficient for propensity score matching. Propensity score matching allowed for easy calculation of the sample size and interpretation of the results; however, the feasibility of this method depended on whether the data of enrolled patients regarding the size of the matched sample and patient background were well balanced. For this reason, although we initially attempted to use propensity score matching, we decided to change the method after half of the patients were enrolled. In terms of bias, we consider that this change in the analysis method was acceptable because it was based on baseline data and not postbaseline data.

As part of the sensitivity analysis, we changed the adjustment method for estimating the propensity score, performed adjusted analysis with propensity score matching, used linear regression models adjusting for clinically significant factors, and performed subgroup analysis by unbalanced factors. These results were consistent with the primary results, and the robustness of the primary analysis was confirmed.

The AEs reported in the present study were in line with those previously reported for TCZ-SC in a real-world setting [31, 32]. Thus, no new safety concerns were raised, and TCZ-SC was considered a safe treatment option for Japanese RA patients.

This study had several limitations. First, the primary adjustment method for confounding was changed from propensity score matching to IPTW based on baseline data and not postbaseline data. However, we cannot deny the possibility of residual confounding effects related to the observational study design. Second, this study was conducted in a real-world clinical practice setting, and no specific criteria to initiate treatment with TCZ were applied at any of the 82 participating centers. Additionally, the dose in the TCZ-SC ± csDMARDs group was prescribed by the treating physician according to the prescribing information in the package insert; thus, we had no control over the doses prescribed. This may have affected the lower limit data of WPAI by causing a "floor effect"; in other words, patients with a low score may not have been able to show sufficient improvement. Third, we did not specifically collect information on whether a treat-to-target approach was used. However, the physicians who participated in this study were internal medicine specialists with extensive experience in the management of RA. They assessed patients at every visit (every 1–3 months). Therefore, we consider that all the patients were managed according to a treat-to-target approach. Fourth, PWs are exposed to compelling power (force) depending on the nature of the work they perform; thus, we could hardly confirm the difference between groups in terms of medical treatment. Conversely, HWs can determine their work activity level at will; thus, differences between groups in terms of the effect of medical treatment on QOL and activity level occurred easily. Fifth, WPAI is not adequate to evaluate the productivity of HWs as it was developed specifically for PWs. WPAI indexes, other than activity impairment, cannot be calculated in HWs. The other indexes are considered valid for all patients regardless of whether they are PWs or HWs. Finally, we hypothesized that the observed differences in QOL outcomes for HWs compared with PWs were related to a worst disease status in this subpopulation at baseline. Given the lack of treatment blinding, we cannot rule out other possible reasons for these outcomes such as the psychological bias and the potential emotional component related to initiating a novel treatment (e.g., biologics) that may be judged more effective than the conventional treatments. This may have affected the objectivity of the responses to the questionnaire measurements for QOL in HWs. Nevertheless, all the subjective components of CDAI and SDAI and physician's global assessment of disease activity, as well as the objective parameters, such as C-reactive peptide (CRP) and patient's global assessment of disease activity, improved with TCZ-SC in addition to csDMARDs.

Conclusions

Despite the lack of differences in OWI between groups at week 52, the overall group (particularly HWs) receiving TCZ-SC in addition to csDMARDs showed significant improvements in activity impairment, disease activity, and QOL compared with individuals receiving csDMARDs alone. The safety of TCZ-SC was acceptable for the treatment of Japanese RA patients in a real-world clinical practice. This study may help promote the evaluation of work productivity improvements in HWs and PWs by RA treatment.

Abbreviations

ACR: American College of Rheumatology; AE: Adverse event; CDAI: Clinical Disease Activity Index; CI: Confidence interval; csDMARD: Conventional synthetic disease-modifying antirheumatic drug; DAS28-ESR: Disease Activity Score 28-erythrocyte sedimentation rate; EQ-5D: EuroQol 5 Dimension; EULAR: European League Against Rheumatism; FAI: Frenchay Activities Index; HAQ-DI: Health Assessment Questionnaire Disability Index; HW: House worker; IL: Interleukin; IPTW: Inverse probability of treatment weighting; K6: 6-Item Kessler psychological distress scale; LOCF: Last observation carried forward; mITT: Modified intention-to-treat; OWI: Overall work impairment; PW: Paid worker; QOL: Quality of life; RA: Rheumatoid arthritis; SD: Standard deviation; SDAI: Simplified Disease Activity Index; TCZ: Tocilizumab; TCZ-SC: Tocilizumab by subcutaneous injection; VAS: Visual analog scale; WFun: Work Functioning Impairment Scale (Presenteeism Questionnaire); WPAI: Work Productivity and Activity Impairment Questionnaire

Acknowledgements
The authors would like to thank Hikari Chiba and Keyra Martinez Dunn, MD, of Edanz Medical Writing for providing medical writing services. Support for study management was provided by EPS Corporation. Finally, we would like to thank all of the study sites and investigators who participated in the present study.

Funding
This study was funded by Chugai Pharmaceutical (UMIN000012306) who were not involved in the design of the study, collection, analysis, and interpretation of data, or in writing the manuscript.

Authors' contributions
All authors contributed to the study protocol development. YT, HK, KS, YK, ET, SY, NT, KF, TF, TK, CH, YF, SM, and HK conducted the study. YT, HK, KS, YK, ET, SY, NT, KF, TF, TK, and HK collected the data. CH and TA performed the statistical analysis. YT, HK, CH, HK, and TA contributed to the development of this manuscript. All authors read and approved the final manuscript.

Competing interests
YT received research grants and/or speaking fees from Abbvie, Asahi Kasei Pharma, Astellas Pharma, Bristol-Myers Squibb, Chugai Pharmaceutical, Daiichi-Sankyo, Eisai, Eli Lilly, GlaxoSmithKline, Janssen, Kyowa Hakko Kirin, Mitsubishi-Tanabe Pharma, MSD, Ono Pharmaceutical, Pfizer, Sanofi, Takeda Pharmaceutical, Teijin Pharma, UCB, and YL Biologics; HK received research grants and/or speaking fees from AbbVie, Astellas Pharma, Bristol-Myers Squibb, Chugai Pharmaceutical, Eisai, Eli Lilly, Janssen, Mitsubishi-Tanabe Pharma, Novartis, Pfizer, Sanofi, and Takeda Pharmaceutical; YK received research grants, consulting fees and/or speaking fees from AbbVie, Astellas Pharma, Bristol-Myers Squibb, Chugai Pharmaceutical, Daiichi-Sankyo, Eisai, Eli Lilly, Janssen, Mitsubishi-Tanabe Pharma, Pfizer, Sanofi, and UCB; ET received consulting fees from AbbVie, Ayumi Pharmaceutical, Bristol Myers Squibb, Chugai Pharmaceutical, Eisai, Nippon Kayaku, Pfizer, Takeda Pharmaceutical, and UCB; SY received research grants and/or speaking fees from Astellas Pharma, Bristol-Myers Squibb, Chugai Pharmaceutical, Mitsubishi-Tanabe Pharma, and MSD; NT received research grants and/or speaking fees from Astellas Pharma, Asahi Kasei Pharma, Ayumi Pharmaceutical, Bristol-Myers Squibb, Chugai Pharmaceutical, Eisai, Janssen, Mitsubishi-Tanabe Pharma, and Takeda Pharmaceutical; KF received research grants, consulting fees, royalties and/or speaking fees from Astellas Pharma, Bristol-Myers Squibb, Chugai Pharmaceutical, Daiichi-Sankyo, Eisai, Integrated Development Associates, Janssen, Mitsubishi-Tanabe Pharma, Pfizer, Santen Pharmaceutical, Takeda Pharmaceutical, Taisho Toyama Pharmaceutical, and UCB; TF received research grants and/or speaking fees from AbbVie, Astellas Pharma, Daiichi Sankyo, Eisai, Mitsubishi-Tanabe Pharma, Ono Pharmaceutical, and Pfizer; TK received research grants and/or speaking fees from Ayumi Pharmaceutical, Bristol-

Myers Squibb, Chugai Pharmaceutical, Eli Lilly, Mitsubishi-Tanabe Pharma, Nippon Kayaku, Novartis, Ono Pharmaceutical, Pfizer, and Takeda Pharmaceutical; TA is an employee of EPS Corporation; CH received consulting fees from Chugai Pharmaceutical; and HK received research grants, consulting fees, and/or speaking fees from AbbVie, Asahi Kasei Pharma, Astellas Pharma, Ayumi Pharmaceutical, Bristol-Myers Squibb, Chugai Pharmaceutical, Daiichi Sankyo, Eisai, Eli Lilly, GlaxoSmithKline, Japan Blood Products Organization, Mitsubishi-Tanabe Pharma, MSD, Nippon Kayaku, Novartis, Ono Pharmaceutical, Pfizer, Takeda Pharmaceutical, and Teijin Pharma. The remaining authors declare that they have no competing interests.

Author details
[1]University of Occupational and Environmental Health, 1-1 Iseigaoka, Yahatanishi-ku, Kitakyushu, Fukuoka 807-0804, Japan. [2]Toho University, 2-22-36 Ohashi, Meguro-ku, Tokyo 153-8515, Japan. [3]Tobata General Hospital, 1-3-33 Fukuryugi, Tobata-ku, Kitakyushu, Fukuoka 804-0025, Japan. [4]Keio University School of Medicine, 35 Shinanomachi, Shinjuku-ku, Tokyo 160-8582, Japan. [5]Tokyo Women's Medical University, 10-22 Kawada-cho, Shinjuku-ku, Tokyo 162-0054, Japan. [6]Hokkaido University, N15, W7, Kita-ku, Sapporo, Hokkaido 060-8638, Japan. [7]Juntendo University School of Medicine, 2-1-1 Hongo, Bunkyo-ku, Tokyo 113-8421, Japan. [8]The University of Tokyo, 7-3-1 Hongo, Bunkyo-ku, Tokyo 113-8654, Japan. [9]Wakayama Medical University, 811-1 Kimiidera, Wakayama 641-8509, Japan. [10]Nagoya University Graduate School of Medicine, 65 Tsurumai-cho, Showa-ku, Nagoya, Aichi 466-8550, Japan. [11]EPS Corporation, 6-29 Shinogawamachi, Shinjuku-ku, Tokyo 162-0814, Japan. [12]Tokyo University of Science, 6-3-1 Niijuku, Katsushika-ku, Tokyo 125-8585, Japan. [13]Tokyo Medical and Dental University, 1-5-45 Yushima, Bunkyo-ku, Tokyo 113-8510, Japan.

References
1. Hone D, Cheng A, Watson C, Huang B, Bitman B, Huang XY, et al. Impact of etanercept on work and activity impairment in employed moderate to severe rheumatoid arthritis patients in the United States. Arthritis Care Res (Hoboken). 2013;65:1564–72.
2. Furuya H, Kasama T, Isozaki T, Umemura M, Otsuka K, Isojima S, et al. Effect of TNF antagonists on the productivity of daily work of patients with rheumatoid arthritis. J Multidiscip Healthc. 2013;6:25–30.
3. Zhang W, Sun H, Emery P, Sato R, Singh A, Freundlich B, et al. Does achieving clinical response prevent work stoppage or work absence among employed patients with early rheumatoid arthritis? Rheumatology (Oxford). 2012;51:270–4.
4. Smolen JS, Breedveld FC, Burmester GR, Bykerk V, Dougados M, Emery P, et al. Treating rheumatoid arthritis to target: 2014 update of the recommendations of an international task force. Ann Rheum Dis. 2016;75:3–15.
5. Takeuchi T, Nakajima R, Komatsu S, Yamazaki K, Nakamura T, Agata N, et al. Impact of adalimumab on work productivity and activity impairment in Japanese patients with rheumatoid arthritis: large-scale, prospective, single-cohort ANOUVEAU study. Adv Ther. 2017;34:686–702.
6. Verstappen SM. Rheumatoid arthritis and work: the impact of rheumatoid arthritis on absenteeism and presenteeism. Best Pract Res Clin Rheumatol. 2015;29:495–511.
7. Bertin P, Fagnani F, Duburcq A, Woronoff AS, Chauvin P, Cukierman G, et al. Impact of rheumatoid arthritis on career progression, productivity, and employability: the PRET study. J Bone Spine. 2016;83:47–52.
8. van Vilsteren M, Boot CR, Knol DL, van Schaardenburg D, Voskuyl AE, Steenbeek R, et al. Productivity at work and quality of life in patients with rheumatoid arthritis. BMC Musculoskelet Disord. 2015;16:107.
9. Almoallim H, Kamil A. Rheumatoid arthritis: should we shift the focus from "treat to target" to "treat to work?". Clin Rheumatol. 2013;32:285–7.
10. Rheumatoid Arthritis (RA) 2017. https://www.cdc.gov/arthritis/basics/rheumatoid-arthritis.html Accessed 2 July 2018.
11. Tanaka E, Inoue E, Hoshi D, Shidara K, Sugimoto N, Inoue Y, et al. Assessment of work productivity and activity impairment in patients with rheumatoid arthritis based on the Institute of Rheumatology Rheumatoid Arthritis (IORRA) cohort database (FRI0124). Ann Rheum Dis. 2013;72:A412.
12. Beaton DE, Dyer S, Boonen A, Verstappen SM, Escorpizo R, Lacaille DV, et al. OMERACT filter evidence supporting the measurement of at-work productivity loss as an outcome measure in rheumatology research. J Rheumatol. 2016;43:214–22.
13. Tang K, Beaton DE, Boonen A, Gignac MA, Bombardier C. Measures of work disability and productivity: rheumatoid arthritis specific work productivity survey (WPS-RA), workplace activity limitations scale (WALS), work instability scale for rheumatoid arthritis (RA-WIS), work limitations questionnaire (WLQ), and work productivity and activity impairment questionnaire (WPAI). Arthritis Care Res (Hoboken). 2011;63(Suppl 11):337–49.
14. Alghasham A, Rasheed Z. Therapeutic targets for rheumatoid arthritis: progress and promises. Autoimmunity. 2014;47:77–94.
15. Tanaka T, Narazaki M, Ogata A, Kishimoto T. A new era for the treatment of inflammatory autoimmune diseases by interleukin-6 blockade strategy. Semin Immunol. 2014;26:88–96.
16. Tocilizumab package insert for Japan, https://chugai-pharm.jp/hc/ss/pr/drug/act_via0200/pi/PDF/act_pi.pdf. Accessed 2 July 2018.
17. Fujino Y, Uehara M, Izumi H, Nagata T, Muramatsu K, Kubo T, et al. Development and validity of a work functioning impairment scale based on the Rasch model among Japanese workers. J Occup Health. 2015;57:521–31.
18. Shiratsuchi M, Saeki S, Hachisuka K. Japanese version of the self-rating Frenchay activities index and its clinical application and standard values. General Rehabilitation. 1999;27:469–74.
19. Tsuchiya A, Ikeda S, Ikegami N, Nishimura S, Sakai I, Fukuda T, et al. Estimating an EQ-5D population value set. The case of Japan. Health Econ. 2002;11:341–53.
20. Matsuda Y, Singh G, Yamanaka H, Tanaka E, Urano W, Taniguchi A, et al. Validation of a Japanese version of the Stanford health assessment questionnaire in 3,763 patients with rheumatoid arthritis. Arthritis Rheum. 2003;49:784–8.
21. Fries JF, Spitz P, Kraines RG, Holman HR. Measurement of patient outcome in arthritis. Arthritis Rheum. 1980;23:137–45.
22. Furukawa TA, Kessler R, Slade T, Andrews G. The performance of the K6 and K10 screening scales for psychological distress in the Australian National Survey of mental health and well-being. Psychol Med. 2003;33:357–62.
23. Smolen JS, Aletaha D, Bijlsma JW, Breedveld FC, Boumpas D, Burmester G, et al. Treating rheumatoid arthritis to target: recommendations of an international task force. Ann Rheum Dis. 2010;69:631–7.
24. Kavanaugh A, Smolen JS, Emery P, Purcaru O, Keystone E, Richard L, et al. Effect of certolizumab pegol with methotrexate on home and work place productivity and social activities in patients with active rheumatoid arthritis. Arthritis Rheum. 2009;61:1592–600.
25. Machado DA, Guzman RM, Xavier RM, Simon JA, Mele L, Pedersen R, et al. Open-label observation of addition of etanercept versus a conventional disease-modifying antirheumatic drug in subjects with active rheumatoid arthritis despite methotrexate therapy in the Latin American region. J Clin Rheumatol. 2014;20:25–33.
26. Bae SC, Gun SC, Mok CC, Khandker R, Nab HW, Koenig AS, et al. Improved health outcomes with etanercept versus usual DMARD therapy in an Asian population with established rheumatoid arthritis. BMC Musculoskelet Disord. 2013;8(14):13.
27. Keystone EC, Taylor PC, Tanaka Y, Gaich C, DeLozier AM, Dudek A, et al. Patient-reported outcomes from a phase 3 study of baricitinib versus placebo or adalimumab in rheumatoid arthritis: secondary analyses from the RA-BEAM study. Ann Rheum Dis. 2017;76:1853–61.
28. Tanaka Y, Yamazaki K, Nakajima R, Komatsu S, Igarashi A, Tango T, et al. Economic impact of adalimumab treatment in Japanese patients with rheumatoid arthritis from the adalimumab non-interventional trial for up-verified effects and utility (ANOUVEAU) study. Mod Rheumatol. 2018;28(1):39–47.
29. Choy EHS, Calabrese LH. Neuroendocrine and neurophysiological effects of interleukin 6 in rheumatoid arthritis. Rheumatology (Oxford). https://doi.org/10.1093/rheumatology/kex391.
30. Radner H, Smolen JS, Aletaha D. Remission in rheumatoid arthritis: benefit over low disease activity in patient-reported outcomes and costs. Arthritis Res Ther. 2014;16:R56.
31. Koike T, Harigai M, Inokuma S, Ishiguro N, Ryu J, Takeuchi T, et al. Effectiveness and safety of tocilizumab: postmarketing surveillance of 7901 patients with rheumatoid arthritis in Japan. J Rheumatol. 2014;41:15–23.
32. Yamamoto K, Goto H, Hirao K, Nakajima A, Origasa H, Tanaka K, et al. Longterm safety of tocilizumab: results from 3 years of follow-up postmarketing surveillance of 5573 patients with rheumatoid arthritis in Japan. J Rheumatol. 2015;42:1368–75.

12

The host cellular immune response to cytomegalovirus targets the endothelium and is associated with increased arterial stiffness in ANCA-associated vasculitis

Dimitrios Chanouzas[1,2]*[iD], Michael Sagmeister[1,2], Lovesh Dyall[2], Phoebe Sharp[1,2], Lucy Powley[2], Serena Johal[1,2], Jessica Bowen[2], Peter Nightingale[3], Charles J. Ferro[2,3], Matthew D. Morgan[2,4], Paul Moss[5] and Lorraine Harper[2,3,4]

Abstract

Background: Cardiovascular disease is a leading cause of death in ANCA-associated vasculitis (AAV). An expansion of $CD4^+CD28^{null}$ T cells is seen mainly in cytomegalovirus (CMV)-seropositive individuals and has been linked to increased cardiovascular disease risk in other conditions. The aims of this study were to phenotype $CD4^+CD28^{null}$ T cells in AAV with respect to their pro-inflammatory capacity and ability to target and damage the endothelium and to investigate their relationship to arterial stiffness, a marker of cardiovascular mortality.

Methods: $CD4^+CD28^{null}$ T cells were phenotyped in 53 CMV-seropositive AAV patients in stable remission and 30 age-matched CMV-seropositive healthy volunteers by flow cytometry following stimulation with CMV lysate. The expression of endothelial homing markers and cytotoxic molecules was evaluated in unstimulated $CD4^+CD28^{null}$ T cells. Arterial stiffness was measured by carotid-to-femoral pulse wave velocity (PWV) in patients with AAV.

Results: $CD4^+CD28^{null}$ T cells were CMV-specific and expressed a T helper 1 (Th1) phenotype with high levels of interferon-gamma (IFN-γ) and tumour necrosis factor-alpha (TNF-α) secretion. They also co-expressed the endothelial homing markers CX3CR1, CD49d and CD11b and cytotoxic molecules perforin and granzyme B. $CD4^+CD28^{null}$ T cells were phenotypically similar in patients with AAV and healthy volunteers but their proportion was almost twice as high in patients with AAV (11.3% [3.7–19.7] versus 6.7 [2.4–8.8]; $P = 0.022$). The size of the $CD4^+CD28^{null}$ T-cell subset was independently linked to increased PWV in AAV (0.66 m/s increase per 10% increase in $CD4^+CD28^{null}$ cells, 95% confidence interval 0.13–1.19; $P = 0.016$).

Conclusion: The host cellular immune response to CMV leads to the expansion of cytotoxic $CD4^+CD28^{null}$ T cells that express endothelial homing markers and are independently linked to increased arterial stiffness, a marker of cardiovascular mortality. Suppression of CMV in AAV may be of therapeutic value in reducing the risk of cardiovascular disease.

Keywords: ANCA, Vasculitis, Cytomegalovirus, Inflammation, T cells, Arterial stiffness, Cardiovascular disease

* Correspondence: d.chanouzas@bham.ac.uk
[1]Institute of Inflammation and Ageing, College of Medical and Dental Sciences, University of Birmingham, Birmingham B15 2TT, UK
[2]Renal Unit, University Hospitals Birmingham NHS Foundation Trust, Mindelsohn Way, Edgbaston, Birmingham B15 2TH, UK
Full list of author information is available at the end of the article

Background

Inflammation is a key factor in the pathophysiology of atherosclerosis [1, 2]. The relationship between inflammation and cardiovascular disease (CVD) is evident in patients with rheumatic disorders such as rheumatoid arthritis, systemic lupus erythematosus and ANCA-associated vasculitis (AAV), in which CVD is a leading cause of death [3–5]. Traditional risk factors do not fully explain the increased incidence of CVD seen in these conditions [6], and it is thought that inflammation and immunopathology may accelerate atherosclerosis [7].

CD4 T cells that do not express the co-stimulatory molecule CD28 (CD4$^+$CD28^{null}) have been implicated in vascular injury [8]. CD4$^+$CD28^{null} T cells are pro-inflammatory and their proportion expands under inflammatory conditions [9–11]. They are found preferentially in unstable rather than stable atherosclerotic plaques [12], suggesting direct involvement in plaque disruption, and they have been shown in in vitro assays to exhibit endothelial cytotoxicity in the context of acute coronary syndrome [13] and AAV [14]. Several studies in patients with inflammatory disorders such as rheumatoid arthritis have demonstrated that expansion of CD4$^+$CD28^{null} T cells is independently associated with increased incidence of CVD and cardiovascular mortality [15–19].

Loss of the co-stimulatory molecule CD28 on CD4 T cells suggests repeated exposure to a persistent antigen [20]. We and others have demonstrated that significant expansion of CD4$^+$CD28^{null} T cells occurs mainly in cytomegalovirus (CMV)-seropositive individuals, and negligible or very low proportions of these cells are seen in the absence of previous CMV infection [11, 21–24]. CMV infection is widely prevalent in the general population [25], and CMV itself has been implicated in the pathogenesis of CVD [26]. CMV infects endothelial and smooth muscle cells where it is able to persist during latency [27]. Infection with CMV is associated with impaired vascular function [28], high blood pressure [29], increased arterial stiffness [30] and cardiovascular mortality [26]. Furthermore, a recent meta-analysis demonstrated that CMV infection is associated with a 22% increased relative risk for CVD in the general population [31].

The aims of this study were to characterise the phenotype of CD4$^+$CD28^{null} T cells in AAV, with respect to their pro-inflammatory capacity and ability to target and damage the endothelium, and to determine whether expansion of this cell subset is associated with arterial stiffness, a marker of cardiovascular mortality.

Methods
Study population

Fifty-three CMV-seropositive patients with AAV in stable remission were recruited from the vasculitis clinic at University Hospitals Birmingham NHS Foundation Trust (Birmingham, UK), and 30 age-matched CMV-seropositive healthy volunteers (HVs) were enrolled from the 1000 Elders Cohort (courtesy of Professor Janet Lord, University of Birmingham, UK) and patient household contacts. CD4$^+$CD28^{null} T-cell percentage and phenotype were assessed in all participants. Arterial stiffness was measured in patients with AAV.

Patients were eligible for inclusion if they had a documented diagnosis of AAV and were in stable remission for at least 6 months, on maintenance immunosuppression with a maximum of two agents, and seropositive for CMV (anti-CMV IgG detected in peripheral blood). Exclusion criteria were estimated glomerular filtration rate of less than 15 mL/minute per 1.73 m^2, B cell–depleting therapy within 12 months or T cell–depleting therapy within 6 months, presence of other chronic infection (HIV, hepatitis B, hepatitis C, or tuberculosis) and treatment with anti-CMV therapies within the previous month.

Thirty-eight of 53 patients with AAV were participants in the 'Cytomegalovirus modulation of the immune system in ANca-associated VASculitis' (CANVAS) clinical trial, a proof-of-concept open-label randomised trial of valaciclovir, or no additional treatment, in CMV-seropositive AAV patients in remission [32]. All immune and arterial stiffness assessments reported here were conducted at baseline prior to commencement of valaciclovir.

The study was approved by the Research Ethics Committee of Yorkshire and the Humber (UK). Written informed consent was obtained from all participants.

Blood collection

Up to 50 mL of peripheral blood was obtained and processed within a maximum of 5 hours following venepuncture. Plasma was isolated by centrifugation and cryopreserved at −80 °C. Peripheral blood mononuclear cells (PBMCs) were isolated from heparinised blood by density gradient centrifugation, used immediately in stimulation experiments with CMV lysate to identify cytokine-producing T cells, or cryopreserved in liquid nitrogen.

Cells for flow cytometry experiments were acquired on a BD LSR II Flow Cytometer and analysed by using FACS DIVA Software Version 8.0 (BD, Franklin Lakes, NJ, USA). Monoclonal antibodies used for flow cytometry experiments are listed in Table S1 of Additional file 1. Gating strategies are shown in Figure S1 and S2 of Additional file 1.

Enumeration of peripheral blood CD4$^+$CD28^{null} T cells

Whole blood was stained with anti-CD3, anti-CD4 and anti-CD28 monoclonal antibodies to determine CD4$^+$CD28^{null} T-cell percentage. Quality control was achieved by using a positive control (Cytofix CD4 Normal Range Positive Control; Cytomark, Caltag Medsystems, Buckingham, UK) with a validated acceptance range for $CD3^+CD4^+$ percentage and a fluorescence minus one control to aid CD28 gating. These were assayed with every analytical run.

Peripheral blood mononuclear cell stimulation

To identify CMV lysate-stimulated cytokine-expressing T cells, $0.5–1 \times 10^6$ PBMCs were re-suspended in supplemented medium—(RPMI), 10% foetal calf serum; sterile filtered and heat inactivated (Sigma-Aldrich, St. Louis, MO, USA), 1% penicillin/streptomycin (P/S) (Gibco, Thermo Fisher Scientific, Waltham, MA, USA—overnight for 16 ($\pm$2) hours at 37 °C, 5% CO_2, in the presence of monensin (2 µmol/L) and phycoerythrin-conjugated anti-CD154 monoclonal antibody as previously described [33]. Cells were stimulated with CMV lysate (1:100) prepared from CMV strain AD169-infected human foetal foreskin fibroblasts. Unstimulated cells served as controls. Following overnight incubation, cells were stained with eFluor-506 viability dye (eBioscience, Thermo Fisher Scientific) for 30 min at 4 °C, washed with phosphate-buffered saline and flow cytometry buffer, and co-stained with saturating amounts of anti-CD3, anti-CD4 and anti-CD28 antibodies for 30 min at 4 °C before washing with flow cytometry buffer. Cells were fixed and permeabilised with an intracellular flow cytometry staining kit (eBioscience) and stained for 30 min at 4 °C with saturating amounts of anti-interferon-gamma (anti-IFN-γ), anti-tumour necrosis factor-alpha (anti-TNF-α), anti-interleukin-2 (anti-IL-2), anti-IL-5, anti-IL-10 and anti-T-bet monoclonal antibodies before washing with flow cytometry buffer.

Identification of Th1-, Th2- and Th17-skewed subsets

The expression of chemokine receptors on unstimulated $CD4^+CD28^{null}$ T cells from 17 patients with AAV was defined by staining whole blood with anti-CXCR3, anti-CCR4, anti-CCR6, anti-CD3, anti-CD4 and anti-CD28 monoclonal antibodies. T helper 1 (Th1)-skewed CD4 T cells were identified as $CXCR3^+CCR6^-$, Th2-skewed as $CCR4^+CCR6^-$ and Th17-skewed as $CCR4^+CCR6^+$ [34].

Identification of endothelial homing receptors and cytotoxic molecules

In order to phenotype unstimulated $CD4^+CD28^{null}$ T cells with respect to their expression of endothelial homing receptors and cytotoxic molecules, cryopreserved PBMCs from 10 patients with AAV were stained with Fixable Viability dye eFluor-506 as described above; co-stained with anti-CD3, anti-CD4, anti-CD28, anti-CX3CR1, anti-CD49d and anti-CD11b antibodies;

and fixed and permeabilised as already described, followed by intracellular staining with anti-perforin and anti-granzyme B antibodies.

Measurement of soluble markers of inflammation

Soluble markers of inflammation (IL-2, TNF-α, IFN-γ, IL-10, IL-17A, IL-6 and highly sensitive C-reactive protein) were measured in plasma by Luminex array (ProcartaPlex, eBioscience) in accordance with the instructions of the manufacturer, read on a Bio-Rad Luminex 200 instrument (Bio-Rad, Hercules, CA, USA) and analysed by using ProcartaPlex Analyst 1.0 Software (eBioscience).

Determination of anti-CMV IgG titre

Plasma anti-CMV IgG titre was assayed by using an enzyme-linked immunosorbent assay as previously described [30]. CMV seropositivity was defined as an anti-CMV IgG titre of more than 10 units.

Arterial stiffness measurement

Arterial stiffness was estimated by measuring carotid-to-femoral pulse wave velocity (PWV) using the non-invasive, non-operator-dependent Vicorder system (Skidmore, Bristol, UK) that employs a volume displacement method, as previously described [32]. Briefly, the patient was allowed to rest for 5 min prior to inflating a 100-mm-wide cuff on the non-dominant arm to measure peripheral blood pressure. A 30-mm-wide cuff was then placed on the neck at the level of the carotid artery and a 100-mm-wide cuff placed around the proximal thigh. The distance between the mid-clavicular point and the mid-point of the thigh cuff, the aortic path length, was measured with the patient supine. With the patient at a supine 30° head-tilt position, the cuffs were inflated to 60 mm Hg. The Vicorder instrument uses the resultant oscillometric signal to extract the pulse waveforms and pulse transit time to calculate carotid-to-femoral PWV. The mean value of three consistent readings was used for subsequent analysis.

Statistical analysis

Continuous variables were summarised as medians and quartiles (unless stated otherwise) and categorical data as counts and percentages. Groups were compared with the Mann–Whitney test, the Kruskal–Wallis and Dunn's multiple comparison test, and the chi-squared or Fisher's exact test. Associations were assessed with Spearman's rank correlation. Univariable and multivariable linear regression models were constructed for variables associated with PWV. Analyses were undertaken by using SPSS Statistics Version 21 (IBM, Armonk, NY, USA) and Prism Version 5

(GraphPad, La Jolla, CA, USA) and were two-tailed; a P value of less than 0.05 was considered significant.

Results

Baseline characteristics of study participants are shown in Table 1.

CD4$^+$CD28^{null} T cells are CMV-specific and display a pro-inflammatory phenotype

We initially undertook a phenotypic analysis of CD4$^+$CD28^{null} T cells from 53 CMV-seropositive AAV patients in stable remission. PBMCs were stimulated *in vitro* with CMV lysate, and the proportion of CMV-specific cells within the CD4$^+$CD28^{null} and CD4$^+$CD28$^+$ subfractions was determined. A greater proportion of CMV-specific T cells was observed within the CD4$^+$CD28^{null} population as determined by expression of the activation marker CD154 and cytokine expression: IFN-γ, TNF-α and IL-2 (Fig. 1a). Neither cell type expressed significant amounts of IL-5 or IL-10.

The percentage of CD4$^+$CD28^{null} T cells was strongly correlated with the total CMV-specific CD4$^+$ response (rho = 0.846, P <0.001; Fig. 1b), indicating that the size of the CD4$^+$CD28^{null} T-cell accumulation is a good measure of the impact of CMV infection on the CD4 compartment in this population. CD4$^+$CD28^{null} T-cell percentage also correlated with the humoral response to CMV, anti-CMV IgG titre (rho = 0.324, P = 0.018; Fig. 1b).

As well as expressing IFN-γ and TNF-α, the majority of CD4$^+$CD28^{null} T cells expressed the Th1 lineage transcription factor T-bet (Fig. 1c) and a Th1-skewed chemokine receptor profile (CXCR3$^+$CCR6$^-$) (Fig. 1d). In contrast, the chemokine receptor staining profile that identifies Th2-skewed (CCR4$^+$CCR6$^-$) and Th17-skewed (CCR4$^+$CCR6$^+$) cells was not seen on CD4+CD28^{null} T cells. Indeed, CD4$^+$CD28^{null} T cells comprised the majority of the Th1 compartment (median 51.6%, 30.0–77.3). In addition, the percentage of CD4$^+$CD28^{null} T cells was strongly correlated with the overall size of the Th1 compartment (Fig. 1c), indicating that the size of the CD4$^+$CD28^{null} T-cell expansion in CMV-seropositive AAV patients determines the relative proportion of Th1 cells, a subset known to exert a strong pro-atherosclerotic effect [35].

There was no difference between AAV patients and age-matched CMV-seropositive HVs in the induction of CD154 expression on CD4$^+$CD28^{null} T cells or their cytokine expression profile following CMV lysate stimulation (Fig. 1e). However, patients with AAV had larger expansions of CD4$^+$CD28^{null} T cells compared with HVs (11.3% [3.7–19.7] versus 6.7 [2.4–8.8]; P = 0.022).

CD4$^+$CD28^{null} T cells are endothelial homing cytotoxic T cells

IFN-γ and TNF-α activate endothelial cells and increase surface expression of chemokines and adhesion molecules such as IFN-γ–inducible protein-10 (IP-10), fractalkine, vascular adhesion molecule-1 (VCAM-1) and intercellular adhesion molecule-1 (ICAM-1) [36]. Having identified high levels of expression of the IP-10 receptor CXCR3 on the surface of CD4$^+$CD28^{null} T cells, we evaluated the surface expression of the receptors for fractalkine, VCAM-1 and ICAM-1 (CX3CR1, CD49d and CD11b) on unstimulated PBMCs from 10 patients with AAV. Co-expression of all three endothelial homing receptors was significantly more common on CD4$^+$

Table 1 Participant baseline characteristics

	AAV (n = 53)	HV (n = 30)
Age, years	69.0 [62.8–75.3]	70.5 [66.8–74.0]*
Gender, male:female	35:18	14:16*
ANCA specificity, PR3:MPO	34:18	–
AAV disease chronicity, years	6.0 [3.2–12.0]	–
Renal function eGFR, mL/min per 1.73 m^2	53 [21]	–
Urine albumin-to-creatinine ratio, mg/mmol	4.4 [1.4–9.9]	–
Steroids, n (%)	39 (73.6)	–
Mycophenolate mofetil, n (%)	14 (26.4)	–
Azathioprine, n (%)	19 (35.8)	–
No current immunosuppression, n (%)	4 (7.5)	–
Ever smoker, n (%)	26 (49.1)	–
Diabetes mellitus, n (%)	11 (20.8)	–
On statin treatment, n (%)	29 (54.7)	

Data are displayed as median [interquartile range] apart from renal function displayed as mean [standard deviation]. Immunosuppressive treatment refers to number and percentage of patients on the respective immunosuppressive agent at the time of study entry.
*Comparison between ANCA-associated vasculitis (AAV) and healthy volunteers (HV): age (Mann–Whitney U test, P = 0.557), gender (Fisher's exact, P = 0.106)
Abbreviations: *eGFR* estimated glomerular filtration rate, *MPO* myeloperoxidase, *PR3* proteinase 3

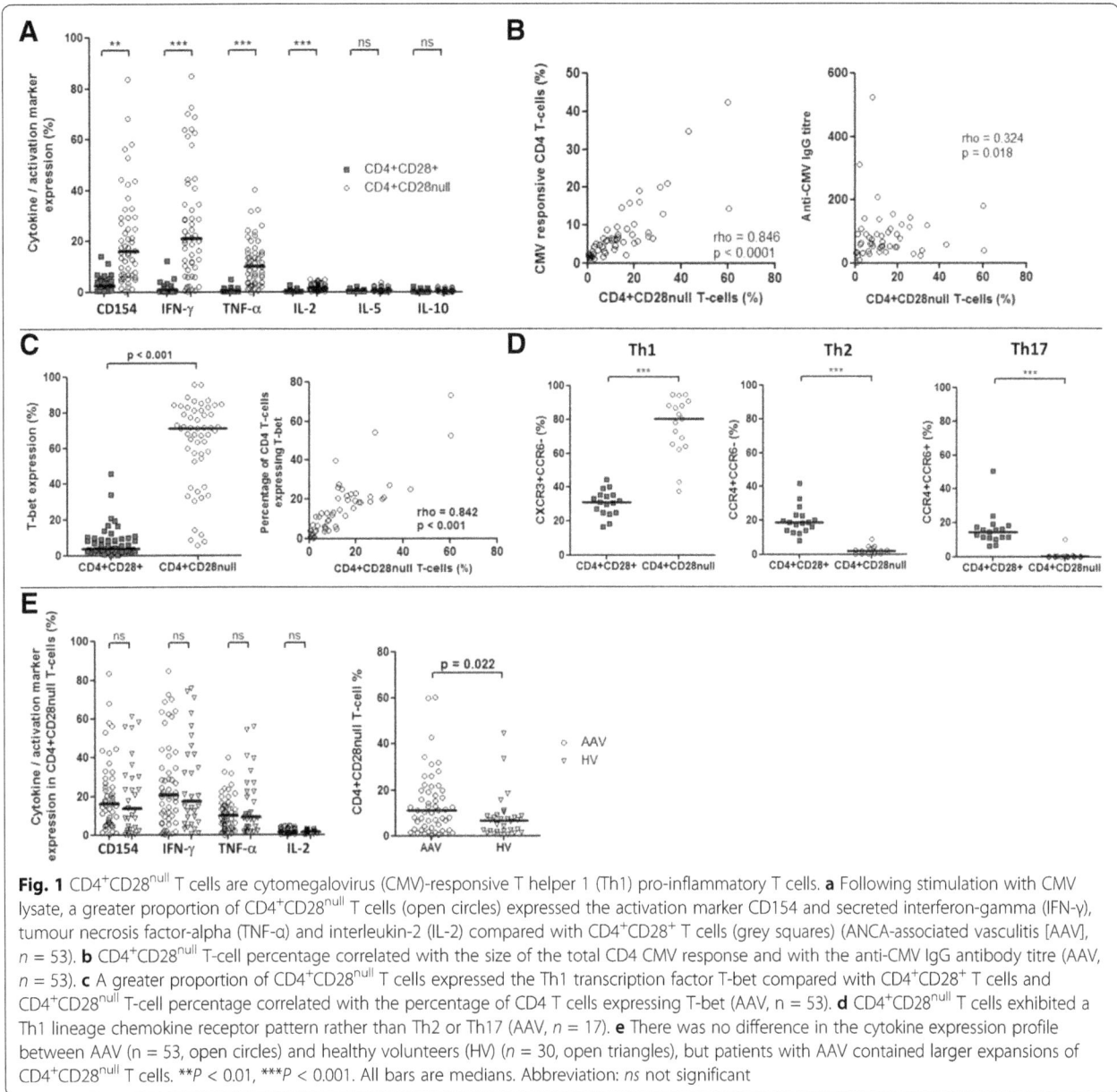

Fig. 1 CD4$^+$CD28^{null} T cells are cytomegalovirus (CMV)-responsive T helper 1 (Th1) pro-inflammatory T cells. **a** Following stimulation with CMV lysate, a greater proportion of CD4$^+$CD28^{null} T cells (open circles) expressed the activation marker CD154 and secreted interferon-gamma (IFN-γ), tumour necrosis factor-alpha (TNF-α) and interleukin-2 (IL-2) compared with CD4$^+$CD28$^+$ T cells (grey squares) (ANCA-associated vasculitis [AAV], n = 53). **b** CD4$^+$CD28^{null} T-cell percentage correlated with the size of the total CD4 CMV response and with the anti-CMV IgG antibody titre (AAV, n = 53). **c** A greater proportion of CD4$^+$CD28^{null} T cells expressed the Th1 transcription factor T-bet compared with CD4$^+$CD28$^+$ T cells and CD4$^+$CD28^{null} T-cell percentage correlated with the percentage of CD4 T cells expressing T-bet (AAV, n = 53). **d** CD4$^+$CD28^{null} T cells exhibited a Th1 lineage chemokine receptor pattern rather than Th2 or Th17 (AAV, n = 17). **e** There was no difference in the cytokine expression profile between AAV (n = 53, open circles) and healthy volunteers (HV) (n = 30, open triangles), but patients with AAV contained larger expansions of CD4$^+$CD28^{null} T cells. ******P < 0.01, *******P < 0.001. All bars are medians. Abbreviation: *ns* not significant

CD28^{null} compared with CD4$^+$CD28$^+$ T cells (51.6% [42.7–64.4] versus 5.0 [1.7–6.3]; P = 0.006; Fig. 2a). In addition, the majority of unstimulated CD4$^+$CD28^{null} T cells contained intracellular stores of both perforin and granzyme B (74.5%, 63.5–92.7; Fig. 2b), suggesting that they have the capacity to target and lyze endothelial cells.

The size of the CD4$^+$CD28^{null} T-cell expansion is independently associated with increased arterial stiffness in AAV

To determine whether the size of the CD4$^+$CD28^{null} T-cell expansion is associated with arterial stiffness, as a clinical marker of cardiovascular pathology, carotid-

to-femoral PWV was measured in the patients with AAV. The CD4$^+$CD28^{null} T-cell percentage was found to be significantly correlated with increased systolic blood pressure (rho = 0.305, P = 0.026), pulse pressure (rho = 0.428, P = 0.001) and PWV (rho = 0.371, P = 0.006; Fig. 3).

On univariable analysis, age, percentage of CD4$^+$CD28^{null} T cells, plasma concentration of TNF-α, and blood pressure parameters (Table 2) were associated with increased PWV. In contrast, we did not observe an association between anti-CMV IgG titre and PWV.

To account for confounding factors, we constructed a multivariable linear regression model including all variables that were associated with PWV on univariable

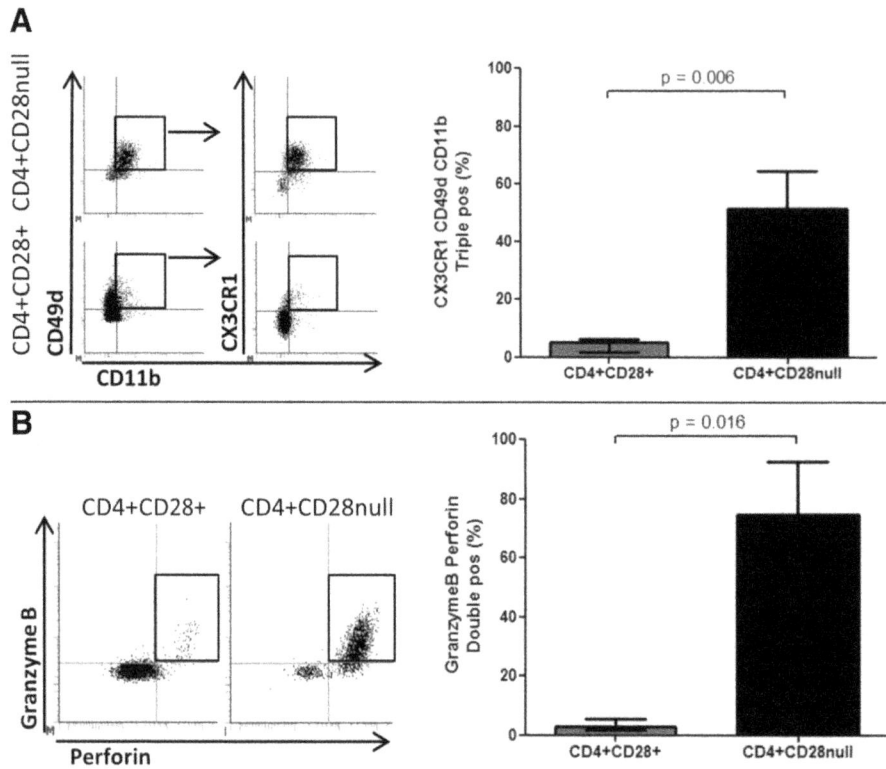

Fig. 2 CD4$^+$CD28^{null} T cells are endothelial homing, cytotoxic T cells. Unstimulated CD4 T cells from patients with ANCA-associated vasculitis (AAV) ($n = 10$) were stained for expression of endothelial homing receptors CX3CR1, CD49d and CD11b and intracellular cytotoxic molecules perforin and granzyme B. **a** Representative staining and summary data for unstimulated CD4 T cells gated on CD4$^+$CD28^{null} (top two flow cytometry plots) and CD4$^+$CD28$^+$ T cells (bottom two flow cytometry plots). Sequential gating was performed as follows: CD49d and CD11b to identify CD49d CD11b double-positive cells, followed by CX3CR1 to identify CD49d CD11b CX3CR1 triple-positive cells. **b** Representative staining and summary data for unstimulated CD4 T cells gated on CD4$^+$CD28$^+$ and CD4$^+$CD28^{null} T cells showing cells double-positive for perforin and granzyme B

analysis with a P value of less than 0.1 (Tables 2 and 3). This demonstrated that the percentage of CD4$^+$CD28^{null} T cells associated with increased arterial stiffness independently of age, proteinuria, peripheral mean arterial blood pressure, and plasma concentration of TNF-α.

There was a 0.66 m/s [95% confidence interval 0.13–1.19] increase in PWV for every 10% increase in CD4$^+$CD28^{null} T cells ($P = 0.016$; Table 3). This relationship did not change when systolic blood pressure or pulse pressure was substituted for mean arterial blood pressure, and the

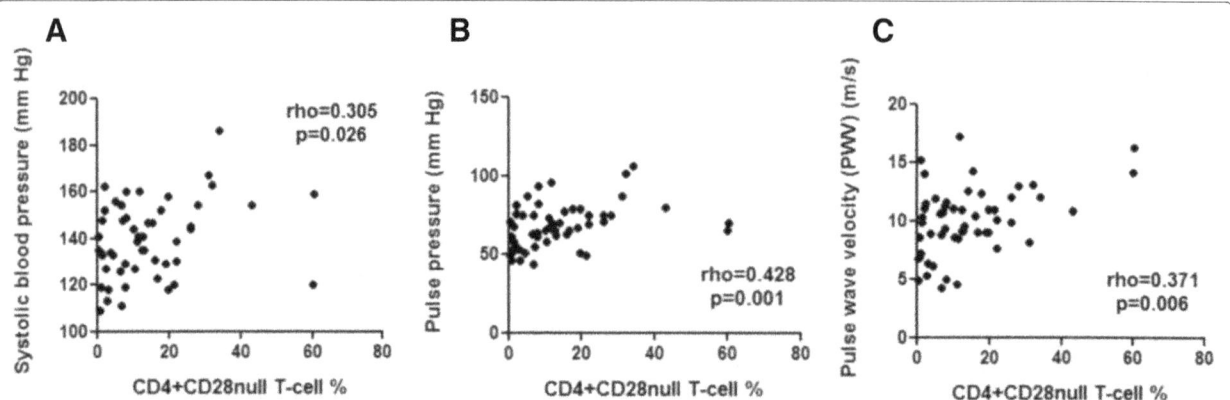

Fig. 3 CD4$^+$CD28^{null} T-cell expansion correlates with increased arterial stiffness and blood pressure parameters. CD4$^+$CD28^{null} T-cell percentage correlated with increased systolic blood pressure (**a**), pulse pressure (**b**), a surrogate marker of arterial stiffness, and carotid-to-femoral pulse wave velocity (**c**) (n = 53)

Table 2 Variables associated with pulse wave velocity on univariable analysis

Variable	Univariable analysis		
	R^2	Regression coefficient [95% CI]	P value
Age, years	0.183	0.131 [0.053, 0.208]	0.001
Gender	0.004	0.393 [− 1.313, 2.100]	0.645
eGFR, mL/min per 1.73 m^2	0.026	− 0.023 [− 0.062, 0.017]	0.252
Urinary albumin-to-creatinine ratio, mg/mmol	0.056	0.019 [−0.003, 0.041]	0.088
Ever smoker	0.017	−0.759 [−2.364, 0.847]	0.347
Presence of diabetes	0.002	0.291 [−1.704, 2.286]	0.771
On statin treatment	0.044	1.208 [−0.383, 2.799]	0.134
Pulse pressure, mm Hg	0.163	0.084 [0.030, 0.137]	0.003
Mean arterial pressure, mm Hg	0.102	0.088 [0.015, 0.161]	0.020
Systolic blood pressure, mm Hg	0.191	0.079 [0.033, 0.124]	0.001
Diastolic blood pressure, mm Hg	0.027	0.056 [−0.039, 0.150]	0.243
CD4$^+$CD28^{null} T-cell proportion (%), per 10% increase	0.182	0.912 [0.368, 1.455]	0.001
C-reactive protein, mg/mL	0.008	−0.234 [− 0.958, 0.490]	0.520
IL-2, pg/mL	0.066	0.007 [0.000, 0.015]	0.065
IFN-γ, pg/mL	0.036	−0.004 [− 0.010, 0.002]	0.179
IL-10, pg/mL	0.025	0.089 [−0.068, 0.245]	0.260
IL-6, pg/mL	0.004	0.002 [−0.007, 0.011]	0.649
TNF-α, pg/mL	0.083	0.015 [0.001, 0.029]	0.039
IL-17, pg/mL	0.015	−0.003 [−0.011, 0.004]	0.389

All variables with a P value of less than 0.1 on univariable analysis were included in the multivariable model shown in Table 3
Abbreviations: CI confidence interval, eGFR estimated glomerular filtration rate, IL interleukin, TNF-α tumour necrosis factor-alpha

size of the CD4$^+$CD28^{null} T-cell expansion remained independently associated with increased PWV.

Discussion

Our findings demonstrate that the host cellular immune response to CMV is associated with the expansion of a subset of pro-inflammatory, endothelial homing, cytotoxic CD4$^+$CD28^{null} T cells in patients with AAV. Furthermore, the size of this expansion is independently linked to increased arterial stiffness, a marker of cardiovascular mortality [37]. This is significant in AAV as

cardiovascular disease is a leading cause of death in this patient group.

Our data provide further insight into the properties of CD4$^+$CD28^{null} T cells and their capacity to cause vascular damage of relevance to AAV. We identified CD4$^+$CD28^{null} T cells in AAV to be Th1-skewed pro-inflammatory T cells that produce IFN-γ and TNF-α in response to stimulation with CMV lysate. These findings are in keeping with previous reports in HVs [38] as well as in AAV where CD4$^+$CD28^{null} T cells have been shown to be a major source of IFN-γ and TNF-α [39].

Table 3 Multivariable linear regression model for pulse wave velocity (meters per second)

Variable	Univariable analysis		Multivariable analysis	
	Regression coefficient [95% CI]	P value	Regression coefficient [95% CI]	P value
CD4$^+$CD28^{null} T-cell percentage, per 10% increase	0.912 [0.368, 1.455]	0.001	0.663 [0.132, 1.194]	0.016
Age, years	0.131 [0.053, 0.208]	0.001	0.080 [0.006, 0.155]	0.035
Proteinuria (urinary ACR), mg/mmol	0.019 [−0.003, 0.041]	0.088	0.013 [−0.007, 0.033]	0.196
Mean arterial pressure, mm Hg	0.088 [0.015, 0.161]	0.020	0.053 [−0.016, 0.122]	0.128
TNF-α, pg/mL	0.015 [0.001, 0.029]	0.039	0.010 [−0.002, 0.022]	0.086

Variables with P value of less than 0.1 on univariable analysis (Table 2) were included in the model. In order to avoid collinearity, only one blood pressure parameter and either plasma concentration of tumour necrosis factor-alpha (TNF-α) or interleukin-2 (IL-2) were added at each iteration of the model. This table shows the final model with mean arterial pressure (MAP) and TNF-α. The size of the CD4$^+$CD28^{null} T-cell expansion remained independently associated with pulse wave velocity with negligible impact on the model characteristics when pulse pressure or systolic blood pressure was substituted for MAP and when plasma concentration of IL-2 was substituted for TNF-α
R value: 0.635, R^2: 0.404
Abbreviations: ACR albumin-to-creatinine ratio, CI confidence interval

Th1 T cells are recognised as important players in the atherosclerotic process with Th1-driven responses exerting detrimental effects [40]. Mice deficient in T-bet, the master regulator of the Th1 transcriptional response, are relatively protected from the development of atherosclerotic lesions [35], and both T-bet and IFN-γ are essential in the generation of angiotensin II–mediated vascular dysfunction [41]. We observed that the CD4 Th1 compartment in AAV CMV-seropositive patients was made up mostly of $CD4^+CD28^{null}$ T cells and that up to 94% of Th1 cells were $CD4^+CD28^{null}$. Taken together, our findings indicate that CMV exerts a powerful influence on the shape and magnitude of the Th1 repertoire.

IFN-γ and TNF-α cytokines mediate inflammation in blood vessel walls through disruption of endothelial junctions and induction of chemokine and adhesion molecule expression on vascular endothelium. This promotes the recruitment and adherence of lymphocytes and monocytes on the inflamed endothelium and facilitates leukocyte transmigration [36]. In our phenotypic analysis, $CD4^+CD28^{null}$ T cells were found to express the chemokine receptors CX3CR1, CD49d, CD11b and CXCR3 that are able to bind their respective adhesion molecule ligands fractalkine, VCAM-1, ICAM-1 and IP-10 on activated endothelial cells [42, 43]. They also co-expressed the cytolytic granules granzyme B and perforin, as previously found by others [44], suggesting that they act as cytotoxic effector cells. The endothelium is an important site for CMV infection [27] and as such endothelial targeting by CMV-specific T cells would be expected to have the capacity to suppress viral reactivation but might also contribute to vascular damage.

Consistent with these observations, our findings revealed that the size of the $CD4^+CD28^{null}$ T-cell expansion in patients with AAV was independently associated with increased arterial stiffness. This is contrary to a recent report in patients with AAV where the size of the $CD4^+CD28^{null}$ T-cell expansion was found not to be related to arterial stiffness [45]. However, the AAV cohort within that study included a substantial proportion of CMV-seronegative patients and only 24 patients were CMV-seropositive. Given that significant expansion of $CD4^+CD28^{null}$ T cells is seen mainly in CMV-seropositive individuals, this may explain the discrepancy between our findings and those of Slot et al. [45]. Furthermore, our data are in agreement with several published studies reporting associations in other patient groups such as rheumatoid arthritis [15] and chronic kidney disease [18], between $CD4^+CD28^{null}$ T cells and markers of atherosclerotic damage.

Previous work by our group has shown that CMV-seropositive patients with chronic kidney disease have stiffer arteries compared with CMV-seronegative chronic kidney disease patients [30]. In the present study, we observed that expansion of $CD4^+CD28^{null}$ T cells in CMV-seropositive AAV patients is associated with increased arterial stiffness in that carotid-to-femoral PWV increases by 0.66 m/s for every 10% increase in the size of the $CD4^+CD28^{null}$ T-cell subset. Such an effect size on PWV is greater than the impact of smoking on arterial stiffness [46] and roughly equivalent to 10 years' worth of ageing [47]. In contrast, we found no correlation between the humoral response to CMV, measured by the anti-CMV IgG titre, and arterial stiffness. Based on our data, we propose that the host cellular immune response to CMV is directly involved in the development of cardiovascular pathology and that this is driven by the expansion of the pro-inflammatory endothelial homing $CD4^+CD28^{null}$ T-cell subset. However, it should be noted that our study was cross-sectional in nature and therefore cannot definitively confirm a longitudinal increase in arterial stiffness driven by $CD4^+CD28^{null}$ T cells.

It is likely that expansion of $CD4^+CD28^{null}$ T cells itself is driven by asymptomatic subclinical reactivation of CMV. Viral reactivation is more likely to occur in an inflammatory milieu, and TNF-α has recently been shown to reverse the transcriptional silencing that maintains CMV latency, leading to lytic reactivation [48]. We recently observed that subclinical CMV reactivation occurs in over a quarter of patients with AAV in remission within a 12-month period [49], indicating that CMV reactivation is a frequent event in this patient group. This could explain our finding that $CD4^+CD28^{null}$ T-cell expansions are almost twice as large in AAV patients compared with age-matched HVs. Subclinical CMV reactivation is likely to be even higher during the acute phase of AAV, when patients are exposed to high levels of systemic inflammation and intensive immunosuppressive treatment. As viral reactivation is expected to act as a potent stimulus for boosting the CMV-specific cellular immune response, anti-viral therapy could act to suppress CMV-specific immune responses and potentially reduce cardiovascular damage. Anti-viral therapy in this context would suppress all herpes viruses. This could be advantageous as recent evidence suggests that concomitant CMV and Epstein–Barr virus infection may be associated with increased expansion of $CD4^+CD28^{null}$ T cells in AAV [50].

Conclusions

In summary, the results presented here support a mechanism for vascular damage secondary to expansion of pro-inflammatory CMV-specific T cells that target the endothelium and are independently linked to arterial stiffness. Our data suggest that suppression of CMV may hold therapeutic potential for patients with AAV, lending support to the design of further studies aiming to determine whether CMV suppression might reduce expansion of CD4[+]CD28[null] T cells, ameliorating surrogate markers of atherosclerotic damage, and ultimately reducing risk of cardiovascular disease, the leading cause of death in this patient group.

Abbreviations
AAV: ANCA-associated vasculitis; ANCA: Anti-neutrophil cytoplasmic antibody; CMV: Cytomegalovirus; CVD: Cardiovascular disease; CX3CR1: CX3C chemokine receptor 1; HV: Healthy volunteer; ICAM-1: Intercellular adhesion molecule 1; IFN-γ: Interferon-gamma; IL: Interleukin; IP-10: IFN-gamma-inducible protein 10; PBMC: Peripheral blood mononuclear cell; PWV: Pulse wave velocity; Th: T helper; TNF-α: Tumour necrosis factor-alpha; VCAM-1: Vascular cell adhesion molecule 1

Acknowledgements
The study was conducted within the Birmingham National Institute for Health Research (NIHR)/Wellcome Trust (WT) Clinical Research Facility (CRF) (Birmingham, UK). The views expressed are those of the authors and not necessarily those of the NHS, the NIHR or the Department of Health. Parts of this work have been presented in abstract form at a scientific meeting or published as a conference abstract or both.

Funding
This research was funded by a Wellcome Trust Research Training Fellowship Grant (097962/Z/11/Z) and by Vasculitis UK. The funding sources had no role in the design and conduct of the study; collection, management, analysis and interpretation of the data; preparation, review, or approval of the manuscript; or decision to submit the manuscript for publication.

Authors' contributions
DC, LH, MDM, PM and CF conceived and designed the study. DC, MS, LD, PS, LP, SJ and JB acquired data. DC, MS, PN, CF and LH analysed and interpreted data. DC drafted the manuscript. All authors critically revised the manuscript and approved the final version.

Consent for publication
Not applicable.

Competing interests
The authors declare that they have no competing interests.

Author details
[1]Institute of Inflammation and Ageing, College of Medical and Dental Sciences, University of Birmingham, Birmingham B15 2TT, UK. [2]Renal Unit, University Hospitals Birmingham NHS Foundation Trust, Mindelsohn Way, Edgbaston, Birmingham B15 2TH, UK. [3]Institute of Translational Medicine Birmingham, Heritage Building, Mindelsohn Way, Edgbaston, Birmingham B15 2TH, UK. [4]Institute of Clinical Sciences, College of Medical and Dental Sciences, University of Birmingham, Birmingham B15 2TT, UK. [5]Institute of Immunology and Immunotherapy, College of Medical and Dental Sciences, University of Birmingham, Birmingham B15 2TT, UK.

References
1. Brown WV, Remaley AT, Ridker PM. JCL roundtable: is inflammation a future target in preventing arteriosclerotic cardiovascular disease. J Clin Lipidol. 2015;9(2):119–28.
2. Ridker PM, Everett BM, Thuren T, MacFadyen JG, Chang WH, Ballantyne C, et al. Antiinflammatory therapy with Canakinumab for atherosclerotic disease. N Engl J Med. 2017;377(12):1119–31.
3. Goodson NJ, Wiles NJ, Lunt M, Barrett EM, Silman AJ, Symmons DP. Mortality in early inflammatory polyarthritis: cardiovascular mortality is increased in seropositive patients. Arthritis Rheum. 2002;46(8):2010–9.
4. Thomas G, Mancini J, Jourde-Chiche N, Sarlon G, Amoura Z, Harle JR, et al. Mortality associated with systemic lupus erythematosus in France assessed by multiple-cause-of-death analysis. Arthritis Rheum. 2014;66(9):2503–11.
5. Flossmann O, Berden A, de Groot K, Hagen C, Harper L, Heijl C, et al. Long-term patient survival in ANCA-associated vasculitis. Ann Rheum Dis. 2011; 70(3):488–94.
6. del Rincon ID, Williams K, Stern MP, Freeman GL, Escalante A. High incidence of cardiovascular events in a rheumatoid arthritis cohort not explained by traditional cardiac risk factors. Arthritis Rheum. 2001;44(12): 2737–45.
7. Hansson GK. Inflammation, atherosclerosis, and coronary artery disease. N Engl J Med. 2005;352(16):1685–95.
8. Liuzzo G, Kopecky SL, Frye RL, O'Fallon WM, Maseri A, Goronzy JJ, et al. Perturbation of the T-cell repertoire in patients with unstable angina. Circulation. 1999;100(21):2135–9.
9. Schmidt D, Goronzy JJ, Weyand CM. CD4+ CD7- CD28- T cells are expanded in rheumatoid arthritis and are characterized by autoreactivity. J Clin Invest. 1996;97(9):2027–37.
10. Ugarte-Gil MF, Sanchez-Zuniga C, Gamboa-Cardenas RV, Aliaga-Zamudio M, Zevallos F, Tineo-Pozo G, et al. Circulating CD4+CD28[null] and extra-thymic CD4+CD8+ double positive T cells are independently associated with disease damage in systemic lupus erythematosus patients. Lupus. 2016; 25(3):233–40.
11. Thewissen M, Somers V, Hellings N, Fraussen J, Damoiseaux J, Stinissen P. CD4+CD28[null] T cells in autoimmune disease: pathogenic features and decreased susceptibility to immunoregulation. J Immunol. 2007;179(10): 6514–23.
12. Liuzzo G, Goronzy JJ, Yang H, Kopecky SL, Holmes DR, Frye RL, et al. Monoclonal T-cell proliferation and plaque instability in acute coronary syndromes. Circulation. 2000;101(25):2883–8.
13. Nakajima T, Schulte S, Warrington KJ, Kopecky SL, Frye RL, Goronzy JJ, et al. T-cell-mediated lysis of endothelial cells in acute coronary syndromes. Circulation. 2002;105(5):570–5.
14. de Menthon M, Lambert M, Guiard E, Tognarelli S, Bienvenu B, Karras A, et al. Excessive interleukin-15 transpresentation endows NKG2D+CD4+ T cells with innate-like capacity to lyse vascular endothelium in granulomatosis with polyangiitis (Wegener's). Arthritis Rheum. 2011;63(7):2116–26.
15. Gerli R, Schillaci G, Giordano A, Bocci EB, Bistoni O, Vaudo G, et al. CD4 +CD28- T lymphocytes contribute to early atherosclerotic damage in rheumatoid arthritis patients. Circulation. 2004;109(22):2744–8.
16. Betjes MG, Meijers RW, de Wit LE, Litjens NH. A killer on the road: circulating CD4(+)CD28[null] T cells as cardiovascular risk factor in ESRD patients. J Nephrol. 2012;25(2):183–91.
17. Lopez P, Rodriguez-Carrio J, Martinez-Zapico A, Caminal-Montero L, Suarez A. Senescent profile of angiogenic T cells from systemic lupus erythematosus patients. J Leukoc Biol. 2016;99(3):405–12.
18. Yadav AK, Banerjee D, Lal A, Jha V. Vitamin D deficiency, CD4+CD28[null] cells and accelerated atherosclerosis in chronic kidney disease. Nephrology. 2012; 17(6):575–81.
19. Pera A, Broadley I, Davies KA, Kern F. Cytomegalovirus as a driver of excess cardiovascular mortality in rheumatoid arthritis: a red herring or a smoking gun? Circ Res. 2017;120(2):274–7.
20. Schmidt D, Martens PB, Weyand CM, Goronzy JJ. The repertoire of CD4+ CD28- T cells in rheumatoid arthritis. Mol Med. 1996;2(5):608–18.
21. Morgan MD, Pachnio A, Begum J, Roberts D, Rasmussen N, Neil DA, et al. CD4 +CD28- T cell expansion in granulomatosis with polyangiitis (Wegener's) is driven by latent cytomegalovirus infection and is associated with an increased risk of infection and mortality. Arthritis Rheum. 2011;63(7):2127–37.
22. Eriksson P, Sandell C, Backteman K, Ernerudh J. Expansions of CD4+CD28- and CD8+CD28- T cells in granulomatosis with polyangiitis and microscopic polyangiitis are associated with cytomegalovirus infection but not with disease activity. J Rheumatol. 2012;39(9):1840–3.
23. Shabir S, Smith H, Kaul B, Pachnio A, Jham S, Kuravi S, et al. Cytomegalovirus-associated CD4(+) CD28[(null)] cells in NKG2D-dependent glomerular endothelial injury and kidney allograft dysfunction. Am J Transplant Off J Am Soc Transplant Am Soc Transplant Surg. 2016;16(4): 1113–28.
24. Hooper M, Kallas EG, Coffin D, Campbell D, Evans TG, Looney RJ. Cytomegalovirus seropositivity is associated with the expansion of CD4 +CD28- and CD8+CD28- T cells in rheumatoid arthritis. J Rheumatol. 1999; 26(7):1452–7.

25. Bate SL, Dollard SC, Cannon MJ. Cytomegalovirus seroprevalence in the United States: the national health and nutrition examination surveys, 1988-2004. Clin Infect Dis. 2010;50(11):1439–47.

26. Spyridopoulos I, Martin-Ruiz C, Hilkens C, Yadegarfar ME, Isaacs J, Jagger C, et al. CMV seropositivity and T-cell senescence predict increased cardiovascular mortality in octogenarians: results from the Newcastle 85+ study. Aging Cell. 2016;15(2):389–92.

27. Pampou S, Gnedoy SN, Bystrevskaya VB, Smirnov VN, Chazov EI, Melnick JL, et al. Cytomegalovirus genome and the immediate-early antigen in cells of different layers of human aorta. Virchows Archiv. 2000;436(6):539–52.

28. Haarala A, Kahonen M, Lehtimaki T, Aittoniemi J, Jylhava J, Hutri-Kahonen N, et al. Relation of high cytomegalovirus antibody titres to blood pressure and brachial artery flow-mediated dilation in young men: the cardiovascular risk in young Finns study. Clin Exp Immunol. 2012;167(2):309–16.

29. Firth C, Harrison R, Ritchie S, Wardlaw J, Ferro CJ, Starr JM, et al. Cytomegalovirus infection is associated with an increase in systolic blood pressure in older individuals. QJM. 2016;109(9):595–600.

30. Wall NA, Chue CD, Edwards NC, Pankhurst T, Harper L, Steeds RP, et al. Cytomegalovirus seropositivity is associated with increased arterial stiffness in patients with chronic kidney disease. PLoS One. 2013;8(2):e55686.

31. Wang H, Peng G, Bai J, He B, Huang K, Hu X, Liu D. Cytomegalovirus infection and relative risk of cardiovascular disease (ischemic heart disease, stroke, and cardiovascular death): a meta-analysis of prospective studies up to 2016. J Am Heart Assoc. 2017;6(7):e005025.

32. Chanouzas D, Dyall L, Nightingale P, Ferro C, Moss P, Morgan MD, et al. Valaciclovir to prevent Cytomegalovirus mediated adverse modulation of the immune system in ANCA-associated vasculitis (CANVAS): study protocol for a randomised controlled trial. Trials. 2016;17(1):338. https://doi.org/10.1186/s13063-13016-11482-13062.

33. Chattopadhyay PK, Yu J, Roederer M. Live-cell assay to detect antigen-specific CD4+ T-cell responses by CD154 expression. Nat Protoc. 2006;1(1):1–6.

34. Becattini S, Latorre D, Mele F, Foglierini M, De Gregorio C, Cassotta A, et al. T cell immunity. Functional heterogeneity of human memory CD4(+) T cell clones primed by pathogens or vaccines. Science. 2015;347(6220):400–6.

35. Buono C, Binder CJ, Stavrakis G, Witztum JL, Glimcher LH, Lichtman AH. T-bet deficiency reduces atherosclerosis and alters plaque antigen-specific immune responses. Proc Natl Acad Sci U S A. 2005;102(5):1596–601.

36. Ait-Oufella H, Taleb S, Mallat Z, Tedgui A. Recent advances on the role of cytokines in atherosclerosis. Arterioscler Thromb Vasc Biol. 2011;31(5):969–79.

37. Chue CD, Townend JN, Steeds RP, Ferro CJ. Arterial stiffness in chronic kidney disease: causes and consequences. Heart. 2010;96(11):817–23.

38. Pachnio A, Ciaurriz M, Begum J, Lal N, Zuo J, Beggs A, et al. Cytomegalovirus infection leads to development of high frequencies of cytotoxic virus-specific CD4+ T cells targeted to vascular endothelium. PLoS Pathog. 2016;12(9):e1005832.

39. Komocsi A, Lamprecht P, Csernok E, Mueller A, Holl-Ulrich K, Seitzer U, et al. Peripheral blood and granuloma CD4(+)CD28(−) T cells are a major source of interferon-gamma and tumor necrosis factor-alpha in Wegener's granulomatosis. Am J Pathol. 2002;160(5):1717–24.

40. Mallat Z, Taleb S, Ait-Oufella H, Tedgui A. The role of adaptive T cell immunity in atherosclerosis. J Lipid Res. 2009;50(Suppl):S364–9.

41. Kossmann S, Schwenk M, Hausding M, Karbach SH, Schmidgen MI, Brandt M, et al. Angiotensin II-induced vascular dysfunction depends on interferon-gamma-driven immune cell recruitment and mutual activation of monocytes and NK-cells. Arterioscler Thromb Vasc Biol. 2013;33(6):1313–9.

42. van de Berg PJ, Yong SL, Remmerswaal EB, van Lier RA, ten Berge IJ. Cytomegalovirus-induced effector T cells cause endothelial cell damage. Clin Vaccine Immunol. 2012;19(5):772–9.

43. Bolovan-Fritts CA, Trout RN, Spector SA. High T-cell response to human cytomegalovirus induces chemokine-mediated endothelial cell damage. Blood. 2007;110(6):1857–63.

44. Dumitriu IE. The life (and death) of CD4+ CD28(^{null}) T cells in inflammatory diseases. Immunology. 2015;146(2):185–93.

45. Slot MC, Kroon AA, Damoiseaux J, Theunissen R, Houben A, de Leeuw PW, et al. CD4+CD28^{null} T cells are related to previous cytomegalovirus infection but not to accelerated atherosclerosis in ANCA-associated vasculitis. Rheumatol Int. 2017;37(5):791–8.

46. Reference Values for Arterial Stiffness C. Determinants of pulse wave velocity in healthy people and in the presence of cardiovascular risk factors: 'establishing normal and reference values'. Eur Heart J. 2010;31(19):2338–50.

47. McEniery CM, Yasmin HIR, Qasem A, Wilkinson IB, Cockcroft JR, Investigators A. Normal vascular aging: differential effects on wave reflection and aortic pulse wave velocity: the Anglo-Cardiff collaborative trial (ACCT). J Am Coll Cardiol. 2005;46(9):1753–60.

48. Rauwel B, Jang SM, Cassano M, Kapopoulou A, Barde I, Trono D. Release of human cytomegalovirus from latency by a KAP1/TRIM28 phosphorylation switch. eLife. 2015;4 https://doi.org/10.7554/eLife.06068.

49. Chanouzas D, Sagmeister M, Faustini S, Nightingale P, Richter A, Ferro CJ, Morgan MD, Moss P, Harper L. Subclinical reactivation of cytomegalovirus drives CD4+CD28null T-cell expansion and impaired immune response to pneumococcal vaccination in ANCA-associated vasculitis. J Infect Dis. 2018.

50. Kerstein A, Schuler S, Cabral-Marques O, Fazio J, Hasler R, Muller A, et al. Environmental factor and inflammation-driven alteration of the total peripheral T-cell compartment in granulomatosis with polyangiitis. J Autoimmun. 2017;78:79–91.

13

NLRP3 inflammasome inhibitor OLT1177 suppresses joint inflammation in murine models of acute arthritis

Carlo Marchetti[1], Benjamin Swartzwelter[1], Marije I. Koenders[2], Tania Azam[1], Isak W. Tengesdal[1,3], Nick Powers[1], Dennis M. de Graaf[1,3], Charles A. Dinarello[1,3] and Leo A. B. Joosten[1,3]*⊙

Abstract

Background: Activation of the NLRP3 inflammasome in gout amplifies the inflammatory response and mediates further damage. In the current study, we assessed the therapeutic effect of OLT1177, an orally active NLRP3 inflammasome inhibitor that is safe in humans, in murine acute arthritis models.

Methods: Zymosan or monosodium urate (MSU) crystals were injected intra-articularly (i.a.) into mouse knee joints to induce reactive or gouty arthritis. Joint swelling, articular cell infiltration, and synovial cytokines were evaluated 25 hours and 4 hours following zymosan or MSU challenge, respectively. OLT1177 was administrated intraperitoneally by oral gavage or in the food by an OLT1177-enriched diet.

Results: OLT1177 reduced zymosan-induced joint swelling ($p < 0.001$), cell influx ($p < 0.01$), and synovial levels of interleukin (IL)-1β, IL-6, and chemokine (C-X-C motif) ligand 1 (CXCL1) ($p < 0.05$), respectively, when compared with vehicle-treated mice. Plasma OLT1177 levels correlated ($p < 0.001$) dose-dependently with reduction in joint inflammation. Treatment of mice with OLT1177 limited MSU crystal articular inflammation ($p > 0.0001$), which was associated with decreased synovial IL-1β, IL-6, myeloperoxidase, and CXCL1 levels ($p < 0.01$) compared with vehicle-treated mice. When administrated orally 1 hour after MSU challenge, OLT1177 reduced joint inflammation, processing of IL-1β, and synovial phosphorylated c-Jun N-terminal kinase compared with the vehicle group. Mice were fed an OLT1177-enriched diet for 3 weeks and then challenged i.a. with MSU crystals. Joint swelling, synovial IL-1β, and expression of *Nlrp3* and *Il1b* were significantly reduced in synovial tissues in mice fed an OLT1177-enriched diet when compared with the standard diet group.

Conclusions: Oral OLT1177 is highly effective in ameliorating reactive as well as gouty arthritis.

Keywords: IL-1β, NLRP3 inflammasome, Gout

Background

Severe inflammation of articular joints is the hallmark of acute arthritides such as gouty arthritis and reactive arthritis. These types of acute inflammatory arthritis are initiated either by sterile triggers, such as in gout, or microbial agents, as in reactive arthritis. In the case of gout, monosodium urate (MSU) crystal deposits and a second signal are needed to trigger joint inflammation [1].

Reactive or septic arthritis is mostly caused by microorganisms such as group A *Streptococcus pyogenes, Chlamydia trachomatis, Campylobacter, Salmonella, Shigella*, or *Yersinia* [2]. Reactive arthritis occurs as a response to infections in the genitals or the gut. Of interest, these forms of acute arthritis occur mainly in males [3]; why males are more susceptible to gouty arthritis or reactive arthritis remains unknown.

A common feature of acute arthritides is the marked influx of neutrophils into the joint cavity [4]. This process is initiated mainly by the production and release of proinflammatory mediators, such as cytokines and chemokines, by the synovial lining cells. Interleukin

* Correspondence: leo.joosten@radboudumc.nl
[1]Department of Medicine, University of Colorado Denver, Aurora, CO, USA
[3]Department of Internal Medicine and Radboud Institute of Molecular Life Sciences (RIMLS), Radboud University Medical Center, Geert Grooteplein Zuid 8, 6525, GA, Nijmegen, The Netherlands
Full list of author information is available at the end of the article

(IL)-1β, IL-6, and IL-8 are the main mediators implicated in the onset of acute arthritis, both in humans and in murine models [5–7]. Decades ago, IL-1β was reported as the prominent cytokine for inducing production of IL-6 and IL-8 [8, 9]. IL-8 is the classical chemokine that drives large numbers of neutrophils into sites of infection or inflammation, and IL-8 has been detected in high concentrations in the synovial fluid of patients with acute arthritis [10]. In murine models of acute arthritis, IL-1β inhibition during onset of arthritis results in effective suppression of joint swelling and influx of inflammatory cells [7, 11]. These observations were further underscored by studies in which models of acute joint inflammation were induced in IL-1β-deficient mice [11].

In gout and several other forms of arthritis, nucleotide-binding oligomerization domain-like receptor (NLR) protein 3 (NACHT, LRR and PYD domains-containing protein 3 [NLRP3], cryopyrin) inflammasome activation is critical in both the inflammatory phase and the progression of disease [12]. Inflammasomes are macromolecular complexes formed in the cytosol of cells in response to various stimuli [13, 14]. Following activation of the NLRP3 inflammasome, the intracellular cysteine protease caspase-1 is activated and generates bioactive IL-1β and IL-18 [15].

We recently reported that OLT1177 (recommended International Nonproprietary Name [rINN] depansutrile) specifically targets the NLRP3 inflammasome and thereby prevents processing and release of IL-1β and IL-18 in vitro [16]. OLT1177 is active in vivo and limits the severity of endotoxin-induced inflammation [16]. The role of IL-1β in rare autoinflammatory diseases, such as familial Mediterranean fever and cryopyrin-associated periodic syndrome, is long established using specific inhibitory strategies to prevent IL-1β activity [17, 18]. Gout is a common inflammatory joint disorder, and specific inhibition of IL-1β is approved by the U.S. Food and Drug Administration and the European Medicines Evaluation Agency for reducing the number of gout attacks [19–21]. Nevertheless, a clinical need, particularly for the refractory cases, remains unmet [22]. In the current study, using two distinct murine models of acute inflammatory arthritis, we validated the rationale for treatment of acute joint inflammation with the NLRP3 inflammasome inhibitor OLT1177.

Methods
OLT1177 treatments
OLT1177 was synthesized as described elsewhere [16]. Crystalline OLT1177 was solubilized with sterile saline for intraperitoneal administrations and with water for oral gavage studies. OLT1177 dosing solutions were prepared fresh before each experiment.

Mice
Animal protocols were approved by the University of Colorado Animal Care and Use Committee. Male C57BL/6 mice (10–12 weeks of age) were purchased from The Jackson Laboratory (Bar Harbor, ME, USA) and housed in the animal facility for at least 7 days before use.

Zymosan-induced arthritis
Knee joints were injected intra-articularly (i.a.) into the synovial space directly under the patella with 180 μg of zymosan from *Saccharomyces cerevisiae* (Sigma-Aldrich, St. Louis, MO, USA). Briefly, 300 mg of zymosan were dissolved in 10 ml of sterile saline, boiled three times, and sonicated to ensure a uniform suspension. Mice were treated with OLT1177 (60, 200, or 600 mg/kg as indicated) in 200 μl of saline for intraperitoneal administration or in water for oral gavage at 24 hours, 12 hours, and 1 hour before zymosan injection. Mice received two additional administrations of the corresponding dose of OLT1177 at 11 and 23 hours after the zymosan challenge. Twenty-five hours after the zymosan instillation, mice were anesthetized, joint swelling was scored, and knee and synovial tissues were collected for histological and cytokine analyses.

MSU crystal-induced arthritis
Gouty arthritis was induced by injecting into the right and left knees of mice 10 μl of a mixture of 300 μg of MSU crystals, 200 μM C16:0 palmitic acid (Sigma-Aldrich), and 1 mg of bovine serum albumin (Sigma-Aldrich). The effect of OLT1177 in the gouty arthritis model was tested using three different OLT1177 treatment protocols.

First protocol
OLT1177 and vehicle were given by oral gavage every 12 hours for five doses. One hour after the last dose, the MSU suspension was administrated in the knees of the mice.

Second protocol
OLT1177 and vehicle were administered orally as a single dose 1 hour after the induction of gouty arthritis.

Third protocol
The third protocol used a special research diet. Mice were fed either an OLT1177-enriched diet or a standard food diet for 3 weeks. The composition of the food was identical (standard mouse chow), except that OLT1177-enriched food contained 7.5 g of OLT1177 per kilogram of food. Food and water were provided ad libitum for the entire length of the study. Standard and OLT1177-enriched diets were prepared by Research Diets (New Brunswick, NJ, USA). Mice that were given i.a. injections with saline and

not subjected to gouty arthritis were used as sham animals for the comparison of the joint swelling.

For each dosing protocol, mice were anesthetized, and the skin over the knee joints was opened so the MSU mixture could be injected i.a. Mice were killed 4 hours following MSU crystal instillation. The joint was exposed and scored macroscopically. Thereafter, knee joints and synovial tissue specimens were collected for histological or molecular analysis.

Joint scoring

After the skin was removed from each knee, the joint (R and L) was scored macroscopically on a scale from 0 to 3, where 0 = no inflammation, 1 = mild inflammation, 2 = moderate inflammation, and 3 = severe inflammation, in increments of 0.25. A score of 0.25 was given when the first signs of swelling and redness were present. Joint swelling scoring was performed by two authors without knowledge of the experimental groups.

Sample collection and cytokine measurement

After macroscopic scoring, the entire right knee joint was removed and fixed in 4% formaldehyde for histological analysis. The synovial tissue specimens from the left knee were removed for cytokine measurements. Briefly, patella with minimal surrounding muscle tissue and maximal synovial membrane was excised from the left knee joint. The synovial tissue explants were placed in 250 µl of 0.5% Triton X-100 (in water) and subjected to three freeze-thaw cycles to increase the extraction process. Cytokines were measured in the lysates of synovial tissues by specific enzyme-linked immunosorbent assays (R&D Systems, Minneapolis, MN, USA) following the manufacturer's instructions. Because of experiment-related variations in cytokine production in some experiments, the raw data were calculated as percent changes of cytokine levels between vehicle-treated and OLT1177-treated mice. For example, in the zymosan-challenged group, each mean value in picograms per milliliter for vehicle-treated mice was set at 100%. For each value of OLT1177-treated mice, percent change was calculated. The ranges of levels in picograms per milliliter are indicated in each figure legend.

Histological analysis

The right knee joints were fixed in 4% formaldehyde for 7 days before decalcification using 5% formic acid and processed for paraffin embedding. Tissue sections (7 µm) were stained with H&E. Histopathological changes in the knee joints were scored in the patellar/femoral region in five semiserial sections by the number of infiltrating cells in the synovial lining and/or joint cavity on a scale ranging from 0 to 3. Joint inflammation was graded on decoded slides by two separate observers.

OLT1177 plasma exposure

OLT1177 was extracted from 50.0 µl of mouse plasma by a liquid-liquid procedure and quantified in plasma using gas chromatography (GC) with detection by MS/MS (Chemic Laboratories, Inc., Canton, MA, USA). OLT1177-D3 was used as the internal standard. Extraction started with the addition of 20.0 µl of the internal standard working solution for all samples. The samples were vortexed gently, and then 2.0 ml of ethyl acetate was added. Samples were vortexed, centrifuged, and placed in an acetone dry ice water bath, where the supernatant was transferred to clean tubes. The supernatant was then evaporated to dryness and reconstituted with N,O-bis(trimethylsilyl)trifluoroacetamide (1:25 vol/vol) with 1% trimethylchlorosilane/ethyl acetate. Samples were covered, vortexed, and transferred to clean amber vials. The extracts were examined by chromatograph on a DB-17 GC column (J&W Scientific, Folsom, CA, USA). OLT1177 was detected and quantified by MS/MS in positive ion mode using an Agilent 7890A GC system (Agilent Technologies, Santa Clara, CA, USA). A method qualification run was performed, and the qualified quantitation range was 20.0–2000 ng/ml.

Whole-blood culture

Blood was collected in ethylenediaminetetraacetic acid-coated tubes, and total white blood cell (WBC) counts and the percentages of monocytes, lymphocytes, and granulocytes were determined using a HemaTrue cell counter (Heska, Loveland, CO, USA). For the whole-blood cultures, blood was diluted in RPMI 1640 medium (Mediatech CellGro; Corning, Corning, NY, USA) (1:), and 200 µl was added to each round-bottomed well. The microtiter plates were incubated for 24 hours at 37 °C. After incubation, the supernatants were removed and frozen at − 80 °C until assayed for cytokines.

Western blotting

The protein concentration of the synovial tissue extracts (L) was determined in the clarified supernatants using a Bio-Rad protein assay (Bio-Rad Laboratories, Hercules, CA, USA). Proteins were electrophoresed on Mini-PROTEAN TGX 4–20% gels (Bio-Rad Laboratories) and transferred to nitrocellulose of 0.45 µm pore size (GE Healthcare Life Sciences, Marlborough, MA, USA). Membranes were blocked in 5% dried milk in PBS-Tween 0.5% for 1 hour at room temperature. Phosphorylated stress-activated protein kinase/c-Jun N-terminal kinase (JNK) (1:500; Cell Signaling Technology, Danvers, MA, USA), IL-1β (1:1000, AF-401; R&D Systems), and NLRP3 (1:1000, Cryo-2; AdipoGen Life Sciences, San Diego, CA, USA) were used as the primary antibodies. Peroxidase-conjugated secondary antibodies and chemiluminescence were used to develop the blots. A primary antibody against β-actin (Santa Cruz Biotechnology, Dallas, TX, USA) was used to assess protein loading.

Statistical analysis

Statistical significance of differences was evaluated with a two-tailed Student's t test using Prism version 6.0 software (GraphPad Software, La Jolla, CA, USA). Statistical significance was set at $p < 0.05$.

Results

OLT1177 reduces the severity of zymosan-induced arthritis

Joint swelling and i.a. neutrophil infiltration were assessed 25 hours after injection of zymosan into the knee joints. Figure 1a depicts the marked knee joint swelling after the zymosan challenge as compared with the saline-injected group. In OLT1177-treated mice, the inflammation was reduced by 45% ($p < 0.0001$) (Fig. 1a and b). We next

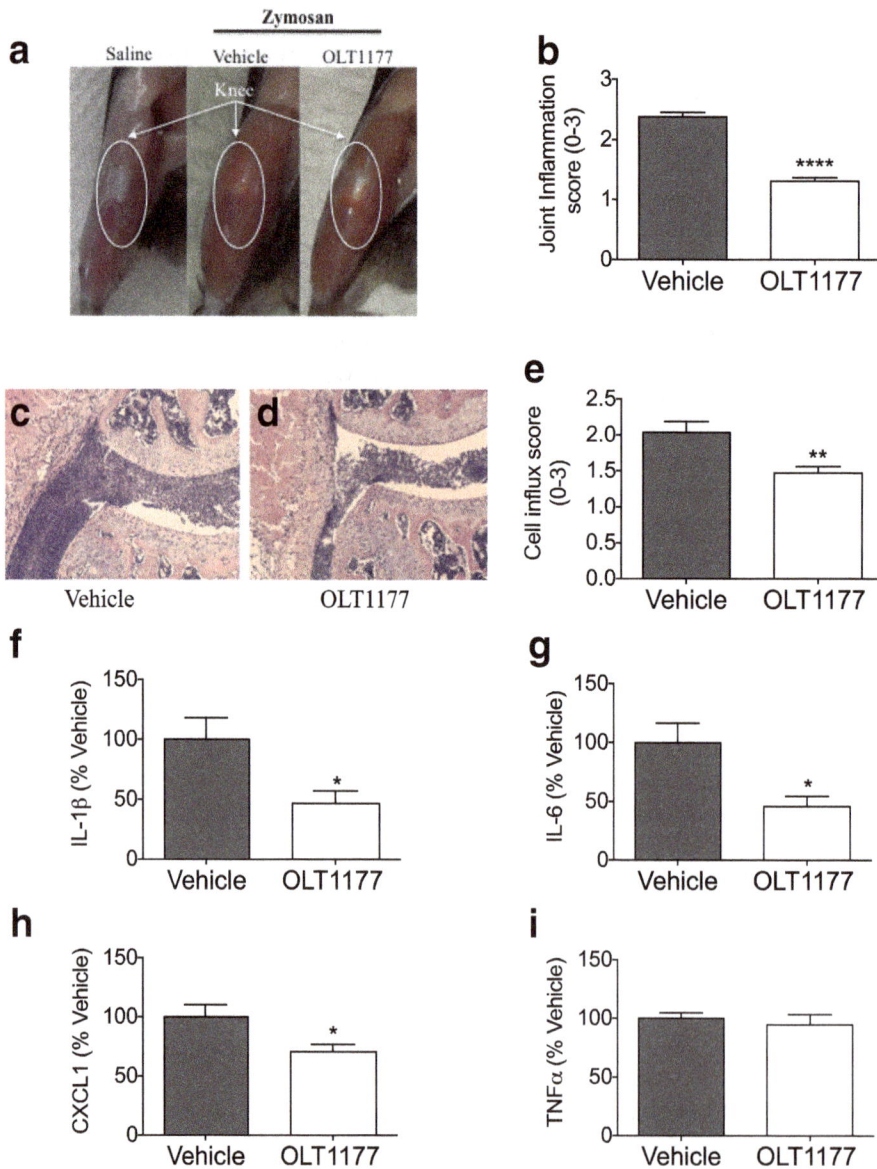

Fig. 1 Effect of OLT1177 on zymosan-induced arthritis. **a** Representative images of knees from saline injected (Saline), vehicle-treated, and OLT1177 (200 mg/kg)-treated mice. **b** Mean ± SEM of joint score ($n = 16$ per group). **c** and **d** H&E-stained histological knee sections from vehicle- and OLT1177-treated mice. Original magnification 100 ×. **e** Mean ± SEM of cell influx ($n = 5$ per group). **f–i** Mean ± SEM percent change of interleukin (IL)-1β (range 189–2488 pg/ml), IL-6 (range 100–843 pg/ml), chemokine (C-X-C motif) ligand 1 (CXCL1) (range 169–472 pg/ml), and tumor necrosis factor (TNF)-α (282–405 pg/ml) in synovial tissue extracts from mice subjected to experimental zymosan-induced arthritis and treated with OLT1177 (200 mg/kg). Percent change was calculated as described in the Methods section of text. $n = 8$ per group; **** $p < 0.0001$, ** $p < 0.01$, * $p < 0.05$

examined cell influx, a hallmark of inflammation and tissue damage, using histological analysis of the knee joint. H&E staining revealed that mice treated with OLT1177 had a visible reduction in infiltrating cells, predominantly neutrophils ($p = 0.006$) (Fig. 1c–e) when compared with vehicle-treated mice.

We next determined the effect of OLT1177 treatment on the levels of inflammatory mediators in inflamed synovial tissue. As depicted in Fig. 1f–h, treatment with OLT1177 (200 mg/kg) reduced synovial tissue concentrations of IL-1β and IL-6 by 55% ($p < 0.05$) and the neutrophil chemokine (C-X-C motif) ligand 1 (CXCL1) by 30% ($p < 0.05$). No significant effect was observed in tumor necrosis factor (TNF)-α levels (Fig. 1i). In addition, OLT1177 was effective in reducing joint inflammation following zymosan instillation when administrated orally. Oral gavage of OLT1177 (600 mg/kg) showed a significant reduction in synovial swelling ($p < 0.001$) and IL-1β level (-70%; $p = 0.01$) (Additional file 1: Figure S1A and B), with no effect on TNF-α (Additional file 1: Figure S1C), when compared with vehicle-treated mice. These data indicate that OLT1177 reduced cytokine levels, which was associated with decreased severity of the zymosan-induced arthritis.

Dose-response suppressive effect of OLT1177 on joint inflammation in mice with zymosan-induced arthritis

The anti-inflammatory effect of different concentrations of OLT1177 was evaluated. As depicted in Fig. 2a, treatment with OLT1177 revealed a dose-dependent reduction of joint inflammation scores following i.a. injection of zymosan, with maximal inhibition at 600 mg/kg (-63%; $p < 0.0001$). The different concentrations used of OLT1177 (60, 200, and 600 mg/kg) corresponded to plasma levels of 9.22 ± 0.55, 16.73 ± 9.89, and 41.4 ± 3.68 μg/ml, respectively (Fig. 2b). This analysis demonstrates a direct correlation ($p < 0.001$) between the reduction in joint inflammation and the circulating concentration of OLT1177.

OLT1177 reduces joint inflammation of MSU crystal-induced gouty arthritis

Next, we examined the effect of OLT1177 in a model of MSU-induced gouty arthritis. Following i.a. administration of MSU crystals, severe swelling of the knee joint was observed in vehicle-treated mice (Fig. 3a). Oral treatment with OLT1177 (600 mg/kg) showed significant reduction in joint scores when compared with the vehicle group (75% reduction; $p < 0.0001$) (Fig. 3b). Histological analyses of the knee joints showed suppression of influx of inflammatory cells (31% reduction; $p < 0.05$) into the joint cavity following OLT1177 treatment (Fig. 3c, d). Synovial tissue extracts were analyzed for cytokine and chemokine concentrations. As depicted in

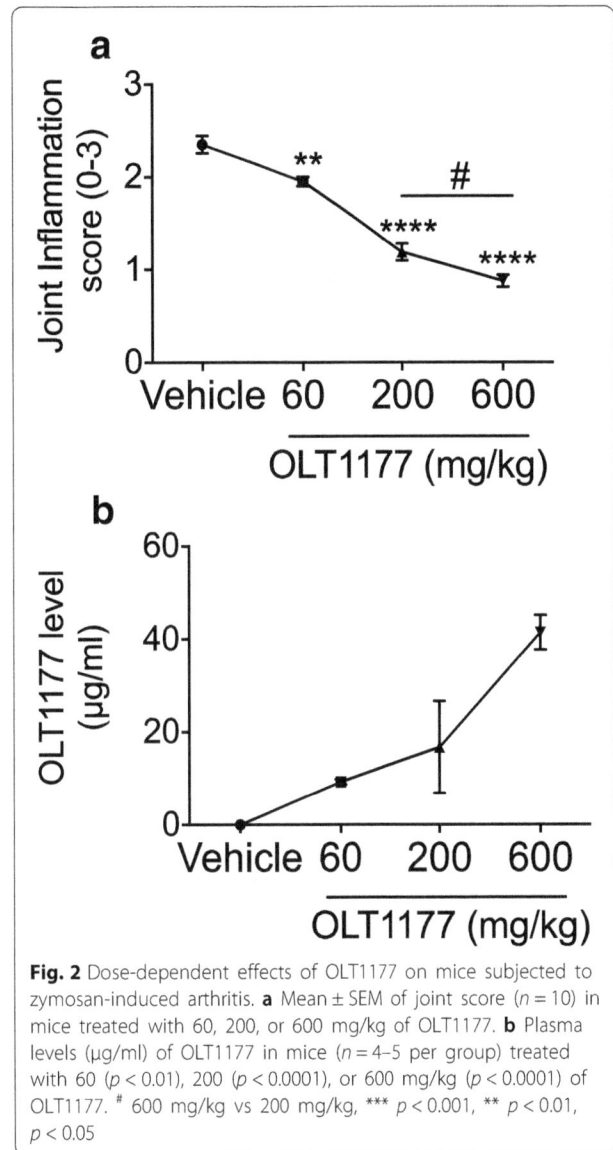

Fig. 2 Dose-dependent effects of OLT1177 on mice subjected to zymosan-induced arthritis. **a** Mean ± SEM of joint score ($n = 10$) in mice treated with 60, 200, or 600 mg/kg of OLT1177. **b** Plasma levels (μg/ml) of OLT1177 in mice ($n = 4$–5 per group) treated with 60 ($p < 0.01$), 200 ($p < 0.0001$), or 600 mg/kg ($p < 0.0001$) of OLT1177. # 600 mg/kg vs 200 mg/kg, *** $p < 0.001$, ** $p < 0.01$, $p < 0.05$

Fig. 3e–h, there were significant reductions in IL-1β (69%; $p = 0.004$), IL-6 (70%; $p < 0.001$), myeloperoxidase (MPO) (39%; $p = 0.006$), and CXCL1 (75%; $p < 0.001$) in OLT1177-treated mice. Thus, OLT1177 reduced the local level of inflammatory mediators, which were associated with a significant amelioration in joint swelling in this model of MSU-induced gouty arthritis.

Therapeutic administration of OLT1177 suppresses MSU-induced gouty arthritis

Next, we evaluated the effect of oral administration of OLT1177 after the onset of arthritis to explore a therapeutic treatment strategy. Mice were injected i.a. with MSU crystals to elicit arthritis. One hour thereafter, mice received a single oral dose of OLT1177 (600 mg/kg) and were killed 3 hours later. As depicted in Fig. 4a and b, OLT1177-treated mice showed a trend toward reduced

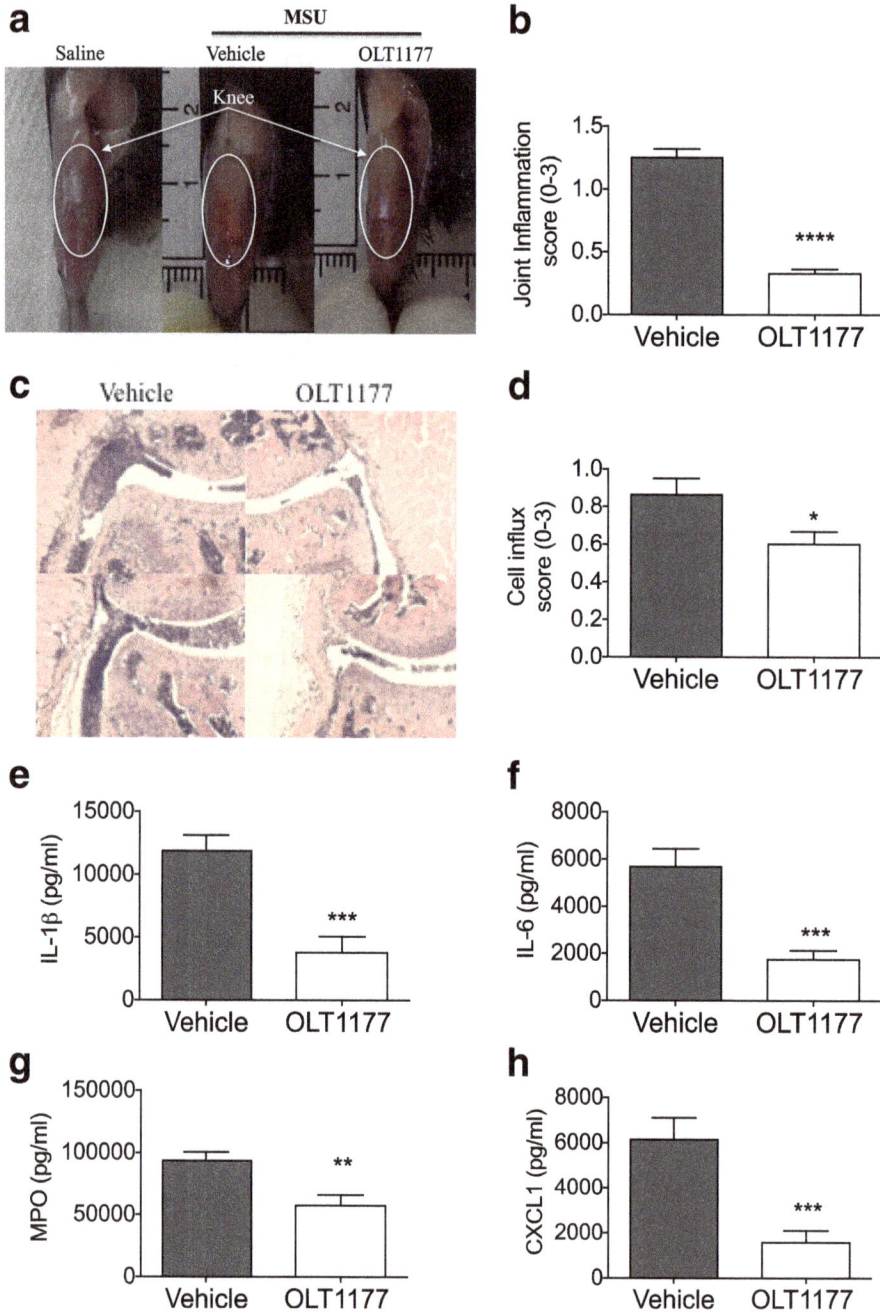

Fig. 3 Effect of oral treatment with OLT1177 in monosodium urate (MSU)-induced arthritis. **a** Representative images of joints of saline-injected knee (Saline) and from vehicle-treated and OLT1177 (600 mg/kg)-treated mice. **b** Mean ± SEM of joint score (n = 20). **c** H&E-stained histological knee joint sections from vehicle- or OLT1177-treated mice. Original magnification 100 ×. **d** Mean ± SEM of cell influx (n = 10). **e–h** Mean ± SEM of interleukin (IL)-1β, IL-6, myeloperoxidase (MPO), and chemokine (C-X-C motif) ligand 1 (CXCL1) in synovial tissue lysates from mice subjected to experimental MSU-induced arthritis. n = 10 per group. **** $p < 0.0001$, *** $p < 0.001$, ** $p < 0.01$, * $p < 0.05$

total circulating leukocytes ($p = 0.09$) and a significant reduction in monocytes (– 45%; $p < 0.01$) and granulocytes (– 38%; $p < 0.05$). Whole-blood cultures revealed that spontaneous IL-6 production by circulating WBCs was lower in OLT1177-treated mice than in the vehicle-treated group (Fig. 4c) ($p < 0.05$).

Joints from mice treated with OLT1177 exhibited markedly reduced macroscopic joint inflammation (Fig. 4d) ($p < 0.0001$). In addition, in the synovial tissue extracts, IL-1β (44%; $p = 0.0002$), IL-6 (30%; $p < 0.001$), and CXCL1 (31%; $p < 0.05$) were reduced (Fig. 4e–g).

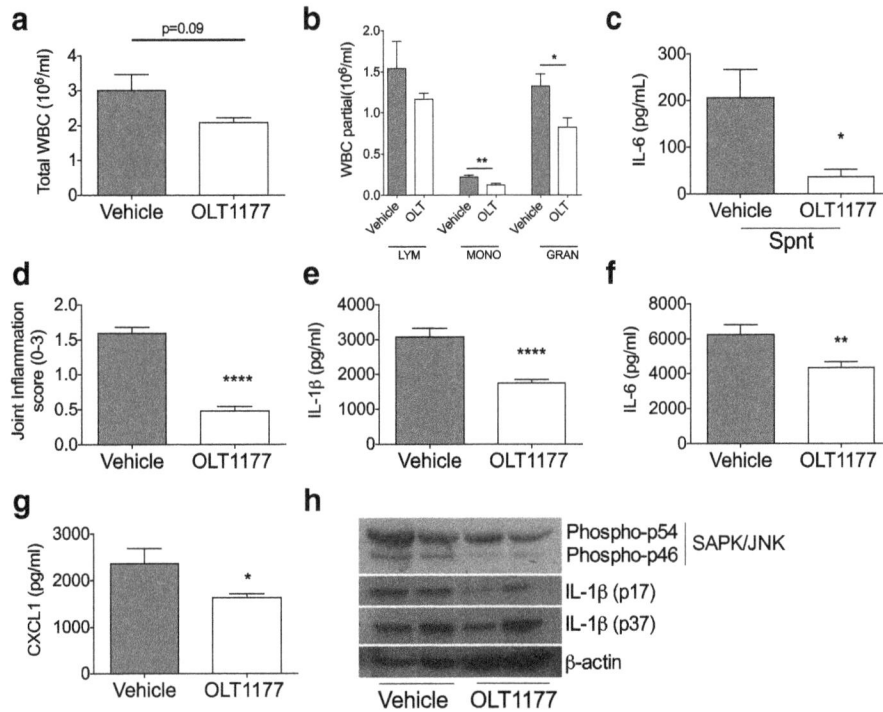

Fig. 4 Effect of posttreatment of oral OLT1177 in monosodium urate-induced arthritis. Total white blood cell (WBC) count (**a**) and differential counts (**b**) in mice treated with vehicle or OLT1177 (600 mg/kg) ($n = 5$). **c** Mean ± SEM of spontaneous (Spnt) interleukin (IL)-6 levels from whole-blood culture in vehicle- and OLT1177-treated mice. **d** Mean ± SEM of joint score ($n = 20$). **e–g** Mean ± SEM of IL-1β, IL-6, and chemokine (C-X-C motif) ligand 1 (CXCL1) in synovial tissue extracts ($n = 10$ per group). **h** Western blot of phospho-c-Jun N-terminal kinase (JNK) and IL-1β (p17 and IL-1β precursor p37) in synovial tissue extracts. Each lane represents a single mouse. **** $p < 0.0001$, ** $p < 0.01$, * $p < 0.05$. *SAPK* Stress-activated protein kinase

We next investigated the effect of OLT1177 treatment on the activation of the mitogen-activated protein kinase family member JNK. As depicted in Fig. 4h, phosphory-lated JNK in synovial extracts from mice treated with OLT1177 was lower than in vehicle-treated mice. Reduction in IL-1β in synovial lysates was also confirmed by Western blot analysis, with reduced levels of the mature form of IL-1β (p17) in OLT1177-treated mice when compared with the vehicle-treated mice (Fig. 4h).

OLT1177 treatment in daily food reduces MSU-induced gouty arthritis

We designed a study of OLT1177 treatment to resemble an option for patients with recurrent gout attacks. Mice were fed an OLT1177-enriched diet (7.5 g of OLT1177 per kilogram of food) or a standard research diet for 3 weeks. All mice were then challenged i.a. with MSU crystals and killed after 4 hours. Figure 5a reveals signifi-cantly lower joint inflammation scores in mice fed the OLT1177 diet than in mice fed standard food. Concen-trations of cytokines in the synovial tissue explants were significantly reduced for IL-1β (− 47%) and IL-6 (− 37%) ($p < 0.05$) in mice fed the OLT1177 diet compared with mice fed the standard diet (Fig. 5b, c). Both the IL-1β

precursor and the active form of IL-1β (p17) were re-duced in OLT1177-treated mice, as shown by Western blot analysis (Fig. 5d). No significant differences were measured in NLRP3 protein level between the two groups (Fig. 5d). Gene expression of *Nlrp3* and *Il1b* from synovial tissue extracts was reduced in the OLT1177 diet-fed mice compared with mice fed the standard diet (Fig. 5e, f).

Comparative analysis of plasma OLT1177 concentrations following food intake in mice and in human phase I study

We next determined the concentration of OLT1177 in the plasma of mice fed the OLT1177-enriched diet for 3 weeks. During the entire duration of the study, mice had access to water and food ad libitum and were not sub-jected to any challenge. Figure 6a shows that mice fed the OLT1177-enriched diet reached a mean plasma OLT1177 concentration of 46.3 ± 3.15 μg/ml. Plasma OLT1177 exposure in humans was measured in a phase I clinical study in healthy subjects as described elsewhere [16]. Following a single oral dose of 1000 mg of OLT1177, the mean maximum plasma concentration (C_{max}) was 32 ± 9.1 μg/ml (Fig. 6b). Plasma OLT1177 ex-posure in human subjects was also measured following

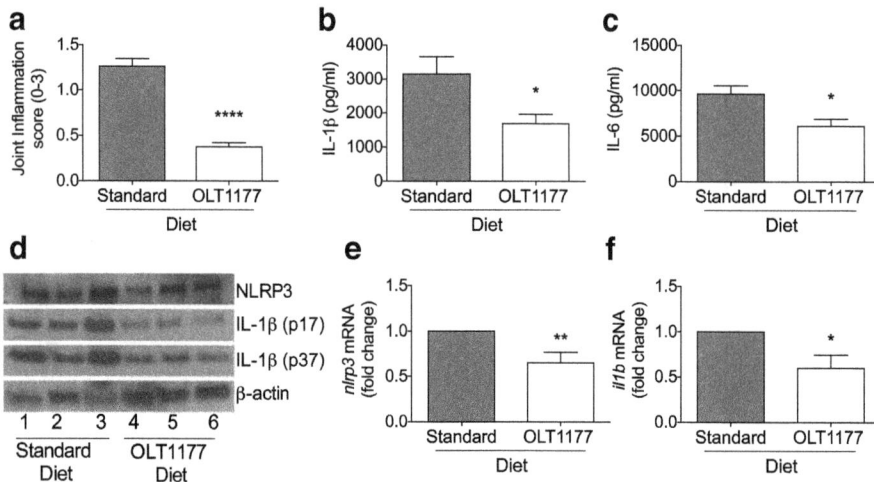

Fig. 5 Effect of OLT1177-enriched diet in monosodium urate (MSU)-induced arthritis. **a** Mean ± SEM of joint score ($n = 9$–10). **b** and **c** Mean ± SEM of interleukin (IL)-1β and IL-6 in synovial tissue lysates from mice subjected to experimental MSU-induced arthritis ($n = 9$–10 per group). **d** Western blot for NLRP3 and IL-1β (p17 and IL-1β precursor p37) in synovial tissue lysates from mice subjected to experimental MSU-induced arthritis and fed a standard diet or an OLT1177-enriched diet. Each lane represents a single mouse. **e** and **f** Fold change of messenger RNA (mRNA) levels of *nlrp3* and *il1b* of synovial tissue extracts from mice treated with OLT1177 ($n = 4$–5 per group). **** $p < 0.0001$, ** $p < 0.01$, * $p < 0.05$

repeated daily oral dosing for 8 consecutive days. The mean group C_{max} after eight consecutive doses of 1000 mg was 41.4 ± 10.8 μg/ml (Fig. 6b). The mean OLT1177 plasma level in mice following 3 weeks of OLT1177-enriched diet reached the same order of magnitude as the level reached in humans.

Discussion

In the current study, we describe the anti-inflammatory effects of the synthetic small molecule sulfonyl nitrile compound OLT1177 in two different mouse models of experimental arthritis representative of reactive arthritis and gouty arthritis. As previously reported, OLT1177 in humans is safe, orally active, and specifically inhibits the NLRP3 inflammasome, preventing processing and release of active IL-1β [16]. The favorable phase I safety

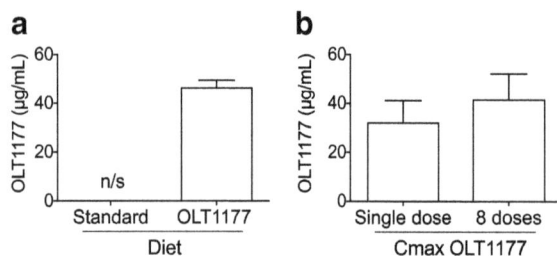

Fig. 6 Comparison of plasma OLT1177 levels in mice and humans. **a** Mean ± SEM of OLT1177 resting plasma level (μg/ml) of mice fed for 3 weeks with standard and OLT1177-enriched diets ($n = 5$). **b** Mean ± SEM of maximum concentration (C_{max}) of resting plasma levels of OLT1177 in healthy human subjects following a single dose ($n = 5$) and after eight daily oral doses ($n = 5$) of OLT1177 (16 mg/kg). Figure 6b is adapted from [16]

profile of OLT1177 combined with the reported inhibitory effects on NLRP3 inflammasome and IL-1β release led to approval of the molecule for phase II development in gout.

OLT1177 treatment administered either intraperitoneally or by oral gavage reduced joint inflammation in zymosan-induced arthritis when compared with vehicle-treated mice. We observed a significant reduction in the level of inflammatory cytokines in synovial tissue explants, including IL-1β and IL-6. Prolonged neutrophil activity, as in chronic inflammatory conditions, leads to detrimental effects [23]. In the present study, we have shown that treatment with OLT1177 suppressed cell infiltration into the joint with reduced levels of the neutrophil chemokine CXCL1 in synovial tissue extracts. These data and the reduced knee swelling in the OLT1177-treated mice are representative of the benefits of IL-1 inhibition, also observed in previous studies of reactive arthritis [7, 24].

OLT1177 is a specific NLRP3 inflammasome inhibitor [16]. Zymosan contains β-glucan from the cell wall of the yeast (*S. cerevisiae*), and this glucan induces NLRP3 inflammasome activation [25]. In the present study, we have demonstrated that OLT1177 reduces the severity of zymosan-induced arthritis in a dose-dependent manner by intraperitoneal administration and via oral gavage in mice. The lack of effect of OLT1177 treatment on TNF-α production supports previously observed data [16] confirming that OLT1177 primarily targets IL-1β.

We observed a direct correlation between the doses 60, 200, and 600 mg/kg of OLT1177 and the reduction in joint inflammation ($- 17$, $p < 0.01$; $- 50$, $p < 0.0001$;

and – 63%, $p < 0.0001$, respectively). In comparison, human exposure after oral administration of OLT1177 led to an average C_{max} of 41.4 ± 10.8 µg/ml after 1000 mg/d for 8 consecutive days [16], which is of the same order of magnitude achieved in the 600 mg/kg dose group. Thus, the OLT1177 exposure used in this study, which was shown to be effective in reducing the severity of zymosan-induced arthritis in a mouse model, reached plasma levels similar to those observed in humans, with no significant adverse effects [16].

Gouty arthritis is a specific form of inflammatory arthritis with elevated urate levels in the bloodstream [3, 26]. In this condition, formation and deposition of MSU crystals in the synovial space cause acute inflammation due to neutrophil infiltration. Acute gout manifestations include attacks of severe pain, stiffness, and swelling of a distal joint, with great impact on patient quality of life [27]. In the present study, we have demonstrated that oral treatment with OLT1177 reduced joint swelling and infiltration of inflammatory cells in a murine model of gouty arthritis simulated by administration of MSU crystals into the articular space. Compared with the vehicle-treated group, mice treated with OLT1177 exhibited significant reductions in IL-1β, IL-6, MPO, and CXCL1 levels in extracted synovial membranes. These data support the therapeutic potential of the use of OLT1177 in gout, an IL-1β-mediated disease [4, 28].

In this study, treatment with OLT1177 was consistently associated with a reduction in IL-6. Although the properties of IL-6 during an acute-phase response are well known, the role of IL-6 in gout remains unclear. Mokuda et al. showed that treatment with tocilizumab improved clinical symptoms in a patient with systemic tophaceous gout [29]. Pinto et al. showed the benefit of tocilizumab treatment in another case of gouty arthritis not responding to the nonsteroidal anti-inflammatory drugs colchicine and allopurinol [30]. However, unlike IL-1β blockade, there are no randomized clinical trials of tocilizumab in refractory gout. It is likely that the increase in IL-6 in gout is a biomarker for active IL-1β. In fact, the ability of IL-1β to induce IL-6 is long established, and elevated IL-6 is often used as a surrogate marker for subpicogram levels of IL-1β in humans. In mice, IL-6 is decreased by genetic and pharmacologic inhibition of IL-1 in gouty arthritis [31]. Further, IL-6 functions as a marker in inflammasome-mediated inflammation with no direct role in MSU-induced inflammation [32]. The acute inflammation of arthritis induced by zymosan is IL-6-independent [33]. In the present study, the reduction in IL-6 is likely due to OLT1177-mediated IL-1β reduction as a consequence of the NLRP3 inflammasome inhibition.

We also evaluated the anti-inflammatory effect of therapeutically administered OLT1177. To this end, we designed a study that mimics a clinical setting where a subject begins treatment after the onset of clinical disease. Mice were subjected to an i.a. injection of MSU crystals, and after 1 hour, vehicle or OLT1177 was administered as a single oral dose. Mice were killed 3 hours following treatment. A single dose of OLT1177 given therapeutically reduced joint inflammation as well as IL-1β, IL-6, and CXCL1 concentrations in the extracted synovial tissue. The anti-inflammatory properties of OLT1177 treatment in the MSU-induced arthritis model were also confirmed with the reduction in the phosphorylation of JNK, which has been implicated in the pathophysiology of several forms of arthritis, such as rheumatoid arthritis and gouty arthritis [34–36].

Patients with recurrent attacks of gout have been treated chronically with IL-1β-blocking therapies (anakinra [37, 38], canakinumab [39, 40], or rilonacept [41, 42]) and have significantly reduced attack rates. Considering the safety profile of oral OLT1177 in humans [16], we designed a study of prolonged oral OLT1177 exposure. Mice were fed a standard diet or an OLT1177-enriched diet for 3 weeks before i.a. injection of MSU crystals into the joints. Joint inflammation and inflammatory markers were reduced in the mice fed an OLT1177 diet when compared with the standard diet group. In addition, Western blot analysis of the synovial membranes revealed a reduction in IL-1β precursor (p37) as well as the mature form of IL-1β (p17) with no change in NLRP3 protein level. These data are consistent with the autopositive feedback of IL-1, where IL-1 induces IL-1 [43]. Thus, we postulate that chronic OLT1177-mediated suppression of active IL-1β production interrupted IL-1β-induced IL-1β precursor synthesis and not solely the NLRP3-dependent release of bioactive IL-1β and the downstream effect of IL-1β.

The unchanged NLRP3 protein level between the two treatment groups indicates that OLT1177 does not reduce inflammasome protein levels in the short-term model (4 hours). We previously reported that there is no reduction in NLRP3 in cells treated in vitro with OLT1177 [16]. However, we did observe reduced Nlrp3 gene expression in the OLT1177-enriched diet group compared with the standard diet mice. Because messenger RNA was extracted from whole synovial tissue, the reduction in Nlrp3 gene expression likely reflects a reduction of cell influx into the synovial membrane in the OLT1177-treated mice. Alternatively, OLT1177 in the food may have reduced gene expression of Nlrp3 during the 3 weeks of the enriched diet. Mean plasma levels of OLT1177 after the 3 weeks was 46.3 ± 3.15 µg/ml (347 µM). In humans, after 8 days of oral OLT1177, the mean plasma level was 41.4 µg/ml (311 µM). In vitro, the half maximal inhibitory concentration of OLT1177 for IL-1β secretion was 1 µM for human blood monocyte-derived macrophages [16]. Thus, on the basis of efficacy in vitro, OLT1177 reaches plasma levels 300-fold greater than those needed to reduce IL-1β secretion in primary human cells.

Conclusions

There is a growing body of research substantiating the mechanism and efficacy of NLRP3 inflammasome inhibitors in experimental animal models, including acute arthritides. However, no approved human agents are available. The small and orally active molecule OLT1777 inhibits the formation of the NLRP3 inflammasome and reduces the severity of reactive and gouty arthritis. On the basis of evidence described in this study and the favorable phase I safety profile, oral OLT1177 has advanced into three phase II development programs, including gout, establishing the translational value of OLT1177 as a safe oral NLRP3 inhibitor.

Abbreviations

C_{max}: Maximum plasma concentration ; CXCL1: Chemokine (C-X-C motif) ligand 1; GC: Gas chromatography; i.a.: Intra-articularly; IL-18: Interleukin 18; IL-1β: Interleukin 1β; IL-6: Interleukin 6; IL-8: Interleukin 8; JNK: c-Jun N-terminal kinase; MPO: Myeloperoxidase; mRNA: Messenger RNA; MSU: Monosodium urate; NLR: Nucleotide-binding oligomerization domain-like receptor; NLRP3: NACHT, LRR and PYD domains-containing protein 3; rINN: Recommended International Nonproprietary Name; SAPK: Stress-activated protein kinase; TNF-α: Tumor necrosis factor-α; WBC: White blood cell

Acknowledgements

The authors thank Niklas Lonnemann.

Funding

These studies are supported by National Institutes of Health grant AI-15614 (to CAD), the Interleukin Foundation for Medical Research, and Olatec Industries.

Authors' contributions

CAD, CM, and LABJ designed the study and wrote the manuscript. BS, CM, NP, DMdG, IWT, MIK, and TA performed research, analyzed or interpreted results, and edited the manuscript. All authors read and approved the final manuscript.

Ethics approval

The animal protocols of this study were approved by the University of Colorado Animal Care and Use Committee.

Consent for publication

Not applicable.

Competing interests

CAD serves as chair of Olatec's Scientific Advisory Board, is co-chief scientific officer, and receives compensation from Olatec. LABJ serves on Olatec's Scientific Advisory Board and receives compensation from Olatec. The other authors declare that they have no competing interests.

Author details

[1]Department of Medicine, University of Colorado Denver, Aurora, CO, USA. [2]Department of Rheumatology, Radboud University Medical Center, Nijmegen, The Netherlands. [3]Department of Internal Medicine and Radboud Institute of Molecular Life Sciences (RIMLS), Radboud University Medical Center, Geert Grooteplein Zuid 8, 6525, GA, Nijmegen, The Netherlands.

References

1. Joosten LA, Netea MG, Mylona E, Koenders MI, Malireddi RK, Oosting M, Stienstra R, van de Veerdonk FL, Stalenhoef AF, Giamarellos-Bourboulis EJ, et al. Engagement of fatty acids with Toll-like receptor 2 drives interleukin-1β production via the ASC/caspase 1 pathway in monosodium urate monohydrate crystal-induced gouty arthritis. Arthritis Rheum. 2010;62(11): 3237–48.
2. Carter JD, Hudson AP. Reactive arthritis: clinical aspects and medical management. Rheum Dis Clin North Am. 2009;35(1):21–44.
3. Dalbeth N, Merriman TR, Stamp LK. Gout. Lancet. 2016;388(10055):2039–52.
4. So AK, Martinon F. Inflammation in gout: mechanisms and therapeutic targets. Nat Rev Rheumatol. 2017;13(11):639–47.
5. Dinarello CA. An expanding role for interleukin-1 blockade from gout to cancer. Mol Med. 2014;20(Suppl 1):S43–58.
6. Kuiper S, Joosten LA, Bendele AM, Edwards CK 3rd, Arntz OJ, Helsen MM, Van de Loo FA, Van den Berg WB. Different roles of tumour necrosis factor α and interleukin 1 in murine streptococcal cell wall arthritis. Cytokine. 1998; 10(9):690–702.
7. van de Loo FA, Joosten LA, van Lent PL, Arntz OJ, van den Berg WB. Role of interleukin-1, tumor necrosis factor α, and interleukin-6 in cartilage proteoglycan metabolism and destruction: effect of in situ blocking in murine antigen- and zymosan-induced arthritis. Arthritis Rheum. 1995;38(2):164–72.
8. Dinarello CA. Interleukin-1 in the pathogenesis and treatment of inflammatory diseases. Blood. 2011;117(14):3720–32.
9. O'Neill LA. The interleukin-1 receptor/toll-like receptor superfamily: 10 years of progress. Immunol Rev. 2008;226:10–8.
10. Bertazzolo N, Punzi L, Pianon M, Cesaro G, Todesco S. Interrelationship between interleukin 8 and neutrophils in synovial fluid of crystal induced arthritis. J Rheumatol. 1994;21(9):1776–7.
11. Joosten LA, Koenders MI, Smeets RL, Heuvelmans-Jacobs M, Helsen MM, Takeda K, Akira S, Lubberts E, van de Loo FA, van den Berg WB. Toll-like receptor 2 pathway drives streptococcal cell wall-induced joint inflammation: critical role of myeloid differentiation factor 88. J Immunol. 2003;171(11):6145–53.
12. Martinon F. Mechanisms of uric acid crystal-mediated autoinflammation. Immunol Rev. 2010;233(1):218–32.
13. Martinon F, Petrilli V, Mayor A, Tardivel A, Tschopp J. Gout-associated uric acid crystals activate the NALP3 inflammasome. Nature. 2006;440(7081):237–41.
14. Schroder K, Zhou R, Tschopp J. The NLRP3 inflammasome: a sensor for metabolic danger? Science. 2010;327(5963):296–300.
15. Franchi L, Eigenbrod T, Munoz-Planillo R, Nunez G. The inflammasome: a caspase-1-activation platform that regulates immune responses and disease pathogenesis. Nat Immunol. 2009;10(3):241–7.
16. Marchetti C, Swartzwelter B, Gamboni F, Neff CP, Richter K, Azam T, Carta S, Tengesdal I, Nemkov T, D'Alessandro A, et al. OLT1177, a β-sulfonyl nitrile compound, safe in humans, inhibits the NLRP3 inflammasome and reverses the metabolic cost of inflammation. Proc Natl Acad Sci U S A. 2018;115(7): E1530–9.
17. Hoffman HM, Throne ML, Amar NJ, Sebai M, Kivitz AJ, Kavanaugh A, Weinstein SP, Belomestnov P, Yancopoulos GD, Stahl N, et al. Efficacy and safety of rilonacept (interleukin-1 trap) in patients with cryopyrin-associated periodic syndromes: results from two sequential placebo-controlled studies. Arthritis Rheum. 2008;58(8):2443–52.
18. Stankovic Stojanovic K, Delmas Y, Torres PU, Peltier J, Pelle G, Jeru I, Colombat M, Grateau G. Dramatic beneficial effect of interleukin-1 inhibitor treatment in patients with familial Mediterranean fever complicated with amyloidosis and renal failure. Nephrol Dial Transplant. 2012;27(5):1898–901.
19. Schlesinger N. Anti-interleukin-1 therapy in the management of gout. Curr Rheumatol Rep. 2014;16(2):398.
20. So A, Dumusc A, Nasi S. The role of IL-1 in gout: from bench to bedside. Rheumatology (Oxford). 2018;57(Suppl 1):i12–9.
21. Schlesinger N, De Meulemeester M, Pikhlak A, Yucel AE, Richard D, Murphy V, Arulmani U, Sallstig P, So A. Canakinumab relieves symptoms of acute flares and improves health-related quality of life in patients with difficult-to-treat gouty arthritis by suppressing inflammation: results of a randomized, dose-ranging study. Arthritis Res Ther. 2011;13(2):R53.
22. Fels E, Sundy JS. Refractory gout: what is it and what to do about it? Curr Opin Rheumatol. 2008;20(2):198–202.
23. Soehnlein O, Steffens S, Hidalgo A, Weber C. Neutrophils as protagonists and targets in chronic inflammation. Nat Rev Immunol. 2017;17(4):248–61.
24. Cavalli G, Koenders M, Kalabokis V, Kim J, Choon Tan A, Garlanda C, Mantovani A, Dagna L, Joosten LAB, Dinarello CA. Treating experimental arthritis with the innate immune inhibitor interleukin-37 reduces joint and systemic inflammation. Rheumatology (Oxford). 2017;56(12):2256.
25. Kumar H, Kumagai Y, Tsuchida T, Koenig PA, Satoh T, Guo Z, Jang MH, Saitoh T, Akira S, Kawai T. Involvement of the NLRP3 inflammasome in innate and humoral adaptive immune responses to fungal β-glucan. J Immunol. 2009;183(12):8061–7.

26. McCarty DJ, Hollander JL. Identification of urate crystals in gouty synovial fluid. Ann Intern Med. 1961;54:452–60.

27. Duff GW, Atkins E, Malawista SE. The fever of gout: urate crystals activate endogenous pyrogen production from human and rabbit mononuclear phagocytes. Trans Assoc Am Phys. 1983;96:234–45.

28. Dinarello CA, Simon A, van der Meer JW. Treating inflammation by blocking interleukin-1 in a broad spectrum of diseases. Nat Rev Drug Discov. 2012; 11(8):633–52.

29. Mokuda S, Kanno M, Takasugi K, Okumura C, Ito Y, Masumoto J. Tocilizumab improved clinical symptoms of a patient with systemic tophaceous gout who had symmetric polyarthritis and fever: an alternative treatment by blockade of interleukin-6 signaling. SAGE Open Med Case Rep. 2014;2: 2050313X13519774.

30. Pinto JL, Mora GE, Fernández-Avila DG, Gutiérrez JM, Díaz MC, Grupo Javeriano de Investigacion en Enfermedades Reumáticas. Tocilizumab in a patient with tophaceous gout resistant to treatment. Reumatol Clin. 2013; 9(3):178–80.

31. Torres R, Macdonald L, Croll SD, Reinhardt J, Dore A, Stevens S, Hylton DM, Rudge JS, Liu-Bryan R, Terkeltaub RA, et al. Hyperalgesia, synovitis and multiple biomarkers of inflammation are suppressed by interleukin 1 inhibition in a novel animal model of gouty arthritis. Ann Rheum Dis. 2009; 68(10):1602–8.

32. McGeough MD, Pena CA, Mueller JL, Pociask DA, Broderick L, Hoffman HM, Brydges SD. Cutting edge: IL-6 is a marker of inflammation with no direct role in inflammasome-mediated mouse models. J Immunol. 2012;189(6): 2707–11.

33. van de Loo FA, Kuiper S, van Enckevort FH, Arntz OJ, van den Berg WB. Interleukin-6 reduces cartilage destruction during experimental arthritis: a study in interleukin-6-deficient mice. Am J Pathol. 1997;151(1):177–91.

34. Guma M, Ronacher LM, Firestein GS, Karin M, Corr M. JNK-1 deficiency limits macrophage-mediated antigen-induced arthritis. Arthritis Rheum. 2011;63(6): 1603–12.

35. Han Z, Boyle DL, Chang L, Bennett B, Karin M, Yang L, Manning AM, Firestein GS. C-Jun N-terminal kinase is required for metalloproteinase expression and joint destruction in inflammatory arthritis. J Clin Invest. 2001; 108(1):73–81.

36. Thalhamer T, McGrath MA, Harnett MM. MAPKs and their relevance to arthritis and inflammation. Rheumatology (Oxford). 2008;47(4):409–14.

37. Ghosh P, Cho M, Rawat G, Simkin PA, Gardner GC. Treatment of acute gouty arthritis in complex hospitalized patients with anakinra. Arthritis Care Res (Hoboken). 2013;65(8):1381–4.

38. So A, De Smedt T, Revaz S, Tschopp J. A pilot study of IL-1 inhibition by anakinra in acute gout. Arthritis Res Ther. 2007;9(2):R28.

39. Schlesinger N, Alten RE, Bardin T, Schumacher HR, Bloch M, Gimona A, Krammer G, Murphy V, Richard D, So AK. Canakinumab for acute gouty arthritis in patients with limited treatment options: results from two randomised, multicentre, active-controlled, double-blind trials and their initial extensions. Ann Rheum Dis. 2012;71(11):1839–48.

40. So A, De Meulemeester M, Pikhlak A, Yucel AE, Richard D, Murphy V, Arulmani U, Sallstig P, Schlesinger N. Canakinumab for the treatment of acute flares in difficult-to-treat gouty arthritis: results of a multicenter, phase II, dose-ranging study. Arthritis Rheum. 2010;62(10):3064–76.

41. Mitha E, Schumacher HR, Fouche L, Luo SF, Weinstein SP, Yancopoulos GD, Wang J, King-Davis S, Evans RR. Rilonacept for gout flare prevention during initiation of uric acid-lowering therapy: results from the PRESURGE-2 international, phase 3, randomized, placebo-controlled trial. Rheumatology (Oxford). 2013;52(7):1285–92.

42. Terkeltaub RA, Schumacher HR, Carter JD, Baraf HS, Evans RR, Wang J, King-Davis S, Weinstein SP. Rilonacept in the treatment of acute gouty arthritis: a randomized, controlled clinical trial using indomethacin as the active comparator. Arthritis Res Ther. 2013;15(1):R25.

43. Dinarello CA, Ikejima T, Warner SJ, Orencole SF, Lonnemann G, Cannon JG, Libby P. Interleukin 1 induces interleukin 1. I. Induction of circulating interleukin 1 in rabbits in vivo and in human mononuclear cells in vitro. J Immunol. 1987;139(6):1902–10.

14

Serum metabolomic profiling predicts synovial gene expression in rheumatoid arthritis

Rekha Narasimhan[1†], Roxana Coras[1,2†], Sara B. Rosenthal[3], Shannon R. Sweeney[4], Alessia Lodi[4], Stefano Tiziani[4], David Boyle[1], Arthur Kavanaugh[1†] and Monica Guma[1,2*†] (iD)

Abstract

Background: Metabolomics is an emerging field of biomedical research that may offer a better understanding of the mechanisms of underlying conditions including inflammatory arthritis. Perturbations caused by inflamed synovial tissue can lead to correlated changes in concentrations of certain metabolites in the synovium and thereby function as potential biomarkers in blood. Here, we explore the hypothesis of whether characterization of patients' metabolomic profiles in blood, utilizing [1]H-nuclear magnetic resonance (NMR), predicts synovial marker profiling in rheumatoid arthritis (RA).

Methods: Nineteen active, seropositive patients with RA, on concomitant methotrexate, were studied. One of the involved joints was a knee or a wrist appropriate for arthroscopy. A Bruker Avance 700 MHz spectrometer was used to acquire NMR spectra of serum samples. Gene expression in synovial tissue obtained by arthroscopy was analyzed by real-time PCR. Data processing and statistical analysis were performed in Python and SPSS.

Results: Analysis of the relationships between each synovial marker-metabolite pair using linear regression and controlling for age and gender revealed significant clustering within the data. We observed an association of serine/glycine/phenylalanine metabolism and aminoacyl-tRNA biosynthesis with lymphoid cell gene signature. Alanine/aspartate/glutamate metabolism and choline-derived metabolites correlated with TNF-α synovial expression. Circulating ketone bodies were associated with gene expression of synovial metalloproteinases. Discriminant analysis identified serum metabolites that classified patients according to their synovial marker levels.

Conclusion: The relationship between serum metabolite profiles and synovial biomarker profiling suggests that NMR may be a promising tool for predicting specific pathogenic pathways in the inflamed synovium of patients with RA.

Keywords: NMR, Metabolomics, Biomarkers, Synovium, Rheumatoid arthritis, Gene expression

Background

The hallmark of rheumatoid arthritis (RA) is chronic synovitis that affects multiple joints and invades cartilage causing bone erosions and joint destruction [1]. As the synovium is the principal target of inflammation in RA, and the resident synoviocytes (fibroblast-like synoviocytes and macrophages-like synoviocytes) along with recruited cells (myeloid cells and lymphocytes) are implicated in the pathogenesis of synovitis, special interest has been given to the study of synovial tissue in this disease. These studies not only aim to clarify RA pathogenesis and provide insight into the mechanisms of action of therapeutic interventions [1, 2], but are also a promising approach to search for biomarkers in the inflamed synovial tissue [1]. Changes in the cellular infiltrate or biomarkers such as cytokines or growth factors in RA-affected synovial tissue have long been known to be associated with the clinical course of disease and have been used to identify specific responses to RA therapies [1–4]. Recently there has been increasing interest in synovial biopsies to obtain inflamed synovial tissue from joints and thereby gain a better

* Correspondence: mguma@ucsd.edu
†Rekha Narasimhan, Roxana Coras, Arthur Kavanaugh and Monica Guma contributed equally to this work.
[1]Division of Rheumatology, University of California, San Diego, 9500 Gilman Drive, San Diego, CA 92093, USA
[2]Department of Medicine, Autonomous University of Barcelona, Plaça Cívica, 08193 Bellaterra, Barcelona, Spain
Full list of author information is available at the end of the article

understanding of the pathogenic events in these diseases [5]. Histopathotype and pathological pathways-based patient stratification prior to therapeutic intervention could be exploited to identify biomarker predictors of clinical outcomes and responses to therapy [6, 7].

Tissue pathology and pathogenic pathways cannot yet be reliably explored through noninvasive circulating or imaging biomarkers. Given the complexity and heterogeneous nature of RA, it is unlikely that a single cytokine will provide sufficient discrimination between patients and thus be a good biomarker [8, 9]. Global biomarker signatures may represent a more appropriate approach for improving treatment protocols and outcomes for patients with RA. Metabolomics is the science of identifying and quantifying the biochemical byproducts of metabolism in a cell, tissue, or organism [10]. Metabolomics is an emerging field of biomedical research that can offer a better understanding of the mechanisms underlying disease and help to develop new strategies for treatment [11]. Unlike genes and proteins, which are epigenetically regulated and post-translationally modified, metabolites are direct signatures of biochemical activity and thus it may be easier to test whether they are correlated with phenotype [12].

The fundamental rationale in metabolomics is that perturbations caused by a disease in a biological system will lead to changes that are correlated with the concentrations of certain metabolites [13, 14]. Metabolite patterns represent the final response of biological systems to disease status, or in response to a medical or external intervention [12]. ^{1}H-nuclear magnetic resonance (NMR) can delineate patterns of changes in biomarkers that are highly discriminatory for the observed disease or intervention [15]. We propose in this work, that the study of metabolomics in serum from patients with RA, using NMR, can be used to predict synovial pathology. We hypothesize that perturbations caused by inflamed synovial tissue will lead to changes that correlate with the concentration of certain metabolites in the synovium. These changes will then be reflected in blood serum and function as potential biomarkers of different synovial markers. Here we describe the first study that defines metabolite signatures in serum that correlate with gene expression profiling in synovial tissue from patients with active RA.

Methods

Patients

The Assessment of rituximab's immunomodulatory synovial effects (ARISE) clinical trial (registered at ClinicalTrials.gov, NCT00147966) has been described in detail [3]. Briefly, the study enrolled people between 18 and 70 years of age with an established diagnosis of RA and a positive serum test for rheumatoid factor (RF). Patients had to have active disease (defined as a tender joint count > 8/68, a swollen joint count > 6/66, and either early morning stiffness > 45 min in duration, or an elevation in erythrocyte sedimentation rate (ESR) > 28 mm/h or C-reactive protein (CRP) > 1.5 mg/dL), despite the concomitant use of methotrexate (MTX) at a dose of > 12.5 mg/week for at least 12 weeks. One of the involved joints had to be a knee or a wrist that could be appropriately examined by arthroscopy. Concomitant use of non-steroidal anti-inflammatory drugs and oral prednisone at doses of 10 mg/day or less were permitted, provided dosing was stable for at least 4 weeks before the study. Patients previously treated with tumor necrosis factor (TNF-α) inhibitors were permitted to enroll in the study provided they had been off therapy for > 2 months for etanercept and > 3 months for adalimumab or infliximab. Patients meeting eligibility criteria underwent baseline arthroscopic synovial biopsy of an affected knee or wrist. Nineteen patients for whom both baseline synovial biopsy gene expression data and baseline serum metabolomics data were available were analyzed in the current study. Clinical disease parameters, including disease activity score (DAS), health assessment questionnaire (HAQ), pain, joint swelling and tenderness, ESR, RF, and anti-cyclic citrullinated peptide (anti-CCP) are described in Additional file 1: Table S1.

Synovial gene expression analysis

Synovial RNA was extracted from pools of six tissue fragments and complementary DNA (cDNA) was synthesized. TaqMan PCR was performed using predeveloped reagents (Applied Biosystems, Foster City, CA, USA) as described previously [3]. Gene expression, utilizing quantitative reverse transcriptase (RT)-PCR, was performed to measure inflammatory mediators and B cell survival factors, including IgM (heavy chain), IgG (heavy chain), IgKappa (light chain), CD3E, TNF-α, interleukin (IL)-1β, IL-6, IL-8, matrix metalloproteinase (MMP)-1, MMP-3, B lymphocyte stimulator (BLyS), stromal cell-derived factor 1 (SDF1), and a proliferation-inducing ligand (APRIL). Synovial gene expression for the 19 patients analyzed in this study are summarized in Additional file 1: Table S2.

ELISA

TNF-α, MMP3 IL-1β, and IL-6 from serum were evaluated by DuoSet enzyme-linked immunosorbent assays following the manufacturer's protocol (R&D systems).

Metabolomics analysis

Frozen serum was obtained from the Division of Rheumatology, Allergy, and Immunology at the University of California (UC) San Diego School of Medicine (San Diego, CA, USA). Lipid and protein fractions were removed via ultrafiltration (Nanosep 3 K OMEGA, Pall Corporation, Ann Arbor, MI, USA) at 4 °C. The filtered biofluid was used for NMR analysis. An aliquot of 160 μL of filtered serum was mixed with 20 μL D₂O and 20 μL of phosphate buffer (100 mM final concentration) containing TMSP-d4 (0.1 mM final concentration) and sodium azide (0.05% (w/v) final concentration). The prepared samples were centrifuged to remove any remaining particulates and a 180 μL aliquot was transferred to a 3 mm NMR tube (Norell, Landisville, NJ, USA) prior to acquisition. NMR spectra were acquired with a 16.4 T (700 MHz) Bruker Avance spectrometer (Bruker BioSpin Corp., Billerica, MA, USA) equipped with a 5 mm TCI cryogenically cooled probe and autosampler at 30 °C. Following acquisition, spectra were processed using NMRlab and MetaboLab [16]. Metabolite assignment and quantification was performed using several databases [16]. Metabolite assignment and quantification was performed using Chenomx NMR Suite (Chenomx Inc., Edmonton, AB, Canada), the Birmingham Metabolite Library [17], and the Human Metabolome Database [18]. The NMR results were recently published [19] and are summarized in Additional file 1: Table S3 for the 19 patients analyzed in this study.

Data analysis

The data, consisting of 19 patient samples measured across 18 synovial markers and 49 metabolites, were processed using Python. Hierarchically clustered heatmaps were generated for correlation between synovial markers and metabolites separately. Hierarchical clustering and visualization was performed using the scientific computing package SciPy, and the visualization package Seaborn (https://seaborn.pydata.org/). Dendrograms were divided into flat clusters using a cophenetic distance metric. Linear regression was performed between each cytokine-metabolite pair, controlling for patient age and gender using the ordinary least squares (OLS) method from the Python package StatsModels. Normally distributed independent variables were standardized so they had a mean of zero and a standard deviation of one. Discriminant analyses were performed to determine coefficients for linear combinations of variables that assigned cluster membership to individual cases. Basic descriptive statistics used to describe the patient population and discriminant analysis were performed using the SPSS software version 15.0.

Results

Synovial marker and blood metabolite clustering

We first analyzed whether synovial markers clustered into different groups (Fig. 1). IL-6, MMP1, and MMP3 are strongly correlated among themselves but are inversely correlated with TNF-α, which interestingly, is strongly correlated with CD3E. MMP1 and MMP3 are also inversely correlated with another cluster that includes IL-1β and IL-8. In addition, there was a big cluster comprising B and plasma cell markers, and growth factors, including SDF1, APRIL, CD138, CD19, CD79A, IgG and IgM heavy chains, and IgKappa.

We also characterized the blood metabolites. As shown in Additional file 1: Table S3 and Fig. 2a, most of the metabolites were downregulated compared to reference values, suggesting that these metabolites might be consumed by the inflamed synovium due to an increase in its metabolic demand. A few metabolites were upregulated compared to reference values, including glycolytic metabolites such as lactate and pyruvate. This likely reflects the increased bioenergetic and biosynthetic demands of sustained inflammation. Choline metabolism has recently been strongly related to inflammation [20]. Dietary intake of choline, through two circulating metabolites, trimethylamine (TMA) and trimethylamine N-oxide (TMAO), are mechanistically linked to cardiovascular inflammation [20]. Interestingly TMA was also elevated in our patients with RA. In addition, 3-hydroxybutyrate, a ketone body, and select amino acids, such as leucine, threonine, tyrosine, and aspartate were upregulated in patients with active RA. We also analyzed whether blood metabolites could be clustered in groups. Metabolites primarily clustered into groups according to their biological function or chemical classification (Fig. 2b). As expected, the group of metabolites that were elevated in patients, namely lactate, methylmalonate, xanthine, and 3-hydroxybutyrate, were inversely correlated with the most of metabolites.

Linear regression analysis between grouped synovial markers and metabolites

Linear regression was analyzed between each synovial marker-metabolite pair; age and gender were controlled for by including these factors as covariates in the model. The regression coefficients for each cytokine-metabolite pair were used to form a clustered heatmap to lend insight into which groups of synovial markers were correlated with which groups of metabolites. We observed significant clustering structures in the data (Fig. 3a). The color bar along the top of Fig. 3 preserves the synovial marker clusters from Fig. 1. Interestingly the clusters of synovial markers almost correspond to the clusters observed within synovial markers (Fig. 1), suggesting that cytokine clusters in the synovial tissue have a similar metabolite signature in blood. The most striking difference is seen in the cluster comprising SDF1, APRIL, CD138, CD19, CD79A, and IgG and IgM heavy chain, and IgKappa in Fig. 1, which is seen split into two groups in Fig. 3. One metabolite signature correlates with CD19, CD79A and IgG heavy chain, markers of B cells; and the other metabolite signature correlates with SDF1, APRIL, CD138 and IgM heavy chain, markers related to plasma cell biology. Of interest BLyS, had a different metabolite profile than the rest of plasma cell

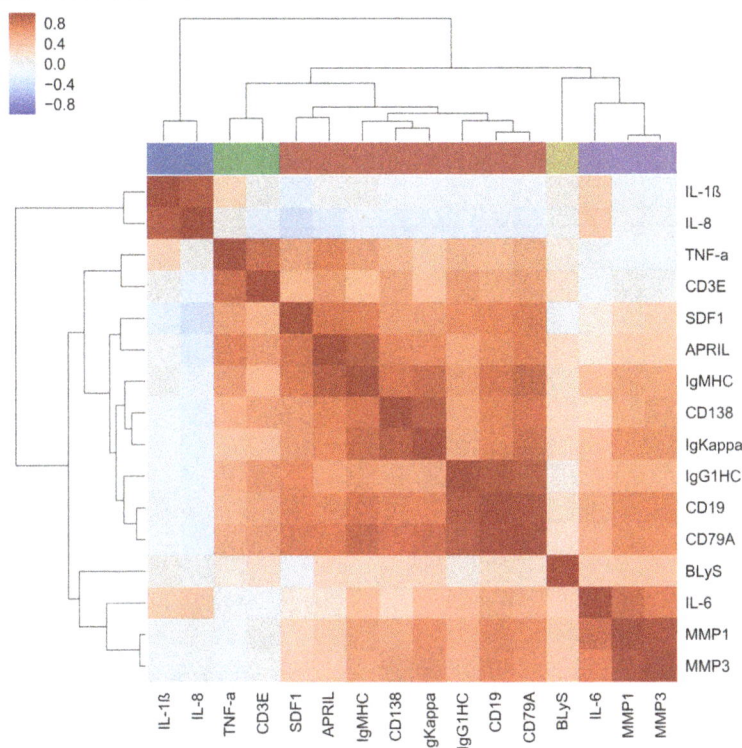

Fig. 1 Synovial markers clustering. Heat map and hierarchical cluster analysis indicates positive relationships between cytokines identified by quantitative PCR in synovial tissue from patients with rheumatoid arthritis. Pearson's correlation coefficients for each metabolite and hierarchical clustering with Euclidean distance metric are included. The color bar along the top indicates cytokine grouping based on hierarchical clustering. APRIL, a proliferation-inducing ligand; BLyS, lymphocyte stimulator; MMP, matrix metalloproteinase; SDF1, S cell-derived factor 1

biomarkers. Metabolite regression p values are displayed in Fig. 3b, where the row and column order are preserved from Fig. 3a and Additional file 2: Figure S1.

As observed in Fig. 3, metabolites can be grouped into five clusters (Fig. 4) that were further analyzed using the MetaboAnalyst [21, 22] web tool for functional enrichment of these groups of metabolites. Both pathway significance and pathway impact were assessed using this tool (Additional file 3: Figure S2).

We then determined the most strongly correlated or anti-correlated serum metabolites for each synovial marker, using linear regression, and controlling for both age and gender. We also included Benjamini-Hochberg false discovery rate (FDR)-adjusted p values to correct for multiple testing. As shown in Fig. 5, the synovial markers TNF-α and CD3E were negatively correlated with several metabolites in serum. The significant polar metabolites were mapped to known metabolic pathways using MetaboAnalyst 3.0 [22, 23]. and ranked by their overall p values (Fig. 5c). Additional file 4: Figure S3, Additional file 5: Figure S4, Additional file 6: Figure S5, and Additional file 7: Figure S6 show correlation between metabolites and the remaining synovial marker clusters.

Discriminant analysis

We then explored whether or not one or more metabolites in serum could discriminate between high or low levels of synovial marker gene expression. At present, no factors have been identified that fully explain or predict response to RA therapy [24], but pre-treatment differences at baseline between patient groups have been identified, including synovial tissue TNF expression and an increased number of synovial macrophages and T cells in patients who subsequently exhibited clinical improvement after initiation of anti-TNF therapy [25]. Therefore, we used stepwise discriminant function analyses to discriminate TNF-α or CD3E levels. Multivariate and cross-validation classification using the "leave-one-out" classification method was used for these calculations. We defined high or low marker levels according to their synovial marker gene expression mean. This stepwise discriminant analysis is presented in Fig. 6. For TNF-α discriminant analysis, three metabolites namely glutamine, TMA, and dimethylsulfone were sufficient to correctly classify 94.7% of TNF-α levels. There was canonical correlation of 0.821 and Wilks' lambda of 0.326 when these three variables were used, with high significance ($p < 0.001$; Fig. 6a). For CD3E discriminant

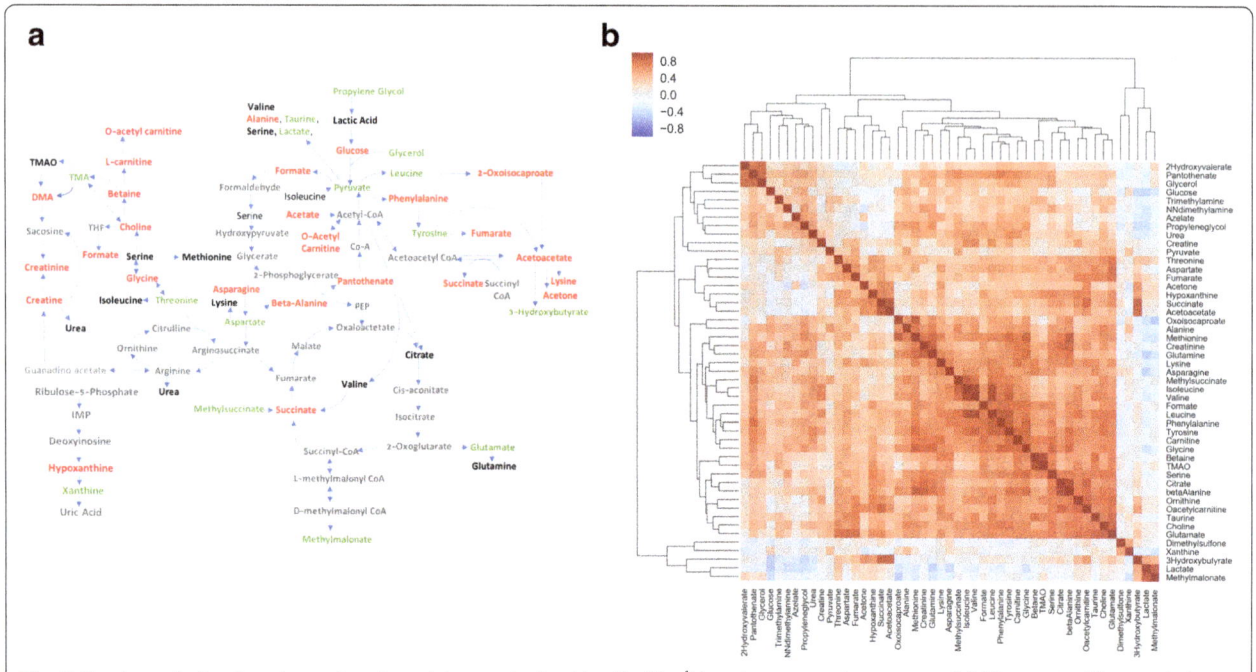

Fig. 2 Blood metabolite clustering. **a** Overview of the metabolites identified by [1]H-nuclear magnetic resonance (NMR) organized by metabolic pathway. Metabolites that were elevated by at least 20% compared to reference values are in green and metabolites that were decreased by more than 20% compared to reference values are in red.. Metabolites not identified by NMR are in gray. Abbreviations: TMA, trimethylamine; TMAO, trimethylamine N-oxide; DMA, NN-dimethylamine; THF, tetrahydrofolate; IMP, inosine monophosphate. **b** Heat map and hierarchical cluster analysis indicate positive relationships between polar metabolites identified by ^{1}H-NMR in serum from patients with rheumatoid arthritis before treatment with rituximab. Pearson's correlation coefficients for each metabolite and hierarchical clustering with Euclidean distance metric are shown

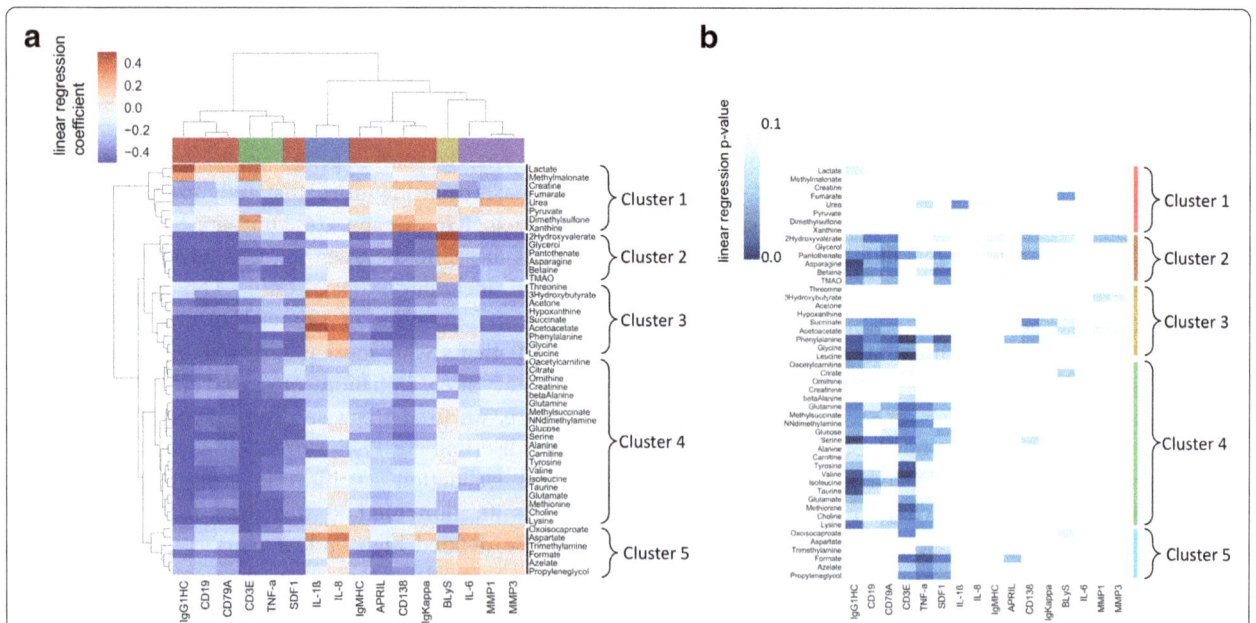

Fig. 3 Correlation of synovial markers with serum metabolites. **a** Linear regression was performed between each synovial marker–serum metabolite pair, controlling for age and gender. The regression coefficients for each pair were used to form a clustered heatmap, to lend insight into which groups of synovial markers were correlated with which groups of metabolites. The color bar along the top is preserved from Fig. 1, and indicates groups of similar cytokines. Row clusters have been identified by cophenetic cutting of the row dendrogram. **b** Metabolite regression *p* values are displayed in Fig. 3b, where the row and column order are preserved from Fig. 3a. APRIL, a proliferation-inducing ligand; BLyS, lymphocyte stimulator; MMP, matrix metalloproteinase; SDF1, S cell-derived factor 1

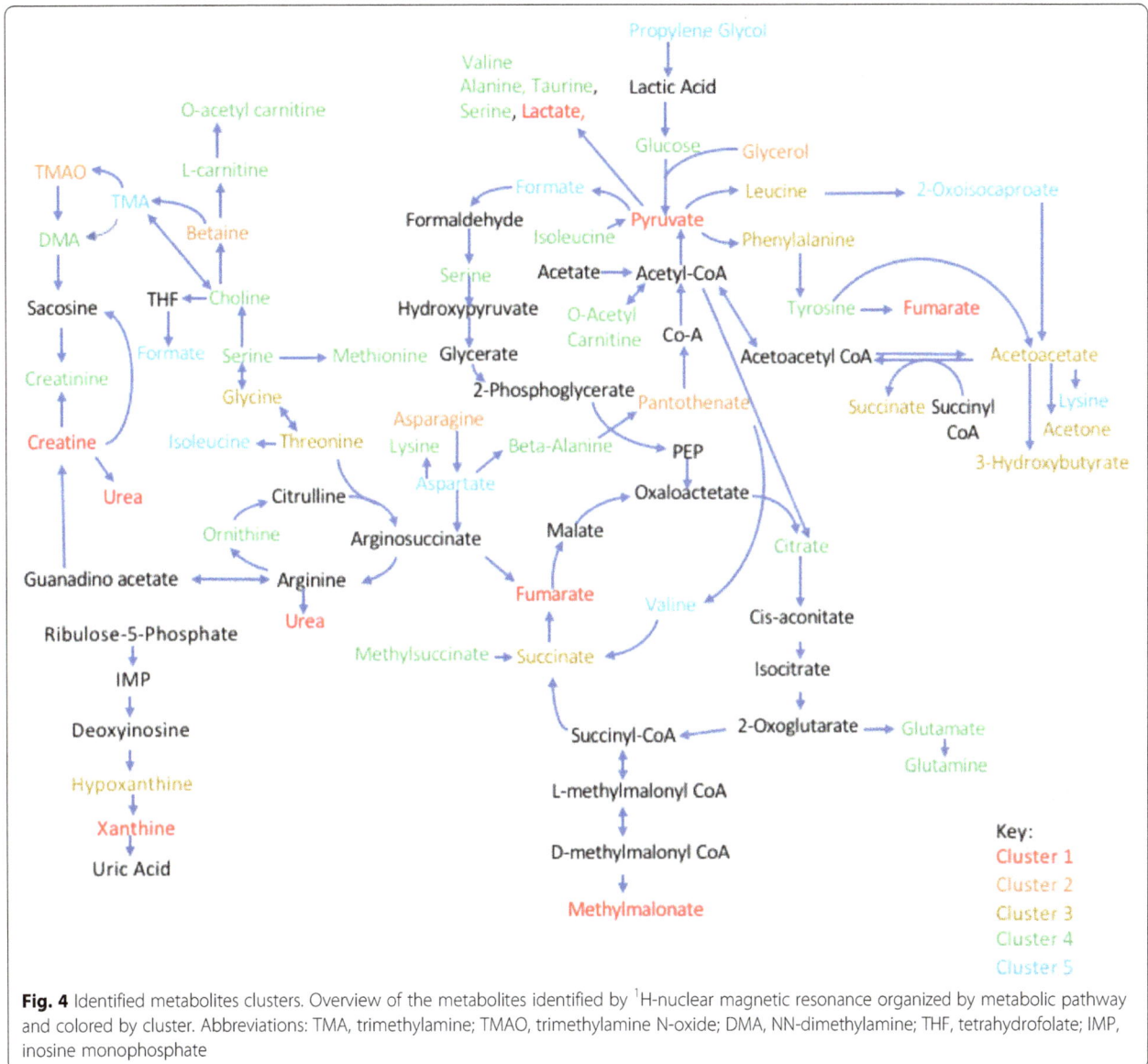

Fig. 4 Identified metabolites clusters. Overview of the metabolites identified by ¹H-nuclear magnetic resonance organized by metabolic pathway and colored by cluster. Abbreviations: TMA, trimethylamine; TMAO, trimethylamine N-oxide; DMA, NN-dimethylamine; THF, tetrahydrofolate; IMP, inosine monophosphate

analysis, two metabolites namely carnitine and methionine were sufficient to correctly classify 89.6% of CD3E levels. There was canonical correlation of 0.765 and Wilks' lambda of 0.414 when these three variables were used, with high significance ($p < 0.001$; Fig. 6b).

Discussion

Our increasing understanding of the pathogenesis of RA has transformed the therapeutic options available for people with this disease. The introduction of newer agents and novel treatment strategies has resulted in improved outcomes for patients. However, these successes have raised the bar for the goals of therapy. At present, disease remission, or low disease activity at the very least, has become the new goal of treatment for all patients. Therefore, there is still an unmet need in RA. Biomarkers employed

in "personalized" medicine might be useful in an attempt to match a patient with the most appropriate biologic therapy, and thereby optimize outcomes. The accessibility of a biological biomarker is an important factor in this approach [8]. Although sampling inflamed synovial tissue from joints might be critical to gain a better understanding of the pathogenic events of inflammatory arthritis, a biomarker that can be obtained in a minimally invasive manner is more attractive, particularly for patients in early stages of the disease, where mostly small joints are involved [8]. In this study, we attempt, for the first time, to find serum metabolomics profiles that correlate with synovial marker gene expression.

Recent studies have indicated that metabolic regulation and cell signaling are tightly and ubiquitously linked with immune responses. Metabolomics studies that aim

a

	TNF-a coef	p value	fdr_bh
Formate	-0.721795512	0.007615349	0.174737158
Propyleneglycol	-0.590410875	0.020238909	0.174737158
Glutamine	-0.573019026	0.023859919	0.174737158
Dimethylamine	-0.568085958	0.029498262	0.174737158
Lysine	-0.561321683	0.033189404	0.174737158
Azelate	-0.55830895	0.033986355	0.174737158
Phenylalanine	-0.545706629	0.038101508	0.174737158
Methionine	-0.528014471	0.040775615	0.174737158
Alanine	-0.557879697	0.041120035	0.174737158
Glucose	-0.530972967	0.045983406	0.174737158
Serine	-0.523916898	0.046117837	0.174737158
Choline	-0.512162739	0.048222123	0.174737158
	CD3E coef	p value	fdr_bh
Leucine	-0.745741039	0.001413016	0.041797774
Phenylalanine	-0.749050081	0.001706032	0.041797774
Valine	-0.703212891	0.003154410	0.051522025
Methionine	-0.639690429	0.009650316	0.083196136
Tyrosine	-0.640469250	0.010182686	0.083196136
Formate	-0.677584891	0.014503087	0.083196136
Dimethylamine	-0.624630481	0.014703349	0.083196136
Glutamine	-0.610377740	0.014876348	0.083196136
Isoleucine	-0.600778315	0.016781132	0.083196136
Serine	-0.609306927	0.016978803	0.083196136
Choline	-0.580601942	0.022115008	0.088324693
Oxoisocaproate	-0.607192712	0.024064158	0.088324693
Methylsuccinate	-0.569425349	0.027376216	0.088324693
Lysine	-0.573228375	0.029603555	0.088324693
Pantothenate	-0.581930411	0.029849975	0.088324693
Propyleneglycol	-0.559864214	0.030360237	0.088324693
Glucose	-0.569707225	0.030643261	0.088324693
Alanine	-0.570902608	0.036569913	0.094348881
Glycine	-0.549685228	0.038154935	0.094348881
Glutamate	-0.540404886	0.038509747	0.094348881
Succinate	-0.530451380	0.045877481	0.107047455

b

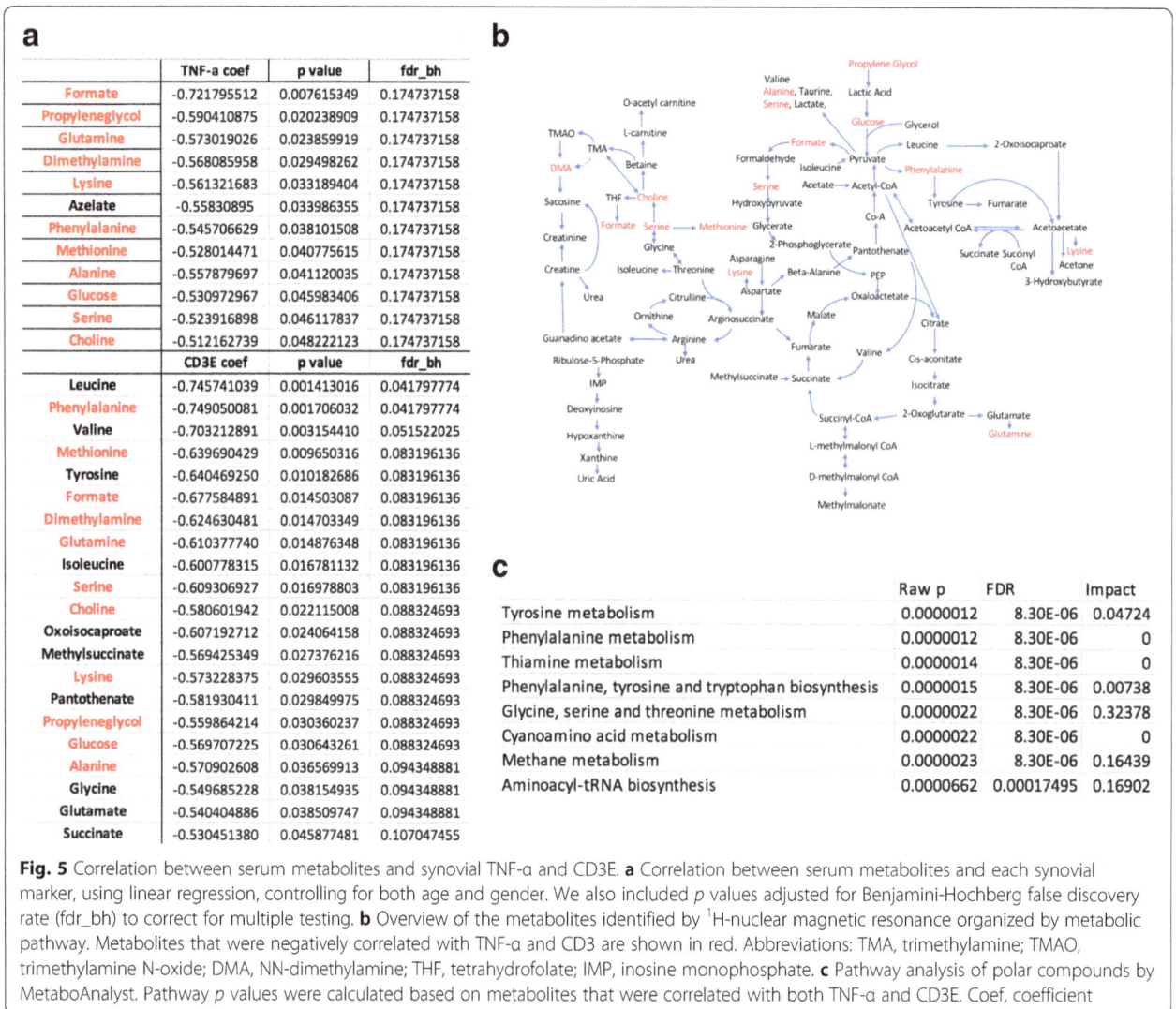

c

	Raw p	FDR	Impact
Tyrosine metabolism	0.0000012	8.30E-06	0.04724
Phenylalanine metabolism	0.0000012	8.30E-06	0
Thiamine metabolism	0.0000014	8.30E-06	0
Phenylalanine, tyrosine and tryptophan biosynthesis	0.0000015	8.30E-06	0.00738
Glycine, serine and threonine metabolism	0.0000022	8.30E-06	0.32378
Cyanoamino acid metabolism	0.0000022	8.30E-06	0
Methane metabolism	0.0000023	8.30E-06	0.16439
Aminoacyl-tRNA biosynthesis	0.0000662	0.00017495	0.16902

Fig. 5 Correlation between serum metabolites and synovial TNF-α and CD3E. **a** Correlation between serum metabolites and each synovial marker, using linear regression, controlling for both age and gender. We also included *p* values adjusted for Benjamini-Hochberg false discovery rate (fdr_bh) to correct for multiple testing. **b** Overview of the metabolites identified by [1]H-nuclear magnetic resonance organized by metabolic pathway. Metabolites that were negatively correlated with TNF-α and CD3 are shown in red. Abbreviations: TMA, trimethylamine; TMAO, trimethylamine N-oxide; DMA, NN-dimethylamine; THF, tetrahydrofolate; IMP, inosine monophosphate. **c** Pathway analysis of polar compounds by MetaboAnalyst. Pathway *p* values were calculated based on metabolites that were correlated with both TNF-α and CD3E. Coef, coefficient

to improve biological understanding through the analysis of metabolite profiles of the underlying biological pathways are certainly relevant and have been successful in other fields, especially oncology. Though the application of metabolomics to RA is still in its infancy, early studies have yielded promising results [19, 26–33]. A small number of metabolomics studies have focused on identifying metabolites associated with rheumatic diseases, primarily in the serum for diagnostic purposes [30–32], but none have attempted to predict synovial pathology.

We hypothesized that perturbations caused by inflamed synovial tissue will lead to changes that correlate with the concentrations of certain metabolites in the synovium that will be then reflected in blood serum. A recent publication on a study of metabolic profiling in the synovial tissue reported altered glucose and choline metabolism [34]. Both pathways have recently been involved in RA pathogenesis [27, 34, 35]. Choline levels in patients from our cohorts are decreased in blood compared to the normal range;

this, along with an increased uptake in the joints on choline C-11 PET scanning in inflammatory arthritis [36] and high expression in fibrocyte-like synoviocytes (FLS) of choline like transporter (CTL)1 (high-affinity) and CTL2 (low-affinity) [37], suggest increased circulating choline uptake and consumption by the inflamed synovium. Glucose levels were decreased, and lactate levels increased in serum from our cohort. Glucose is consumed through upregulation of aerobic glycolysis and when metabolized, gives rise to production of copious amounts of lactate, which must be extruded from the cell to prevent lactic acidosis [38]. Several studies have highlighted the increase in glucose metabolism in the hypoxic joint [27, 35]. Thus, our results in serum seem to agree well with recently described synovial studies [34]. Of interest, both choline and glucose levels in the blood negatively correlated with TNF-α and CD3E gene expression in the synovium.

Literature in the field of oncology can help us to interpret some of our results. For instance, we observed an

a

Variables	Unstandardized coefficients	Standardized coefficients	Structure matrix	Centroids	Constant
Dimethylsulfone	-38.842	-.627	-.237	Low:-2.002 High:.924	-4.422
Glutamine	6.701	.748	.661		
Trimethylamine	1225.244	.689	.518		

b

Variables	Unstandardized coefficients	Standardized coefficients	Structure matrix	Centroids	Constant
Carnitine	-127.906	-1.178	.185	Low:-1.319 High: .959	-3.143
Methionine	338.898	1.681	.725		

Fig. 6 Discriminant analysis. Unstandardized and standardized discriminant function coefficients, structure matrix, centroids, and constant for direct discriminant function for TNF-α (**a**) and CD3E (**b**)

association of serine/glycine metabolism and aminoacyl-tRNA biosynthesis with TNF-α/CD3E and B/plasma cell signatures that suggest that lymphoid cells could be using these pathways after activation in the rheumatoid synovium. Although alterations in glucose and glutamine metabolism are central to metabolic transformation, recent studies have focused on the role of the nonessential amino acids serine and glycine in supporting tumor growth [39]. In addition to their role in protein synthesis, serine and glycine contribute to anabolic pathways important for the generation of glutathione, nucleotides, phospholipids, and other metabolites [40]. The requirement for intracellular serine and glycine for the support of cell growth and proliferation is clear. Other amino acids are also critical substrates that fuel mitochondrial metabolism and the biosynthesis of proteins, lipids, and other molecules. Of particular interest in cancer are key mitochondrial enzymes in the metabolism of glutamine, glutamate, proline, aspartate, and alanine [41]. The branched chain amino acids (BCAAs) valine, leucine, and isoleucine are also highly metabolized by transaminases. By coordinating cellular bioenergetics and biosynthesis through the tricarboxylic acid (TCA) cycle, amino acid metabolism could be critical not only in tumor cells but also in lymphoid cell proliferation and survival as described recently [42].

Another metabolite that correlates with several of our cytokine pathways is succinate. Succinate is an intermediate of the TCA cycle and plays a crucial role in adenosine triphosphate (ATP) generation in mitochondria. Recently, new roles for succinate outside metabolism have emerged. Succinate promotes expression of the pro-inflammatory cytokine IL-1β by inhibiting prolyl hydroxylases and stabilizing the transcription factor hypoxia-inducible factor-1α (HIF-1α) in activated macrophages, and stimulates dendritic cells via succinate receptor 1 [38, 43]. Furthermore, succinate has been shown to post-translationally modify proteins. Of interest, the succinate level in blood positively associated with synovial IL-1β gene expression although it did not reach statistical significance.

The cluster comprising MMP1/MMP3/IL-6, which could represent a fibroblast-driven phenotype, was negatively correlated with ketone bodies. Acetoacetate is the common precursor of the two other circulating ketone bodies, acetone and 3-hydroxybutyrate [44]. 3-hydroxybutyrate is the most abundant circulating ketone body and is less likely to degrade spontaneously into acetone than acetoacetate. One can speculate that rheumatoid fibroblasts require intracellular ketone bodies for the support of their invasive phenotype and that the increase in 3-hydroxybutyrate uptake and/or enzymes in this pathway could explain the negative correlation. Of note, the positive correlation between 3-hydroxybutyrate and IL-1β and IL-8 is also of interest, as 3-hydroxybutyrate, long viewed as a simple carrier of energy from the liver to peripheral tissues, also possesses signaling activities and is also an endogenous inhibitor of histone deacetylases (HDACs) [45]. Moreover, recent research has shown that 3-hydroxybutyrate can block the NOD-like receptor pyrin containing 3 (NLRP3) inflammasome [46]. Further studies are needed to understand the effect of these metabolites in the synovium in RA.

As mentioned above, metabolites can not only be biomarkers of perturbations caused by inflamed synovial tissue but also can have a pathogenic effect that would amplify synovial inflammation. Secondary roles have emerged for glucose metabolites, metabolic enzymes, and TCA cycle intermediates outside of metabolism. Not only succinate but also other metabolites including α-ketoglutarate, fumarate, and acetyl-CoA might be expected to accumulate in macrophages and FLS under hypoxic conditions, and are involved in eliciting important epigenetic changes, with unexplored potential for driving chronic inflammation [47, 48]. Also, essential glycolytic enzymes have been shown to translocate to the nucleus or mitochondria where they function independently of their canonical metabolic roles in the regulation of cytokines and anti-apoptotic responses [49, 50]. Thus, metabolomics studies have also the potential of defining the elements of synovial metabolic pathobiology.

Although NMR spectroscopy has less sensitivity compared to mass spectrometry instrumentation, NMR requires minimal sample preparation, and is not only non-destructive, inherently untargeted, highly reproducible [51, 52], and intrinsically quantitative, but is also cheaper and more accessible than mass spectrometry [53–55]. Depending on the biological samples, NMR can identify and quantify more than 200 metabolites in an untargeted fashion and more than 100 metabolites are uniquely identified by NMR [56]. In this work, we also showed that the combination of only two or three metabolites identified in serum by NMR could discriminate between high or low levels of synovial TNF-α and CD3E gene expression. Studies in other cohorts of patients with active RA are needed to validate these results, yet the relationship between serum metabolic profiles and synovial biomarker profiling suggests that NMR may be a promising tool for predicting specific pathogenic pathways in the inflamed synovium in RA.

Although these findings are certainly promising, this study is not without limitations. Most importantly, we evaluated a small number of clinical samples. Despite similar clinical parameters for patient inclusion, large biological variance is expected in primary samples. In addition, patients had long-standing disease and were exposed to various therapies prior to the study, and were on methotrexate at the time of the study, which is reported to change several metabolic pathways including adenosine metabolism [57]. Confirmation of our results in a larger sample size from a cohort of patients with new onset inflammatory arthritis before treatment initiation, studied prospectively, is necessary to strengthen our conclusions. Comparison with other arthritides or other systemic inflammatory diseases to determine if these changes in metabolite levels come from the joints or from different sources is also critical to interpret our results. One other confounder is the microbiome, which is altered in RA and can potentially cause metabolic changes in both serum and synovial tissues [58–60]. In addition, further studies are needed to evaluate the relationship between circulating metabolites and synovial pathology. Metabolite profiles in blood, if they correlate with metabolic changes in synovial tissue, will certainly reveal more about RA etiology. We did not identify correlation between cytokine serum levels and cytokine synovial gene expression (Additional file 8: Figure S7), yet it remains unknown whether or not metabolic changes will display stronger correlation between blood and synovium.

Conclusions

The relationship between serum metabolite profiles and synovial biomarker profiling suggests that NMR may be a promising tool for predicting specific pathogenic pathways in the inflamed synovium of patients with RA. Further studies will help to better test the correlation and understand the metabolic profiles between cytokine and cell signatures, and address whether or not NMR metabolomics can be used to stratify patients with RA by predicting specific cellular infiltrates or other synovial biomarkers, and to identify specific responses to RA therapies.

Abbreviations
APRIL: A proliferation-inducing ligand; ARISE: Assessment of rituximab's immunomodulatory synovial effects; ATP: Adenosine triphosphate; BLySB: Lymphocyte stimulator; CRP: C-reactive protein; CTL: Choline like transporter; DAS: Disease activity score; FLS: Fibroblast-like synoviocytes; HAQ: Health assessment questionnaire; HIF-1α: Hypoxia-inducible factor-1α; IL-1β: Interleukin; MMP: Matrix metalloproteinase; MTX: Methotrexate; NMR: ^{1}H-nuclear magnetic resonance; RA: Rheumatoid arthritis; RF: Rheumatoid factor; SDF1: S cell-derived factor 1; TCA: Tricarboxylic acid; TMA: Trimethylamine; TMAO: Trimethylamine N-oxide; TNF-α: Tumor necrosis factor

Funding
This work was supported by grants from the National Institutes of Arthritis and Musculoskeletal and Skin (to MG, 1K08AR064834 and R03AR068094), and the Spanish Society of Rheumatology to RC.

Authors' contributions
MG designed and supervised the overall project. DB and AK designed and conducted the ARISE trial. RN, RC, AK, SBR, and MG analyzed the data. ST, AL, and SS acquired and analyzed NMR data. SBR, AK, and MG wrote the manuscript. All authors read and approve the final manuscript.

Consent for publication
N/A

Competing interests
The authors declare that thet have no competing interest.

Author details
[1]Division of Rheumatology, University of California, San Diego, 9500 Gilman Drive, San Diego, CA 92093, USA. [2]Department of Medicine, Autonomous University of Barcelona, Plaça Cívica, 08193 Bellaterra, Barcelona, Spain. [3]Center for Computational Biology and Bioinformatics, University of California, San Diego, 9500 Gilman Drive, San Diego, CA 92093, USA. [4]Department of Nutritional Sciences & Dell Pediatric Research Institute, Dell Medical School, University of Texas at Austin, 1400 Barbara Jordan Blvd, Austin, TX, USA.

References

1. Orr C, Vieira-Sousa E, Boyle DL, Buch MH, Buckley CD, Canete JD, et al. Synovial tissue research: a state-of-the-art review. Nat Rev Rheumatol. 2017;13(8):463–75.
2. Vieira-Sousa E, Gerlag DM, Tak PP. Synovial tissue response to treatment in rheumatoid arthritis. Open Rheumatol J. 2011;5:115–22.
3. Kavanaugh A, Rosengren S, Lee SJ, Hammaker D, Firestein GS, Kalunian K, et al. Assessment of rituximab's immunomodulatory synovial effects (ARISE trial). 1: clinical and synovial biomarker results. Ann Rheum Dis. 2008;67(3):402–8.
4. Dennis G Jr, Holweg CT, Kummerfeld SK, Choy DF, Setiadi AF, Hackney JA, et al. Synovial phenotypes in rheumatoid arthritis correlate with response to biologic therapeutics. Arthritis Res Ther. 2014;16(2):R90.
5. Kelly S, Humby F, Filer A, Ng N, Di Cicco M, Hands RE, et al. Ultrasound-guided synovial biopsy: a safe, well-tolerated and reliable technique for obtaining high-quality synovial tissue from both large and small joints in early arthritis patients. Ann Rheum Dis. 2015;74(3):611–7.
6. Astorri E, Nerviani A, Bombardieri M, Pitzalis C. Towards a stratified targeted approach with biologic treatments in rheumatoid arthritis: role of synovial pathobiology. Curr Pharm Des. 2015;21(17):2216–24.
7. Pitzalis C, Kelly S, Humby F. New learnings on the pathophysiology of RA from synovial biopsies. Curr Opin Rheumatol. 2013;25(3):334–44.
8. Burska A, Boissinot M, Ponchel F. Cytokines as biomarkers in rheumatoid arthritis. Mediat Inflamm. 2014;2014:545493.
9. Burska AN, Roget K, Blits M, Soto Gomez L, van de Loo F, Hazelwood LD, et al. Gene expression analysis in RA: towards personalized medicine. Pharmacogenomics J. 2014;14(2):93–106.
10. Eckhart AD, Beebe K, Milburn M. Metabolomics as a key integrator for "omic" advancement of personalized medicine and future therapies. Clin Transl Sci. 2012;5(3):285–8.
11. Patti GJ, Yanes O, Siuzdak G. Innovation: metabolomics: the apogee of the omics trilogy. Nat Rev Mol Cell Biol. 2012;13(4):263–9.
12. Semerano L, Romeo PH, Boissier MC. Metabolomics for rheumatic diseases: has the time come? Ann Rheum Dis. 2015;74(7):1325–6.
13. Patti GJ, Tautenhahn R, Rinehart D, Cho K, Shriver LP, Manchester M, et al. A view from above: cloud plots to visualize global metabolomic data. Anal Chem. 2013;85(2):798–804.
14. Patti GJ, Yanes O, Shriver LP, Courade JP, Tautenhahn R, Manchester M, et al. Metabolomics implicates altered sphingolipids in chronic pain of neuropathic origin. Nat Chem Biol. 2012;8(3):232–4.
15. Priori R, Scrivo R, Brandt J, Valerio M, Casadei L, Valesini G, et al. Metabolomics in rheumatic diseases: the potential of an emerging methodology for improved patient diagnosis, prognosis, and treatment efficacy. Autoimmun Rev. 2013;12(10):1022–30.
16. Ludwig C, Gunther UL. MetaboLab–advanced NMR data processing and analysis for metabolomics. BMC Bioinformatics. 2011;12:366.
17. Ludwig CEJ, Lodi A, Tiziani S, Manzoor SE, et al. Birmingham metabolite library: a publicly accessible database of 1-D H-1 and 2-D H-1 J-resolved NMR spectra of authentic metabolite standards (BML-NMR). Metabolomics. 2012;8:8–18.
18. Wishart DS, Tzur D, Knox C, Eisner R, Guo AC, Young N, et al. HMDB: the human metabolome database. Nucleic Acids Res. 2007;35(Database):D521–6.
19. Sweeney SR, Kavanaugh A, Lodi A, Wang B, Boyle D, Tiziani S, et al. Metabolomic profiling predicts outcome of rituximab therapy in rheumatoid arthritis. RMD Open. 2016;2(2):e000289.
20. Smallwood T, Allayee H, Bennett BJ. Choline metabolites: gene by diet interactions. Curr Opin Lipidol. 2016;27(1):33–9.
21. Xia J, Wishart DS. Using MetaboAnalyst 3.0 for comprehensive metabolomics data analysis. Curr Protoc Bioinformatics. 2016;55:14. 0 1–0 91
22. Xia J, Psychogios N, Young N, Wishart DS. MetaboAnalyst: a web server for metabolomic data analysis and interpretation. Nucleic Acids Res. 2009; 37(Web Server issue):W652–60.
23. Xia J, Mandal R, Sinelnikov IV, Broadhurst D, Wishart DS. MetaboAnalyst 2.0–a comprehensive server for metabolomic data analysis. Nucleic Acids Res. 2012;40(Web Server issue):W127–33.
24. Wijbrandts CA, Tak PP. Prediction of response to targeted treatment in rheumatoid arthritis. Mayo Clin Proc. 2017;92(7):1129–43.
25. Wijbrandts CA, Dijkgraaf MG, Kraan MC, Vinkenoog M, Smeets TJ, Dinant H, et al. The clinical response to infliximab in rheumatoid arthritis is in part dependent on pretreatment tumour necrosis factor alpha expression in the synovium. Ann Rheum Dis. 2008;67(8):1139–44.
26. Kapoor SR, Filer A, Fitzpatrick MA, Fisher BA, Taylor PC, Buckley CD, et al. Metabolic profiling predicts response to anti-tumor necrosis factor alpha therapy in patients with rheumatoid arthritis. Arthritis Rheum. 2013;65(6):1448–56.
27. Garcia-Carbonell R, Divakaruni AS, Lodi A, Vicente-Suarez I, Saha A, Cheroutre H, et al. Critical role of glucose metabolism in rheumatoid arthritis fibroblast-like synoviocytes. Arthritis Rheumatol. 2016;68(7):1614–26.
28. Guma M, Sanchez-Lopez E, Lodi A, Garcia-Carbonell R, Tiziani S, Karin M, et al. Choline kinase inhibition in rheumatoid arthritis. Ann Rheum Dis. 2015; 74(7):1399–40.
29. Hugle T, Kovacs H, Heijnen IA, Daikeler T, Baisch U, Hicks JM, et al. Synovial fluid metabolomics in different forms of arthritis assessed by nuclear magnetic resonance spectroscopy. Clin Exp Rheumatol. 2012;30(2):240–5.
30. Kim S, Hwang J, Xuan J, Jung YH, Cha HS, Kim KH. Global metabolite profiling of synovial fluid for the specific diagnosis of rheumatoid arthritis from other inflammatory arthritis. PLoS One. 2014;9(6):e97501.
31. Kosinska MK, Liebisch G, Lochnit G, Wilhelm J, Klein H, Kaesser U, et al. Sphingolipids in human synovial fluid–a lipidomic study. PLoS One. 2014;9(3):e91769.
32. Madsen RK, Lundstedt T, Gabrielsson J, Sennbro CJ, Alenius GM, Moritz T, et al. Diagnostic properties of metabolic perturbations in rheumatoid arthritis. Arthritis Res Ther. 2011;13(1):R19.
33. Guma M, Tiziani S, Firestein GS. Metabolomics in rheumatic diseases: desperately seeking biomarkers. Nat Rev Rheumatol. 2016;12(5):269–81.
34. Volchenkov R, Dung Cao M, Elgstoen KB, Goll GL, Eikvar K, Bjorneboe O, et al. Metabolic profiling of synovial tissue shows altered glucose and choline metabolism in rheumatoid arthritis samples. Scand J Rheumatol. 2017;46(2):160–1.
35. Biniecka M, Canavan M, McGarry T, Gao W, McCormick J, Cregan S, Gallagher L, Smith T, Phelan JJ, Ryan J, O'sullivan J. Dysregulated bioenergetics: a key regulator of joint inflammation. Annals of the rheumatic diseases. 2016;75(12):2192-200.
36. Roivainen A, Parkkola R, Yli-Kerttula T, Lehikoinen P, Viljanen T, Mottonen T, et al. Use of positron emission tomography with methyl-11C-choline and 2-18F-fluoro-2-deoxy-D-glucose in comparison with magnetic resonance imaging for the assessment of inflammatory proliferation of synovium. Arthritis Rheum. 2003;48(11):3077–84.
37. Beckmann J, Schubert J, Morhenn HG, Grau V, Schnettler R, Lips KS. Expression of choline and acetylcholine transporters in synovial tissue and cartilage of patients with rheumatoid arthritis and osteoarthritis. Cell Tissue Res. 2015;359(2):465–77.
38. Corcoran SE, O'Neill LA. HIF1alpha and metabolic reprogramming in inflammation. J Clin Invest. 2016;126(10):3699–707.
39. Amelio I, Cutruzzola F, Antonov A, Agostini M, Melino G. Serine and glycine metabolism in cancer. Trends Biochem Sci. 2014;39(4):191–8.
40. Labuschagne CF, van den Broek NJ, Mackay GM, Vousden KH, Maddocks OD. Serine, but not glycine, supports one-carbon metabolism and proliferation of cancer cells. Cell Rep. 2014;7(4):1248–58.
41. Ahn CS, Metallo CM. Mitochondria as biosynthetic factories for cancer proliferation. Cancer Metab. 2015;3(1):1.
42. Ma EH, Bantug G, Griss T, Condotta S, Johnson RM, Samborska B, et al. Serine is an essential metabolite for effector T cell expansion. Cell Metab. 2017;25(2):345–57.
43. Mills EL, Kelly B, O'Neill LAJ. Mitochondria are the powerhouses of immunity. Nat Immunol. 2017;18(5):488–98.
44. Newman JC, Verdin E. Ketone bodies as signaling metabolites. Trends Endocrinol Metab. 2014;25(1):42–52.
45. Shimazu T, Hirschey MD, Newman J, He W, Shirakawa K, Le Moan N, et al. Suppression of oxidative stress by beta-hydroxybutyrate, an endogenous histone deacetylase inhibitor. Science. 2013;339(6116):211–4.
46. Youm YH, Nguyen KY, Grant RW, Goldberg EL, Bodogai M, Kim D, et al. The ketone metabolite beta-hydroxybutyrate blocks NLRP3 inflammasome-mediated inflammatory disease. Nat Med. 2015;21(3):263–9.
47. Li Y, Zheng JY, Liu JQ, Yang J, Liu Y, Wang C, et al. Succinate/NLRP3 Inflammasome induces synovial fibroblast activation: therapeutical effects of clematichinenoside AR on arthritis. Front Immunol. 2016;7:532.
48. Mills E, O'Neill LA. Succinate: a metabolic signal in inflammation. Trends Cell Biol. 2014;24(5):313–20.
49. Chang CH, Curtis JD, Maggi LB Jr, Faubert B, Villarino AV, O'Sullivan D, et al. Posttranscriptional control of T cell effector function by aerobic glycolysis. Cell. 2013;153(6):1239–51.

50. Yu X, Li S. Non-metabolic functions of glycolytic enzymes in tumorigenesis. Oncogene. 2017;36(19):2629.

51. Dumas M-E, Maibaum EC, Teague C, Ueshima H, Zhou B, Lindon JC, et al. Assessment of analytical reproducibility of 1H NMR spectroscopy based metabonomics for large-scale epidemiological research: the INTERMAP study. Anal Chem. 2006;78(7):2199–208.

52. Viant MR, Bearden DW, Bundy JG, Burton IW, Collette TW, Ekman DR, et al. International NMR-based environmental metabolomics intercomparison exercise. Environ Sci Technol. 2008;43(1):219–25.

53. Zhang S, Nagana Gowda GA, Ye T, Raftery D. Advances in NMR-based biofluid analysis and metabolite profiling. Analyst. 2010;135(7):1490–8.

54. Wishart DS. Quantitative metabolomics using NMR. TrAC Trends Anal Chem. 2008;27(3):228–37.

55. Whitfield PD, German AJ, Noble PJM. Metabolomics: an emerging post-genomic tool for nutrition. Br J Nutr. 2004;92(4):549–55.

56. Bouatra S, Aziat F, Mandal R, Guo AC, Wilson MR, Knox C, et al. The human urine metabolome. PLoS One. 2013;8(9):e73076.

57. Brown PM, Pratt AG, Isaacs JD. Mechanism of action of methotrexate in rheumatoid arthritis, and the search for biomarkers. Nat Rev Rheumatol. 2016;12(12):731–42.

58. Jubair WK, Hendrickson JD, Severs EL, Schulz HM, Adhikari S, Ir D, et al. Modulation of inflammatory arthritis by gut microbiota through mucosal inflammation and autoantibody generation. Arthritis Rheumatol. 2018.

59. Maeda Y, Kurakawa T, Umemoto E, Motooka D, Ito Y, Gotoh K, et al. Dysbiosis contributes to arthritis development via activation of autoreactive T cells in the intestine. Arthritis Rheumatol. 2016;68(11):2646–61.

60. Scher JU, Abramson SB. The microbiome and rheumatoid arthritis. Nat Rev Rheumatol. 2011;7(10):569–78.

15

Loss of Gαq impairs regulatory B-cell function

Yan He[1], Xiaoqing Yuan[1,2], Yan Li[1], Chunlian Zhong[1], Yuan Liu[1], Hongyan Qian[1], Jingxiu Xuan[1], Lihua Duan[1*] and Guixiu Shi[1*]

Abstract

Background: Recent studies have shown a crucial role of Gαq in immune regulation, but how Gαq modulates regulatory B-cell (Breg) function is still unclear. We address this here.

Methods: $CD19^+IL-10^+$ Bregs of wild-type (WT) and $Gnaq^{-/-}$ mice were analyzed by flow cytometry after stimulation by lipopolysaccharide. The WT and $Gnaq^{-/-}$ Bregs were isolated and cocultured with WT $CD4^+CD25^-$ T cells in the presence of T-activator, and the proliferation of T cells and differentiation of regulatory T cells (Tregs) were analyzed by flow cytometry. We used inhibitors of PI3 kinase (PI3K), extracellular regulated protein kinases 1/2 (Erk1/2), and p38 mitogen-activated protein kinase (p38 MAPK) to detect the pathways involved in the regulation of Gαq on Breg differentiation, which were confirmed by western blot analysis. Furthermore, the expression level of Gαq was assessed by quantitative real-time PCR in peripheral blood mononuclear cells (PBMCs) from healthy controls and rheumatoid arthritis patients. The frequency of $CD19^+CD24^{hi}CD38^{hi}$ B cells in PBMCs was detected by flow cytometry, and the association of the Gαq mRNA expression level and the frequency of $CD19^+CD24^{hi}CD38^{hi}$ B cells was analyzed by Spearman test.

Results: The differentiation of $CD19^+IL-10^+$ Bregs was inhibited in the $Gnaq^{-/-}$ mice. In addition, Gαq depletion showed an impaired suppressive function of Bregs on T-cell proliferation, which might be due to the decreased Treg expansion. Mechanically, our data demonstrated that the PI3K, Erk1/2, and p38 MAPK signaling pathways were required for regulation of Gαq on Bregs, and blockage of these signaling pathways impaired Breg differentiation. Consistent with our previous studies, we also found a decreased frequency of $CD19^+CD24^{hi}CD38^{hi}$ Bregs in rheumatoid arthritis patients. As expected, a significantly positive correlation was investigated between $CD19^+CD24^{hi}CD38^{hi}$ Bregs with Gαq mRNA expression.

Conclusions: Our results indicate that Gαq plays a critical role in the differentiation and immunosuppression of Bregs, and it may provide a new therapeutic target for autoimmune diseases.

Keywords: Gαq, Regulatory B cells, IL-10, Regulation

Background

B cells are best known for their capacity to produce antibodies. In addition, they also exert a variety of other functions during the immune response, including antigen presentation and production of various cytokines, which are involved in the early and late stages of T-cell-mediated immune responses [1]. However, B-cell-deficient mice were observed to be susceptible to experimental autoimmune encephalitis (EAE), and to be unable to recover from it [2]. Furthermore, adoptive transfer of IL-10[+] B cells can suppress inflammation of EAE [3]. A new population of B cells, regulatory B cells (Bregs), has increasingly gained attention for restraining inflammation [4, 5]. Bregs can suppress the differentiation of T helper 1 (Th1) and T helper 17 (Th17) cells, and promote regulatory T-cell (Treg) induction [6, 7]. It was also reported that Bregs support the maintenance of invariant nature killer T (iNKT) cells [8]. Bregs have been shown to inhibit autoreactive and pathogen-driven immune response mainly through the production of interleukin-10 (IL-10), interleukin-35

* Correspondence: lh-duan@163.com; gshi@xmu.edu.cn
[1]Department of Rheumatology and Clinical Immunology, The First Affiliated Hospital of Xiamen University, Xiamen, China
Full list of author information is available at the end of the article

(IL-35), and transforming growth factor beta (TGF-β) [9]. Until now, the production of immune-suppressive cytokine IL-10 was thought to be a hallmark of Breg function [10]. In some human autoimmune diseases, it has been reported that Breg function is impaired and does not prevent the development of human autoimmune diseases, such as RA [7], relapsing–remitting multiple sclerosis [11], systemic lupus erythematosus (SLE) [12], and so on [13]. However, the mechanism of impaired Breg function in autoimmune diseases remains unclear.

The heterotrimeric guanine nucleotide-binding proteins (G proteins) are important signal transducers, which when attached to the cell surface plasma membrane receptors, G protein-coupled receptors (GPCRs), can communicate with signals from a large number of hormones, neurotransmitters, chemokines, sensory stimuli, and autocrine and paracrine factors. The heterotrimeric G proteins are composed of three subunits (α, β, and γ subunits) that cycle between inactive and active signaling states in response to guanine nucleotides [14, 15]. On the basis of downstream signaling targets of α subunits, these α subunits are divided into four classes: Gαi/0, Gαs, Gαq/11, and Gα12/13. Gαq is a member of the Gαq/11 subfamily encoded by GNAQ [16]. Gαq is ubiquitously expressed in mammalian cells and nearly 40% of all GPCRs rely upon Gαq family members to stimulate inositol lipid signaling [15]. It is well known that Gαq plays an essential role in the nervous system, endocrine system, and cardiovascular system [16–20]. Many studies have also established the physiological importance of Gαq in the immune system. A previous study showed that Gαq-deficient ($Gnaq^{-/-}$) mice exhibited impaired eosinophil recruitment to the lung after antigenic challenge, probably due to an impaired production of granulocyte macrophage colony stimulating factor (GM-CSF) by resident airway leukocytes [21]. Our previous study reported that $Gnaq^{-/-}$ dendritic cells were defective in migrating from the skin to draining lymph nodes after fluorescein isothiocyanate sensitization, and $Gnaq^{-/-}$ monocytes were defective in migrating from the bone marrow into inflamed skin after contact sensitization [22]. The functional involvement of Gαq in TCR-induced immune responses was also investigated [23]. In addition, $Gnaq^{-/-}$ chimeras could spontaneously develop manifestations of systemic autoimmune disease with high titer antinuclear antibody and inflammatory arthritis, which was observed in our previous study [24]. In humans, our previous work also showed that Gαq mRNA expression was decreased in peripheral blood lymphocyte cells (PBMCs) and T cells from SLE patients compared to that from healthy individuals. What is more, the Gαq expression in T cells from SLE patients was associated with disease severity, the presence of lupus nephritis,

and expression of Th1, Th2, and Th17 cytokines [25]. We also found that B cells from mice lacking the Gαq subunit of trimeric G proteins have an intrinsic survival advantage over normal B cells, suggesting that Gαq is critically important for maintaining control of peripheral B-cell tolerance induction and repressing autoimmunity [24]. Whether Gαq regulates Breg function is still unknown.

In this study, we found a critical role of Gαq in Breg differentiation and $Gnaq^{-/-}$ Bregs showed an impaired suppressive function on T-cell proliferation. Our human data also showed that the decreased frequency of Bregs showed a significantly positive correlation with Gαq mRNA expression in RA patients. Taken together, our work reveals a novel function of Gαq in regulating Breg function.

Methods
Patients and controls
Peripheral blood was obtained from 34 RA patients and 24 healthy controls from the inpatient clinic of the Department of Rheumatology, The First Affiliated Hospital of Xiamen University, Xiamen, China. The criteria used for RA diagnosis were based on those of the American Rheumatism Association (1987) [26] and the new criteria from the ACR/EULAR (2010) [27]. Gαq mRNA expressions were detected by RT–PCR, the frequency of CD19$^+$CD24^{hi}CD38^{hi} B cells in PBMCs was detected by flow cytometry, and the association of Gαq mRNA expression level and frequency of CD19$^+$CD24^{hi}CD38^{hi} B cells was studied. The clinical characteristics of the RA patients are summarized in Table 1. Informed consent was obtained from all recruits to this study. This study was approved by the Ethics Committee of the First Affiliated Hospital of Xiamen University in accordance with the World Medical Association Declaration of Helsinki.

Table 1 Demographic data and clinical characteristics of RA patients in the study

Characteristic	RA ($n = 34$)	HC ($n = 24$)
Age (years), mean (range)	56 (34–78)	45 (29–68)
Sex (n), female/male	26/8	17/7
CRP (mg/L), mean (range)	30.35 (0.5–75.1)	
ESR (mm/h), mean (range)	47.29 (7–117)	
RF (IU/ml), mean (range)	223.35 (9.69–991)	
Anti-CCP (RU/ml), mean (range)	52.50 (1–200)	
Tender joint count, mean (range) of 68 joints	6.35 (0–26)	
Swollen joint count, mean (range) of 68 joints	4.47 (0–22)	

RA rheumatoid arthritis, *HC* healthy controls, *CRP* C-reaction protein, *ESR* erythrocyte sedimentation rate, *RF* rheumatoid factor, *anti-CCP* anti-cyclic citrullinated peptide antibody

Animals

All experimental procedures involving mice were approved by the institutional animal care committee of Xiamen University. C57BL/6 J (B6) mice were purchased from Xiamen University Laboratory Animal Center. C57BL/6 J (B6) mice and $Gnaq^{-/-}$ ($n > 8$ backcrossed to C57BL/6 J) mice were bred in Xiamen University Laboratory Animal Center. The mice used in this study were 6–8 weeks age.

Cell isolation

The purification of CD4$^+$CD25$^-$ T cells from the spleen of mice was performed using the CD4$^+$CD25$^-$ T Cell Isolation Kit (Miltenyi Biotec, Bergisch-Gladbach, Germany), LS Columns (Miltenyi Biotec), and MidiMACS™ Separators (Miltenyi Biotec) according to the manufacturer's instructions. Briefly, $1*10^7$ cells from the mice spleen were stained with biotin-antibody cocktail in buffer (PBS/2 mM EDTA/0.5% BSA) for 5 min at 4 °C. After that, the anti-Biotin MicroBeads and CD44 MicroBeads were sequentially added and incubated for 10 min at 4 °C. Cells were washed, centrifuged, and resuspended in 0.5 ml of buffer, and applied onto the column. The CD4$^+$CD25$^-$ T cells in flow-through fluids were collected. The isolation of B cells and Tregs from the spleen of mice was performed using the corresponding Pan B Cell Isolation Kit II (Miltenyi Biotec) and the CD4$^+$CD25$^+$ Regulatory T cell Isolation Kit (Miltenyi Biotec) according to the manufacturer's instructions. Purity of the target cells was > 90% in all experiments assessed by flow cytometry. CD1d^{hi}CD5$^+$ B cells were isolated using a MoFlo High-Performance Cell Sorter (Beckman Coulter, Fullerton, CA, USA) with purities of 90–95%. Human PBMCs were isolated from 4 ml sodium heparin-treated venous blood samples by Ficoll density-gradient centrifugation using Lymphoprep™ (Axis-Shied PoC AS, Oslo, Norway). Washed and resuspended, the PBMCs were cryopreserved for future real-time polymerase chain reaction.

Cell culture

Purified B cells were planted in complete RPIM 1640 with 2.05 mM L-glutamine (GE Healthcare Life Sciences, Logan, UT, USA) supplement with 10% fetal bovine serum (PAN Seratech, Aidan Bach, Germany) and maintained in standard cell culture environment (95% humidity, 5% CO$_2$ at 37 °C). For Breg induction, B cells were stimulated with LPS (*Escherichia coli* 0111:B4; Sigma-Aldrich, St. Louis, MO, USA) (10 μg/ml) for 48 h. PMA (50 ng/ml), ionomycin (250 ng/ml) (Sigma-Aldrich), and brefeldin A (10 μg/ml) (BD Biosciences, San Jose, CA, USA) were added for the last 5 h of culture before flow cytometry. For analysis of CD4$^+$ T-cell proliferation and Treg differentiation, purified LPS-induced Bregs from the spleen of WT mice or $Gnaq^{-/-}$ mice and sorted CD4$^+$CD25$^-$ T cells

from the spleen of WT mice were 1:1 cocultured and activated with Dynabeads™ Mouse T-Activator CD3/CD28 (Life Technologies AS, Oslo, Norway) at a bead-to-cell ratio of 1:2 in 200 μl medium in a 96-well U-bottom plate for 72 h.

Antibodies

Anti-human antibodies included: anti-CD19-FITC from BD Biosciences; anti-CD24-PE (ML5) and anti-CD38-PE /Cy7 (HIT2) from Biolegend (San Diego, CA, USA); and Human FcR Binding Inhibitor from eBioscience (San Diego, CA, USA). Anti-mouse antibodies included: anti-CD4-FITC (RM4–5), anti-CD19-PE/Cy5, anti-CD19-APC (6D5), anti-CD25-APC (3C7), anti-IL-10-PE (JES5-16E3), PE Rat IgG2b, κ Isotype Ctrl (RTK4530), and anti-PD-L1-APC (10.F.9G2) from Biolegend; anti-CD1d-PE (1B1), anti-CD5-FITC (53–7.3), anti-CD16/CD32 (mouse Fc block), anti-Annexin-V-APC, and 7-AAD from BD Biosciences; and anti-CD25-PE/Cy5.5 (PC61.5), anti-Foxp3-PE (NRRF-30), anti-TLR4-Alexa Fluor® 488(UT41), and anti-FasL-FITC (MFL3) from eBioscience. Phosho-p38 MAPK (Thr180/ Tyr182) (28B10) mouse mAb, p38 MAPK (D13E1) XP® rabbit mAb, phosho-p44/42 MAPK (Erk1/2) (Thr202/ Tyr204) (D13.14.4E) XP® rabbit mAb, p44/42 MAPK (Erk1/2) (137F5) rabbit mAb, phosho-PI3K p85 (Tyr458)/ p55 (Tyr199) antibody, PI3K p85α (6G10) mouse mAb, phospho-STAT1 (Thr701) (58D6) rabbit mAb, STAT1 (D1K9Y) rabbit mAb, GAPDH (14C10) rabbit mAb, β-Tubulin (9F3) rabbit mAB, anti-mouse IgG, HRP-linked antibody, anti-rabbit IgG, and HRP-linked antibody were obtained from Cell Signaling Technology (MA, USA); and anti-MyD88 antibody was obtained from Abcam (Cambridge, UK).

Real-time polymerase chain reaction

Total RNA was extracted from PBMCs with TriPure Isolation Reagent (Roche Diagnostics GmbH, Mannheim, Germany) and the concentration of RNA was determined by measuring the absorbance at 260 nm in a UV–Vis spectrophotometer (Quawell, San Jose, CA, USA). Reverse transcription was performed by the Bio-Rad Systems (Bio-Rad, Hercules, CA, USA) according to standard protocols using the Transcriptor First Strand cDNA Synthesis Kit (Roche Diagnostics GmbH). The expression level of Gαq was measured by real-time quantitative PCR. β-actin was simultaneously amplified and used as an internal control. The primer sequences were as follows: β-actin forward, 5′-AGAAAATCT GGCACCACACC-3′; β-actin reverse, 5′-AGAGGCG TACAGGGATAGCA-3′; Gαq forward, 5′-GTTGAT GTGGAGAAGGTGTCTG-3′; and Gαq reverse, 5′-G TAGGCAGGTAGGCAGGGT-3′. Amplification was performed with the 7500 Real Time PCR Systems (Applied Biosystems, CA, USA). Gene expression levels were normalized by comparing to β-actin and relative expression was calculated by the $2^{-\Delta\Delta Ct}$ method.

Enzyme-linked immunosorbent assay

The concentration of mouse IL-10 (BD Biosciences), IL-35 (Wuhan Huamei, China), TGF-β, IL-23 (Invitrogen, Carlsbad, CA, USA), and IL-6 (R&D, Minneapolis, MN, USA) were measured using commercially available ELISA kits according to the manufacturer's instructions. Absorbance at 450 nm was measured with an ELISA microplate reader (Molecular Devices, Sunnyvale, CA, USA).

Flow cytometry

Fc receptors were blocked with mouse Fc block and the dead cells were detected using Fixable Viability Dye eFlour™ 506 or 510 (eBioscience) before cell surface staining. For Breg staining, CD19-FITC or PE/Cy5, CD24-PE, CD38-PE/Cy7, CD1d-PE, and CD5-FITC mAbs were used. For intracellular IL-10 staining, cells were stained with CD19-PE/Cy5 or APC mAbs. Cells were washed, fixed with IC Fixation Buffer (eBioscience), permeabilized with Permeabilization Buffer (eBioscience), and stained with IL-10-PE. For Treg staining, cells were stained with combinations of CD4-FITC and CD25-PE/Cy5.5 or APC mAbs, fixed and permeabilized with Fixation/Permeabilization solution (eBioscience) and Permeabilization Buffer, and stained for detection of intracellular Foxp3-PE mAbs. For apoptotic cell detection, cells were washed twice with cold PBS and then resuspended in 1× Binding Buffer (BD Biosciences), and then the cells were stained with CD4-FITC, APC Annexin-V, and 7-AAD and incubated for 15 min at RT in the dark. Last, 400 μl of 1× Binding Buffer was added. Data were acquired using Cytomic FC500 or Cytoflex (Beckman Coulter) and analyzed using CXP Analysis and Cytexpert (Beckman Coulter).

Western blot analysis

Single-cell suspensions were lysed after stimulation in cOmplete Lysis-M (Roche Diagnostics GmbH) containing protease inhibitor cocktail (Roche Diagnostics GmbH) and phosphatase inhibitor cocktail (Roche Diagnostics GmbH) for 10 min with gentle shaking. The lysates were centrifuged at $14,000 \times g$ for 15 min, and frozen at – 80 °C until use. For western blotting assays, the protein concentrations were determined using the BCA Protein Assay Kit (Thermo Scientific, Rockford, IL, USA), and equal amounts of protein (20 μg) per lane were separated by 10% SDS-PAGE gels and transferred to PVDF membranes. Membranes were blocked and then probed with primary antibodies against p-p38 MAPK (1:1000), p-Erk1/2 (1:2000), p-PI3K (1:1000), p-STAT1 (1:1000), or MyD88 (1:1000) at 4 °C overnight. After washing, the membranes were incubated with the appropriate HRP-conjugated secondary antibodies for 1 h at room temperature. After extensive washing, signals were visualized using the chemiluminescent HRP substrate system (Millipore, Billerica, MA, USA). Band quantification was performed on the Molecular Imager® ChemiDoc™ XRS+ system with Image Lab™ Software (Bio-Rad, Hercules, CA, USA). Thereafter, membranes were stripped with stripping buffer before reprobing with anti-p38 MAPK (1:1000), Erk1/2 (1:1000), PI3K (1:1000), and STAT1 (1:1000) to ensure equal loading. GAPDH or β-Tubulin was also detected as the loading control. The level of protein phosphorylation was normalized to the loading control (total protein).

Statistical analysis

All data were obtained from at least three independent experiments and shown as mean ± standard deviation (SD). All data were analyzed using GraphPad Prism 5.01 software (GraphPad, San Diego, CA, USA). Statistical significance was determined by Student's t test and the Mann–Whitney U test. Correlation was analyzed using Spearman's test. A probability value of $p < 0.05$ was considered statistically significant.

Results

Gαq regulates Breg differentiation

We and others have reported that Gαq plays a critical role in immune disorders via regulating immune cell function. Recently, a crucial role of Bregs has been described in many studies. Nevertheless, whether Gαq regulates Breg function remains unknown. The $Gnaq^{-/-}$ mice were used to address this question. The flow cytometry analysis showed that there was no difference between WT and $Gnaq^{-/-}$ mice on the percentage of $CD19^+CD1d^{hi}CD5^+$ Bregs (Fig. 1a, b) and $CD19^+IL-10^+$ Bregs (Fig. 1d, e), both of which are considered Breg markers in mice [9]. Additionally, no marked difference in the absolute number of Bregs was observed (Fig. 1c, f). Interestingly, a significantly higher expression of IFN-γ and IL-17 was observed in $Gnaq^{-/-}$ $CD19^+CD1d^{hi}CD5^+$ Bregs (see Additional file 1: Figure S1A–D). Although increased production of IFN-γ by $Gnaq^{-/-}$ Bregs was observed, the STAT1 phosphorylation after LPS stimulation showed no difference between WT and $Gnaq^{-/-}$ Bregs (see Additional file 1: Figure S1E). In order to address whether Gαq has a role in regulating Breg differentiation, splenic B cells were isolated from WT and $Gnaq^{-/-}$ mice, and then stimulated with lipopolysaccharide (LPS) for 48 h, which was shown to induce $IL-10^+$ Breg differentiation [4]. After stimulation, the percentage of $CD19^+IL-10^+$ Bregs was significantly lower in $Gnaq^{-/-}$ mice (Fig. 1g, h). In addition, the expression of IL-10 in culture supernatant was also lower in $Gnaq^{-/-}$ mice when compared with that in WT mice

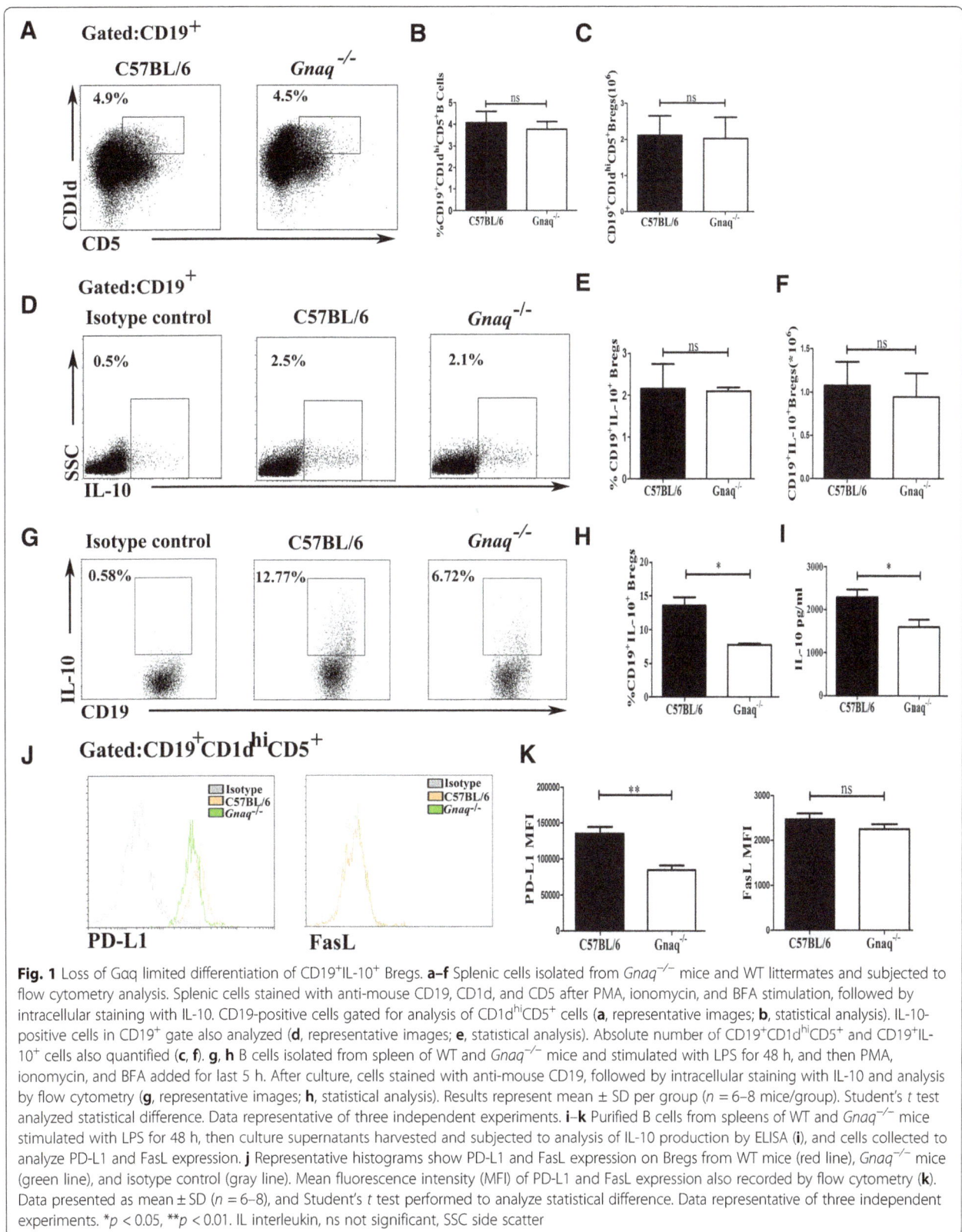

Fig. 1 Loss of Gαq limited differentiation of CD19⁺IL-10⁺ Bregs. **a–f** Splenic cells isolated from *Gnaq*⁻/⁻ mice and WT littermates and subjected to flow cytometry analysis. Splenic cells stained with anti-mouse CD19, CD1d, and CD5 after PMA, ionomycin, and BFA stimulation, followed by intracellular staining with IL-10. CD19-positive cells gated for analysis of CD1d^hiCD5⁺ cells (**a**, representative images; **b**, statistical analysis). IL-10-positive cells in CD19⁺ gate also analyzed (**d**, representative images; **e**, statistical analysis). Absolute number of CD19⁺CD1d^hiCD5⁺ and CD19⁺IL-10⁺ cells also quantified (**c**, **f**). **g**, **h** B cells isolated from spleen of WT and *Gnaq*⁻/⁻ mice and stimulated with LPS for 48 h, and then PMA, ionomycin, and BFA added for last 5 h. After culture, cells stained with anti-mouse CD19, followed by intracellular staining with IL-10 and analysis by flow cytometry (**g**, representative images; **h**, statistical analysis). Results represent mean ± SD per group (*n* = 6–8 mice/group). Student's *t* test analyzed statistical difference. Data representative of three independent experiments. **i–k** Purified B cells from spleens of WT and *Gnaq*⁻/⁻ mice stimulated with LPS for 48 h, then culture supernatants harvested and subjected to analysis of IL-10 production by ELISA (**i**), and cells collected to analyze PD-L1 and FasL expression. **j** Representative histograms show PD-L1 and FasL expression on Bregs from WT mice (red line), *Gnaq*⁻/⁻ mice (green line), and isotype control (gray line). Mean fluorescence intensity (MFI) of PD-L1 and FasL expression also recorded by flow cytometry (**k**). Data presented as mean ± SD (*n* = 6–8), and Student's *t* test performed to analyze statistical difference. Data representative of three independent experiments. *$p < 0.05$, **$p < 0.01$. IL interleukin, ns not significant, SSC side scatter

(Fig. 1i). The IL-17 expression was slightly decreased in both groups, which might due to Breg differentiation by LPS stimulation (see Additional file 1: Figure S1F). Due to a critical role of IL-35 and TGF-β in Breg suppressive function, we also detected the expression of IL-35 and TGF-β. TGF-β production was lower in

Gnaq$^{-/-}$ mice, while IL-35 expression was comparable with that in WT mice (see Additional file 2: Figure S2). Additionally, the inhibitory ligand PD-L1 on *Gnaq*$^{-/-}$ Bregs was also decreased. No different change was observed in FasL expression (Fig. 1j, k).

To rule out the effect of cell death on the decreased percentages of *Gnaq*$^{-/-}$ Bregs after 48 h LPS stimulation, the rates of dead cells were analyzed in the WT and *Gnaq*$^{-/-}$ Bregs. We found that Gαq deficiency did not promote cell death, while a decreased rate of cell death in *Gnaq*$^{-/-}$ Bregs was observed (Fig. 2a, b), which was in keeping with our previous published data [24]. Previous studies have shown the role of Toll-like receptors (TLRs) in B cell-mediated regulation [28–30]. Since we induced Bregs using LPS, the agonist of TLR4, we next detected TLR4 expression on both WT and *Gnaq*$^{-/-}$ B-cell surfaces. As shown in Fig. 2, there was no difference between them.

Furthermore, myeloid differentiation primary response 88 (MyD88), a key signaling molecule downstream of TLRs, was also analyzed by immunoblotting. Consistently, no marked differences were observed (Fig. 2c, d). These data indicated that Gαq has no effect on the TLR4/MyD88 signal pathway.

Gαq is required for Breg immunosuppression

To verify whether *Gnaq*$^{-/-}$ Bregs have an inhibitory effect on T-cell proliferation, CD1d^{hi}CD5^{+} B cells were sorted from both WT and *Gnaq*$^{-/-}$ mice, and then we cocultured with purified CD4^{+}CD25^{-} T cells from the WT mice for 72 h under the stimulation of Mouse T-Activator CD3/CD28 Dynabeads™. Although it was weaker than that of Tregs, the inhibitory effect of WT Bregs on T-cell proliferation was significantly strong when compared to that of *Gnaq*$^{-/-}$ Bregs (Fig. 3a–c). Furthermore, there was no

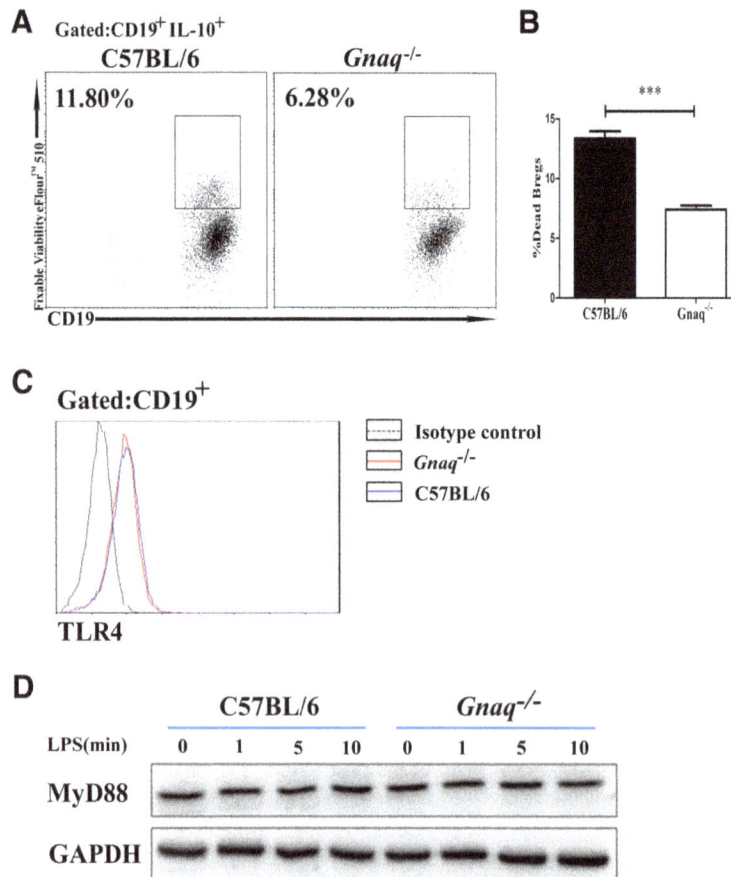

Fig. 2 Gαq deficiency did not affect TLR4 signaling in B cells. **a, b** B cells purified from WT and *Gnaq*$^{-/-}$ mice stimulated with LPS for 48 h, and PMA, ionomycin, and BFA added for last 5 h. Fixable Viability Dye eFlour™ 510 used to analyze B-cell death by flow cytometry. Data presented as mean ± SD of five mice. Results shown are one from three independent experiments. Student's *t* test analyzed statistical difference. ***$p < 0.001$. **c** Splenic cells from WT and *Gnaq*$^{-/-}$ mice stained with anti-mouse CD19 and anti-mouse TLR4, followed by flow cytometry analysis (*n* = 5). Representative histogram shown. Blue line, WT mice; red line, *Gnaq*$^{-/-}$ mice. Data representative of three independent experiments. **d** WT and *Gnaq*$^{-/-}$ B cells treated with LPS, then harvested to analyze Myd88 expression by western blot analysis at indicated times. Data representative of three independent experiments. Breg regulatory B cell, IL interleukin, LPS lipopolysaccharide, MyD88 myeloid differentiation primary response 88, TLR Toll-like receptor

difference among control Bregs, WT Bregs, and $Gnaq^{-/-}$ Bregs in the viability of T cells (Fig. 3d, e), which indicated that the different T-cell proliferation was not due to different cell apoptosis. Previous studies have revealed that Bregs can restrain inflammation by promoting differentiation of Tregs [6, 7]. To evaluate the contribution of Gαq in this function of Bregs, we cocultured Bregs purified from WT or $Gnaq^{-/-}$ mice with WT CD4$^+$CD25$^-$ T cells. As expected, an increased frequency of CD4$^+$CD25$^+$Foxp3$^+$ Tregs was detected in the WT group after stimulation, whereas there was no significant change of Foxp3 expression in the $Gnaq^{-/-}$ group when compared with the no Breg experimental group (Fig. 4a, b). Lots of studies have demonstrated that the cytokines IL-6, IL-23, and TGF-β act a crucial role in the regulation of Treg differentiation. Next, we analyzed these cytokines in the supernatants of cocultured WT or $Gnaq^{-/-}$ Bregs with activated CD4$^+$CD25$^-$ T cells. As expected, IL-6 was increased in $Gnaq^{-/-}$ Bregs, whereas TGF-β production was decreased (Fig. 4c). Unfortunately, the IL-23 concentration was lower than the sensitivity of the test kit. These data showed that Gαq modulated Breg immunosuppression by

regulating Breg cytokine production, which might affect Treg differentiation.

Involvement of PI3K, Erk1/2, and p38 MAPK pathways in the regulation of Gαq on Breg differentiation

Numerous reports indicate that Gαq was implicated in regulating the MAPK pathways, PI3K/Akt pathways, and PLC-β activation [15, 31]. Interestingly, these pathways were also involved in production of IL-10 [32]. Therefore, we supposed that there might be crosstalk between Gαq and IL-10 signaling pathways. To address this hypothesis, we first confirmed these signal pathways in Breg differentiation. The differentiation of WT Bregs was significantly decreased in the presence of LY294002 (PI3K inhibitor), U0126 (Erk1/2 inhibitor), or SB203580 (p38 MAPK inhibitor). However, no significant changes were observed in $Gnaq^{-/-}$ Bregs (Fig. 5a, b), which may be related to a significantly reduced activation of these signaling pathways in $Gnaq^{-/-}$ Bregs. Consistently, we found that the levels of phospho-PI3K, phospho-Erk1/2, and phospho-p38 MAPK were lower after LPS stimulation in $Gnaq^{-/-}$ B cells when compared with those in WT B cells (Fig. 5c, d). In conclusion, the decreased

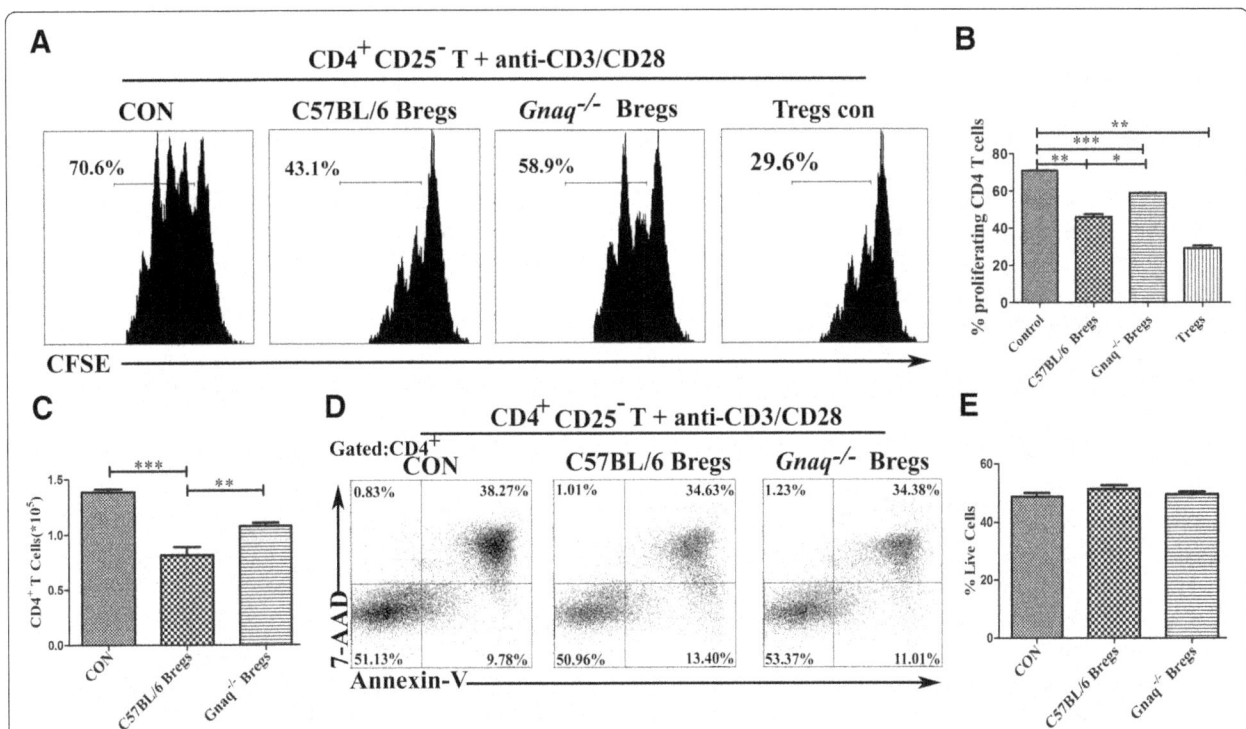

Fig. 3 Lack of Gαq impairs ability of Bregs to suppress CD4$^+$ T-cell proliferation. CFSE-labeled WT CD4$^+$CD25$^-$ T cells cocultured (1:1) with sorting-purified WT Bregs, $Gnaq^{-/-}$ Bregs, or WT Tregs in presence of Mouse T-Activator CD3/CD28 Dynabeads™ for 72 h. Percentage of proliferated CD4$^+$ T cells detected by flow cytometry (a, b), and total number of T cells also investigated (c). d, e Culture cells also harvested to analyze viability of T cells. Cells labeled with anti-mouse CD4, Annexin-V, and 7-AAD, and then analyzed by flow cytometry. Results represent mean ± SD per group (n = 5 mice/group). Data representative of three independent experiments. Student's t test analyzed statistical difference. *p < 0.05, **p < 0.01, ***p < 0.001. Breg regulatory B cell, CON control, Treg regulatory T cell

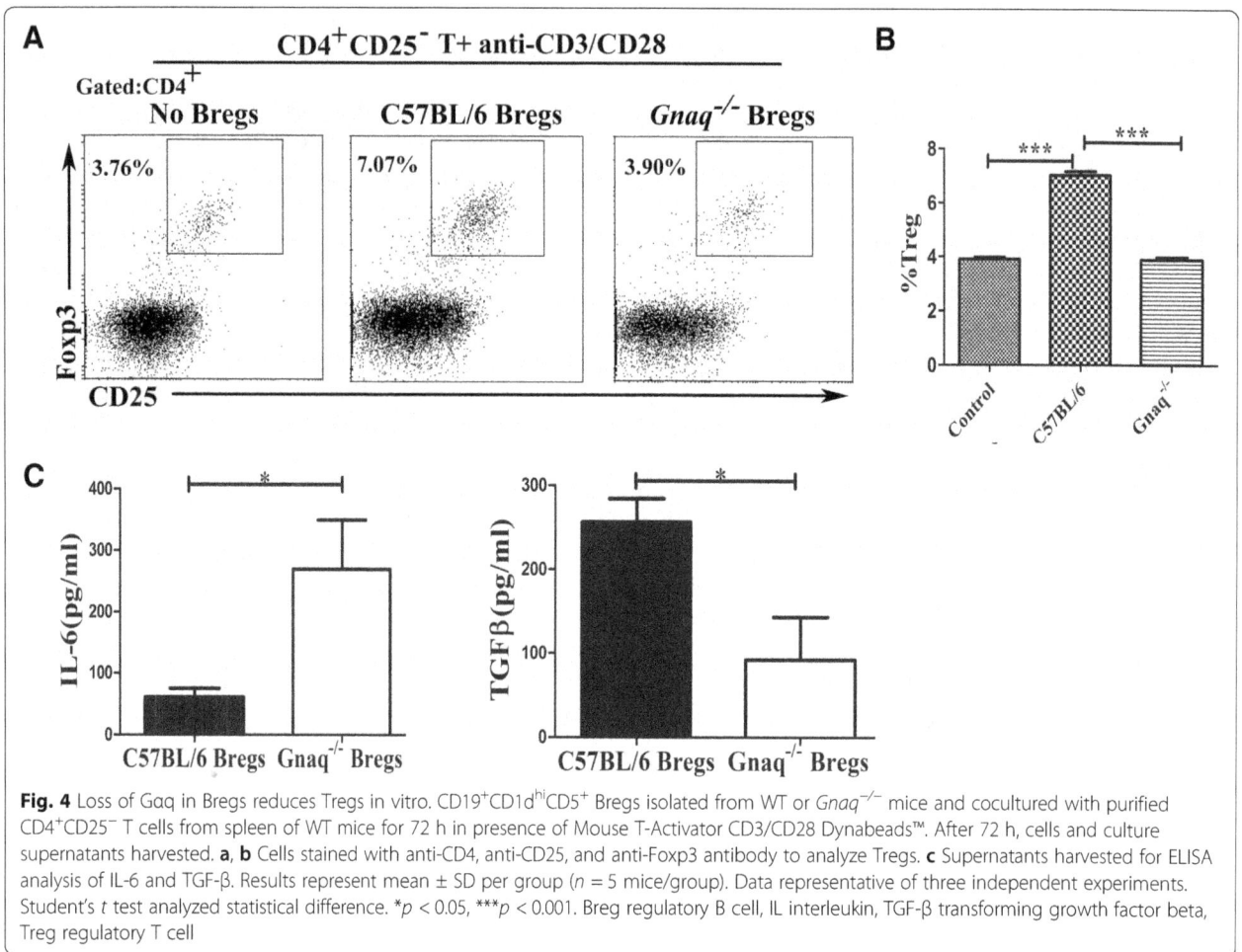

Fig. 4 Loss of Gαq in Bregs reduces Tregs in vitro. CD19+CD1d^hi^CD5+ Bregs isolated from WT or *Gnaq*^−/−^ mice and cocultured with purified CD4+CD25− T cells from spleen of WT mice for 72 h in presence of Mouse T-Activator CD3/CD28 Dynabeads™. After 72 h, cells and culture supernatants harvested. **a, b** Cells stained with anti-CD4, anti-CD25, and anti-Foxp3 antibody to analyze Tregs. **c** Supernatants harvested for ELISA analysis of IL-6 and TGF-β. Results represent mean ± SD per group (*n* = 5 mice/group). Data representative of three independent experiments. Student's *t* test analyzed statistical difference. *$p < 0.05$, ***$p < 0.001$. Breg regulatory B cell, IL interleukin, TGF-β transforming growth factor beta, Treg regulatory T cell

activation of PI3K, Erk1/2, and p38 MAPK contributed to the impaired differentiation of *Gnaq*^−/−^ Bregs.

Decreased frequency of CD19+CD24^hi^CD38^hi^ Bregs was correlated with Gαq mRNA expression in RA patients

Our presented experiments demonstrated that Gαq exerted a role in regulating Bregs in mice. Previous studies have shown that the frequency of CD19+CD24^hi^CD38^hi^ Bregs was decreased in RA patients. Human CD19+CD24^hi^CD38^hi^ Breg subsets have been shown to maintain tolerance in immune disorders via the release of IL-10 [9]. Here, to further address the regulation of Gαq in Breg function, we analyzed the correlation between Gαq mRNA expression and frequency of regulatory B cells in PBMCs from RA patients. In comparison to HC, a decreased frequency of CD19+CD24^hi^CD38^hi^ B cells was observed in RA patients (Fig. 6a, b), and the mRNA expression of Gαq was also significantly lower in the RA group (Fig. 6c). Consistent with the animal results, we observed a significant positive correlation between the frequency of CD19+CD24^hi^CD38^hi^ B cells and the expression of Gαq mRNA in PBMCs from patients with RA and HC (Fig. 6d). These data further confirm that

Gαq plays a critical role in immune tolerance via regulation of Bregs.

Discussion

Recent studies have shown that Bregs play a crucial role in autoimmune diseases through suppressing the differentiation of Th1 and Th17 cells, and promoting Treg induction [9]. However, the mechanism of Breg differentiation still remains unknown. Our previous studies demonstrated that Gαq exerts an important role in immune regulation, including Th1 and Th17 function, while the role of Gαq in Breg regulation is still unclear. Here, we found that the differentiation and immunosuppressive effect of Bregs were inhibited in the *Gnaq*^−/−^ mice. In addition, our data demonstrated that the PI3K, Erk1/2, and p38 MAPK signaling pathways were involved in the regulation of Breg function by Gαq. Furthermore, we also showed a decreased frequency of CD19+CD24^hi^CD38^hi^ Bregs in RA patients, which positively correlated with Gαq mRNA expression. These data suggest that Gαq was involved in the immune tolerance via regulating Breg function.

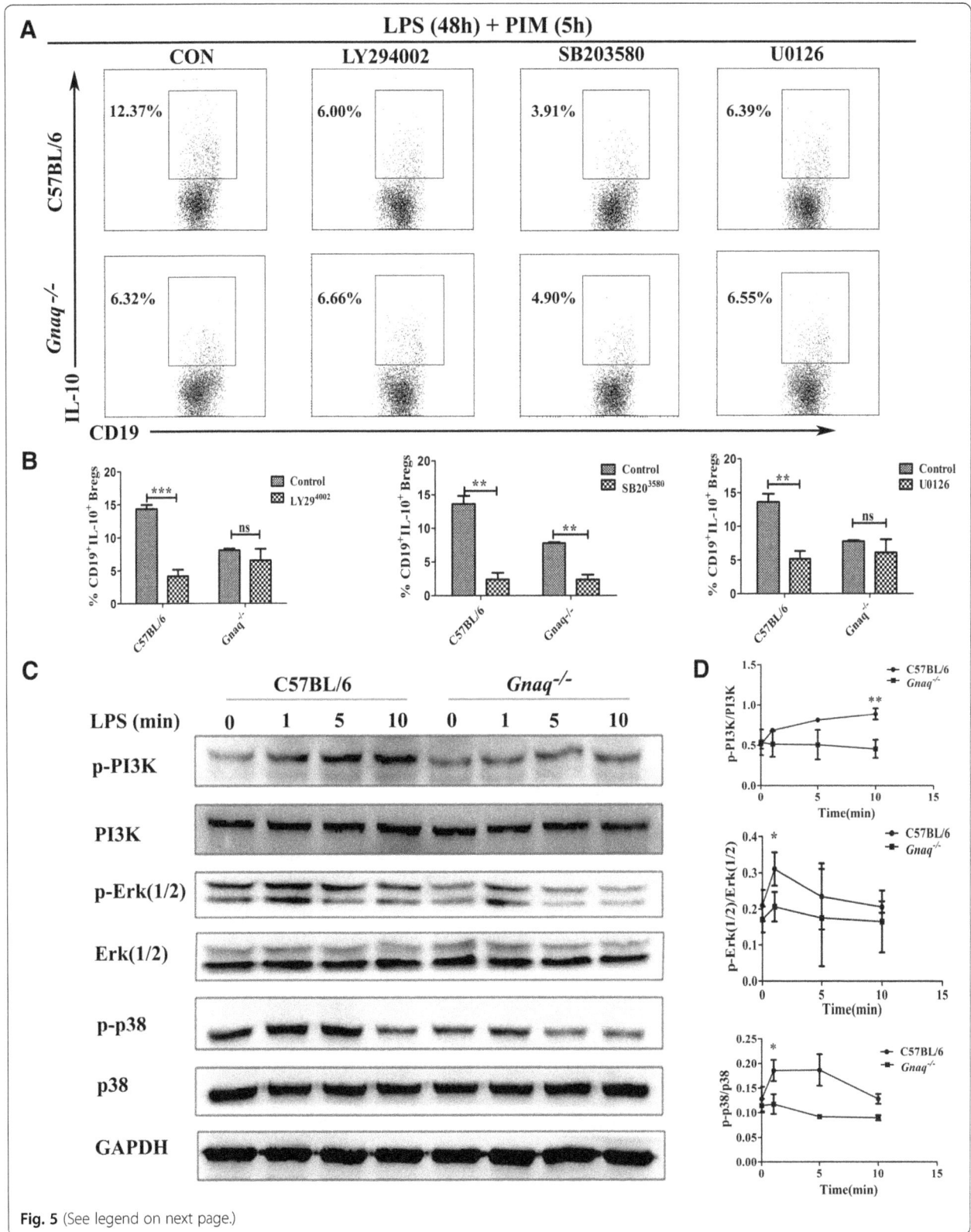

A LPS (48h) + PIM (5h)

CON · LY294002 · SB203580 · U0126

C57BL/6

CON 12.37%
LY294002 6.00%
SB203580 3.91%
U0126 6.39%

Gnaq-/-

CON 6.32%
LY294002 6.66%
SB203580 4.90%
U0126 6.55%

IL-10 / CD19

B

% CD19+IL-10+ Bregs

Control / LY29⁴⁰⁰² *** ns C57BL/6 Gnaq-/-

Control / SB20³⁵⁸⁰ ** ** C57BL/6 Gnaq-/-

Control / U0126 ** ns C57BL/6 Gnaq-/-

C

C57BL/6   Gnaq-/-

LPS (min)   0   1   5   10   0   1   5   10

p-PI3K
PI3K
p-Erk(1/2)
Erk(1/2)
p-p38
p38
GAPDH

D

p-PI3K/PI3K — C57BL/6, Gnaq-/- ** Time(min)

p-Erk(1/2)/Erk(1/2) — C57BL/6, Gnaq-/- * Time(min)

p-p38/p38 — C57BL/6, Gnaq-/- * Time(min)

Fig. 5 (See legend on next page.)

(See figure on previous page.)

Fig. 5 Decreased activation of PI3K, Erk1/2 MAPK, and p38 MAPK signaling pathways in $Gnaq^{-/-}$ Bregs. Isolated B cells from WT and $Gnaq^{-/-}$ mice cultured in presence of SB203580 (p38 inhibitor) (2.65 μM), U0126 (Erk1/2 inhibitor) (26 μM), or LY294002 (PI3K inhibitor) (6.4 μM) for 1 h, then cells stimulated by LPS for 48 h, and PMA, ionomycin, and brefeldin A added for last 5 h of culture. After culture, cells stained with anti-mouse CD19 and intracellular staining with IL-10, followed by flow cytometry analysis (**a**, representative images; **b**, statistical analysis). **c** Splenic B cells purified from WT and $Gnaq^{-/-}$ mice and stimulated with LPS for 0–10 min. Protein from cell lysates exacted for analysis of phospho-PI3K, PI3K, phospho-Erk1/2, Erk1/2, phospho-p38 MAPK, and p38 MAPK by western blot analysis with specific antibodies individually. GAPDH used as loading control. **d** Protein expression levels quantified with Image Lab software. Ratios of phosphor-specific proteins versus total proteins obtained. Results represent mean ± SD per group ($n = 4$–5 mice/group). Data representative of three independent experiments. Student's t test analyzed statistical difference. *$p < 0.05$, ***$p < 0.001$, ***$p < 0.001$. Breg regulatory B cell, CON control, Erk1/2 extracellular regulated protein kinases 1/2, GAPDH glyceraldehyde 3-phosphate dehydrogenase, IL interleukin, LPS lipopolysaccharide, ns not significant, PI3K PI3 kinase, PIM PMA/ionomycin/brefeldin A

The existence of B cells with a suppressive capacity was initially reported in the study of guinea pigs in the mid-1970s [33, 34]. In the past 40 years, lots of studies have been focused on regulatory B cells and their mechanisms of action. Mizoguchi et al. [35] defined the B cells that produce IL-10 as regulatory B cells. Through producing IL-10, IL-35, and TGF-β, Bregs suppress immunopathology by prohibiting the expansion of pathogenic T cells and maintaining the pool of Tregs [9]. In our study, we also showed that the impaired immunosuppression of $Gnaq^{-/-}$ Bregs might be due to the decreased production of IL-10 and TGF-β. Bregs have been considered an important immune regulatory cell in many diseases, such as EAE, type 1 diabetes,

collagen-induced arthritis, inflammatory bowel diseases, lupus, and so on [36]. Similarly, $CD19^+CD24^{hi}CD38^{hi}$ B cells, which were considered Bregs in human, can limit the differentiation of naïve $CD4^+$ T cells into Th1 and Th17 populations, and maintain Treg function [7]. RA patients with active disease have reduced numbers of $CD19^+CD24^{hi}CD38^{hi}$ B cells in PBMCs compared with healthy individuals [7]. Our data also found a remarkable decrease in the frequency of $CD19^+CD24^{hi}CD38^{hi}$ Bregs in RA patients. Although the number of $CD19^+CD24^{hi}CD38^{hi}$ B cells was increased in SLE patients, they lacked the suppressive capacity due to their failure to produce IL-10 [12]. Previous studies showed that IL-10 production of human B cells was associated

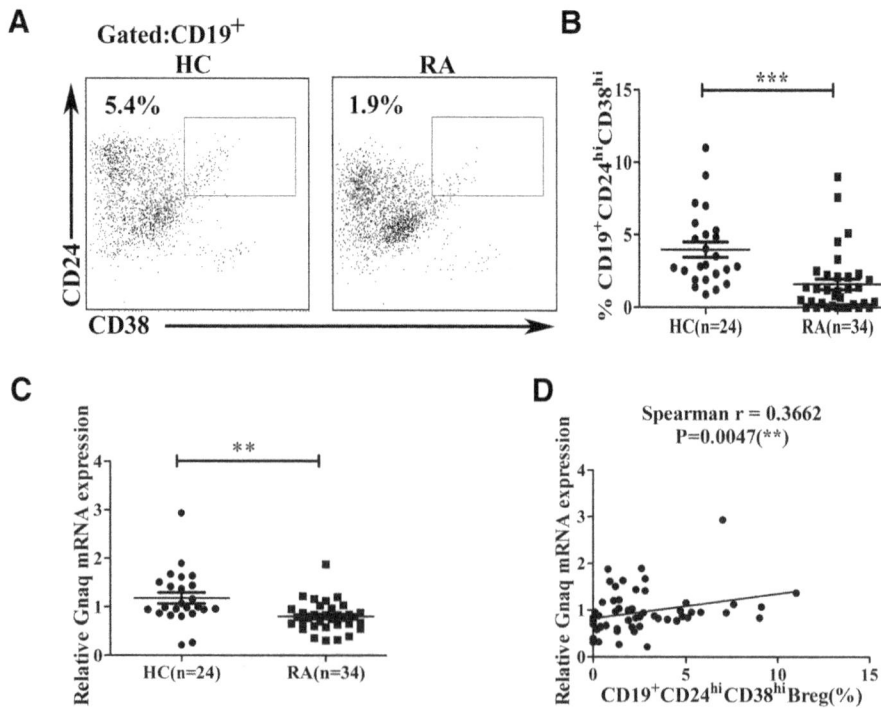

Fig. 6 Correlation of frequencies of $CD19^+CD24^{hi}CD38^{hi}$ B cells with Gαq mRNA expression in PBMCs from RA patients. PBMCs isolated from patients with RA and healthy individuals stained with CD19, CD24, and CD38. Representative flow cytometry plots showed $CD19^+CD24^{hi}CD38^{hi}$ B-cell subpopulations in PBMCs from healthy individuals ($n = 24$) and RA patients ($n = 34$) (**a**, representative images; **b**, statistical analysis). **c** Expression level of Gαq assessed by qPCR and normalized to β-actin in PBMCs from HC and RA patients. Mann–Whitney test compared data between two groups. **d** Correlation coefficient between Gαq expression and $CD19^+CD24^{hi}CD38^{hi}$ B-cell frequencies analyzed using the Spearman test ($n = 58$). **$p < 0.01$, ***$p < 0.001$. Breg regulatory B cell, HC healthy controls, RA rheumatoid arthritis

with the activation of STAT3 and ERK [37]. Our current findings showed that IL-10 production was also impaired in Bregs in the absence of Gαq.

Activation of the ERK pathway is a common requirement for IL-10 expression by T cells, macrophages, and myeloid dendritic cells [32]. Abrogation of either ERK or p38 activation after TLR stimulation leads to a reduced IL-10 expression, which suggests that these two pathways might cooperate in TLR-induced IL-10 production [32]. Consistently, inhibition of PI3K, Erk1/2, or p38 MAPK significantly ablates the Breg differentiation in our study here. As expected, we found that the basal levels of phospho-PI3K, phospho-Erk1/2, and phospho-p38 MAPK in response to LPS were lower in $Gnaq^{-/-}$ B cells than in WT B cells. These data suggest that Gαq was involved in the differentiation of Bregs partly through regulation of PI3K, Erk1/2, or p38 MAPK signaling. That IL-10 can be induced by LPS in many cells has been demonstrated. However, we here observed no marked differences of TLR4 and MyD88 expression between B cells from WT and $Gnaq^{-/-}$ mice, which further confirms the regulation of Gαq in the PI3K, Erk1/2, and p38 MAPK signaling pathways of Breg function.

In a previous study we demonstrated that $Gnaq^{-/-}$ chimeras could spontaneously develop manifestations of systemic autoimmune disease with high titer antinuclear antibody and inflammatory arthritis, and B cells from $Gnaq^{-/-}$ mice have an intrinsic survival advantage over normal B cells, suggesting that Gαq is critically important for maintaining control of peripheral B-cell tolerance induction and repressing autoimmunity [24]. However, the role of Gαq in Breg regulation remains unknown. Actually, the percentage of Bregs was significantly lower in the spleen of $Gnaq^{-/-}$ mice. Consistent with the animal experiments, our data here showed a significant positive correlation between the frequency of CD19$^+$CD24^{hi}CD38^{hi} Bregs and the expression of Gαq mRNA in PBMCs from patients with RA and HC. Our current findings showed that Gαq deficiency limited the differentiation of Bregs. Several studies demonstrated that Bregs were important for the generation and maintenance of Tregs [4]. Bregs could induce the differentiation of type 1 regulatory T (Tr1) cells [38, 39]. Moreover, Bregs might promote the differentiation of other type of regulatory T-cell subsets [40]. Consistent with prior studies, purified WT Bregs could convert CD4$^+$CD25$^-$ T cells into Tregs, but this function of $Gnaq^{-/-}$ Bregs was impaired. Indeed, we also observed an impaired inhibition of T-cell expansion in $Gnaq^{-/-}$ Bregs. This might be the reason for impaired suppressive function of $Gnaq^{-/-}$ Bregs on T-cell proliferation. Some studies suggested that CD40 mAb-stimulated CD1d^{hi}CD5$^+$ B cells could not regulate T-cell proliferation in vitro [41]. TLRs and CD40 activation are well-characterized signals in Breg

differentiation [4, 9]. However, LPS but not CD40 activator can induce IL-10 secretion [36], which might be the reason for no effect on T-cell proliferation inhibition being observed.

Conclusions

Although we do not yet know whether Gαq deficiency in Bregs alone is sufficient to induce autoimmune disease, our work showed a critical intrinsic role for Gαq in the maintenance of Breg differentiation and function. Furthermore, our data suggested that the regulation of Gαq on Breg differentiation might occur partly via the PI3K, Erk1/2, and p38 MAPK signaling pathways. Our study here provides new insights into the mechanisms of Breg immune tolerance.

Abbreviations
Breg: Regulatory B cell; EAE: Experimental autoimmune encephalitis; Erk1/2: Extracellular regulated protein kinases 1/2; G protein: Guanine nucleotide-binding protein; GPCR: G protein-coupled receptor; HC: Healthy controls; IL: Interleukin; LPS: Lipopolysaccharide; MyD88: Myeloid differentiation primary response 88; p38 MAPK: p38 mitogen-activated protein kinase; PBMC: Peripheral blood mononuclear cell; PI3K: PI3 kinase; qPCR: Quantitative real-time PCR; RA: Rheumatoid arthritis; SD: Standard deviation; SLE: Systemic lupus erythematosus; TGF-β: Transforming growth factor beta; Th1: T helper 1; Th17: T helper 17; TLR: Toll-like receptor; Treg: Regulatory T cell; WT: Wild type

Acknowledgements
The authors thank Dr Junhui Zhang and Xue Zhao for the genotyping of $Gnaq^{-/-}$ mice.

Funding
This work was partly supported by the National Natural Science Foundation of China (NFSC, No. 81701556, U1605223, 81671544, and 8151407), the National Key Basic Research Program of China (973 Program, No. 2014CB541903), and the Xiamen Science and Technology Bureau (Project No. 3502Z20174066, 3502Z20164006).

Authors' contributions
YH, XY, LD, and GS conceived and designed this study, were responsible for integrity of the work, interpretation of data, and drafting the manuscript, and gave final approval to the version of the paper to be published. YLi, CZ, and HQ participated in clinical material collection, cell culture, and ELISA test. YH and LD performed flow cytometric experiments and analysis. XY and YLiu performed qPCR and western blot analysis. JX helped with statistical analysis of the data. All authors reviewed and approved the submission.

Ethics approval
Animal studies were approved by the institutional animal care committee of Xiamen University (Xiamen, Fujian, China). Patient consent was obtained. This study was approved by the Ethics Committee of the First Affiliated Hospital of Xiamen University in accordance with the World Medical Association Declaration of Helsinki.

Consent for publication
Not applicable.

Competing interests
The authors declare that they have no competing interests.

Author details

[1]Department of Rheumatology and Clinical Immunology, The First Affiliated Hospital of Xiamen University, Xiamen, China. [2]Ningbo City Medical Treatment Center Lihuili Hospital, No. 57 Xingning Road, Ningbo 315000, China.

References

1. Lund FE, Randall TD. Effector and regulatory B cells: modulators of CD4+ T cell immunity. Nat Rev Immunol. 2010;10(4):236–47.
2. Wolf SD, Dittel BN, Hardardottir F, Janeway CA Jr. Experimental autoimmune encephalomyelitis induction in genetically B cell-deficient mice. J Exp Med. 1996;184(6):2271–8.
3. Fillatreau S, Sweenie CH, McGeachy MJ, Gray D, Anderton SM. B cells regulate autoimmunity by provision of IL-10. Nat Immunol. 2002;3(10):944–50.
4. Mauri C, Bosma A. Immune regulatory function of B cells. Annu Rev Immunol. 2012;30:221–41.
5. Berthelot JM, Jamin C, Amrouche K, Le Goff B, Maugars Y, Youinou P. Regulatory B cells play a key role in immune system balance. Joint Bone Spine. 2013;80(1):18–22.
6. Carter NA, Vasconcellos R, Rosser EC, Tulone C, Munoz-Suano A, Kamanaka M, Ehrenstein MR, Flavell RA, Mauri C. Mice lacking endogenous IL-10-producing regulatory B cells develop exacerbated disease and present with an increased frequency of Th1/Th17 but a decrease in regulatory T cells. J Immunol. 2011;186(10):5569–79.
7. Flores-Borja F, Bosma A, Ng D, Reddy V, Ehrenstein MR, Isenberg DA, Mauri C. CD19+CD24hiCD38hi B cells maintain regulatory T cells while limiting TH1 and TH17 differentiation. Sci Transl Med. 2013;5(173):173ra123.
8. Bosma A, Abdel-Gadir A, Isenberg DA, Jury EC, Mauri C. Lipid-antigen presentation by CD1d(+) B cells is essential for the maintenance of invariant natural killer T cells. Immunity. 2012;36(3):477–90.
9. Rosser EC, Mauri C. Regulatory B cells: origin, phenotype, and function. Immunity. 2015;42(4):607–12.
10. Candando KM, Lykken JM, Tedder TF. B10 cell regulation of health and disease. Immunol Rev. 2014;259(1):259–72.
11. Ramgolam VS, Sha Y, Marcus KL, Choudhary N, Troiani L, Chopra M, Markovic-Plese S. B cells as a therapeutic target for IFN-beta in relapsing-remitting multiple sclerosis. J Immunol. 2011;186(7):4518–26.
12. Blair PA, Norena LY, Flores-Borja F, Rawlings DJ, Isenberg DA, Ehrenstein MR, Mauri C. CD19(+)CD24(hi)CD38(hi) B cells exhibit regulatory capacity in healthy individuals but are functionally impaired in systemic lupus erythematosus patients. Immunity. 2010;32(1):129–40.
13. Kalampokis I, Venturi GM, Poe JC, Dvergsten JA, Sleasman JW, Tedder TF. The regulatory B cell compartment expands transiently during childhood and is contracted in children with autoimmunity. Arthritis Rheumatol. 2017;69(1):225–38.
14. Neves SR, Ram PT, Iyengar R. G protein pathways. Science. 2002;296(5573):1636–9.
15. Hubbard KB, Hepler JR. Cell signalling diversity of the Gqalpha family of heterotrimeric G proteins. Cell Signal. 2006;18(2):135–50.
16. Wettschureck N, Offermanns S. Mammalian G proteins and their cell type specific functions. Physiol Rev. 2005;85(4):1159–204.
17. Offermanns S, Toombs CF, Hu YH, Simon MI. Defective platelet activation in G alpha(q)-deficient mice. Nature. 1997;389(6647):183–6.
18. Offermanns S, Hashimoto K, Watanabe M, Sun W, Kurihara H, Thompson RF, Inoue Y, Kano M, Simon MI. Impaired motor coordination and persistent multiple climbing fiber innervation of cerebellar Purkinje cells in mice lacking Galphaq. Proc Natl Acad Sci U S A. 1997;94(25):14089–94.
19. Wettschureck N, Moers A, Wallenwein B, Parlow AF, Maser-Gluth C, Offermanns S. Loss of Gq/11 family G proteins in the nervous system causes pituitary somatotroph hypoplasia and dwarfism in mice. Mol Cell Biol. 2005;25(5):1942–8.
20. Borchers MT, Biechele T, Justice JP, Ansay T, Cormier S, Mancino V, Wilkie TM, Simon MI, Lee NA, Lee JJ. Methacholine-induced airway hyperresponsiveness is dependent on Galphaq signaling. Am J Physiol Lung Cell Mol Physiol. 2003;285(1):L114–20.
21. Borchers MT, Justice PJ, Ansay T, Mancino V, McGarry MP, Crosby J, Simon MI, Lee NA, Lee JJ. Gq signaling is required for allergen-induced pulmonary eosinophilia. J Immunol. 2002;168(7):3543–9.
22. Shi G, Partida-Sanchez S, Misra RS, Tighe M, Borchers MT, Lee JJ, Simon MI, Lund FE. Identification of an alternative G{alpha}q-dependent chemokine receptor signal transduction pathway in dendritic cells and granulocytes. J Exp Med. 2007;204(11):2705–18.
23. Ngai J, Methi T, Andressen KW, Levy FO, Torgersen KM, Vang T, Wettschureck N, Tasken K. The heterotrimeric G-protein alpha-subunit Galphaq regulates TCR-mediated immune responses through an Lck-dependent pathway. Eur J Immunol. 2008;38(11):3208–18.
24. Misra RS, Shi G, Moreno-Garcia ME, Thankappan A, Tighe M, Mousseau B, Kusser K, Becker-Herman S, Hudkins KL, Dunn R, et al. G alpha q-containing G proteins regulate B cell selection and survival and are required to prevent B cell-dependent autoimmunity. J Exp Med. 2010;207(8):1775–89.
25. He Y, Huang Y, Tu L, Luo J, Yu B, Qian H, Duan L, Shi G. Decreased Galphaq expression in T cells correlates with enhanced cytokine production and disease activity in systemic lupus erythematosus. Oncotarget. 2016;7(52):85741–9.
26. Arnett FC, Edworthy SM, Bloch DA, McShane DJ, Fries JF, Cooper NS, Healey LA, Kaplan SR, Liang MH, Luthra HS, et al. The American Rheumatism Association 1987 revised criteria for the classification of rheumatoid arthritis. Arthritis Rheum. 1988;31(3):315–24.
27. Aletaha D, Neogi T, Silman AJ, Funovits J, Felson DT, Bingham CO 3rd, Birnbaum NS, Burmester GR, Bykerk VP, Cohen MD, et al. 2010 rheumatoid arthritis classification criteria: an American College of Rheumatology/European League Against Rheumatism collaborative initiative. Arthritis Rheum. 2010;62(9):2569–81.
28. Yanaba K, Bouaziz JD, Matsushita T, Tsubata T, Tedder TF. The development and function of regulatory B cells expressing IL-10 (B10 cells) requires antigen receptor diversity and TLR signals. J Immunol. 2009;182(12):7459–72.
29. Lampropoulou V, Hoehlig K, Roch T, Neves P, Calderon Gomez E, Sweenie CH, Hao Y, Freitas AA, Steinhoff U, Anderton SM, et al. TLR-activated B cells suppress T cell-mediated autoimmunity. J Immunol. 2008;180(7):4763–73.
30. Neves P, Lampropoulou V, Calderon-Gomez E, Roch T, Stervbo U, Shen P, Kuhl AA, Loddenkemper C, Haury M, Nedospasov SA, et al. Signaling via the MyD88 adaptor protein in B cells suppresses protective immunity during Salmonella typhimurium infection. Immunity. 2010;33(5):777–90.
31. Lattin J, Zidar DA, Schroder K, Kellie S, Hume DA, Sweet MJ. G-protein-coupled receptor expression, function, and signaling in macrophages. J Leukoc Biol. 2007;82(1):16–32.
32. Saraiva M, O'Garra A. The regulation of IL-10 production by immune cells. Nat Rev Immunol. 2010;10(3):170–81.
33. Katz SI, Parker D, Turk JL. B-cell suppression of delayed hypersensitivity reactions. Nature. 1974;251(5475):550–1.
34. Neta R, Salvin SB. Specific suppression of delayed hypersensitivity: the possible presence of a suppressor B cell in the regulation of delayed hypersensitivity. J Immunol. 1974;113(6):1716–25.
35. Mizoguchi A, Mizoguchi E, Takedatsu H, Blumberg RS, Bhan AK. Chronic intestinal inflammatory condition generates IL-10-producing regulatory B cell subset characterized by CD1d upregulation. Immunity. 2002;16(2):219–30.
36. Tedder TF. B10 cells: a functionally defined regulatory B cell subset. J Immunol. 2015;194(4):1395–401.
37. Liu BS, Cao Y, Huizinga TW, Hafler DA, Toes RE. TLR-mediated STAT3 and ERK activation controls IL-10 secretion by human B cells. Eur J Immunol. 2014;44(7):2121–9.
38. Sayi A, Kohler E, Toller IM, Flavell RA, Muller W, Roers A, Muller A. TLR-2-activated B cells suppress helicobacter-induced preneoplastic gastric immunopathology by inducing T regulatory-1 cells. J Immunol. 2011;186(2):878–90.
39. Ahangarani RR, Janssens W, VanderElst L, Carlier V, VandenDriessche T, Chuah M, Weynand B, Vanoirbeek JA, Jacquemin M, Saint-Remy JM. In vivo induction of type 1-like regulatory T cells using genetically modified B cells confers long-term IL-10-dependent antigen-specific unresponsiveness. J Immunol. 2009;183(12):8232–43.
40. Wei B, Velazquez P, Turovskaya O, Spricher K, Aranda R, Kronenberg M, Birnbaumer L, Braun J. Mesenteric B cells centrally inhibit CD4+ T cell colitis through interaction with regulatory T cell subsets. Proc Natl Acad Sci U S A. 2005;102(6):2010–5.
41. Matsushita T, Horikawa M, Iwata Y, Tedder TF. Regulatory B cells (B10 cells) and regulatory T cells have independent roles in controlling experimental autoimmune encephalomyelitis initiation and late-phase immunopathogenesis. J Immunol. 2010;185(4):2240–52.

16

Impact of oral osteoarthritis therapy usage among other risk factors on knee replacement: a nested case-control study using the Osteoarthritis Initiative cohort

Marc Dorais[1], Johanne Martel-Pelletier[2], Jean-Pierre Raynauld[2], Philippe Delorme[2] and Jean-Pierre Pelletier[2*]

Abstract

Background: The aim of this study was to measure the association between exposure to commonly used oral osteoarthritis (OA) therapies and relevant confounding risk factors on the occurrence of knee replacement (KR), using the Osteoarthritis Initiative (OAI) database.

Methods: In this nested case-control design study, participants who had a KR after cohort entry were defined as "cases" and were matched with up to four controls for age, gender, income, Western Ontario and McMaster Universities Osteoarthritis Index (WOMAC) pain, Kellgren-Lawrence grade, and duration of follow up. Exposure to oral OA therapies (acetaminophen, non-steroidal anti-inflammatory drugs (NSAIDs), cyclooxygenase-2 (COX-2) inhibitors, narcotics, and glucosamine/chondroitin sulfate) was determined within the 3 years prior to the date of the KR. Conditional regression analyses were performed to estimate the association between KR and exposure to oral OA therapies and other potential confounding risk factors.

Results: A total of 218 participants who underwent a KR (cases) were matched to 540 controls. The median time to KR was 4.3 years among cases. The majority in both groups were Caucasian with mean age of 69 years and 61% were female. Numerically, cases were more exposed to acetaminophen, NSAIDs, and COX-2 inhibitors. Exposure to narcotics and glucosamine/chondroitin sulfate was relatively similar between cases and controls. No significant association was found between the occurrence of KR and exposure to any of the oral OA therapies within the 3 years prior to KR. A significantly higher occurrence of KR was found in Caucasian subjects (OR 1.84; 95% CI, 1.13–2.99; $p = 0.015$) and subjects with body mass index (BMI) ≥ 27 kg/m^2 (OR 1.65; 95% CI, 1.06–2.58; $p = 0.027$).

Conclusion: This study provides evidence that the main risk factors leading to KR are disease severity, symptoms and high BMI. Importantly, exposure to oral OA therapies was not associated with the occurrence of KR.

Keywords: Nested case-control, Osteoarthritis, Osteoarthritis Initiative, Knee replacement, Acetaminophen, NSAIDs, Coxibs, Narcotics, Glucosamine/chondroitin sulfate

* Correspondence: dr@jppelletier.ca
[2]Osteoarthritis Research Unit, University of Montreal Hospital Research Centre (CRCHUM), Montreal, Quebec, Canada
Full list of author information is available at the end of the article

Background

Osteoarthritis (OA) is one of the arthritis conditions most often associated with chronic pain and disability [1]. As such, patients with OA are in need of treatment that includes a number of different pharmacological classes of agents. They are most commonly oral agents and are very often prescribed for chronic administration over an extended period of time. In recent years there has been concern about the safety of some of drug treatments, mainly related to potential detrimental systemic effects such as cardiovascular risks and morbidity associated, for instance, with non-steroidal anti-inflammatory drugs (NSAIDs) and coxibs [2]. Moreover, the use of narcotics by patients with OA has also been associated with an increased risk of morbidity and even mortality [3]. Concerns have also been raised about the effects of these drug treatments on the evolution of OA structural changes, particularly in weight-bearing joints such as the hip and knee [4–11]. The impact of such oral treatments, especially NSAIDs, on OA disease progression and outcome, whether negative or positive, remains at this time an open question that needs to be further explored.

Studying the effects of different therapeutic classes of drugs used for the treatment of OA and their potential impact on disease progression is not an easy task. However, the use of observational cohorts provides a real-life scenario [8, 10, 11]. The Osteoarthritis Initiative (OAI) cohort presents several advantages for such purpose owing to its size, duration, and very large amount of comprehensive demographic and clinical information available on the study participants, including drug treatment. Structural changes are also assessed by imaging using knee x-rays and magnetic resonance imaging (MRI). The latter has proven to be extremely reliable, sensitive, and very useful for studying disease outcomes [10–15]. Joint replacement is considered a clinically relevant disease outcome in knee OA, which is related to both disease symptoms and structural damage [14–18]. Using the OAI cohort, the objective of this nested case-control study was to explore the potential effects of the most commonly used drug treatments for knee OA, while controlling for the most relevant confounding risk factors on the occurrence of knee replacement (KR). One of the main reasons for choosing a nested case-control design was that, in addition to the robustness of this approach, the exposure to oral OA therapies could be measured in different time windows before the KR.

Methods

Study population

Participants were selected from the OAI database, which is publicly available at https://oai.epi-ucsf.org/datarelease/. The OAI established and maintains a natural history database for knee OA that includes clinical evaluation data and radiological and magnetic resonance (MR) images of 4796 (including the controls) men and women aged 45–79 years at the time of enrolment (cohort entry) between February 2004 and May 2006. The participants selected for the study were from both the progression and the incidence subcohorts. In brief, the participants in the progression subcohort ($n = 1389$) were subjects with symptomatic tibiofemoral knee OA at baseline who had both of the following in at least one knee at baseline: frequent knee symptoms in the past 12 months defined as "pain, aching or stiffness in or around the knee on most days" for at least 1 month during the past 12 months, and radiographic tibiofemoral knee OA, defined as definite tibiofemoral osteophytes (Osteoarthritis Research Society International (OARSI) atlas grades 1–3), equivalent to Kellgren-Lawrence (KL) grade ≥ 2 on the fixed-flexion radiograph. The participants in the incidence subcohort ($n = 3285$) did not have symptomatic knee OA, as defined above, in either knee at baseline. However, they had characteristics that placed them at increased risk of developing symptomatic knee OA during the study. The specific eligibility risk factor criteria for the incidence subcohort were: knee symptoms in a native knee in the past 12 months; being overweight defined using gender and age-specific cut-off points for weight; knee injury defined as a history of knee injury causing difficulty walking for at least a week; knee surgery including meniscal and ligamentous repairs and unilateral total KR for OA; family history defined as a knee replacement for OA in a biological parent or sibling; Heberden's nodes; repetitive knee bending at work or outside work; and age 70 to 79 years.

In this nested case-control study, participants are defined as subjects presenting a first occurrence of a KR procedure between February 2004 and October 2015. The date on which the KR was reported is defined as the index date. For each case, up to four control subjects [19] without a history of KR before the index date were matched for age (± 1 year), gender, and index date information on income level ($\pm 40,000$ USD), Western Ontario and McMaster Universities Osteoarthritis Index (WOMAC) pain ($\pm 10\%$), KL grade (same grade), and duration of follow up. Subjects who had missing information on KR or matching variables were excluded.

Definition of exposure to oral OA therapies

The oral OA therapies included acetaminophen, NSAIDs, cyclooxygenase-2 (COX-2) inhibitors, narcotics, and glucosamine/chondroitin sulfate. The information concerning the use of these therapies was obtained from the medical history in the OAI database (typical question: "During the past 6 months (or 30 days), did you use *(specific therapy)* for joint pain or arthritis on most days?") For the primary objective, exposure to each of these classes of oral OA therapies was measured within the 3 years preceding the index date. Exposure was defined as the percentage (%) of all available follow ups at which the subjects reported currently using, at the time of the query, oral OA therapies. Hence, categories of exposure were defined as "no exposure", "exposure of 1–79%", and "exposure of 80% or more". For the secondary objectives, different time periods were employed to measure the exposure to oral OA therapies: 2 years, 4 years, and 5 years before the index date. Subjects who had missing information on exposure to oral OA therapies were excluded.

Covariates

The covariates were race, education level, body mass index (BMI), WOMAC scores (stiffness, function, total), knee injury and osteoarthritis outcome scores (KOOS) (pain, symptoms, and quality of life (QoL)), joint space width (JSW), cartilage volume, bone marrow lesions (BML) size, and presence of meniscal extrusion. The WOMAC [20] and KOOS [21] questionnaires are self-administered: higher WOMAC scores and lower KOOS scores indicate more pain/symptoms and greater functional impairment. Covariates were measured at the index date or at the last available visit before the index date.

Clinical and demographics data

The clinical data were extracted from the OAI database. These included variables used for the matching (age, gender, income level, WOMAC pain, KL), covariates, and arthritis drug treatment taken by the patients, which included acetaminophen, NSAIDs, COX-2 inhibitors, narcotics, and glucosamine/chondroitin sulfate.

Imaging characteristics

The KL grade and the JSW data were obtained from the OAI database (central reading). The MR images were acquired from 3.0 T apparatus (Magnetom Trio, Siemens) at the four OAI clinical centers using a double-echo steady-state imaging protocol. Fully automated and validated quantitative MRI technology was used to assess the cartilage volume [12, 22] and the BMLs [23], and a validated scoring method for the meniscal extrusion [24].

Cartilage volume was analyzed in the knee (femur and plateau) and in the medial and lateral compartments. The change over time was assessed as previously described [12]. Quantitative BML assessment was expressed as a percentage (%) of the lesion in the bone volume in each region of interest [23]. Meniscal extrusion was scored as absence or presence of partial or complete extrusion detected in any of the three segments of the meniscus [24, 25].

Statistical analyses

Descriptive analyses of sociodemographic and clinical characteristics were conducted for case and control patients.

These included matching variables (gender and, at index date, age, income level, WOMAC pain, and KL grade), the aforementioned covariates, and exposure to the different classes of oral OA therapies in the 3 years prior to KR. Proportions were calculated for categorical variables, and median and interquartile range (IQR) for continuous variables.

The association between the occurrence of KR and sociodemographic/clinical characteristics (not those used in the matching between cases and controls) was measured using crude conditional logistic regression. An adjusted regression model including significant covariates and pertinent clinical variables was employed to determine the association between exposure to oral OA therapies and occurrence of KR. Odds ratios (OR) and 95% confidence interval (CI) were calculated. Only data with sufficient patient number ($n > 10$) per time exposure were analyzed and presented. A two-tailed p value <0.05 was considered significant. All statistical analyses were performed using SAS software, V.9.3 (SAS Institute, Cary, NC, USA).

Results

Of the 4674 participants from the incidence and progression subcohorts enrolled in the OAI, 393 had a KR during the follow up. After exclusions for follow up less than 1 year, missing information for matching variables, or no possible match with at least one control, a total of 218 cases were matched to 540 controls for age, gender, income level, WOMAC pain, KL grade, and duration of follow up (Fig. 1).

Characteristics at index date

For the cases (Table 1) the mean age was 68.9 years, 60.6% were female, and the median (IQR) time from cohort entry to having a KR was 4.3 years (1.0–8.9). The majority of cases and controls were white/Caucasian, had an income level greater than $50,000, and had either some college education or a graduate degree. The proportion of cases with a BMI of 27 kg/m² or higher was 75% compared to 71% in controls (Table 2). Compared to controls, cases had higher WOMAC scores (except stiffness), smaller joint space width (JSW), and globally had more BMLs in the knee. Cases and controls had similar characteristics in terms of cartilage volume and meniscal extrusion.

Exposure to narcotics and glucosamine/chondroitin sulfate treatment in the 3 years prior to index date was similar between cases and controls (Table 3). Cases were, however, numerically more exposed to acetaminophen, NSAIDs, and COX-2 inhibitors. Due to absence of specific NSAID description in the OAI database, it was not possible to analyze the effects of the different NSAIDs separately.

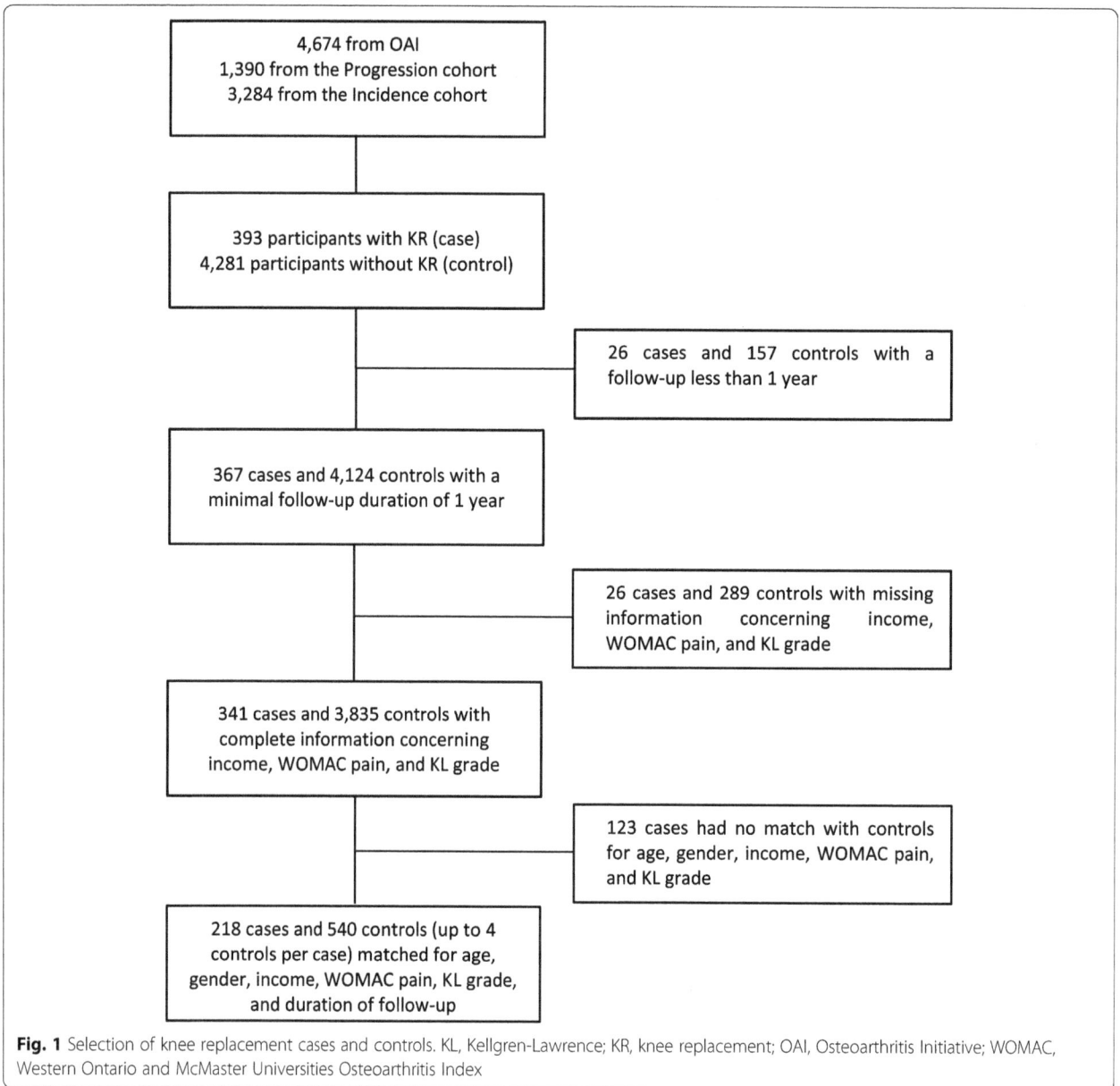

Fig. 1 Selection of knee replacement cases and controls. KL, Kellgren-Lawrence; KR, knee replacement; OAI, Osteoarthritis Initiative; WOMAC, Western Ontario and McMaster Universities Osteoarthritis Index

Occurrence of KR

The risk of KR occurrence (Table 4) was significantly greater in participants who were white/Caucasian, had a BMI of 27 kg/m^2 or higher, and had higher WOMAC scores (function, stiffness, total). The KOOS score (pain, symptoms, QoL) was significantly associated with KR occurrence.

Table 5 presents the adjusted OR of KR occurrence for both primary and secondary analyses according to each class of the oral OA therapies. In the primary analysis (exposure measured in the 3 years prior to index date), none of the oral OA therapeutic classes was significantly associated with the occurrence of KR. Secondary analyses (Table 5) were performed to evaluate the impact of varying time windows of exposure on the occurrence of KR in the

adjusted regression analyses. KR occurrence was not associated with exposure to any of the oral OA therapies.

Discussion

This study demonstrated, using the OAI database and a nested case-control study design, that exposure to some of the most commonly used oral OA therapies, i.e. acetaminophen, NSAIDs, COX-2 inhibitors, narcotics, or glucosamine/chondroitin sulfate, in a range of 2– 5 years, was not associated with the occurrence of KR when compared to no exposure to such medications. However, a number of risk factors were identified as being linked to KR, including race, level of symptoms, and BMI.

Table 1 Sociodemographics at index date

	Knee replacement	
	Case (n = 218)	Control (n = 540)
Time to KR after cohort entry, % (n)		
Between year 1 and year 2	10.6% (23)	–
Between year 2 and year 3	15.1% (33)	–
Between year 3 and year 4	18.8% (41)	–
Between year 4 and year 5	17.9% (39)	–
Between year 5 and year 6	12.8% (28)	–
Between year 6 and year 7	7.8% (17)	–
Between year 7 and year 8	8.3% (18)	–
Between year 8 and year 9	8.7% (19)	–
Median (IQR) (years)	4.3 (1.0–8.9)	
OAI subcohort, % (n)		
Progression	61.9% (135)	58.5% (316)
Incidence	38.1% (83)	41.5% (224)
Age (years), median (IQR)	68.9 (61.8–74.3)	68.6 (61.6–73.8)
Female, % (n)	60.6% (132)	61.1% (330)
Race, % (n)	(n = 217)	
White or Caucasian	83.9% (182)	78.0% (421)
Black or African American	12.5% (27)	19.4% (105)
Asian	1.8% (4)	0.4% (2)
Other non-white	1.8% (4)	2.2% (12)
Income level USD, % (n)		
Less than $25,000	10.6% (23)	12.4% (67)
$25,000 to < $50,000	28.0% (61)	30.6% (165)
$50,000 to < $100,000	38.0% (83)	38.9% (210)
$100,000 or greater	23.4% (51)	18.1% (98)
Education level, % (n)		
Less than high school graduate	0.9% (2)	4.1% (22)
High school graduate	19.3% (42)	10.9% (59)
Some college	26.6% (58)	30.7% (166)
College graduate	18.3% (40)	18.2% (98)
Some graduate school	6.9% (15)	7.2% (39)
Graduate degree	28.0% (61)	28.9% (156)

Data shown are proportion of patients (%), number of patients (n), age in years, or median (interquartile range (IQR))

KR knee replacement, *OAI* Osteoarthritis Initiative

Our study also revealed that the oral medications studied had a "neutral" effect on KR while controlling for the most important confounding factors known to promote such occurrences: demographics, socioeconomic status, symptom severity, radiographic grading, and structural changes assessed by quantitative MRI. These results are in contrast to those of Hafezi-Nejad et al. [11], also using the same OAI cohort, showing that long-term use of analgesics comprising NSAIDs, acetaminophen, and narcotics alone or in combination may be associated with radiographic progression of knee OA and increased risk of KR. Similar results on the potential deleterious effects of NSAIDs on the evolution of OA structural changes and disease outcome have already been suggested. Early studies based on the radiographic evaluation of disease progression (joint space narrowing (JSN)) in patients with OA treated with NSAIDs reported a negative impact of long-term use of diclofenac or indomethacin in hip and knee OA [4–8]. Another report on the effects of regular use of prescription NSAID treatment in patients with knee OA identified a reduction in JSN compared to non-users over a 4-year follow-up period [10], although the difference between groups was not statistically significant. However, recent observational studies and randomized controlled trials in patients with knee OA using MRI technology to assess disease progression have shown that treatment with NSAIDs such as naproxen or celecoxib (a cyclooxygenase-2 (COX-2) selective inhibitor) has a neutral effect on cartilage loss [26, 27]. Studies from our group, also using MRI technology, and the participants from the incidence and progression subcohorts of the Osteoarthritis Initiative (OAI) database have also explored the effects of NSAIDs/analgesics and glucosamine/chondroitin sulfate on disease progression by assessing the change in cartilage volume [12, 13]. The findings of these studies showed that the extent of progression of cartilage volume loss was driven by disease severity and meniscal extrusion. NSAID/analgesic treatment had no significant effect on cartilage volume loss. In the latter study [13], glucosamine/chondroitin sulfate treatment reduced the cartilage volume loss in participants with meniscal extrusion regardless of whether or not they were receiving NSAID/analgesic treatment.

Interestingly, the findings of Hafezi-Nejad et al. [11] were also not confirmed in the study of Lapane et al. [10] using the same OAI cohort and exploring the effects of long-term use of NSAIDs on knee OA progression also using x-rays. The greater loss of JSW in the NSAID users compared to the non-users was not statistically significant on multivariate adjusted analysis. In another study using the OAI cohort, assessment of disease progression using x-rays and MRI did not demonstrate any effects of long-term use of NSAIDs/analgesics on knee OA disease progression [12, 13]. Finally, in another population-based study, Klop et al. [28] also showed that long-term users of non-selective NSAIDs and coxibs did not have a different risk of KR.

The sociodemographic and clinical data from our study population, being quite similar to those from previous studies exploring the role of disease treatment on KR [8, 10, 11, 28, 29], do not explain the discrepancy in the impact of such NSAIDs. Moreover, studies in preclinical animal models of OA have provided a number of

Table 2 Clinical characteristics at index date

	Knee replacement	
	Case (*n* = 218)	Control (*n* = 540)
	(*n* = 204)	(*n* = 537)
BMI ≥ 27 kg/m², % (*n*)	75.0% (153)	70.6% (379)
WOMAC, median (IQR)		
Pain (0–20)	6.0 (4.0–9.0)	5.0 (3.0–8.0)
Function (0–68)	22.2 (14.9–31.0)	18.0 (8.5–25.5)
Stiffness (0–10)	3.0 (2.0–4.0)	3.0 (2.0–4.0)
Total (0–98)	31.2 (21.8–43.0)	25.0 (13.0–37.0)
KOOS, median (IQR)		
Pain (0–100)	61.1 (47.2–72.2)	66.7 (55.6–79.3)
Symptoms (0–100)	64.3 (50.0–78.6)	75.0 (58.9–85.7)
QoL (0–100)	43.8 (31.3–56.3)	56.3 (43.8–68.8)
Kellgren-Lawrence grade, % (*n*)		
0	1.4% (3)	1.7% (9)
1	3.7% (8)	3.7% (20)
2	19.3% (42)	23.9% (129)
3	31.6% (69)	29.8% (161)
4	44.0% (96)	40.9% (221)
	(*n* = 211)	(*n* = 524)
JSW (mm), median (IQR)	2.0 (0.8–4.6)	2.8 (1.1–4.6)
Cartilage volume (mm³), median (IQR)	(*n* = 201)	(*n* = 510)
Global knee	11,037 (9127 - 13,634)	11,058 (9351 - 13,508)
Medial compartment	5127 (3971 - 6482)	5219 (4176 - 6502)
Lateral compartment	6028 (4864 - 7480)	6043 (4970 - 7265)
BML	(*n* = 201)	(*n* = 511)
Global		
Median (IQR)	2.0 (0.6–4.4)	1.7 (0.4–3.8)
BML ≥ 1%, % (*n*)	65.7% (132)	61.5% (314)
Medial compartment		
Median (IQR)	0.014 (0.0–0.058)	0.021 (0.0–0.057)
BML ≥ 1%, % (*n*)	34.9% (76)	42.2% (228)
Lateral compartment		
Median (IQR)	0.005 (0.0–0.025)	0.0 (0.0–0.018)
BML ≥ 1%, % (*n*)	23.9% (52)	20.7% (112)
	(*n* = 215)	(*n* = 532)
Meniscal extrusion, % (*n*)	39.5% (85)	38.5% (205)

Data shown are proportion of patients (%), number of patients (n), or median (interquartile range (IQR))

BMI body mass index, *BML* bone marrow lesions, *JSW* joint space width, *KOOS* Knee injury and Osteoarthritis Outcome Score, *QoL* quality of life, *WOMAC* Western Ontario and McMaster Universities Osteoarthritis Index

positive as well as negative findings with regard to the potential beneficial or deleterious effects of such drugs on OA structural changes [7, 9], which does not help to settle this debate.

A very important distinction of the present study compared to most others, is the use of a nested case-control design that we chose for a number of reasons. The well-recognized advantage of such a study design is that it allowed us to assess patients' characteristics as risk factors to be evaluated at the very date of KR surgery. This is in sharp contrast to a cohort study design, in which the patient profiles are assessed at entry (baseline) into

Table 3 Exposure to different oral OA therapies in the 3 years prior to index date

Oral OA therapies, % (n)	Knee replacement	
	Case (n = 161)[a]	Control (n = 360)[a]
Acetaminophen		
No exposure	70.2% (113)	75.0% (270)
Exposure 1–79%	26.7% (43)	22.5% (81)
Exposure ≥ 80%	3.1% (5)	2.5% (9)
NSAIDs		
No exposure	37.3% (60)	51.4% (185)
Exposure 1–79%	38.5% (62)	33.3% (120)
Exposure ≥ 80%	24.2% (39)	15.3% (55)
COX-2 inhibitors		
No exposure	86.3% (139)	91.1% (328)
Exposure 1–79%	7.5% (12)	4.7% (17)
Exposure ≥ 80%	6.2% (10)	4.2% (15)
Narcotics		
No exposure	88.8% (143)	89.7% (323)
Exposure 1–79%	10.0% (16)	7.5% (27)
Exposure ≥ 80%	1.2% (2)	2.8% (10)
Glucosamine/chondroitin sulfate		
No exposure	45.3% (73)	45.8% (165)
Exposure 1–79%	23.0% (37)	23.1% (83)
Exposure ≥ 80%	31.7% (51)	31.1% (112)

Data shown are proportion of patients (%) and number of patients (n)

COX-2 cyclooxygenase-2, *NSAIDs* non-steroidal anti-inflammatory drugs, *OA* osteoarthritis

[a]Of the total number of cases (218) and controls (540), 161 cases and 360 controls had complete information for the 3 years prior to index date

the cohort [10, 11, 30]. During the elapsed time between cohort entry and date of KR, which may be several years in most cases, the profiles of patients who undergo KR, such as symptoms, function, and medication usage, may change substantially. The nested case-control design thus allowed evaluation of patient characteristics that best represent the patient status at the time of the KR occurrence, not several years before. It is therefore important to recognize that such a study design will probably impact findings when assessing a relationship between drug exposure and risk of KR, in turn potentially explaining results different from those of recent longitudinal cohort study designs using the same OAI database [11], as mentioned previously.

Another important issue of our study is the use of KR as the sole marker of disease progression, which has already been established as a valid outcome in a number of studies [11, 15–18, 30, 31]. Indeed, there is a general consensus that MRI parameters assessed in knee OA, such as the medial compartment cartilage volume/thickness, can predict outcomes such as KR in a consistent manner [14–18]. However, findings of the present and

previous studies [17, 29, 32] also indicate that the ultimate decision of the patient to undergo KR is likely multifactorial in origin and involves a large number of confounding factors that extend well beyond the severity of knee OA structural changes. In our study, however, the cartilage volume at index (KR) time as assessed by MRI was similar in both groups, suggesting that over time the factors leading to progression of cartilage volume loss up to the KR were globally balanced in both groups. One must be cautious with the interpretation that drug treatment that can accelerate disease progression, if true, may have exerted its effects on both control and KR groups. Although the effect of drug treatment on rate of disease progression was not assessed in this study, several previous studies have addressed this very specific issue, a number of which used the OAI cohort [10–13]. Based on the findings of these studies, one may be tempted to conclude that factors in addition to disease progression are very likely to influence the patient's decision to undergo KR. The results of the present study showing that JSW at index time was not linked to the occurrence of KR certainly support this view.

In the present study we also explored the cumulative exposure to oral OA therapies measured in different time windows, from 2 to 5 years before the date of the KR, to evaluate their impact in different scenarios to yield robustness of our analyses. Interestingly, these analyses did not show any time frame trends, shorter or longer, that would significantly promote greater risk of KR. Windows of 6 to 8 years of exposure to oral OA therapies were also considered, but the number of available patients was too small for statistical inference.

The results of the study are reassuring and clinically relevant since they tackle the confounding role of any oral intervention to treat pain as a "last resort" prior to inevitable surgery, creating a spurious association between drug usage and the risk of KR, in turn suggesting a deleterious role of the medication via a channeling bias. Moreover, presence of severe comorbidities, frequently encountered with severe OA, are usually perceived by orthopedic surgeons as promoting perioperative risks and, as such, they are less inclined to recommend surgery for these patients. These same comorbidities may also preclude the use of NSAIDs and narcotics for these "morbid" patients, hence yielding spurious correlation between use of these medications and more KRs being performed.

Our study has a number of strengths. First, it was conducted using the large OAI database, representative of a North American population with fairly open access to usual care for knee OA, including KR, based on patient and physician preferences in a context of a real-world scenario. Second, to our knowledge, this is among the first studies that allowed stratification of risk of KR by

Table 4 Association between sociodemographic/clinical characteristics[a] at the index date and occurrence of knee replacement

	Crude OR	95% CI	p[b]
Race: white or Caucasian (reference other race)	1.84	(1.13–2.99)	**0.015**
Education level: college graduate or above (reference less than college graduate)	0.95	(0.65–1.38)	0.778
BMI ≥ 27 kg/m² (reference < 27 kg/m²)	1.65	(1.06–2.58)	**0.027**
WOMAC			
Function	1.04	(1.02–1.06)	**< 0.001**
Stiffness	1.25	(1.12–1.40)	**0.001**
Total	1.03	(1.02–1.04)	**< 0.001**
KOOS			
Pain	0.98	(0.97–0.99)	**< 0.001**
Symptoms	0.98	(0.97–0.99)	**< 0.001**
QoL	0.97	(0.96–0.98)	**< 0.001**
X-ray (JSW)	0.93	(0.85–1.01)	0.092
MRI			
BML			
By increase of 1%	1.04	(0.99–1.09)	0.144
BML ≥ 1% (reference < 1%)	1.41	(0.95–2.11)	0.091
Meniscal extrusion (reference no extrusion)	1.18	(0.80–1.73)	0.404

BMI body mass index, *BML* bone marrow lesion, *CI* confidence interval, *JSW* joint space width, *KOOS* Knee injury and Osteoarthritis Outcome Score, *OR* odds ratio, *QoL* quality of life, *WOMAC* Western Ontario and McMaster Universities Osteoarthritis Index
[a]Excluding characteristics used in the matching between cases and controls (i.e. age, gender, income, WOMAC pain, and KL grade)
[b]Crude conditional logistic regression. Bold indicates statistical significance ($p < 0.05$)

extent of exposure to oral OA medication versus no exposure, which is paramount when trying to establish a cause-effect of medication on an ultimate outcome such as KR. We chose a priori a 3-year window of oral OA medication exposure based on a clinical rationale and the design of previous studies [17, 30, 31]. Third, per the OAI design, we have great certainty about the knee OA diagnosis and its KR indication based on detailed information on demographics, symptoms, imaging, and drug use for both patients and their matched controls. Fourth, medical data were routinely recorded by investigators including rheumatologists and orthopedic surgeons without a study hypothesis, yielding a "nested" case-control study, hence minimizing the possibility of recall bias, which plagues conventional retrospective chart review studies. Last, the excellent matching yielded from our control selection strategy, as shown in the baseline characteristics comparison, is reassuring, as control selection is always an important issue for nested case-control designs as poor choices may yield very different conclusions.

Limitations of this study include the fact that it did not allow identification of any specific drug class. For instance, the impossibility of defining a specific NSAID name within the database is a limitation as some NSAIDs, such as for example indomethacin, may prove to be more deleterious than others [4–9]. The data provided on drug usage were obtained by self-administered questionnaire and not by a traditional pill count, which is used to assess adherence and persistence to medication in most clinical trials. This could underestimate true prolonged and cumulative usage of these medications. We have nonetheless tried to establish a "dose-effect" response using categories we have coined levels of "exposure": no exposure, occasional (exposure 1–79%), or regular (≥ 80%) medication usage, acknowledging such limitation.

The study design also did not allow comprehensive assessment of the influence of confounding factors, as some of the data used were only available at baseline and not at the index time of KR. Despite attempts to adjust for several confounders, causal interpretation of the findings is restricted, and residual confounding must be considered when interpreting the results.

Furthermore, this study focused on patients with severe OA in need of surgery; other beneficial or deleterious associations with chronic use of oral OA drugs and subclinical structural damage, as seen using quantitative MRI for example, may be found in subjects with less severe OA.

It was also impossible to assess the knee OA disease duration since onset of symptoms or date of OA diagnosis was not collected in the OAI dataset. Knee OA duration could have a significant impact on the cumulative and progressive joint damage, but we were unfortunately unable to control for it.

Statistical power may also be an issue since, by selecting subjects that had a KR but also had almost all demographic, clinical and MRI information, patient number was reduced from more than 4674 subjects to a mere 218 cases of KR, which is somewhat limited for performing multivariate analyses.

Finally, actual KR occurrences may be considered by some as an inadequate outcome for a comprehensive severe progressive OA definition. In fact, in the present work, we did not assess knee OA progression using imaging outcomes such as JSW or cartilage thickness/volume loss prior to the KR. The rate of such progression might accelerate while nearing the KR occurrence, which may or may not be associated with oral OA medication use. However, as already mentioned, the cartilage volume at index (KR) time as assessed by MRI was similar in both groups, suggesting that over time the factors leading to progression of cartilage volume loss up to the KR were globally balanced in both groups. Despite the great clinical success of KR, the criteria on which surgery is performed are not uniform. Apart from symptoms and radiographic

Table 5 Association between exposure to different oral osteoarthritis therapies and occurrence of knee replacement

	Acetaminophen				NSAIDs				COX-2 inhibitors				Narcotics				Glucosamine/chondroitin sulfate			
	n	OR[b]	95% CI	p[c]	n	OR[b]	95% CI	p[c]	n	OR[b]	95% CI	p[c]	n	OR[b]	95% CI	p[c]	n	OR[b]	95% CI	p[c]
Primary analysis																				
In the 3 years prior to index date (n = 521: 161 KR/360 controls)																				
Exposure 1–79%[a]	124	1.09	(0.66–1.78)	0.745	313	1.05	(0.64–1.72)	0.839	68	1.13	(0.48–2.67)	0.784	67	1.00	(0.48–2.09)	0.995	120	0.85	(0.50–1.48)	0.573
Exposure ≥ 80%[a]	14	1.11	(0.30–4.09)	0.872	44	1.66	(0.93–2.95)	0.086	21	1.15	(0.47–2.83)	0.761			ND		163	0.73	(0.43–1.23)	0.236
Secondary Analyses																				
In the 2 years prior to index date (n = 642: 193 KR/449 controls)																				
Exposure 1–79%[a]	210	1.10	(0.66–1.84)	0.722	369	0.96	(0.60–1.54)	0.853	88	1.40	(0.57–3.48)	0.465	77	1.19	(0.54–2.58)	0.670	255	0.70	(0.39–1.26)	0.235
Exposure ≥ 80%[a]	20	1.46	(0.69–3.11)	0.322	58	1.41	(0.88–2.26)	0.159	27	1.18	(0.55–2.52)	0.671			ND		166	1.00	(0.65–1.55)	0.989
In the 4 years prior to index date (n = 363: 121 KR/242 controls)																				
Exposure 1–79%[a]	113	1.34	(0.74–2.41)	0.333	234	1.40	(0.78–2.52)	0.256	50	1.63	(0.64–4.13)	0.303	50	1.43	(0.62–3.33)	0.405	156	0.65	(0.33–1.25)	0.191
Exposure ≥ 80%[a]			ND		26	1.65	(0.75–3.66)	0.215			ND				ND		83	0.63	(0.32–1.21)	0.165
In the 5 years prior to index date (n = 228: 82 KR/146 controls)																				
Exposure 1–79%[a]	60	1.38	(0.66–2.88)	0.397	110	1.88	(0.85–4.20)	0.121	18	1.35	(0.41–4.49)	0.623	33	1.19	(0.48–2.93)	0.706	54	0.90	(0.37–2.14)	0.803
Exposure ≥ 80%[a]	15	1.66	(0.44–6.35)	0.457	45	2.27	(0.90–5.71)	0.081			ND				ND		70	0.73	(0.33–1.64)	0.445

CI confidence interval, COX-2 cyclooxygenase-2, KR knee replacement, ND not determinable, n value too small, NSAIDs non-steroidal anti-inflammatory drugs, OA osteoarthritis, OR odds ratio

[a]Compared to the "no exposure" category

[b]Adjusted for race, body mass index, other medication for pain, joint space width, Western Ontario and McMaster Universities Osteoarthritis Index (WOMAC) stiffness, meniscal extrusion, bone marrow lesions, and Knee Injury and Osteoarthritis Outcome Score (KOOS)

[c]Conditional logistic regression

status, surgical indication depends on willingness, comorbidity, access to health care, socioeconomic status, etc. A validated KR "indication" as a clinical outcome, as suggested by the OARSI/Outcome Measures in Rheumatology (OMERACT) group [32] could help in that regard for future studies.

Conclusion

The present study indicates that patients chronically taking the most commonly used oral OA therapies do not have an increased risk of KR. In an era of OA therapeutic choice paucity, our study is somewhat reassuring and repositions chronic symptomatic OA treatment as safe. However, longer-term and controlled studies and safety assessments should also be performed in the context of longitudinal follow up to further probe our initial findings.

Abbreviations

BMI: Body mass index; BML: Bone marrow lesion; CI: Confidence interval; COX-2: Cyclooxygenase-2; IQR: Interquartile range; JSW: Joint space width; KL: Kellgren-Lawrence; KOOS: Knee injury and osteoarthritis outcome score; KR: Knee replacement; MRI: Magnetic resonance image; NSAIDs: Nonsteroidal anti-inflammatory drugs; OA: Osteoarthritis; OAI: Osteoarthritis Initiative; OARSI: Osteoarthritis Research Society International; OR: Odds ratio; QoL: Quality of life score; WOMAC: Western Ontario and McMaster Universities Osteoarthritis Index

Acknowledgements

The authors thank the OAI participants and Coordinating Center for their work in generating the clinical and radiological data from the OAI cohort and for making them publicly available. The OAI is a public-private partnership comprising five contracts (N01-AR-2-2258; N01-AR-2-2259; N01-AR-2-2260; N01-AR-2-2261; N01-AR-2-2262) funded by the National Institutes of Health, a branch of the Department of Health and Human Services, and conducted by the OAI Study Investigators. Private funding partners include Merck Research Laboratories; Novartis Pharmaceuticals Corporation, GlaxoSmithKline; and Pfizer, Inc. Private sector funding for the OAI is managed by the Foundation for the National Institutes of Health. This manuscript was prepared using an OAI public use data set and does not necessarily reflect the opinions or views of the OAI investigators, the NIH, or the private funding partners. We also thank Virginia Wallis for her assistance with the manuscript preparation.

Funding

The study conception was funded by grants from Bioibérica (Barcelona, Spain), the Osteoarthritis Research Unit and the Chair in Osteoarthritis of the University of Montreal (Montreal, Quebec, Canada).

Authors' contributions

J-PP and JMP have full access to all data in the study and take responsibility for the integrity of the data and the accuracy of the data analysis. MD, J-PR, and PD are responsible for statistical analyses for this study. Study concept and design: MD, JMP, J-PR, and J-PP. Acquisition of data: MD, JMP, PD, and J-PP. Drafting of the manuscript: MD, JMP, J-PR, and J-PP. Critical revision of the manuscript for important intellectual content: MD, JMP, J-PR, PD, and J-PP. JMP and J-PP obtained funding. Study supervision: JMP and J-PP. All authors read and approved the final manuscript.

Consent for publication

Not applicable

Competing interests

Although funded in part by Bioibérica (see *Funding* above), the sponsor had no role in the design and conduct of the study; the collection, management, analysis, and interpretation of the data; or the preparation, review, or approval of the manuscript. The sponsor had no access to the data and did not perform any of the study analysis. Drs Martel-Pelletier and Pelletier are consultants for Bioibérica and shareholders in ArthroLab Inc. M Dorais and Dr Raynauld are consultants for ArthroLab Inc. None of the authors are part of the OAI investigative team.

Author details

[1]StatSciences Inc., Notre-Dame-de-l'Île-Perrot, Quebec, Canada. [2]Osteoarthritis Research Unit, University of Montreal Hospital Research Centre (CRCHUM), Montreal, Quebec, Canada.

References

1. Hagen KB, Smedslund G, Moe RH, Grotle M, Kjeken I, Kvien TK. The evidence for non-pharmacological therapy of hand and hip OA. Nat Rev Rheumatol. 2009;5(9):517–9.
2. FDA Drug Safety Communication. FDA strengthens warning that non-aspirin nonsteroidal anti-inflammatory drugs (NSAIDs) can cause heart attacks or strokes (7-9-2015). Available at: https://www.fda.gov/Drugs/DrugSafety/ucm451800.htm (Accessed 23 May 2018).
3. Solomon DH, Rassen JA, Glynn RJ, Lee J, Levin R, Schneeweiss S. The comparative safety of analgesics in older adults with arthritis. Arch Intern Med. 2010;170(22):1968–76.
4. Milner JC. Osteoarthritis of the hip and indomethacin. J Bone Joint Surg (Br). 1972;54B:752–6.
5. Ronningen H. Indomethacin hips. Acta Orthop Scand. 1977;48:556–61.
6. Huskisson EC, Berry H, Gishen P, Jubb RW, Whitehead J. Effects of antiinflammatory drugs on the progression of osteoarthritis of the knee. LINK study group. Longitudinal investigation of nonsteroidal antiinflammatory drugs in knee osteoarthritis. J Rheumatol. 1995;22:1941–6.
7. Ding C. Do NSAIDs affect the progression of osteoarthritis? Inflammation. 2002;26(3):139–42.
8. Reijman M, Bierma-Zeinstra SM, Pols HA, Koes BW, Stricker BH, Hazes JM. Is there an association between the use of different types of nonsteroidal antiinflammatory drugs and radiologic progression of osteoarthritis? The Rotterdam study. Arthritis Rheum. 2005;52(10):3137–42.
9. Hauser RA. The acceleration of articular cartilage degeneration in osteoarthritis by nonsteroidal anti-inflammatory drugs. J Prolotherapy. 2010;2(1):305–22.
10. Lapane KL, Yang S, Driban JB, Liu SH, Dube CE, McAlindon TE, Eaton CB. Effects of prescription nonsteroidal antiinflammatory drugs on symptoms and disease progression among patients with knee osteoarthritis. Arthritis Rheumatol. 2015;67(3):724–32.
11. Hafezi-Nejad N, Guermazi A, Roemer FW, Eng J, Zikria B, Demehri S. Long term use of analgesics and risk of osteoarthritis progressions and knee replacement: propensity score matched cohort analysis of data from the osteoarthritis initiative. Osteoarthr Cartil. 2016;24(4):597–604.
12. Martel-Pelletier J, Roubille C, Abram F, Hochberg MC, Dorais M, Delorme P, Raynauld JP, Pelletier JP. First-line analysis of the effects of treatment on progression of structural changes in knee osteoarthritis over 24 months: data from the osteoarthritis initiative progression cohort. Ann Rheum Dis. 2015;74(3):547–56.
13. Roubille C, Martel-Pelletier J, Abram F, Dorais M, Delorme P, Raynauld JP, Pelletier JP. Impact of disease treatments on the progression of knee osteoarthritis structural changes related to meniscal extrusion: data from the OAI progression cohort. Semin Arthritis Rheum. 2015;45(3):257–67.
14. Eckstein F, Boudreau RM, Wang Z, Hannon MJ, Wirth W, Cotofana S, Guermazi A, Roemer F, Nevitt M, John MR, et al. Trajectory of cartilage loss

within 4 years of knee replacement–a nested case-control study from the osteoarthritis initiative. Osteoarthr Cartil. 2014;22(10):1542–9.

15. Eckstein F, Kwoh CK, Boudreau RM, Wang Z, Hannon MJ, Cotofana S, Hudelmaier MI, Wirth W, Guermazi A, Nevitt MC, et al. Quantitative MRI measures of cartilage predict knee replacement: a case-control study from the osteoarthritis initiative. Ann Rheum Dis. 2013;72(5):707–14.

16. Pelletier JP, Cooper C, Peterfy C, Reginster JY, Brandi ML, Bruyere O, Chapurlat R, Cicuttini F, Conaghan PG, Doherty M, et al. What is the predictive value of MRI for the occurrence of knee replacement surgery in knee osteoarthritis? Ann Rheum Dis. 2013;72(10):1594–604.

17. Raynauld JP, Martel-Pelletier J, Haraoui B, Choquette D, Dorais M, Wildi LM, Abram F, Pelletier JP. Risk factors predictive of joint replacement in a 2-year multicentre clinical trial in knee osteoarthritis using MRI: results from over 6 years of observation. Ann Rheum Dis. 2011;70(8):1382–8.

18. Cicuttini FM, Jones G, Forbes A, Wluka AE. Rate of cartilage loss at two years predicts subsequent total knee arthroplasty: a prospective study. Ann Rheum Dis. 2004;63(9):1124–7.

19. Breslow NE, Day NE. Chapter 7. Design considerations. Table 7.9. In: Breslow NE, Day NE, editors. Statistical methods in cancer research. Volume II–the design and analysis of cohort studies. Oxford: IARC Sci Publ; 1987. p. 297–300.

20. Bellamy N, Buchanan WW, Goldsmith CH, Campbell J, Stitt LW. Validation study of WOMAC: a health status instrument for measuring clinically important patient relevant outcomes to antirheumatic drug therapy in patients with osteoarthritis of the hip or knee. J Rheumatol. 1988;15:1833–40.

21. Roos EM, Roos HP, Lohmander LS, Ekdahl C, Beynnon BD. Knee injury and osteoarthritis outcome score (KOOS)–development of a self-administered outcome measure. J Orthop Sports Phys Ther. 1998;28(2):88–96.

22. Dodin P, Pelletier JP, Martel-Pelletier J, Abram F. Automatic human knee cartilage segmentation from 3D magnetic resonance images. IEEE Trans Biomed Eng. 2010;57:2699–711.

23. Dodin P, Abram F, Pelletier J-P, Martel-Pelletier J. A fully automated system for quantification of knee bone marrow lesions using MRI and the osteoarthritis initiative cohort. J Biomed Graph Comput. 2013;3(1):51–65.

24. Berthiaume MJ, Raynauld JP, Martel-Pelletier J, Labonté F, Beaudoin G, Bloch DA, Choquette D, Haraoui B, Altman RD, Hochberg M, et al. Meniscal tear and extrusion are strongly associated with the progression of knee osteoarthritis as assessed by quantitative magnetic resonance imaging. Ann Rheum Dis. 2005;64:556–63.

25. Raynauld JP, Martel-Pelletier J, Berthiaume MJ, Beaudoin G, Choquette D, Haraoui B, Tannenbaum H, Meyer JM, Beary JF, Cline GA, et al. Long term evaluation of disease progression through the quantitative magnetic resonance imaging of symptomatic knee osteoarthritis patients: correlation with clinical symptoms and radiographic changes. Arthritis Res Ther. 2006;8(1):R21.

26. Raynauld JP, Martel-Pelletier J, Beaulieu A, Bessette L, Morin F, Choquette D, Haraoui B, Abram F, Pelletier JP. An open-label pilot study evaluating by magnetic resonance imaging the potential for a disease-modifying effect of celecoxib compared to a modelized historical control cohort in the treatment of knee osteoarthritis. Semin Arthritis Rheum. 2010;40(3):185–92.

27. Raynauld JP, Martel-Pelletier J, Bias P, Laufer S, Haraoui B, Choquette D, Beaulieu AD, Abram F, Dorais M, Vignon E, et al. Protective effects of licofelone, a 5-lipoxygenase and cyclo-oxygenase inhibitor, versus naproxen on cartilage loss in knee osteoarthritis: a first multicentre clinical trial using quantitative MRI. Ann Rheum Dis. 2009;68(6):938–47.

28. Klop C, de Vries F, Lalmohamed A, Mastbergen SC, Leufkens HG, Noort-van der Laan WH, Bijlsma JW, Welsing PM. COX-2-selective NSAIDs and risk of hip or knee replacements: a population-based case-control study. Calcif Tissue Int. 2012;91(6):387–94.

29. Riddle DL, Kong X, Jiranek WA. Two-year incidence and predictors of future knee arthroplasty in persons with symptomatic knee osteoarthritis: preliminary analysis of longitudinal data from the osteoarthritis initiative. Knee. 2009;16(6):494–500.

30. Bruyere O, Pavelka K, Rovati LC, Gatterova J, Giacovelli G, Olejarova M, Deroisy R, Reginster JY. Total joint replacement after glucosamine sulphate treatment in knee osteoarthritis: results of a mean 8-year observation of patients from two previous 3-year, randomised, placebo-controlled trials. Osteoarthr Cartil. 2008;16(2):254–60.

31. Raynauld JP, Pelletier JP, Abram F, Dodin P, Delorme P, Martel-Pelletier J. Long-term effects of glucosamine and chondroitin sulfate on the progression of

structural changes in knee osteoarthritis: six-year follow up data from the osteoarthritis initiative. Arthritis Care Res (Hoboken). 2016;68(10):1560–6.

32. Gossec L, Paternotte S, Bingham CO 3rd, Clegg DO, Coste P, Conaghan PG, Davis AM, Giacovelli G, Gunther KP, Hawker G, et al. OARSI/OMERACT initiative to define states of severity and indication for joint replacement in hip and knee osteoarthritis. An OMERACT 10 special interest group. J Rheumatol. 2011;38(8):1765–9.

17

The risk of clinically diagnosed gout by serum urate levels: results from 30 years follow-up of the Malmö Preventive Project cohort in southern Sweden

Meliha C. Kapetanovic[1*], Peter Nilsson[2,3], Carl Turesson[4], Martin Englund[5], Nicola Dalbeth[6] and Lennart Jacobsson[7]

Abstract

Background: Hyperuricemia (HU) is in the causal pathway for developing clinical gout. There are few population-based assessments of the absolute and relative risk of clinically diagnosed incident gout in subjects with HU. We aimed to explore the long-term risk of developing incident gout among asymptomatic adults with different levels of serum urate (SU).

Methods: Malmö Preventive Project was a population-based screening program for cardiovascular risk factors, alcohol abuse, and breast cancer in Malmö, Sweden. The study population was screened between 1974 and 1992. At baseline, subjects were assessed with a questionnaire, physical examination, and laboratory tests. Follow-up ended at first gout diagnosis, death, moving from area, or December 31, 2014. Incident gout (using ICD10 codes) was diagnosed based on national registers for specialized inpatient and outpatient care, and from 1998 onward in the Skåne Healthcare Register including primary healthcare. Incidence rates, absolute risk, hazard ratios (HRs) and potentially associated factors were analyzed by baseline SU levels, i.e. normal levels (≤ 360 μmol/L); 361–405 (levels below tissue solubility of SU); and > 405 (HU), overall, and by sex.

Results: Overall, 1275 individuals [3.8%; 1014 men (4.5%) and 261 women (2.4%)] of the 33,346 study participants (mean age: 45.7 (SD: 7.4), 67% men), developed incident gout during follow-up (mean 28.2 years). Of those with HU, 14.7% of men and 19.5% of women developed gout. Compared to subjects in the lowest SU category, the age-adjusted HR in men increased from 2.7 to 6.4, and in women from 4.4 to 13.1 with increasing baseline SU category, and with a statistically significant interaction of sex ($p < 0.001$). Body mass index, estimated glomerular filtration rate (negative), triglycerides, alcohol risk behavior (only in men), and comorbidities such as hypertension, cardiovascular disease, and diabetes were strongly associated with SU at baseline in both sexes.

Conclusions: The absolute risk for developing clinically diagnosed gout over 30 years in middle-aged subjects was 3.8%, and increased progressively in both men and women in relation to baseline SU. This risk increase was significantly higher in women than in men, whereas the associations between baseline risk markers and SU levels were similar in both sexes.

Keywords: Hyperuricemia, Incident gout, Risk factors

* Correspondence: meliha.c_kapetanovic@med.lu.se
[1]Department of Clinical Sciences Lund, Section of Rheumatology, Lund University and Skåne University Hospital, Kioskgatan 5, SE-221 85 Lund, Sweden
Full list of author information is available at the end of the article

Background

Hyperuricemia (HU) is defined as serum urate concentrations above its levels of solubility in the serum [1–9], which is considered to be at approximately 405 mmol/L (6.8 mg/dL) [10]. We have previously reported a prevalence of 1.7% for clinically diagnosed gout among adults in two regions in Sweden [11, 12], but there are limited data regarding the risk of incident gout in individuals with asymptomatic HU [9]. Asymptomatic HU is common and, depending on the chosen cutoff value, figures of 10–20% have been reported in Western populations [1–3]. Unpublished data from the ongoing Swedish CArdioPulmonary BioImage Study (SCAPIS) in Sweden suggest that 20% of men and 12% of women with mean age 57 years have HU (personal communication, Mats Dehlin). A systematic review and meta-analysis of studies conducted in China reported pooled prevalence of HU and gout being 13.3% and 1.1%, respectively [7]. HU and gout have repeatedly been reported to be associated with the metabolic syndrome, several comorbidities, and unhealthy lifestyle factors in non-European and European populations [13]. It is commonly referenced that 10–20% of subject with HU will develop clinically relevant gout, the most established adverse health outcome of HU [1, 5, 6, 9], whereas it still debated whether HU is causally related to other chronic diseases such as cardiovascular disease (CVD), kidney disease, dementia, or cancer [13], or not. At present, asymptomatic HU is therefore not considered as an indication for urate-lowering therapy (ULT) [14]. The risk of incident gout has been reported to increase with duration of HU and degree of increased SU levels [1, 3, 4, 7–9, 13, 15]. These estimates are all based on population outside Europe and often on relatively small samples [1, 3, 4, 7]. Population-based studies from northern Europe are lacking.

Thus, the aims of the present study were: (1) to determine the long-term absolute and relative risks of incident clinically diagnosed gout among adults without gout by different levels of baseline HU; and (2) to describe the relation between SU levels and potentially associated factors. For the analyses we used participants in the Malmö Preventive Project (MPP), a large-scale population based screening and case-finding program for cardiovascular risk factors, alcohol abuse, and breast cancer in Sweden.

Methods
Malmö Preventive Project (MPP)
Setting
In the city of Malmö, a screening program for cardiovascular risk factors, alcohol abuse, and breast cancer was started in 1974 at the Department of Preventive Medicine, University Hospital, Malmö, Sweden [16]. At the study start, the city population comprised approximately 250,000 inhabitants. The aim of MPP was to screen large strata of the adult population in order to find high-risk individuals for preventive interventions directed against cardiovascular risk and alcohol abuse. No specific intervention was offered to subjects with HU.

A total of 33,346 subjects participated in the health survey and their data constitute baseline information. The study population was screened between 1974 and 1992, with a total of 22,444 men and 10,902 women attending. The overall attendance was 71% (range 64–78% for different years). Men were mostly screened in the first half of the period (1974–1982), and women in the latter half (1981–1992), thus with different length of follow-up time. The main results of this survey were described previously [16].

Baseline information from survey
Subjects were invited to participate in a health screening which included: a self-administered questionnaire with 260 questions gathering information on socioeconomic factors, history of CVD, hypertension and diabetes mellitus (DM) (including family history for these conditions), smoking habits, alcohol consumption behavior, physical activity at work and during leisure time, dietary habits and weight gain, presence of signs and symptoms of CVD and history of malignancies); a physical examination (including weight, height, body mass index (BMI), and blood pressure), and laboratory testing (including serum urate level [SU], s-cholesterol; fs-triglycerides, s-creatinine, fasting blood glucose).

Estimated glomerular filtration rate (eGFR) was calculated using the Malmö-Lund revised equation based on the Swedish population [17].

Alcohol consumption behavior was studied using the Malmö modified brief Michigan Alcohol Screening Test (Mm-MAST) comprising nine questions regarding alcohol habits [18, 19]. These were: "Do you take a drink before going to a party?", "Do you usually drink a bottle of wine or corresponding amounts of alcohol over the weekend?", "Do you drink a couple of drinks (beers) a day to relax?", "Do you tolerate more alcohol now than you did 10 years ago?", "Have you difficulties not drinking more than your friends?", "Do you fall asleep after moderate drinking without knowing how you got to bed", "Do you have a bad consciousness after a party?", "Do you take a drink (a beer) after the party?" and "Do you try to avoid alcoholic beverage for a determined period of time e.g. a week?" Confirming answers to at least two of these questions was used to identify the alcohol risk consumption behavior in the present study according to previous studies [18–20]. Mm-MAST could not be analyzed for women due the high frequency of missing data.

A question regarding history of gout was included in the questionnaire. In the present study, concomitant CVD (yes/no) at baseline was defined as history of angina pectoris, myocardial infarction (MI) or concomitant medication for heart disease, and DM at baseline (yes/no) as fasting blood glucose ≥6.7 mmol/L (in blood, according to contemporary reference levels in the 1970s) or history of DM. All individuals with a systolic blood pressure ≥ 160 mmHg at baseline, or those who reported being on antihypertensive treatment, were considered to have hypertension.

Data on marital status, retrieved from the Swedish population and housing census were categorized in five categories: "unmarried", "married", "divorced", "widow/widower", and "not specified" [21].

Identification of incident gout and follow-up

In order to identify all gout diagnoses (using International Classification of Diseases version 10 [ICD10] codes) given at visits to physicians within primary care (from 1998), specialized inpatient (from 1974) and outpatient specialized care (from 2001) the MPP cohort was linked to regional healthcare register (The Skåne Healthcare Register; SHR) and to National Patient Register (NPR), respectively.

Follow-up started at the time point of baseline screening that could vary between 1973 and 1992. Participants were followed until date of first gout diagnosis, death, moving from area, or December 31, 2014. Since the method for identifying incident gout was based on inpatient care up to 1998 and all types of care thereafter (including primary care), results are presented also for the two time periods separately; screening up through 1997 (or end of follow-up if before) and from 1998 until end of follow-up.

Baseline SU levels were stratified into three categories: i.e. normal levels (≤ 360; 361–405 (levels below tissue solubility of UA) and > 405 μmol/L, based on the conception that urate saturation occurs at levels > 405 μmol/L at physiological pH and body temperature and that levels ≤360 μmol/L is the treatment target for ULT [10]. HU was defined as SU > 405 μmol/L.

Statistical analysis

Pearson correlation, Mann-Whitney U test and chi-squared test were used to analyze the associations between, on one hand, comorbidities, socioeconomic and lifestyle-related factors, with SU levels and HU on the other.

Cox regression models, stratified by sex, were applied to determine the hazard ratio (HR), with 95% confidence intervals (95% CI) of incident gout during the two time periods, i.e. date of baseline screening through December 31, 1998, and from January 1, 1999 through December 31,

2014; unadjusted and age-adjusted. The proportional hazard (PH) assumptions for Cox regression analysis were evaluated graphically in survival curves and log-minus-log plots and were found to be valid for the two time periods separately. Interactions between SU category and sex were tested in models separately for the time periods that included all subjects.

Incidence rates of gout in patients with different SU levels were calculated separately for men and women, both for the whole period of follow-up and stratified for the two time periods. Incidence was computed as number of individuals with first-time diagnosis of gout divided by the sum of follow-up time (person-years at risk) by sex and SU level category. A Poisson distribution was assumed when estimating 95% CIs for incidence rates. All analyses were performed by use of IBM SPSS Statistics 24 (IBM Corp., Armonk, NY, USA).

Ethical considerations

The ethical approval was obtained from the Regional Ethics Committee at Lund University (Dnr 85/2004).

Results
Study participants

In total, 33,346 individuals (67% men, mean age 45.7 years at inclusion, mean follow-up 28.2 years; SD 8.4 years) participated in the MPP, and contributed overall with 936,826 person-years at risk (men: 647,114 person-years, women: 289,712 person-years). Patients with gout prior to inclusion ($n = 11$) were excluded from the analysis.

Table 1 summarizes the baseline characteristics of all participants MPP, stratified by sex.

Baseline HU

In total, 33,335 individuals (22,433 men and 10,902 women) were included and SU data were available in the vast majority of participants (22,368 men, 10,848 women). Altogether 2191 (9.8%) men and 164 (1.5%) women had HU (> 405 μmol/L) at baseline.

Relation between baseline SU and other baseline characteristics

In men, SU at baseline correlated with higher BMI ($r = 0.32$), systolic blood pressure ($r = 0.14$), triglycerides ($r = 0.25$), Mm-MAST ≥2 ($p < 0.001$; Mann-Whitney test), lower estimated glomerular filtration rate (eGFR) ($r = - 0.18$), as well as with hypertension and CVD history ($p < 0.001$, Mann-Whitney test). Significant but weaker associations were seen between SU and total cholesterol ($r = 0.11$), Mm-MAST score ($r = 0.08$), fasting blood glucose ($r = 0.04$), erythrocyte sedimentation ratio (ESR) ($r = 0.03$), and history of one or several kidney stone attacks ($p < 0.009$ and $p = 0.03$, respectively; Mann-Whitney test).

Table 1 Baseline characteristics of participants in the Malmö Preventive Project (MPP) stratified by sex

	All	Men	Women
Sex, men n (%)	33,335	22,433 (67.3)	10,902 (32.7)
Age* (years)	45.7 (7.4)	43.7 (6.6)	49.7 (7.4)
BMI (kg/m²)	24.6 (3.6)	24.7 (3.3)	24.4 (4.2)
Serum urate (micromol/L)	300.8 (70.1)	323.2 (64.2)	254.4 (57.8)
Seum urate > 405, n (%)	2455 (7.1%)	2191 (9.8%)	164 (1.5%)
SBP in individuals with non-treated hypertension at baseline (mmHg)**	149 (21)	150 (20)	148 (21)
Fasting glucose (millimol/L) in non-DM individuals at baseline	4.9 (0.5)	4.9 (0.5)	4.8 (0.5)
eGFR (ml/min/1.73m²)	77.9 (10.8)	79.1 (10.5)	75.6 (10.9)
Cholesterol (milimol/L)	5.7 (1.1)	5.6 (1.1)	5.8 (1.1)
Triglycerides (milimol/L)	1.4 (0.9)	1.5 (1.1)	1.1 (0.6)
Hypertension at baseline n (%)§	6070 (17.2)	3672 (16.4)	2398 (22)
Diabetes mellitus at baseline, n (%)§§	828 (2.5)	575 (2.6)	253 (2.3)
Family history of any sibling having hypertension, n (%)	2519 (7.6)	1102 (4.9)	1417 (13)
History of kidney stone attack, n (%)	2729 (8.2)	2003 (8.9)	726 (6.7)
History of several kidney stone attacks, n (%)	1359 (4.1)	1046 (4.7)	313 (2.9)
Mm-MAST ≥ 2, n (%)#	21.7	30.8	2.8
ESR (mm/hour)	7.1 (6.9)	5.7 (6.0)	9.9 (7.7)
Current smoker, n (%)	14,846 (44.5)	11,038 (49.2)	3808 (37.1)

*Values for continuous variables denote mean (SD)
**Number of patients are 2780 male and 1416 female)
#Number of subjects are 6920 (male) and 310 (female)
§Hypertension was defined as systolic BTP ≥ 160 mmHg or using antihypertensive treatment on the regular basis
§§Diabetes mellitus at baseline was defined as f-glucose ≥ 6.7 or history of DM.
SBP systolic blood pressure, Mm-MAST Malmö-modified brief Michigan Alcohol Screening Test, ESR erythrocyte sedimentation rate

In women, SU at baseline correlated with higher BMI ($r = 0.38$), age ($r = 0.20$), systolic blood pressure (r = 0.20), triglycerides ($r = 0.30$), lower eGFR ($r = -0.27$), total cholesterol ($r = 0.18$), ESR ($r = 0.17$), fasting blood glucose ($r = 0.13$), and occurrence of hypertension, CVD and diabetes ($p < 0.001$; Mann-Whitney test).

Table 2 summarizes the baseline characteristics and comorbidities among participants in MPP stratified by sex and category of baseline SU levels (normal levels, i.e. ≤ 360; 361–405; and > 405 µmol /L).

Both men and women with SU > 405 µmol/L had at baseline higher occurrence of hypertension, DM, CVD ($p < 0.001$, chi-squared test) and higher levels of BMI, total cholesterol, triglycerides, fasting blood glucose, systolic blood pressure, but lower levels of eGFR ($p < 0.001$, Mann-Whitney test) compared to those with SU levels ≤ 405 µmol/L.

A family history of hypertension among siblings was also significantly associated with SU > > 405 µmol/L ($p < 0.001$ and $p = 0.017$ in men and women, respectively).

Marital status did not differ statistically between individuals with SU > 405 µmol l/L and those with lower levels (data not shown).

Lifestyle factors
Tobacco smoking
Men with HU were less often smokers at baseline and also a lower proportion of these patients had smoked for at least 10 years prior to baseline screening compared to those with SU levels ≤ 405 µmol/L ($p = 0.001$ and $p = 0.004$, respectively). Women with SU > 405 µmol/L did not differ significantly in smoking status compared to those with SU levels ≤ 405 µmol/L.

Alcohol consumption – Risk behavior
Men with SU > 405 µmol/L had significantly higher Mm-MAST score at baseline (mean score = 1.6 vs 1.3; $p < 0.001$ Mann-Whitney test) and higher occurrence of risk behavior for alcohol consumption, i.e. Mm-MAST ≥2 ($p < 0.001$, chi-squared test) compared to those with SU levels ≤ 405 µmol/L.

Risk of developing gout
Overall, 1275 individuals (3.8%), i.e. 1014 men (4.5%) and 261 women (2.4%) of these middle-aged subjects developed incident gout during the follow up.

The absolute risks for incident gout, and the unadjusted and age-adjusted HRs, stratified by sex and

Table 2 Baseline characteristics and comorbidities among participants in MPP stratified by sex and SU levels

SU at baseline (µmol/L) (n of persons)	Age at baseline (years)	BMI (kg/m2)	Systolic blood pressure (pts not treated for hypertension #) (mmHg)	eGFR (ml/min/ 1.73m²)	s-cholesterol (mmol/L)	s-triglycerides (mmol/L)	Hypertension n (%)	Sibling with hypertension; n (%)	CVD n (%)	DM n (%)	Kidney stone attacks ever; n (%)	Mm-MAST ≥ 2*§; n (%)	ESR (mm/h)	Smoking at baseline (n, %)
Men n = 22,433	Men with available SU at baseline													
≤360 n = 16,824	43.6 (6.5)	24.2 (3.1)	129 (15.5)	80.0 (10.3)	5.6 (1.1)	1.4 (0.8)	2287 (13.6)	739 (4.4)	306 (1.8)	398 (2.4)	1461 (8.7)	4858 (28.9)	5.7 (6.0)	8688 (51.6)
361–405 n = 3353	43.8 (6.6)	25.7 (3.3)	132 (16.2)	77.0 (10.5)	5.7 (1.2)	1.7(1.2)	712 (21.2)	181 (5.4)	83 (2.5)	90 (2.7)	305 (9.1)	1181(35.2)	5.7 (5.4)	1463 (43.6)
>405 n = 2191	44.5 (7.0)	26.9 (3.7)	134(16.6)	75.7 (11.0)	5.8 (1.1)	2.1 (1.8)	662 (30.2)	177 (8.1)	84 (3.8)	86 (3.9)	203 (10.6)	867 (39.6)	6.4 (6.6)	861 (39.3)
Women n = 10,902	Women with available SU at baseline													
≤360 n = 10,357	49.5 (7.5)	24.2 (4.0)	126 (17.6)	75.9 (10.8)	5.8 (1.1)	1.1 (0.5)	2130 (20.6)	1323 (12.8)	326 (3.1)	209 (2)	675 (6.5)	299 (2.9)	9.7 (7.5)	3636 (35.1)
361–405 n = 327	53 (4.8)	29.0 (5.6)	136 (20.0)	70.2 (10.1)	6.4 (1.1)	1.7 (0.4)	173 (52.9)	56 (17.1)	23 (7.0)	27 (8.3)	33 (10.1)	**	13.4 (9.8)	105 (32.1)
>405 n = 164	53.1(4.6)	29.3 (5.3)	137 (18.2)	67.9 (14.6)	6.4 (1.1)	1.9 (1.1)	81 (49.4)	33 (20.1)	15 (9.1)	16 (9.8)	15 (9.1)	**	14.5(9.3)	53 (32.3)

*Mm-MAST = Malmö modified brief Michigan Alcohol Screening Test

**Calculations were not performed due to few observations

#Number of subjects with missing information were in different groups of SU were in men 13/2/2 and in women 434/11/5

§Number of subjects with missing information were in different groups of SU were in men 2521/314/201

MPP Malmö Preventive Project, SU serum urate, BMI body mass index, eGFR estimated glomerular filtration rate, CVD cardiovascular disease, DM diabetes mellitus, Mm-MAST Malmö-modified brief Michigan Alcohol Screening Test, ESR erythrocyte sedimentation rate

baseline SU levels over the whole period of follow-up, are displayed in Table 3. Incidence rates and absolute risks increased substantially and progressively with increasing baseline SU levels. In the group with HU (> 405 µmol/L) at baseline the corresponding absolute risks were 13.3% (95% CI: 12.2–14.8) in men and 17.7% (95% CI: 12.4–24.6) in women, respectively.

Since identifying a first-time gout diagnosis up to 1998 was based only on diagnosis given in inpatient care (probably more severe disease events) in contrast to the period after 1998 until end of study, when it was based on all visits to physician in the healthcare system, incidence rates and HRs are also presented by these two time periods (Table 4). In the first time period incidence rates and HRs (for men) were substantially lower compared to the second period. During both time periods there was a progressive increase in risk for being diagnosed with gout with higher baseline SU levels in both men and women. In the latter period this resulted in an age-adjusted increased risk in women of 4.4 (95% CI: 2.9–6.7; SU 361–405 vs ≤ 360 µmol/L) to 13.1 (95% CI: 8.8–19.4; SU > 405 vs ≤ 360 µmol/L) and in men of 2.7 (95% CI: 2.3–3.2; SU 361–405 vs ≤ 360) to 6.4 (95% CI: 5.6–7.5; SU > 405 vs ≤ 360 µmol/L). In this latter period there was a significant interaction between SU category and sex, with women having a significantly larger increase in HRs for incident gout compared to men with increasing SU levels categories (*p* < 0.001).

Discussion

In the present prospective, observational study we report that the risk for incident gout over on average 28 years (mean follow-up 28.2 years and overall 936,826 person-years at risk) among middle-aged city residents was 3.8% (4.5% in men and 2.4% in women). The risk increased substantially with increasing levels of SU, and among individuals with HU the risk of being diagnosed with gout was 6- and 13-fold higher women in men and

women, respectively. In this urban cohort with a mean age of 47 years at baseline, 10% of men and 1.5% of women had asymptomatic HU.

There are no European, and only few American [1, 15, 22] or non-Caucasian [8, 23], population-based cohort studies on the association between SU and risk of incident gout. Our study has the longest total follow-up of all such studies and a high participation rate. Only a Taiwanese study [23] is based on larger sample (but with a mean follow-up of only 7.2 years). Only the Framingham study [22] has a similar length of follow-up (based on 4427 subjects). Both these previous studies and ours have a balanced sex ratio and comparable mean age at baseline.

Comparison of risk for gout between these studies is possible only for subjects in the SU < 360 µmol/L category due to differences on categorization (i.e. quartiles or fixed other cutoff values) of SU in the different studies. In this subgroup, similar incidence rates as in our study where reported in a meta-analyses (including the above studies, 80 cases/100,000 person-years at risk) [24]. In the Framingham study, which had a similar length of follow-up as our study, the incidence rates were twice as high in men (195 cases/100,000 person-years at risk), but similar in women (103 cases/100,000 person-years at risk) compared to our results [22].

Another difference between studies relates to sex differences in the risk increase for incident gout with increasing baseline SU levels, where both the Taiwanese and the Framingham study showed a higher increase in men, whereas we showed the opposite. In analogy with this, the cumulative risk in those with baseline HU was comparable for men in the MPP and the Framingham study (15 vs 13%) but higher in the MPP for women (20 vs 6%).

Taken together, our results, in accordance with those of other studies, show that SU levels are strongly, and to a similar degree, associated with incident gout. Possible

Table 3 Incidence per 100,000 person years (p-yrs) at risk for developing incident gout in men and women by different levels of SU at baseline screening

No of individuals by sex and s-UA	SU at baseline (µmol/L)	Incident gout (n)	Person years at risk	Incidence (95% CI) per 100,000 person-years at risk	Absolute risk (%)*
Men (n = 22,368)					
16,824	≤360	447	493,612	90 (82.2–99)	2.7 (2.4–2.9)
3353	361–405	227	95,408	238 (208.5–270.5)	6.8 (6.0–7.7)
2191	> 405	292	58,094	527.4 (471.4–588.1)	13.3 (12.0–14.8)
Women (n = 10,902)					
10,357	≤ 360	200	278,493	70.6 (61.2–81.1)	1.9 (1.7–2.2)
327	361–405	25	7655	340.9 (224.6–496)	7.6 (5.1–10.9)
164	> 405	29	3564	828.6 (566.7–1170)	17.7 (12.4–24.6)

*Mean follow-up (SD) for men 29.9 (8.7); 29.3 (8.9); and 27.9 (9.4); and for women 27.5 (7.3); 24.2 (7.5); and 23.5 (8.1) years
*SU levels were missing in two men and one woman, which explains the difference in number of incident gout

Table 4 Incidence per 100,000 person-years at risk and hazard ratios (HRs) for developing incident gout in men and women by different levels of urate at baseline healthcare screening. Results are presented separately for the two time periods; (a) baseline screening until 1998; and (b) from 1998 to end of study period

SU at baseline, µmol/L	Time period from baseline screening to 1998					Time period from 1998 to end of study				
	Incident gout (n)	Person-years at risk	Inc. (95% CI)*	HR unadjusted (95%CI)	HR age adjusted (95%CI)	Incident gout (n)	Person-years at risk	Inc. (95% CI)*	HR un-adjusted (95%CI)	HR age adjusted (95%CI)
Men										
≤ 360	8	322,368	2.5 (1.1–4.9)	1	1	447	188,039	237.7 (216.2–260.8)	1	1
361–405	7	63,617	11.0 (4.4–22.7)	4.4 (1.6–12.2)	4.4 (1.6–12.2)	227	35,336	642.4 (561.5–731.67)	2.7 (2.3–3.2)	2.7(2.3–3.2)
>405	31	41,172	75.3 (51.2–106.9)	30.2 (13.9–65.8)	28.6 (13.1–62.3)	292	19,714	1481 (1316–1661)	6.5 (5.6–7.5)	6.4 (5.6–7.5)
Women										
≤ 360	1	143,968	0.7 (0.009–0.4)	n.a.	n.a.	200	137,282	145.7 (126.2–167.3)	1	1
361–405	2	4026	49.7 (5.6–179.3)	n.a.	n.a.	25	3735	669.3 (433.1–981.1)	4.7(3.1–7.2)	4.4 (2.9–6.7)
>405	3	2048	146.5 (29.5–428)	n.a.	n.a.	29	1589	1825 (1222–2621)	14.0 (9.4–20.6)	13.1 (8.8–19.4)

*Per 100,000 person-years at risk

explanations for the modest difference in incidence and effect of sex on risk for gout with higher baseline SU between studies could be differences between populations with regard to genetics, comorbidities, lifestyle, or other exposures.

We also observed positive cross-sectional associations for both men and women between SU levels at baseline and systolic blood pressure and hypertension, BMI, fasting blood glucose, total cholesterol and triglyceride levels. SU levels were significantly higher in individuals with impaired kidney function determined by eGFR in both sexes. The lowest mean eGFR was observed in both men and women with the highest SU levels. These studies are largely in accordance with previous publications [24–29].

In a previously published meta-analysis, asymptomatic HU was associated with the development of hypertension independently of other traditional risk factors [24]. Furthermore, a recent Japanese study suggested that individuals with asymptomatic HU without other comorbidities were at an increased risk of developing cardiometabolic conditions such as hypertension, dyslipidemia, overweight/obesity, and chronic kidney disease, with a similar trend for development of DM [25]. On the other hand, several of these comorbidities, such as obesity [25, 26] and kidney function [27, 28], have convincingly been shown to predict the risk of both HU and gout [13]. In addition, an association between higher number of ideal cardiovascular health metrics (such as no smoking status, lower BMI, physiological fasting blood glucose level, healthy diet, better physical activity, normal blood pressure) and lower risk of asymptomatic HU was reported in a large longitudinal, population-based study from China [29]. Interestingly, this association was stronger in women than in men [29]. These results are in accordance with our observations and illustrate the close and complex relation between SU and these factors. Causality is not possible to conclude from epidemiological cohort studies as these and in studies using other techniques, i.e. Mendelian randomization, causality has been questioned for many of these associations [30, 31].

The association between alcohol overconsumption and gout is well-known [32, 33]. Since MPP was initiated as a screening program for identifying subjects where prevention through lifestyle changes (including alcohol use) might improve long-term health outcomes, a validated questionnaire, i.e. Mm-MAST [18–20] was used in order to identify alcohol risk consumption. We confirmed a significant positive correlation between alcohol risk consumption behavior (Mm-MAST) in men and HU at baseline.

Gout and HU are common in patients with chronic kidney disease although to what extent HU is the cause, consequence, or both, is still unclear [31, 34]. There is growing evidence that HU may potentially be involved in the initiation and progression of chronic kidney disease [28, 31, 34]. The inverse association between SU and eGFR at baseline was relatively strong in the MPP. In addition, men with increased levels of SU had significantly more often had nephrolitiasis. These results are in accordance with recently published data from a cohort study on approximately 240,000 healthy men where HU was independently associated with increased risk of kidney stones [35]. In addition, a recent Swedish study reported a 60% increased risk for kidney stones in patients with gout [36].

Another interesting observation in the present study is that SU levels at baseline correlated significantly with ESR, in particular in women. This association could possibly be confounded by BMI, which is known to be associated with low-grade inflammation [37]. On the other hand, other results support an association between SU and inflammation adjusting for BMI [37–40].

In the present study, we have deliberately focused on describing the risk for incident gout by different levels of SU and avoided analyzing the effect of other possible predictors, or adjusting for such. The temporal and causal relations between several of such factors and SU are complex and in some cases, as for example kidney function, possibly bi-directional. This is a challenge when attributing risk to individual factors/markers using traditional techniques for cohort analyses. Methods using, for example using Mendelian randomization based on genetic data, may be more suitable for this purpose [41]. However, there is a scarcity of large long-term studies determining the absolute risk for incident gout diagnosis in relation to levels of SU. Our report adds important information on this topic.

Other strengths of this study include its long follow-up time, high participation rate, the large sample size comprising over 33,000 healthy individuals from the same urban area, and the extent of data collection at baseline on several factors and comorbidities possibly associated with both HU and the development of gout.

There are also some important limitations of our study; first, no primary healthcare data were available from the time point of baseline screening and 1998. On the other hand, due to the expected increasing frequency of gout attacks in most patients over time and the documented low use of and adherence to ULT in southern Sweden [42], the vast majority of patients diagnosed with their first gout attack before 1998, are expected to seek healthcare help again and hence be identified as patients with gout at later time points. Second, we did not assess the proportion receiving ULT, but do not think this substantially affects our results, since there were no written initiatives to act upon notification of HU at the time for screening and the use of ULT has continued to be relatively low in this catchment area up through 2012 [42].

Conclusions

Asymptomatic HU is common among healthy middle-aged individuals and is associated with an increased risk for incident gout in both sexes. In contrast to previous studies the risk to develop clinical gout at comparable SU values was found to be higher in women than in men. The close association between HU and several common comorbidities such as CVD, kidney disease, and hypertension, emphasizes the need to establish their causal relationships and whether ULT can decrease the risk for these comorbidities. To address these questions other types of designs such as randomized controlled trials (RCTs) and cohort studies using Mendelian randomization based on genetic markers of HU, will be crucial.

Abbreviations

BMI: Body mass index; CI: Confidence interval; CVD: Cardiovascular disease; DM: Diabetes mellitus; eGFR: Estimated glomerular filtration rate; ESR: Erythrocyte sedimentation ratio; HR: Hazard ratio; HU: Hyperuricemia; ICD10: International Classification of Diseases version 10; Mm-MAST: Malmö-modified brief Michigan Alcohol Screening Test; MPP: Malmö Preventive Project; SHR: Skåne Healthcare Register; SU: Serum urate level; ULT: Urate-lowering therapy

Acknowledgements

The authors thank to biostatistician Jan-Åke Nilsson for his skillful help with the statistical calculations.

Funding

This study was supported by grants from the Swedish Rheumatism Association, Alfred Österlund's Foundation, Greta and Johan Kock's Foundation, Anna-Greta Crafoord Foundation and Professor Nanna Svartz Foundation.

Authors' contributions

The study was conceived by MCK and LJ. All authors have interpreted the results. MCK drafted the manuscript, and PN, CT, ND, ME and LJ have revised it for important intellectual content. All authors read and approved the final manuscript.

Consent for publication

Not applicable.

Competing interests

The authors declare that they have no competing interests.

Author details

[1]Department of Clinical Sciences Lund, Section of Rheumatology, Lund University and Skåne University Hospital, Kioskgatan 5, SE-221 85 Lund, Sweden. [2]Department of Clinical Sciences, Lund University, Malmö, Sweden. [3]Department of Emergency and Internal Medicine, Skåne University Hospital, Malmö, Sweden. [4]Department of Clinical Sciences, Malmö, Lunds University and Skåne University Hospital, Malmö, Sweden. [5]Clinical Epidemiology Unit, Orthopaedics, Department of Clinical Sciences, Lund University, Lund, Sweden. [6]Department of Medicine, University of Auckland, Auckland, New Zealand. [7]Department of Rheumatology and Inflammation Research, Sahlgrenska Academy at University of Gothenburg, Gothenburg, Sweden.

References

1. Campion EW, Glynn RJ, DeLabry LO. Asymptomatic hyperuricemia. Risks and consequences in the normative aging study. Am J Med. 1987;82:421–6.
2. Mikuls TR, Farrar JT, Bilker WB, Fernandes S, Schumacher HR Jr, Saag KG. Gout epidemiology: results from the UK general practice research database 1990-1999. Ann Rheum Dis. 2005;64(2):267–72.
3. Zhu Y, Pandya BJ, Choi HK. Prevalence of gout and hyperuricemia in the US general population: the National Health and nutrition examination survey 2007-2008. Arthritis Rheum. 2011;63(10):3136–41.
4. Lin KC, Lin HY, Chou P. Community based epidemiological study on hyperuricemia and gout in kin-Hu. Kinmen J Rheumatol. 2000;27(4):1045–50.
5. Smith E, Hoy D, Cross M, Merriman TR, Vos T, Buchbinder R, Woolf A, March L. The global burden of gout: estimates from the global burden of disease 2010 study. Ann Rheum Dis. 2014;73(8):1470–6.
6. Kuo C, Grainge MJ, Zhang W, et al. Global epidemiology of gout: prevalence, incidence and risk factors. Nat Publ Gr. 2015;(Box 1):1–14.
7. Liu R, Han C, Wu D, Xia X, Gu J, Guan H, Shan Z, Teng W. Prevalence of Hyperuricemia and gout in mainland China from 2000 to 2014: a systematic review and meta-analysis. Biomed Res Int. 2015;2015:762820.
8. Duskin-Bitan H, Cohen E, Goldberg E, Shochat T, Levi A, Garty M, Krause I. The degree of asymptomatic hyperuricemia and the risk of gout. A retrospective analysis of a large cohort. Clin Rheumatol. 2014;33:549–53.
9. Shiozawa A, Szabo SM, Bolzani A, Cheung A, Choi HK. Serum uric acid and the risk of incident and recurrent gout: a systematic review. J Rheumatol. 2017;44(3):388–96.
10. Loeb JN. The influence of temperature on the solubility of monosodium urate. Arthritis Rheum. 1972;15(2):189–92.
11. Dehlin M, Drivelegka P, Sigurdardottir V, Svärd A, Jacobsson L. Incidence and prevalence of gout in western Sweden. 2016. Arthritis Res Ther. 2016; 18:164.
12. Kapetanovic MC, Adel M, Turkiewicz A, Noegi T, Saxne T, Jacobsson L, Englund M. Prevalence and incidence of gout in southern Sweden from the socioeconomic perspective. RMD Open. 2016;2(2):e00032.
13. Johnson RJ. Why focus on uric acid? Curr Med Res Opin. 2015;31(Suppl 2):3–7.
14. Stamp L, Dalbeth N. Urate-lowering therapy for asymptomatic hyperuricaemia: a need for caution. Semin Arthritis Rheum. 2017 Feb;46(4): 457–64.
15. Dalbeth N, Phipps-Green A, Frampton C, Neogi T, Taylor WJ, Merriman TR. Relationship between serum urate concentration and clinically evident incident gout: an individual participant data analysis. Ann Rheum Dis. 2018 Jul;77(7):1048–52.
16. Berglund G, Nilsson P, Nilsson J-A, et al. Long-term outcome of the Malmö preventive project. Total mortality and cardiovascular morbidity. J Intern Med. 2000;244:19–29.
17. Grubb A, Sterner G, Nyman U. Revised equations for estimating glomerular filtration rate based on the Lund-Malmö study cohort. Scand J Clin Lab Invest. 2011;71(3):232–9.
18. Fex G, Kristenson H, Trell E. Correlations of serum lipids and lipoproteins with gammaglutamyltransferase and attitude to alcohol consumption. Ann Clin Biochem. 1982;19:345–9.
19. Trell E. Community-based preventive medical department for individual risk factor assessment and intervention in an urban population. Prev Med. 1983; 12:397–402.
20. Kristenson H, Trell E. Indicators of alcohol consumption: comparisons between a questionnaire (mm-MAST), interviews and serum gamma-glutamyl transferase (GGT) in a health survey of middle-aged males. Br J Addict. 1982;77(3):297–304.
21. Statistics Sweden. The Swedish population and housing census (folk-och bostadsräkningen) 1965-1990. Available at https://www.scb.se/sv_/Hitta-statistik/Historisk-statistik/Digitaliserat%2D%2D-Statistik-efter-serie/Sveriges-officiella-statistik-SOS-utg-1912-/Folk%2D%2Doch-bostadsrakningarna-1860-1990/. Accessed 26 Feb 2018.
22. Bhole V, de Vera M, Rahman MM, Krishnan E, Choi H. Epidemiology of gout in women: fifty-two-year follow-up of a prospective cohort. Arthritis Rheum. 2010;62(4):1069–76.
23. Chen JH, Yeh WT, Chuang SY, Wu YY, Pan WH. Gender-specific risk factors for incident gout: a prospective cohort study. Clin Rheumatol. 2012;31:239–45.

24. Grayson PC, Kim SY, LaValley M, Choi HK. Hyperuricemia and incident hypertension: a systematic review and meta-analysis. Arthritis Care Res (Hoboken). 2011;63:102–10.

25. Kuwabara M, Niwa K, Hisatome I, Nakagawa T, Roncal-Jimenez CA, Andres-Hernando A, Bjornstad P, Jensen T, Sato Y, Milagres T, Garcia G, Ohno M, Lanaspa MA, Johnson RJ. Asymptomatic hyperuricemia without comorbidities predicts cardiometabolic diseases: five-year Japanese cohort study. Hypertension. 2017;69(6):1036–44.

26. Maglio C, Peltonen M, Neovius M, Jacobson P, Jacobsson L, Rudin A, Carlsson LM. Effects of bariatric surgery on gout ins-cidence in the Swedish Obese Subjects study: a non-randomised, prospective, controlled intervention trial. Ann Rheum Dis. 2017;76(4):688–93.

27. Carlsson LM, Romeo S, Jacobson P, Burza MA, Maglio C, Sjöholm K, Svensson PA, Haraldsson B, Peltonen M, Sjöström L. The incidence of albuminuria after bariatric surgery and usual care in Swedish Obese Subjects (SOS): a prospective controlled intervention trial. Int J Obes. 2015; 39(1):169–75.

28. Wang W, Bhole VM, Krishnan E. Chronic kidney disease as a risk factor for incident gout among men and women: retrospective cohort study using data from the Framingham heart study. BMJ Open. 2015;5(4):e006843.

29. Li Z, Meng L, Huang Z, Cui L, Li W, Gao J, Wang Z, Zhang R, Zhou J, Zhang G, Chen S, Zheng X, Cong H, Gao X, Wu S. Ideal cardiovascular health metrics and incident hyperuricemia. Arthritis Care Res (Hoboken). 2016;68(5):660–6.

30. Robinson PC, Choi HK, Do R, Merriman TR. Insight into rheumatological cause and effect through the use of Mendelian randomization. Nat Rev Rheumatol. 2016;12(8):486–96.

31. Johnson RJ, Bakris GL, Borghi C, Chonchol MB, Feldman D, Lanaspa MA, Merriman TR, Moe OW, Mount DB, Sanchez Lozada LG, Stahl E, Weiner DE, Chertow GM. Hyperuricemia, acute and chronic kidney disease, hypertension, and cardiovascular disease: report of Scientific Workshop organized by the National Kidney Foundation. Am J Kidney. 2018;71(6):851–65.

32. Choi HK, Atkinson K, Karlson EW, Willett W, Curhan G. Alcohol intake and risk of incident gout in men: a prospective study. Lancet. 2004;363(9417): 1277–81.

33. Wandell P, Carlsson AC, Ljunggren G. Gout and its comorbidities in the total population of Stockholm. Prev Med. 2015;81:387–91.

34. Li L, Yang C, Zhao Y, Zeng X, Liu F, Fu P. Is hyperuricemia an independent risk factor for new-onset chronic kidney disease? A systematic review and meta-analysis based on observational cohort studies. BMC Nephrol. 2014;15: 122. https://doi.org/10.1186/1471-2369-15-122.

35. Kim S, Chang Y, Yun KE, Jung HS, Lee SJ, Shin H, Ryu S. Development of nephrolithiasis in asymptomatic hyperuricemia: a cohort study. Am J Kidney Dis. 2017;70(2):173–81.

36. Landgren AJ, Jacobsson LTH, Lindström U, Sandström TZS, Drivelegka P, Björkman L, Fjellstedt E, Dehlin M. Incidence of and risk factors for nephrolithiasis in patients with gout and the general population, a cohort study. Arthritis Res Ther. 2017;19(1):173.

37. Maurizi G, Della Guardia L, Maurizi A, Poloni A. Adipocytes properties and crosstalk with immune system in obesity-related inflammation. Cell Physiol. 2018;233(1):88–97.

38. Lyngdoh T, Marques-Vidal P, Paccaud F, Preisig M, Waeber G, Bochud M, Vollenweider P. Elevated serum uric acid is associated with high circulating inflammatory cytokines in the population-based Colaus study. PLoS One. 2011;6(5):e19901.

39. Kono H, Chen CJ, Ontiveros F, Rock KL. Uric acid promotes an acute inflammatory response to sterile cell death in mice. J Clin Invest. 2010;120(6):1939–49.

40. Krishnan E. Interaction of inflammation, hyperuricemia, and the prevalence of hypertension among adults free of metabolic syndrome: NHANES 2009-2010. J Am Heart Assoc. 2014;3(2):e000157.

41. Zheng J, Baird D, Borges MC, Bowden J, Hemani G, Haycock P, Evans DM, Smith GD. Recent developments in Mendelian randomization studies. Curr Epidemiol Rep. 2017;4(4):330–45.

42. Dehlin M, Ekström EH, Petzold M, Strömberg U, Telg G, Jacobsson LT. Factors associated with initiation and persistence of urate-lowering therapy. Arthritis Res Ther. 2017;19(1):6.

18

Functional consultation and exercises improve grip strength in osteoarthritis of the hand – a randomised controlled trial

Michaela A. Stoffer-Marx[1,2], Meike Klinger[2,3], Simone Luschin[2,3], Silvia Meriaux-Kratochvila[3,4], Monika Zettel-Tomenendal[3], Valerie Nell-Duxneuner[5], Jochen Zwerina[6], Ingvild Kjeken[7,8], Marion Hackl[9], Sylvia Öhlinger[10], Anthony Woolf[11], Kurt Redlich[2], Josef S. Smolen[2] and Tanja A. Stamm[1]*

Abstract

Background: Evidence for non-pharmacological interventions in hand osteoarthritis is promising but still scarce. Combined interventions are most likely to best cover the clinical needs of patients with hand osteoarthritis (OA). The aim of this study was to evaluate the effect of a combined, interdisciplinary intervention feasible in both primary and specialist care compared to routine care plus placebo in patients with hand OA.

Methods: This was a randomised, controlled 2-month trial with a blinded assessor. In the combined-intervention group, rheumatology-trained health professionals from different disciplines delivered a one-session individual intervention with detailed information on functioning, activities of daily living, physical activity, nutrition, assistive devices, instructions on pain management and exercises. Telephone follow up was performed after 4 weeks. The primary outcome was grip strength after 8 weeks. Secondary outcomes were self-reported pain, satisfaction with treatment, health status, two of the Jebsen-Taylor Hand Function subtests and the total score of the Australian/Canadian Hand Osteoarthritis Index (AUSCAN). Statistical significance was calculated by Student's t test or the Mann-Whitney U test depending on data distribution. Binominal logistic regression models were fitted, with the primary outcome being the dependent and the group allocation being the independent variable.

Results: There were 151 participating patients (74 in the combined-intervention and 77 in the routine-care-plus-placebo group) with 2-month follow-up attendance of 84% ($n = 128$). Grip strength significantly increased in the combined-intervention group and decreased in the routine-care group (dominant hand, mean 0.03 bar (SD 0.11) versus − 0.03 (SD 0.13), p value = 0.001, baseline corrected values) after 8 weeks.

Conclusion: The combined one-session individual intervention significantly improved grip strength and self-reported satisfaction with treatment in patients with hand OA. It can be delivered by different rheumatology-trained health professionals and is thus also feasible in primary care.

Keywords: Osteoarthritis, Hand, Occupational therapy, Physiotherapy, Pain management, Quality of healthcare

* Correspondence: tanja.stamm@meduniwien.ac.at
[1]Section for Outcomes Research, Center for Medical Statistics, Informatics, and Intelligent Systems, Medical University of Vienna, Spitalgasse 23, 1090 Vienna, Austria
Full list of author information is available at the end of the article

Key message

A combined intervention feasible in primary and specialist care improves grip strength.

Background

The prevalence of rheumatic diseases rises with age and with increasing longevity of the population [1]. Osteoarthritis (OA) is one of the most common rheumatic diseases and is associated with damage of the articular cartilage and changes in subchondral bone [2]. OA affects 60–70% of the population above the age of 65 years [3–5]. Today, almost 80% of the population can expect to live through most of their seventh decade of life, thus the impact of OA is likely to increase even further in the future [3]. Hand OA leads to a reduction of grip strength [6], difficulties when performing tasks of everyday life [7], loss of productive work time [8] and a decreased ability to perform manual activities [9]. Given the importance of being able to use the hands in daily life, it is apparent that hand OA affects not only body functions and structures but also several activities of daily living and societal participation [10, 11]. Thus, hand OA is a burden not only for the individual but also for society [12].

Management recommendations advise applying pharmacological and non-pharmacological methods for hand OA [13]. Drug treatment recommended for hand OA includes analgesics, non-steroidal anti-inflammatory drugs (NSAIDs) and topical active components [14]. Patients with OA, including hand OA, are frequently managed in primary care and are commonly referred to non-physician health professionals such as occupational therapists and physiotherapists to improve their health and functional performance [13, 15–17].

Based on existing guidelines, patient perspectives and expert opinion, the eumusc.net-working group developed user-focused European standards of care for OA [18]. From a recent focus group study also undertaken within the eumusc.net project, it is known that patients wish to have the possibility to contact a health professional experienced in the care of OA directly over the phone for a follow-up consultation [19].

Recent trials on multidisciplinary interventions in hand, knee, hip [20, 21] and generalised OA [22] showed significance in the subjective self-reported satisfaction of the patients but failed to show effects on clinical outcomes [23, 24]. Furthermore, multidisciplinary approaches were tested only in group settings. Given that the number of OA patients will increase in future, time efficient and individualised treatment options that can be delivered by different health professionals are desirable in OA. As hand OA patients have individual and subjective treatment requirements, combined interventions that take different treatment options into account may be superior to interventions that focus on just one particular component, e.g.

exercises only or orthoses only. However, there is a lack of evidence on these approaches, especially those feasible in primary care.

Thus, high-quality studies on the effect of a brief interdisciplinary, individualized, intervention that is community-applicable in both primary and specialist care are warranted.

The aim of the study was to compare the effect of a combined intervention feasible in both, primary and specialist care, compared with routine care plus placebo in patients with hand OA.

Methods

Study design

The present study was an assessor-blinded randomised controlled trial (RCT) (Table 1) to evaluate functional outcome and personal satisfaction in patients undergoing a combined interdisciplinary intervention, compared with routine clinical care plus a massage ball as placebo intervention. Patients were allocated at a rate of 1:1 to the two groups. Assessments were performed at baseline and the follow-up visit in outpatient clinics 2 months later. Principles of good clinical practice, the Declaration of Helsinki, Consolidated Standards of Reporting Trials (CONSORT) statement 2010 [25] and CONSORT guidelines for non-pharmacological interventions [26] have been taken into consideration in the planning, realisation and reporting of this trial. According to the Declaration of Helsinki the ethical committee of the Medical University of Vienna approved the study (number 1083/2012). Participants gave their written informed consent. The trial was registered at www.controlled-trials.com with the trial registration number ISRCTN62513257.

Participants

Participants diagnosed with hand OA according to the American College of Rheumatology criteria [27] were recruited from the rheumatology outpatient clinic of the Medical University in Vienna, Austria. In order to not exclude patients with hand OA at an early stage, patients with bony swelling of at least one interphalangeal joint of the second to the fifth finger and/or pain or bony swelling of at least one carpometacarpal 1 joint (CMC 1) have also been considered eligible to participate in the study. In addition, eligible patients had to score having hand pain of at least 3 points on an 11-point Likert scale at two time points, at baseline and at the intervention session.

Patients diagnosed with a rheumatic disease other than hand OA, including rheumatoid arthritis, or patients with elevated C-reactive protein levels (> 0.5 mg/dl) were excluded. Patients who had received steroid injections within the last 4 weeks, who had undergone hand surgery within the last year or who planned to receive

Table 1 Content of the combined-intervention delivered to participants according to the patient-centred standards of care for osteoarthritis [18]

Flow chart combined intervention compared to RC group

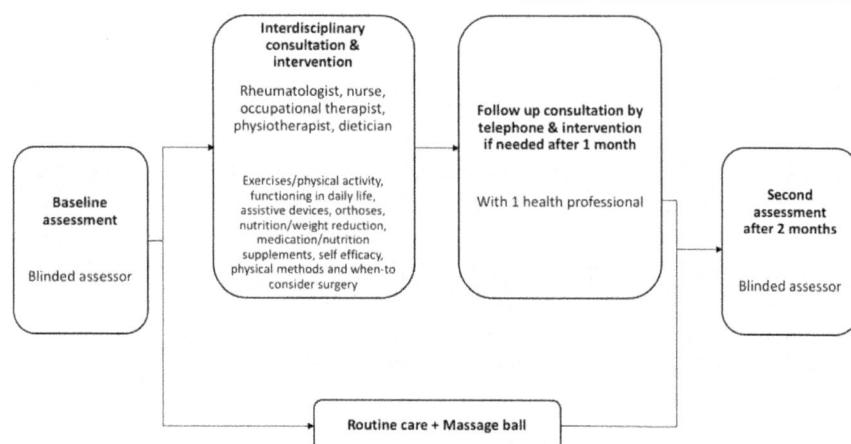

	All mentioned health professionals developed the intervention together. The combined intervention was delivered by an occupational therapist, physiotherapist, dietician and/or nurse according to their availability and the needs of the patient
Pain and difficulties with ADL assessment	Patients have been asked in detail about the pain they experience and asked to report three activities of daily living that are difficult to perform for them
Information and functioning consultation	The diagnosis made by the rheumatologist was explained to the patient in an easy and lay understandable format.
	Information on an active and healthy lifestyle, physical activity, nutrition supplements, nutrition and if necessary (BMI > 27) information about the benefit of an optimal bodyweight was given
	Possibilities of surgery were discussed briefly
	Strategies for self-efficacy, ergonomic principles and pacing strategies were explained to maximise physical functioning
Pain management	Information about medication, the resulting benefit and risks according to available guidelines was given. The value of thermotherapy was explained, especially the benefit of heat during stable periods and cold during inflamed periods. A hot and cold pack to apply hot and cold packing at home was provided free of charge for the patients
Assistive devices	According to the difficulties in daily living reported by the patient, aids and devices were discussed and shown to the patient. Opening screw-caps is a commonly reported problem. If a patient mentioned having problems with this task a non-slip mat (Dycem) was provided and patients were trained in opening glasses/bottles with this device
	All patients were assessed for the need of a CMC 1 joint orthosis (Additional file 1: Material 1 pictures of the CMC 1 orthosis). If required it was custom-made during the consultation
Hand exercises	Patients in the combined-intervention group received instructions for a home-exercise programme to enhance range of motion and grip strength. Detailed information about the hand exercise programme is given in Fig. 1. The therapy putty necessary for the exercise programme was directly provided from the interdisciplinary team free of charge for the patient
	Participants were instructed to exercise daily for 8 weeks with 10 repetitions during weeks 1–2, 12 repetitions in weeks 3–4 and 15 repetitions in weeks 5–8. Beside access to a web-based interactive online video showing the exercises for the hands, the programme was given in paper format to the participants. The programme is accessible following the link: https://elearning.fh-campuswien.ac.at/WBT/Fingerpolyarthrose/2014.html
Follow up	An appointment was scheduled for 8 weeks after the baseline intervention. Patients received a telephone number/email address to contact the therapist if they need further instructions after the consultation. After 1 month, patients received a follow-up telephone call from the therapist, who asked questions according to a standardised protocol, answered emerging questions and encouraged the patient to follow the advice given and the exercise regime
	Patients were advised to bring the used therapy putty to the follow-up session in order to examine the exercise adherence of the individuals in the intervention group

Patients received a booklet with general information, exercises, contact details from the health professionals and the link for the exercise video
ADL activities of daily living, *BMI* body mass index, *CMC* carpometacarpal, *OT* occupational therapist, *PT* physiotherapist, *RC* routine care

steroid injections or surgery during the study period were also excluded.

The combined intervention

The intervention was delivered by two rheumatology-trained health professionals who were present at the same time (either an occupational therapist, a physiotherapist, a nurse and/or a dietician), each of them having clinical expertise either in a primary or specialised care setting or both. They had to have at least 2 years of clinical experience in treating patients with rheumatic diseases. The assignment of the two health professionals was variable and depended on their availability at a specified patient visit.

The combined intervention, which is shown in detail in Table 1, Fig. 1 and Additional file 1: Material 1, included strengthening and mobility exercises and information about physical activity; a consultation on functioning in daily life; the provision of and information on assistive devices and orthoses; information on nutrition and weight reduction, if necessary (defined by body mass index > 27), information on medication and nutrition supplements; strategies for self-efficacy, self-application of physical methods and when-to consider surgery (Table 1).

Patients in the combined intervention group were informed in detail about medications for pain management but were encouraged to use as little analgesic medication as possible. Patients were advised to try topical substances before using oral ones if they required pain medication.

After the face-to-face intervention, which was done on an individual basis, patients could contact the health professionals via email or telephone. Apart from this possibility, a structured telephone follow-up intervention in the form of a consultation was scheduled one month after the initial session. A standardised telephone protocol was used for the follow ups; additionally, patients had the opportunity to ask questions and discuss matters relevant to them during the telephone call.

Routine care plus placebo

Patients in routine care received a massage ball as placebo intervention. Patients were instructed to roll the ball gently at the palmar and dorsal sides of their hands. In the routine care (RC) group, the decision about possible treatments or interventions was at the discretion of the rheumatologist, primary care physician or health professional seeing the patient. If considered necessary, patients were also allowed to be referred to occupational therapy, physiotherapy and a dietician for further instructions; however, these interventions were not structured according to the pre-specified protocol mentioned above. All participants in the study were allowed to use supportive medication during the trial. All interventions

and visits related to the patients' hand OA were documented during the study period.

Assessments, endpoints and sample size calculation

Assessments were carried out at baseline and after 2 months. Participants' sociodemographic data were obtained at baseline. Hand function is a complex concept including several motor, sensory and cognitive abilities of a person. While hand strength represents only one aspect of hand function [28], it is often used as an indicator of overall fitness and the level of physical activity. Hand strength, consisting of grip and pinch strength, is a reliable core outcome measurement for hand OA [29, 30]. Furthermore, the sensitivity to change for grip strength was found to be good [31]. We selected grip strength of the dominant hand as the primary outcome measure of our study in order to choose only one indicator. Grip strength was measured using a Martin Vigorimeter with a 43-mm rubber bulb [32, 33] (Vigorimeter, Martin Tuttlingen Germany). Three measurements were taken for both hands, and mean values were calculated for each hand.

Secondary Outcomes Were Hand Function Measured By Two Subtests Of The Jebsen-Taylor Hand Function Test (JTHFT) [34] (subtest 3 "picking up small common objects" and subtest 7 "picking up large heavy cans"), a self-report questionnaire of function - the Australian/ Canadian Hand Osteoarthritis Index (AUSCAN) [35, 36] and self-reported assessment of pain and satisfaction of patients with their health care and health status (on an 11-point Likert scale). Based on results from an earlier study [15], we calculated that group sizes of 64 were needed to achieve 80% power with an alpha level of 0.05 to detect a potentially significant difference between the null hypothesis that grip strength in both groups would not significantly change and the alternative hypothesis that grip strength would change with a medium effect size (Cohen's d of 0.5). We further estimated that 10% of the participants ($n = 6$) would drop out and therefore aimed at recruiting 70 participants for each group.

Randomisation

Patients were randomised to the combined-intervention group or the RC group with an allocation ratio of 1:1 based on stratification of baseline scores for grip strength. A person from the administrative staff who neither saw patients in the clinic nor was otherwise involved in the study, performed the randomisation. To ensure comparability of the two groups, randomisation was performed in blocks of 10 patients with a similar baseline grip-strength value. The allocation of the patients was determined by a randomisation number.

No.	Exercise illustration	Instructions
1.	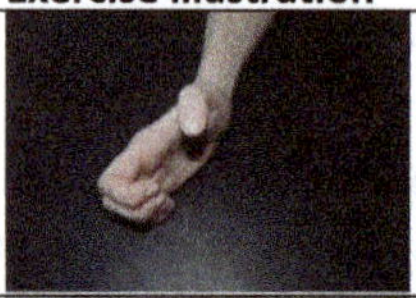	**Small fist** Flex the DIP and PIP joints of the 2nd to the 5th finger, the MCP joints of these fingers remain straight.
2.	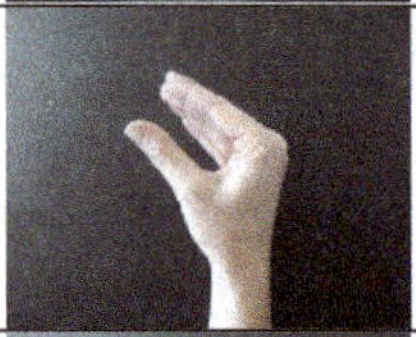	**Build a housetop** Flex the MCP of the 2nd to the 5th finger. The DIP and PIP joints of these fingers remain straight.
3.	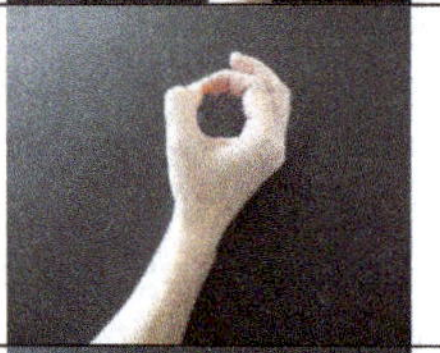	**Make O signs** Form a ring by touching with the thumb and each of the fingertips. It is important to form a ring that is really round.
4.	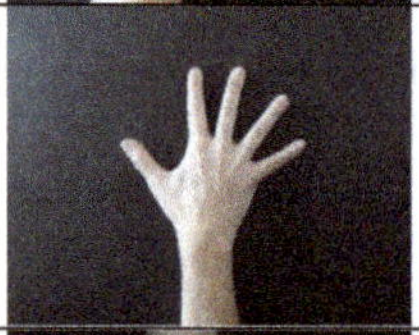	**Spread fingers** Lay down the hand on the table and spread the fingers. (All fingers stay in touch with the surface and stay extended.)
5.	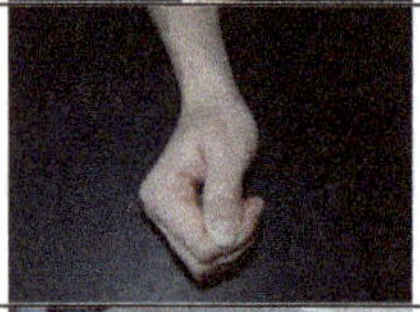	**Lateral pinch** The hand is positioned in a medial position. Touch with the tip of the thumb the index finger in the area of the PIP – press shortly and relax alternately.
6.		**Exercise with therapy putty** Build a ball with the therapy putty with one hand. Subsequently, build a roll with the therapy putty with one hand. "Pincer grip": Squeeze the roll with the thumb and the index finger. All fingertips touch each other. Wrap the roll around all fingers to form it to a ring. Open the hand against the resistance of the therapy putty.

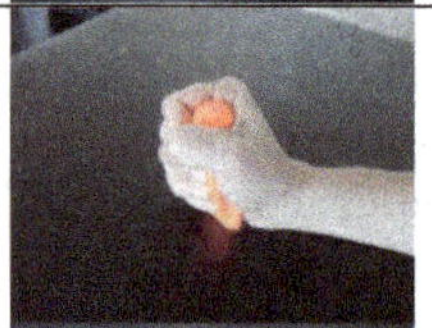

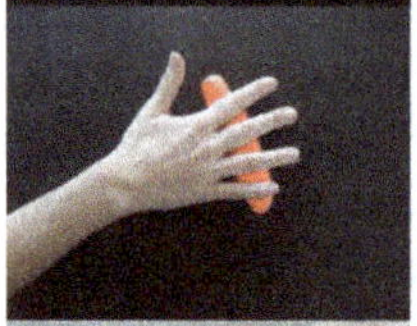

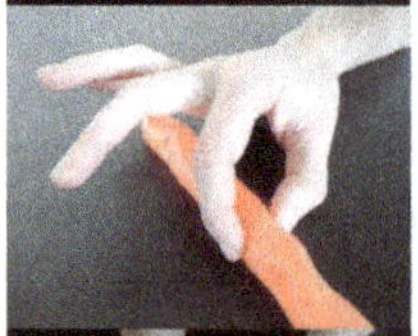

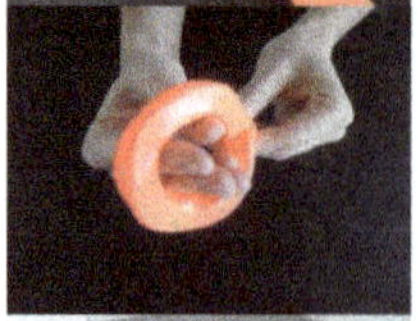

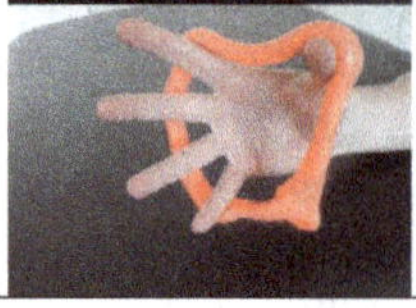

Fig. 1 The hand exercise programme. DIP, distal interphalangeal joint; MCP, metacarpophalangeal joint; PIP, proximal interphalangeal joint

Blinding

Assessors were blinded to all details of the study. Health professionals involved in the intervention did not collect clinical data from participants in this study. According to ethical and legal regulations, patients had to be informed in detail about the study, e.g. that a patient would be randomly allocated to one of two groups. However, we did not discuss with patients our assumption that the combined intervention might be preferable when compared to the placebo intervention. The health professionals who delivered the intervention saw only those patients who had been allocated to the intervention session. Nevertheless, it is a limitation of the study that, due to the nature of the method used, patients and health professionals delivering the intervention were not fully blinded.

Statistical methods

Descriptive statistics were used to describe the sample. Furthermore, data were assessed for normal/non-normal distribution using the Kolmogorov-Smirnov test. Differences in assessments between the groups at baseline and at month 2 were calculated by Students' t test for data with normal distribution and by the Mann-Whitney U test for variables with non-normal distribution. Analyses were performed according to an intention-to-treat approach. Missing data were imputed using the method of last observation carried forward. Due to multiple testing and therefore a larger risk of type 1 error, the significance level was adjusted according to Bonferroni (p value of 0.05/10 outcomes) leading to a new p value of 0.005. We adjusted for baseline values in the analysis in that we used differences between baseline and follow-up values of grip strength for each patient.

Furthermore, we fitted logistic regression models to explore the accuracy of our results: we explored the influence of the group allocation as an independent binary variable on the primary outcome, namely a potential improvement in grip strength of the (non-) dominant hand(s) from baseline to week 8. For this analysis, each patient was classified as either having improved or not. Any positive change in grip strength was classified as improvement as we expected small to moderate effects. IBM SPSS Statistics for Macintosh (Armonk, NY, USA), Version 24.0 was used for statistical analyses.

Results

Demographic data and patient flow

The whole sample was recruited between June 2012 and August 2014. One hundred and seventy-one individuals were informed about the study and were assessed for eligibility. Thereof, three patients declined to participate, six had other reasons for not participating in the study (e.g. long travelling distance to the hospital), and nine patients indicated a pain level < 3 on the day of the baseline assessment and did therefore not fulfil the inclusion criteria. One hundred and fifty-three individuals were randomised; of these, two individuals had a pain level < 3 at the second point in time (day of the intervention) and, therefore, were not included in the study.

The 151 patients fulfilling the inclusion/exclusion criteria were randomly assigned to the combined-intervention (n = 74) or the routine-care-plus-placebo (n = 77) groups (Fig. 2). There were no significant differences in baseline characteristics between the two groups (Table 2).

At the baseline assessment, 24 patients in the combined-intervention group and 27 in the routine-care-plus-placebo group indicated they had taken non-steroidal antirheumatics (NSAR). At the follow-up assessment, this number decreased to 13 patients in the combined-intervention group and 18 in the routine-care-plus-placebo group.

The follow-up assessment was completed by 59 participants (77%) in the intervention group and 69 participants (89%) in the routine-care-plus-placebo group: 12 patients in the intervention group and seven in the routine-care-plus-placebo group withdrew consent (Fig. 1). In each group, one serious adverse event occurred: in the intervention group one patient had hand surgery because of pre-existing carpal tunnel syndrome, and in the routine-care-plus-placebo group, one patient had a hand cast applied after an accident. Neither of the adverse events were considered to be related to the study intervention. Furthermore, two adverse events occurred in the intervention group (common cold and tendovaginitis, Additional file 1: Material 2). The tendovaginitis was considered possibly related to the intervention.

Primary and secondary endpoints

The primary endpoint, grip strength of the dominant hand improved in the combined intervention group and deteriorated in the routine-care-plus-placebo group compared to baseline values; the difference in change from baseline between the two groups at the end of the study was statistically significant (Table 3). A total of 28 patients (38%) improved in the combined-intervention group while in the routine-care group only 15 patients (19%) improved. There were 33 participants in both groups (routine-care group 45%, combined-intervention group 43%) with a grip strength value of 0 at the baseline assessment. At the follow-up assessment, this number increased to 37 (48%) in the routine-care group, but decreased in the combined-intervention group to 17 (23%).

Among the secondary outcomes, there was significant improvement in self-reported satisfaction with treatment and in the JTHFT subtests 7 for the non-dominant hand. There was no significant difference between the groups in change in the JTHFT subtest 3 for both hands and subtest

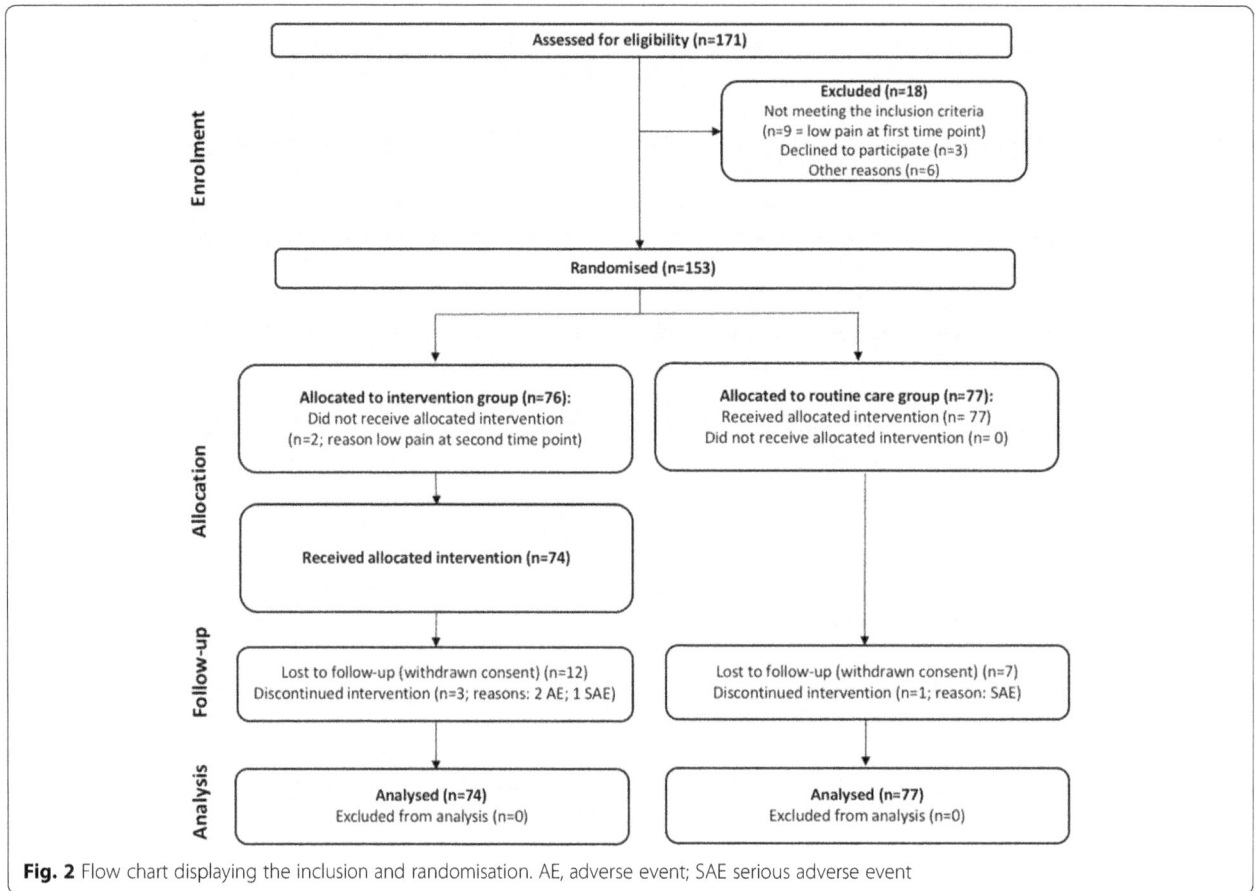

Fig. 2 Flow chart displaying the inclusion and randomisation. AE, adverse event; SAE serious adverse event

7 for the dominant hand, in the total AUSCAN score or in change in self-reported pain and health status.

The binominal univariate logistic regression models showed a significant contribution of the treatment/group allocation to the primary outcome (improved versus non-improved, model 1, $p = 0.012$; model 2, $p = 0.005$). The Nagelkerke R square (Table 4) indicated how much of the total variance was explained by each model. The chance to improve grip strength was 2.572 higher in model 1 (dominant hand) and 3.282 higher for model 2 (non-dominant hand) in the intervention group compared to the controls.

To obtain information about the compliance in the combined intervention group, we asked the patients to bring the therapy putty (used to perform the exercises) to the second assessment. After performing the follow-up assessment, assessors scored traces of usage in the therapy putty. In the combined intervention group, four patients (5%) had not used the therapy putty at all according to the judgement of the assessor. In 28 patients (38%), the therapy putty showed substantial traces of usage; the other patients did not bring the therapy putty to the second appointment. However, the combined intervention did not only consist of hand exercises with therapy putty, but also involved functional exercises

and exercises without therapy putty; we therefore included all patients in the analysis.

Patients not completing the study had lower grip strength values for both hands and a higher AUSCAN index (meaning poorer function) at baseline (Additional file 1: Material 4). This was seen in both treatment groups.

Discussion

The combined intervention in our study included several domains that may be important to individual patients. Combined interventions have the advantage of taking individual issues of patients into account. Patients are presented all options and can then make an informed decision about their preferences, main concerns and symptoms. "Exercise-only interventions" for example may not reach patients whose primary concern is not physical activity or loss of function, but pain and aesthetic changes related to hand OA. Combined interventions may be an option to cover all necessary issues and allow patients to set individual priorities. Furthermore, the effect of the intervention may be due to one or two or more components of the combined intervention. Individual combinations of components of interventions could maximize

Table 2 Baseline characteristics

Characteristics	All patients	Combined intervention	RC
Demographics			
Patient, n	151	74	77
Female, n (%)	127 (84)	59 (79.7)	68 (88.3)
Age, mean (SD), years	59.6 (10.6)	60.1 (10.9)	59.1 (10.4)
Disease duration, mean (SD), years	7.6 (9.4)	6.5 (9.2)	9.0 (9.6)
CMC 1 OA (in one or both hands), n (%)	75 (50)	36 (48.6)	39 (50.6)
Education (persons obtaining more than compulsory schooling), n (%)	74 (49)	37 (50)	37 (48)
Handedness, right handed, n (%)	134 (89)	62 (83.8)	72 (93.5)
BMI, mean (SD)	26.3 (4.8)	25.7 (4.4)	26.9 (5.1)
Self-reported satisfaction with appearance of hands on a LS[a], mean (SD)	1.50 (1.29)	1.47 (1.26)	1.53 (1.32)
Grip strength (Vigorimeter), dominant hand, mean (SD), bar	0.13 (0.19)	0.14 (0.18)	0.13 (0.20)
Grip strength (Vigorimeter), non-dominant hand, mean (SD), bar	0.13 (0.20)	0.14 (0.19)	0.12 (0.21)
Self-reported pain on a LS[a], mean (SD)	5.16 (2.095)	5.22 (1.96)	5.10 (2.23)
Self-reported satisfaction with treatment on a LS[a], mean (SD)	7.17 (2.96)	7.26 (2.53)	7.10 (3.30)
Self-reported health status on a LS[a], mean (SD)	3.99 (2.40)	3.78 (2.35)	4.18 (2.44)
JT Subtest 3, dominant hand, mean (SD)	8.04 (3.82)	7.79 (3.05)	8.28 (4.44)
JT Subtest 3, non-dominant hand, mean (SD)	8.01 (2.75)	7.98 (2.49)	8.05 (2.99)
JT Subtest 7, dominant hand	5.02 (1.49)	5.02 (1.26)	5.02 (1.69)
JT Subtest 7, non-dominant hand, mean (SD)	5.14 (2.23)	5.34 (2.68)	4.94 (1.67)
AUSCAN, mean (SD)	15.71 (4.87)	15.85 (4.08)	15.57 (5.53)

There were no statistically significant differences in baseline characteristics between the combined intervention group and the routine care group

AUSCAN Australian/Canadian Hand Osteoarthritis Index, *CMC 1* Carpometacarpal 1 joint, *JT* Jebsen-Taylor Hand Function Test, *OA* osteoarthritis, *RC* routine care

[a]LS = value examined on a Likert scale from 0 to 10

treatment effects without having an approach of "one intervention fits all" and without having to determine precise profiles/subgroups of patients who benefit most from the specific intervention components, e.g. active exercises. The effects of interventions such as exercises, joint protection, self-management strategies or orthoses in hand OA trials are often studied together, as they were in our study protocol [15, 24, 37]. Another approach was taken by Dziedizic et al. who tested the effect of independent components of hand OA interventions with a positive outcome for joint protection [38].

Table 3 Effect of intervention: differences within the groups

	Combined intervention difference (FU - BL) (mean (SD))	RC difference (FU - BL) (mean (SD))	p value
Grip strength (Vigorimeter), dominant hand, bar	0.03 (0.11)	−0.03 (0.13)	*0.001*
Grip strength (Vigorimeter), non-dominant hand, bar	0.01 (0.10)	−0.03 (0.13)	*0.002*
Self-reported pain on a LS[ab]	−1.35 (2.38)	−0.88 (2.12)	0.339
Self-reported satisfaction with treatment on a LS[ab]	−3.50 (3.37)	− 0.92 (2.95)	*0.002*
Self-reported health status on a LS[ab]	−0.04 (2.00)	−0.44 (2.20)	0.291
JT Subtest 3, dominant hand	−0.55 (1.79)	−0.47 (2.65)	0.193
JT Subtest 3, non-dominant hand	−0.41 (1.96)	0.19 (2.85)	0.010
JT Subtest 7, dominant hand	−0.32 (1.01)	−0.06 (1.30)	0.134
JT Subtest 7, non-dominant hand	−0.39 (1.12)	0.33 (1.27)	*0.000*
AUSCAN[b]	−1.55 (4.95)	−0.63 (4.12)	0.316

Bonferroni adjustment 0.05/10 = 0.005. Mean change - 95% CI - *p*-value

AUSCAN Australian/Canadian Hand Osteoarthritis Index, *BL* baseline, *FU* follow up, *JT* Jebsen-Taylor Hand Function Test, *RC* routine care

p values set in italics indicate statistical significance

[a]LS = on a Likert scale from 0 to 10

[b]Information on both hands is shown due to how the test/questionnaire is administered

Table 4 Binominal logistic regression models

#	Primary outcome grip strength Vigorimeter	Nagelkerke R square	Significance	Odds ratio	Confidence interval
Model 1	Dominant hand	0.062	0.012	2.572	1.233–5.365
Model 2	Non-dominant hand	0.085	0.005	3.282	1.439–7.485

In our study, we developed a time-efficient and personnel-efficient standardised intervention that could be delivered by different non-physician health professionals who were all trained in rheumatology. Our intervention was standardised and was delivered according to a protocol (Table 1) that can be used by health professionals in primary and specialist care settings. Given the number of patients with hand OA and the limited clinical resources, having an intervention that may be delivered by multiple health professionals could be very beneficial. One individual session might have the advantage, compared to a group session, that health professionals can focus explicitly on the needs of the patient and tailor the information according to the patient's personal needs.

Grip strength was chosen as the primary endpoint because strength is an integral part of hand function, although other aspects may be equally relevant [15, 39, 40]. Osteras et al. concluded that further studies should focus on optimal grip strength exercises [41]. In another RCT, significant improvement in grip strength and activity performance was attained with a home-based hand exercise programme for hand OA [42]. On the other hand, a study involving a multidisciplinary group-based treatment for patients with hand OA showed no effect on grip strength and other outcomes, potentially due to a non-directive approach (patients should select and also develop their own treatment goals and treatment plans) [24].

The difference in grip strength compared to baseline in the intervention group was smaller than expected; however, we consider this result to be clinically significant for three reasons: (1) grip strength deteriorated in the control group over the time period more than it improved in the intervention group, (2) non-pharmacological interventions in rehabilitation in general produce small effects and (3) an intervention with a low, but for the patients acceptable (and satisfying) intensity such as our combined intervention may be used to stabilize rather than to largely improve grip strength.

Some of our secondary outcomes did not show significant effects. The self-reported questionnaire for function probably assesses items that are not relevant to all patients, and some assessed activities are important for selected patients only. While pain may be the main concern of one patient, loss of function may be more important for other patients. Personalized outcome measures, such as the Canadian Occupational Performance Measure [43] in which patients can select certain activities for some domains - e.g. self-care, productivity and leisure - may be an option in future clinical trials, especially if the intervention is tailored to improve occupational performance. There was a reduction in self-reported pain between baseline and follow-up examinations in both groups (Table 3). One possible explanation for this finding may be the greater attention received by patients in both groups.

The results from the two logistic models also confirmed that participants in the combined intervention group had a greater chance of improving grip strength. However, a large number of participants in both groups had a grip strength value of 0 in both the baseline assessment and in follow up. It remains an important issue for further research as to how this group of participants can be effectively treated.

The drop-out rate in the routine-care-group was lower compared to the combined intervention group. This could be related to the fact that the combined intervention was offered to the patients in the routine-care group after the second assessment and that the symptoms in the control group did not improve much with the placebo intervention. Therefore, there may have been greater motivation to return for another assessment.

Existing guidelines and standards of care are frequently not implemented. Our intervention was based on the EUMUSC.net standards of care for OA and can therefore be seen as an example of how the standards can be implemented.

There is currently no disease-modifying drug available for hand OA, and to our knowledge, there is no gold standard design for a programme of non-pharmacological interventions (intervention selection, duration and the intensity/frequency). We focused on interdisciplinary care. To this end, health professionals were trained to cover parts of the interventions that were developed by professionals from other health professions, e.g. physiotherapists and nurses were trained to custom-fabricate a thumb splint. In addition, the intervention was delivered by two health professionals present at the same time to ensure a well-coordinated, effective intervention in different areas of expertise.

While a strength of our study is the detailed and feasible treatment approach for hand OA, our study has limitations as well: one is the choice of instrument to measure grip strength, which had floor effects. Another is that the presence of two health professionals to deliver the intervention might reduce cost-effectiveness. Third, it is evident that due to the type of study, the blinding of patients and the professionals delivering the intervention is lacking. We cannot fully eliminate the possibility that this might have influenced our results e.g. the self-reported outcome measures completed by the patient. However, assessments were made by blinded assessors, the primary outcome was grip strength and data were analysed by the first and last authors, who were not involved in randomisation, nor in the assessment of the patients.

In our study, we applied the combined intervention to patients with finger and/or thumb symptoms. As the aetiology of finger and thumb symptoms may also differ, the response to treatment could also be diverse. This should be investigated in further research.

Conclusion

The combined, interdisciplinary, individual, one-session intervention significantly improved grip strength and self-reported satisfaction when compared to treatment with routine care plus placebo. This may be an effective and satisfying time-efficient approach in busy clinical settings in both primary and specialised care, which can be delivered by rheumatology-trained non-physician health professionals.

Abbreviations
AUSCAN: Australian/Canadian Hand Osteoarthritis Index; CMC 1: Carpometacarpal 1 joint; JTHFT: Jebsen-Taylor Hand Function Test; OA: Osteoarthritis; RC: Routine care; RCT: Randomised controlled trial

Acknowledgements
We thank Martina Durechova, Marion Skobek, Stefanie Haider, Michaela Lehner, Mona Dür and Regina Fellner for their support during the study.

Funding
This study was supported by the following organisations:

1. The EU Commission with the project number 20081301EU Grant Agreement
2. The professional organisation for occupational therapists "Ergotherapie Austria" and the professional organisation for physiotherapists "Physio Austria"
3. A restricted grant of the Austrian Science Fund (P21912-B09) and
4. The randomised controlled trial was awarded with the "Projektförderpreis" of the "Österreichische Gesellschaft für Rheumatologie & Rehabilitation" in the year 2012.

The funding bodies did not influence the content of the study.
Role of the funding sources
The Sponsor of the study, the Department of Medicine 3, Medical University of Vienna (MUW), Austria designed the study with all authors involved. The funding sources did not influence the design, the results or the reporting of this study.

Authors' contributions
Conception and design: MAS, MK, SL, SMK, MZT, VN, JZ, IK, MH, SÖ, AW, KR, JSS, TAS; analysis and interpretation of data: MAS, MK, SL, TAS; drafting the article and revising it critically for content: MAS, MK, SL, SMK, MZT, VN, JZ, IK, MH, SÖ, AW, KR, JSS, TAS. All authors approved the final version.

Consent for publication
The present manuscript does not contain any individual person's data, such as individual details, images or videos.

Competing interests
MAS has received speaker fees from MSD; none of them relate to this work.
MK has received speaker fees from AbbVie; none of them relate to this work.
SL has received speaker fees from MSD; none of them relate to this work.
SMK has no competing interests.
MZT has no competing interests.
VN has received speaker's fees from Eli Lilly, Novartis and Pfizer. None of these relate to this work.
JZ has received honoraria/speaker's fees from AbbVie, Astra Zeneca, AstroPharma, BMS, Celgene, MSD, Pfizer and Roche; none of them relate to this work.
IK has no competing interests.
MH has no competing interests.
SÖ has no competing interests.
AW has no competing interests.
KR has received honoraria from AbbVie, Amgen, BMS, Wyeth, Jansen, Roche, Schering-Plough and Sanofi-Aventis; none of them relate to this work.
JSS has received honoraria from AbbVie, Amgen, BMS, Wyeth, Jansen, Roche, Schering-Plough and Sanofi-Aventis; none of them relate to this work.
TAS has received speaker's fees from AbbVie, Janssen, MSD and Roche; none of them relate to this work.

Author details
[1]Section for Outcomes Research, Center for Medical Statistics, Informatics, and Intelligent Systems, Medical University of Vienna, Spitalgasse 23, 1090 Vienna, Austria. [2]Division of Rheumatology, Department of Medicine 3, Medical University of Vienna, Vienna, Austria. [3]Department of Health Sciences, University of Applied Sciences FH Campus Wien, Favoritenstraße 226, 1100 Vienna, Austria. [4]Physio Austria, Lange Gasse 30/1, Vienna, Austria. [5]Klinikum Peterhof of NOEGKK with Ludwig Boltzmann Department of Epidemiology of Rheumatic Diseases, Sauerhofstraße 9-15, Baden bei Wien, Austria. [6]Ludwig Boltzmann Institute of Osteology, 1st Medical Department at Hanusch Hospital, Hanusch Hospital of the WGKK and AUVA Trauma Center, Heinrich Collin Str. 30, 1140 Vienna, Austria. [7]National advisory unit on rehabilitation in rheumatology, Department of rheumatology, Diakonhjemmet Hospital, Oslo, Norway. [8]Program of Occupational Therapy, Prosthetics and Orthotics, Oslo Metropolitan University, Oslo, Norway. [9]Ergotherapie Austria, Bundesverband der Ergotherapeutinnen und Ergotherapeuten Österreichs, Holzmeistergasse 7-9/2/1, Vienna, Austria. [10]University of Applied Sciences for Health Professions Upper Austria, Semmelweisstraße 34, Linz, Austria. [11]Bone and Joint Research Group, Royal Cornwall Hospital, Truro, UK.

References
1. WHO. The world health report 2004. Available from: http://www.who.int/whr/2004/en/report04_en.pdf?ua=1. 31 Oct 2018.
2. Altman R, et al. Development of criteria for the classification and reporting of osteoarthritis. Classification of osteoarthritis of the knee. Diagnostic and Therapeutic Criteria Committee of the American Rheumatism Association. Arthritis Rheum. 1986;29(8):1039–49.

3. Kraus VB. Pathogenesis and treatment of osteoarthritis. Med Clin North Am. 1997;81(1):85–112.

4. Dahaghin S, et al. Prevalence and pattern of radiographic hand osteoarthritis and association with pain and disability (the Rotterdam study). Ann Rheum Dis. 2005;64(5):682–7.

5. Dahaghin S, et al. Prevalence and determinants of one month hand pain and hand related disability in the elderly (Rotterdam study). Ann Rheum Dis. 2005;64(1):99–104.

6. Bagis S, et al. The effect of hand osteoarthritis on grip and pinch strength and hand function in postmenopausal women. Clin Rheumatol. 2003;22(6):420–4.

7. Bukhave EB, Huniche L. Activity problems in everyday life—patients' perspectives of hand osteoarthritis: "try imagining what it would be like having no hands". Disabil Rehabil. 2014;36(19):1636–43.

8. Ricci JA, et al. Pain exacerbation as a major source of lost productive time in US workers with arthritis. Arthritis Rheum. 2005;53(5):673–81.

9. Cimmino MA, et al. Clinical presentation of osteoarthritis in general practice: determinants of pain in Italian patients in the AMICA study. Semin Arthritis Rheum. 2005;35(1 Suppl 1):17–23.

10. Stamm T, et al. Patient perspective of hand osteoarthritis in relation to concepts covered by instruments measuring functioning: a qualitative European multicentre study. Ann Rheum Dis. 2009;68(9):1453–60.

11. Michon M, Maheu E, Berenbaum F. Assessing health-related quality of life in hand osteoarthritis: a literature review. Ann Rheum Dis. 2011;70(6):921–8.

12. Zhang Y, et al. Prevalence of symptomatic hand osteoarthritis and its impact on functional status among the elderly: The Framingham Study. Am J Epidemiol. 2002;156(11):1021–7.

13. Kloppenburg M. Hand osteoarthritis-nonpharmacological and pharmacological treatments. Nat Rev Rheumatol. 2014;10(4):242–51.

14. Zhang W, et al. EULAR evidence based recommendations for the management of hand osteoarthritis: report of a Task Force of the EULAR Standing Committee for International Clinical Studies Including Therapeutics (ESCISIT). Ann Rheum Dis. 2007;66(3):377–88.

15. Stamm TA, et al. Joint protection and home hand exercises improve hand function in patients with hand osteoarthritis: a randomized controlled trial. Arthritis Rheum. 2002;47(1):44–9.

16. Kjeken I, et al. Systematic review of design and effects of splints and exercise programs in hand osteoarthritis. Arthritis Care Res (Hoboken). 2011; 63(6):834–48.

17. Kloppenburg M, et al. 2018 Update of the EULAR recommendations for the management of hand osteoarthritis. Ann Rheum Dis. 2018. https://doi.org/10. 1136/annrheumdis-2018-213826. [Epub ahead of print].

18. Stoffer MA, et al. Development of patient-centred standards of care for osteoarthritis in Europe: the eumusc.net-project. Ann Rheum Dis. 2015;74(6): 1145–9.

19. Moe RH, et al. Facilitators to implement standards of care for rheumatoid arthritis and osteoarthritis: the EUMUSC.NET project. Ann Rheum Dis. 2014; 73(8):1545–8.

20. Loza E, et al. Feasibility and efficacy of a multidisciplinary health care programme for patients with knee osteoarthritis. Clin Exp Rheumatol. 2011; 29(6):913–20.

21. Smink AJ, et al. "Beating osteoARThritis": development of a stepped care strategy to optimize utilization and timing of non-surgical treatment modalities for patients with hip or knee osteoarthritis. Clin Rheumatol. 2011; 30(12):1623–9.

22. Cuperus N, et al. Randomized trial of the effectiveness of a non-pharmacological multidisciplinary face-to-face treatment program on daily function compared to a telephone-based treatment program in patients with generalized osteoarthritis. Osteoarthr Cartil. 2015;23(8):1267–75.

23. Moe RH, et al. Effectiveness of an Integrated Multidisciplinary Osteoarthritis Outpatient Program versus Outpatient Clinic as Usual: a randomized controlled trial. J Rheumatol. 2016;43(2):411–8.

24. Stukstette MJ, et al. No evidence for the effectiveness of a multidisciplinary group based treatment program in patients with osteoarthritis of hands on the short term; results of a randomized controlled trial. Osteoarthr Cartil. 2013;21(7):901–10.

25. Schulz KF, Altman DG, Moher D. CONSORT 2010 statement: Updated guidelines for reporting parallel group randomised trials. J Pharmacol Pharmacother. 2010;1(2):100–7.

26. Boutron I, et al. Extending the CONSORT statement to randomized trials of nonpharmacologic treatment: explanation and elaboration. Ann Intern Med. 2008;148(4):295–309.

27. Altman R, et al. The American College of Rheumatology criteria for the classification and reporting of osteoarthritis of the hand. Arthritis Rheum. 1990;33(11):1601–10.

28. Stamm TA, et al. Content comparison of occupation-based instruments in adult rheumatology and musculoskeletal rehabilitation based on the International Classification of Functioning, Disability and Health (ICF). Arthritis Rheum. 2004;51(6):917–24.

29. Kloppenburg M, et al. OARSI clinical trials recommendations: design and conduct of clinical trials for hand osteoarthritis. Osteoarthr Cartil. 2015;23(5): 772–86.

30. Visser AW, et al. Instruments measuring pain, physical function, or patient's global assessment in hand osteoarthritis: a systematic literature search. J Rheumatol. 2015;42(11):2118–34.

31. Dominick KL, et al. Relationship of radiographic and clinical variables to pinch and grip strength among individuals with osteoarthritis. Arthritis Rheum. 2005;52(5):1424–30.

32. Kleven T, Russwurm H, Finsen V. Tendon interposition arthroplasty for basal joint arthrosis. 38 thumbs followed for 4 years. Acta Orthop Scand. 1996; 67(6):575–7.

33. Jones E, et al. Strength and function in the normal and rheumatoid hand. J Rheumatol. 1991;18(9):1313–8.

34. Jebsen RH, et al. An objective and standardized test of hand function. Arch Phys Med Rehabil. 1969;50(6):311–9.

35. Bellamy N, et al. Clinimetric properties of the AUSCAN Osteoarthritis Hand Index: an evaluation of reliability, validity and responsiveness. Osteoarthr Cartil. 2002;10(11):863–9.

36. Bellamy N, et al. Dimensionality and clinical importance of pain and disability in hand osteoarthritis: development of the Australian/Canadian (AUSCAN) Osteoarthritis Hand Index. Osteoarthr Cartil. 2002;10(11):855–62.

37. Boustedt C, Nordenskiold U, Lundgren Nilsson A. Effects of a hand-joint protection programme with an addition of splinting and exercise: one year follow-up. Clin Rheumatol. 2009;28(7):793–9.

38. Dziedzic K, et al. Self-management approaches for osteoarthritis in the hand: a 2x2 factorial randomised trial. Ann Rheum Dis. 2015;74(1):108–18.

39. Bohannon RW. Hand-grip dynamometry provides a valid indication of upper extremity strength impairment in home care patients. J Hand Ther. 1998;11(4):258–60.

40. Nordenskiold U, Grimby G. Assessments of disability in women with rheumatoid arthritis in relation to grip force and pain. Disabil Rehabil. 1997; 19(1):13–9.

41. Osteras N, et al. Limited effects of exercises in people with hand osteoarthritis: results from a randomized controlled trial. Osteoarthr Cartil. 2014;22(9):1224–33.

42. Hennig T, et al. Effect of home-based hand exercises in women with hand osteoarthritis: a randomised controlled trial. Ann Rheum Dis. 2015;74(8):1501–8.

43. Law M, et al. The Canadian occupational performance measure: an outcome measure for occupational therapy. Can J Occup Ther. 1990;57(2):82–7.

19

Effects of a 15-month anti-TNF-α treatment on plasma levels of glycosaminoglycans in women with rheumatoid arthritis

Anna Szeremeta[1*], Agnieszka Jura-Półtorak[1], Ewa Maria Koźma[1], Andrzej Głowacki[1], Eugeniusz Józef Kucharz[2], Magdalena Kopeć-Mędrek[2] and Krystyna Olczyk[1]

Abstract

Background: In this study, the effect of 15-month anti-tumor necrosis factor alpha (TNF-α) treatment on circulating levels of plasma sulfated glycosaminoglycans (GAGs) and the nonsulfated GAG hyaluronic acid (HA) in female rheumatoid arthritis (RA) patients was assessed.

Methods: Plasma was obtained from healthy subjects and RA women treated with TNF-α antagonists (etanercept or adalimumab or certolizumab pegol) in combination with methotrexate. GAGs were isolated from plasma samples using ion exchange low-pressure liquid chromatography. Total sulfated GAGs were quantified using a hexuronic acid assay. Plasma levels of keratan sulfate (KS) and HA were measured using immunoassay kits.

Results: Total sulfated GAGs and HA levels were higher in female RA patients before treatment in comparison to healthy subjects. KS levels did not differ between RA women and controls. Anti-TNF-α treatment resulted in normalization of plasma total GAG and HA levels in RA patients, without any effect on KS levels.

Conclusions: Our results suggest that anti-TNF-α therapy has a beneficial effect on extracellular matrix remodeling in the course of RA.

Keywords: Rheumatoid arthritis, Tumor necrosis factor-alpha inhibitors, Glycosaminoglycans, Keratan sulfate, Hyaluronic acid

Background

Rheumatoid arthritis (RA) is a chronic, systemic, autoimmune connective tissue disease characterized by nonspecific arthritis of symmetric joints, as well as progressive articular cartilage degradation and bone erosion [1]. In the course of the disease there are numerous extra-articular organ manifestations which are the major causes of fast-growing patient disability. RA is associated with a higher mortality rate compared to that of the general population. RA affects approximately 0.5–1.5% of the world's population at any age. The incidence peaks in the 40–50 age group and women suffer from RA nearly two or three times more frequently than men [2–4].

Despite many studies, the causes of RA are still not completely known [3–5]. Tumor necrosis factor alpha (TNF-α) is one of the main proinflammatory cytokines, playing a key role in the pathogenesis of the disease. It has been shown that TNF-α stimulates catabolic processes in the cartilage tissue and periarticular structures and significantly affects the induction and persistence of inflammation [4–7]. Some of the integral elements of chronic inflammation are the structural and functional changes in extracellular matrix (ECM) compounds, including proteoglycans (PGs) and their sugar constituents—that is, glycosaminoglycans (GAGs) [8, 9]. The latter are negatively charged unbranched polysaccharides consisting of repeating disaccharide units of hexosamine and uronic acid or galactose. Chondroitin/dermatan sulfate (CS/DS), heparan sulfate/heparin (HS/H), keratan sulfate (KS), and hyaluronic acid (HA) represent the major species of GAGs. All GAG types, except HA, are

* Correspondence: aszeremeta@sum.edu.pl
[1]Department of Clinical Chemistry and Laboratory Diagnostics, School of Pharmacy with the Division of Laboratory Medicine in Sosnowiec, Medical University of Silesia in Katowice, Jedności 8, 41-200 Sosnowiec, Poland
Full list of author information is available at the end of the article

covalently attached to the core protein, forming PGs, and exhibit various degrees of sulfation along the polysaccharide chain [10–12]. This structural heterogeneity allows GAGs to interact with and modify the actions of numerous cell-adhesion molecules, growth factors, cytokines, chemokines, components of ECM, proteases, and their inhibitors, which underlie their important biological functions, including cellular communication, cell signaling, and regulation of other biochemical pathways [10, 13]. Hence, every modification of GAG metabolism may play a crucial role in RA pathogenesis. The disturbed balance between biosynthesis and degradation of PGs/GAGs as a consequence of chronic inflammation during RA should be reflected in the concentration of plasma GAGs. Friman et al. [14] suggested that in patients suffering from an active, erosive form of RA, the total plasma GAG content is not different as compared to controls. On the other hand, Jura-Półtorak et al. [15] described an increase in the total plasma GAG level in patients with RA.

The introduction of biologic drugs which neutralize TNF-α activity was a breakthrough in RA treatment. The results of clinical trials revealed a significant reduction of disease activity and inhibition of radiological progression, as well as improvement in the quality of life and physical function in RA patients treated with TNF-α inhibitors (TNFαI) [16–18]. However, the effect of anti-TNF therapy on PG/GAG metabolism in RA is still unknown. Therefore, the main objective of this study was the quantitative evaluation of total plasma sulfated and nonsulfated GAGs in female RA patients, both before and during 15 months of anti-TNF-α therapy.

Methods
Patients and samples
Forty-five female patients (mean ± SD age 47.42 ± 13.70 years) meeting the 1987 revised criteria and the 2010 American College of Rheumatology (ACR)/European League Against Rheumatism (EULAR) diagnostic criteria for RA [19, 20] were recruited for this study. All subjects had a Disease Activity Score of 28 joints (DAS28) > 5.1 despite application of at least two disease-modifying anti-rheumatic drugs at trial entry. Exclusion criteria included previous treatment with biologic agents, withdrawing from the biologic therapy during the study period, presence of illnesses (other autoimmune diseases, infections, heart failure, diabetes mellitus, thyroid disorders, kidney, and liver disease or malignancies), pregnancy, and breast-feeding. Moreover, all of the female RA patients participated in Polish National Health Fund Therapeutic Programs employing TNF blockers—that is, B.33: "Treatment of aggressive forms of rheumatoid arthritis (RA) and juvenile idiopathic arthritis (JIA)" (03.0000.333.02), or B.45: "Treatment of an aggressive

form of rheumatoid arthritis (03.0000.345.02)"—which were valid during 2012–2014. Twenty-two patients received adalimumab 40 mg subcutaneously every other week and 19 patients self-administered etanercept 50 mg by subcutaneous injection once a week, and four patients received certolizumab pegol 400 mg subcutaneously at weeks 0, 2, and 4 followed by 200 mg every 2 weeks thereafter for a period of 15 months. Patients were continuing current antirheumatic therapy, including methotrexate (25 mg/week) and prednisone (≤ 7.5 mg/day). All subjects were given folic acid in the dose of 5 mg/day. Concomitant medications remained unchanged for the duration of the study. Baseline characteristics of patients are presented in Table 1.

The effectiveness of TNFαI treatment was assessed at the baseline of the study and 3, 9, and 15 months after starting anti-TNF-α therapy using the DAS28 indicator, calculated on the basis of the number of swollen and tender joints from among the 28 joints included, the erythrocyte sedimentation rate (ESR), and the patient's global assessment of disease activity on a visual analog scale (VAS) of 100 mm. Furthermore, at each visit, patients were submitted to laboratory tests, such as complete blood count, markers of inflammation including the ESR and C-reactive protein (CRP), creatinine, and liver enzymes. Changes in clinical characteristics during the 15-month TNFαI therapy are summarized in Table 2. Patients who did not experience an

Table 1 Baseline characteristics of female RA patients treated with TNFαI

Characteristic	Value
All women with RA, n (%)	45 (100)
Age (years), mean (SD)	47.42 (13.70)
Disease duration (years), median (IQR)	7 (4–16)
BMI (kg/m²), mean (SD)	21.99 (2.26)
RF positive, n (%)	44 (97.78)
Anti-CCP positive, n (%)	45 (100)
SJC28, median (IQR)	8 (5–10)
TJC28, median (IQR)	14 (10–19)
VAS, median (IQR)	80 (80–80)
DAS28 ESR, mean (SD)	6.10 (0.58)
ESR (mm/h), median (IQR)	18.0 (11.0–33.0)
CRP (mg/l), median (IQR)	5.0 (4.0–14.9)
TNFαI therapy, n (%)	
Etanercept (Enbrel)	19 (42.22)
Adalimumab (Humira)	22 (48.89)
Certolizumab pegol (Cimzia)	4 (8.89)

anti-CCP anti-cyclic citrullinated peptide antibody, *BMI* body mass index, *CRP* C-reactive protein, *DAS28* Disease Activity Score based on evaluation of 28 joints, *ESR* erythrocyte sedimentation rate, *IQR* interquartile range, *RA* rheumatoid arthritis, *RF* rheumatoid factor, *SD* standard deviation, *SJC28* swollen joint count of 28 joints, *TJC28* tender joint count of 28 joints, *TNFαI* tumor necrosis factor-alpha inhibitors, *VAS* visual analog scale

adequate treatment response were excluded from the study. Adequate treatment response in accordance with the principles of the Polish National Health Fund Therapeutic Programs was defined as reduction in DAS28 > 1.2 after the first 3 months of therapy with a TNF-α inhibitor, and further reduction in DAS28 by 1.2 recorded during subsequent medical examinations performed 9 and 15 months after administration of the first dose of TNFαI.

Twenty age-matched healthy female volunteers from the Medical University of Silesia in Katowice, Poland were investigated as controls. Subjects were selected after their medical history, clinical examination, and laboratory screening had been obtained. All volunteers enrolled in this study did not have any diseases that required hospitalization and did not undergo surgical procedures during the previous 3 years. Furthermore, the results of their routine laboratory tests (i.e., complete blood count, ESR, fasting glucose, fasting lipid profile, creatinine, liver enzymes, rheumatoid factor (RF), and CRP) were within the reference range. Subjects were excluded if they took steroidal or nonsteroidal anti-inflammatory drugs. None of the volunteers smoked cigarettes or had any history of drug or alcohol abuse. We selected women who could maintain a healthy body weight and had a body mass index (BMI) < 25 kg/m^2.

On the day of collecting the plasma, prior to that procedure, patients met with rheumatologists for clinical visits, during which assessment of the patient, the physical visual analog scale of disease (VAS), the tender joint count of 28 joints (TJC28), the swollen joint count of 28 joints (SJC28), and the DAS28 were made. Venous blood samples were drawn between 7.00 and 9.00 am after overnight fasting, and were collected into citrate-treated (extraction and determination of plasma GAGs) and heparin-treated (measurement of plasma KS and HA levels) tubes. Plasma samples obtained from healthy subjects and RA patients were separated and stored at −80 °C until the time of analysis.

Table 2 Time-course changes in biochemical, clinical, and functional measures during 15-month anti-TNF-α therapy

	Time after starting anti-TNF-α therapy			
	T$_0$ (baseline)	T$_1$ (3 months)	T$_2$ (9 months)	T$_3$ (15 months)
Women with RA, n (%)	29 (100)			
Age (years), mean (SD)	44.38 (14.17)			
Disease duration (years), median (IQR)	5 (3–8)			
BMI (kg/m^2), mean (SD)	21.25 (2.28)			
RF positive, n (%)	29 (100)			
Anti-CCP positive, n (%)	29 (100)			
SJC28, median (IQR)	6 (5–10)	3 (2–3)[a, c, d]	0 (0–1)[a, b]	0 (0–0)[a, b]
TJC28, median (IQR)	14 (10–20)	5 (3–7)[a, c, d]	2 (1–2)[a, b, d]	0 (0–1)[a, b, c]
VAS, median (IQR)	80 (80–80)	50 (35–55)[a, c, d]	25 (10–30)[a, c, d]	10 (5–20)[a, b, c]
DAS28 ESR, mean (SD)	5.99 (0.50)	4.00 (0.73)[a, c, d]	2.74 (0.72)[a, b, d]	2.06 (0.64)[a, b, c]
Disease activity, n (%)				
High (> 5.1)	29 (100)	2 (6.90)	0	0
Moderate (> 3.2 and ≤ 5.1)	0	24 (82.76)	6 (20.69)	0
Low (≤ 3.2 and > 2.6)	0	3 (10.34)	12 (41.38)	6 (20.69)
Remission (≤ 2.6)	0	0	11 (37.93)	23 (79.31)
ESR (mm/h), median (IQR)	15.0 (10.0–31.0)	10.0 (8.0–17.0)	10.0 (8.0–14.0)[a]	11.0 (8.0–14.0)[a]
CRP (mg/l), median (IQR)	5.0 (4.0–9.2)	4.0 (2.0–4.0)	3.0 (1.30–4.0)[a]	2.0 (1.0–4.0)[a]
TNFαI therapy, n (%)				
Etanercept (Enbrel)	13 (44.83)			
Adalimumab (Humira)	14 (48.27)			
Certolizumab pegol (Cimzia)	2 (6.90)			

Differences noted for all variables (except DAS28 ESR) considered significant at $p < 0.0083$ by applying Bonferroni correction. Differences noted for DAS28 ESR considered significant at $p < 0.001$

anti-CCP anti-cyclic citrullinated peptide antibody, *BMI* body mass index, *CRP* C-reactive protein, *DAS28* Disease Activity Score based on evaluation of 28 joints, *ESR* erythrocyte sedimentation rate, *IQR* interquartile range, *RA* rheumatoid arthritis, *RF* rheumatoid factor, *SD* standard deviation, *SJC28* swollen joint count of 28 joints, *TJC28* tender joint count of 28 joints, *TNF-α* tumor necrosis factor alpha, *TNFαI* tumor necrosis factor-alpha inhibitors, *VAS* Visual analog scale
[a]Statistically significant differences compared to T$_0$
[b]Statistically significant differences compared to T$_1$
[c]Statistically significant differences compared to T$_2$
[d]Statistically significant differences compared to T$_3$

During the entire investigation period we followed the guidelines and regulations of the Helsinki Declaration in 1975, as revised in 1983. The Ethical Committee of the Medical University of Silesia in Katowice approved the research protocol used in this study. All healthy volunteers and RA patients provided written informed consent.

Extraction and determination of total plasma GAG levels

Sulfated GAGs were isolated using the methods of Lu et al. [21] and Capobianco et al. [22]. Firstly, plasma samples (1 ml) were pretreated for 24 h at 37 °C with Benzonase (E1014; Sigma) for the removal of nucleic acids. Next, plasma samples were submitted to exhaustive digestion with *Streptomyces griseus* protease (P0652; Sigma) in order to release GAG chains from plasma PG core proteins. This proteolysis was performed in 20 mM Tris–HCl, pH 9.0, containing 4 mM $CaCl_2$, at 56 °C for 24 h. After incubation, the samples were centrifuged at $19,000 \times g$ for 30 min and the pellet was washed twice with the same buffer. The combined supernatants were applied to DEAE-Sephacel columns equilibrated with 0.1 M NaCl buffered with 20 mM Tris–HCl, pH 8.6, and columns were washed with the same buffer. GAGs were eluted with 2 M LiCl in 20 mM Tris–HCl, pH 8.6. Subsequently, GAGs were exhaustively dialyzed against water at 4 °C for 24 h and lyophilized before further analysis.

The total amount of GAGs was quantified as a hexuronic acid by the carbazole methods of Volpi et al. [23] and Filisetti-Cozzi and Carpita [24] as well as van den Hoogen et al. [25]. Then, 4.0 M ammonium sulfamate was added to each sample containing an aqueous solution of GAGs. The hydrolysis of GAGs to their monosaccharide constituents with simultaneous conversion of the glucuronic acid and/or iduronic acid residues to the corresponding furan derivative was carried out in concentrated sulfuric acid (95%) containing 0.025 M sodium tetraborate by heating the samples at 100 °C for 10 min. The contents of the tubes were then chilled in an ice bath and the background absorbance of the samples was measured at 525 nm with a microplate reader (Infinite M200; Tecan). In the next stage, furan derivatives present in the tested samples were coupled with 0.125% carbazole that was dissolved in absolute ethanol. The tubes were heated to 100 °C for 15 min and left to cool to ambient temperature. Afterward, the absorbance of the pink-colored samples was read again at 525 nm. For hexuronic acid quantification, a calibration curve was constructed using D-(+) glucuronolactone standard series (0–70 μg/ml). The background absorbance was subtracted from the second absorbance reading and the hexuronic acid concentrations were interpolated from the corresponding reference curve. The sensitivity of the reaction was approximately 1.5 μg for glucuronic acid. Testing of all samples was completed in 1 day, so interassay variation was insignificant. The intraassay variability of total GAGs was less than 3%.

Measurement of KS and HA plasma levels

KS levels in plasma samples were measured in duplicate using an enzyme-linked immunosorbent assay (ELISA) from BlueGene Biotech (Shanghai, China) according to the manufacturer's instructions. The minimal detectable KS level was 0.1 ng/ml. All samples were tested within 1 day, and thus interassay variation was insignificant. The intraassay variation of the KS levels was < 10%.

Plasma concentrations of HA were determined in duplicate using a TECO® Hyaluronic Acid Plus Test Kit provided by TECOmedical Group (Sissach, Switzerland), according to the manufacturer's directions. This ELISA uses a highly specific hyaluronic acid binding protein (HABP) to capture HA and an enzyme-conjugated version of the HABP to detect and measure the HA captured from plasma samples. In brief, all plasma samples were diluted 50-fold with Sample Diluent. The analytical sensitivity was at 2.7 ng/ml. Testing of all samples was completed within 1 day to eliminate the effects of interassay variation. The intraassay coefficient of variation was < 2.9%.

Statistical analysis

Data analyses were performed using STATISTICA version 12 (https://www.statsoft.pl). The normality of the distribution was verified using the Shapiro–Wilk test. Data not normally distributed were log-transformed prior to analyses. Variables are summarized as mean (SD) (for normal distribution) or median and interquartile (25th–75th percentile) range (for abnormal distribution). The homogeneity of variance was assessed using Levene's test. Data were evaluated using a repeated-measures analysis of variance (RM-ANOVA) (normal distributed data) with a check for sphericity employing Mauchly's test of sphericity, or using the RM-ANOVA Friedman's test (nonnormal data). In the case of significant differences between subgroups, post-hoc analyses were based on the Tukey test ($p < 0.05$) or the Mann–Whitney U test (p value obtained after applying Bonferroni correction, $p < 0.05$; six possible comparisons).

Results

Clinical response

Out of a total of 45 female RA patients recruited for the study, 16 patients were excluded and the remaining 29 patients completed 15 months of treatment with TNFαI. In the excluded patients, TNFαI were discontinued due to the following reasons: no response in two patients, loss of response in three patients, intolerance in three patients, surgical procedures in four patients, and withdrawal of consent for participation in the therapy by four patients. Overall, 29 female RA patients who continued the TNFαI therapy for 15 months were included in our analysis and are presented in this study.

During the treatment with TNFαI, a significant clinical improvement in all RA patients was observed. Over the course of 3 months, 29 patients (100%) qualified as good responders in accordance with the EULAR response criteria [26]. What is more, this effect was sustained up to the 15th month. Remission of RA occurred in 38% of patients at the 9th month and in 80% at the 15th month of treatment, while the remaining patients experienced low activity. The DAS28 score was significantly reduced 3, 9, and 15 months after the initiation of TNFαI therapy when compared with baseline. Furthermore, CRP and ESR levels decreased significantly after 9 and 15 months of treatment (Table 2).

Plasma levels of total GAGs, KS, and HA

The results regarding evaluation of plasma glycosaminoglycans (total GAGs, KS, and HA) were analyzed only in female RA patients who completed the whole 15-month TNFαI therapy ($n = 29$).

The concentrations of total plasma GAGs, KS, and HA in female RA patients before treatment with TNFαI and in healthy individuals are presented in Fig. 1a–c. Total GAGs and HA levels were significantly higher in RA women before anti-TNF-α therapy than in healthy subjects (both $p < 0.001$; Fig. 1a, c). KS levels were not different in RA women before biological treatment in comparison to those of the controls ($p = 0.862$; Fig. 1b).

Three months after the initiation of TNFαI therapy, a statistically significant decrease in total GAG levels was observed in RA patients ($p < 0.001$; Fig. 2a). Continued therapy resulted in a further decline ($p < 0.001$; Fig. 2a), reaching total GAG levels characteristic of the age-matched healthy controls after 15 months of treatment ($p = 0.183$; Fig. 3a). Similarly, HA levels decreased significantly in response to anti-TNF-α therapy ($p < 0.001$; Fig. 2c). Furthermore, anti-TNF-α treatment also led to normalization of HA in RA patients ($p = 0.826$; Fig. 3c). In contrast, KS levels in RA women were not affected by the treatment ($p = 0.744$; Fig. 2b) and were not significantly different from those in healthy subjects after 15 months of TNFαI therapy ($p = 0.788$; Fig. 3b).

Discussion

TNF-α inhibitors provide a new standard in the treatment of RA. TNFαI administration for 15 months resulted in improvement in terms of disease activity, as shown by the decrease of DAS28 and CRP and the achievement of full remission or low disease activity in all RA patients. We also showed that this beneficial effect was associated with improvement in metabolism of ECM components, assessed through plasma sulfated and nonsulfated GAG levels in

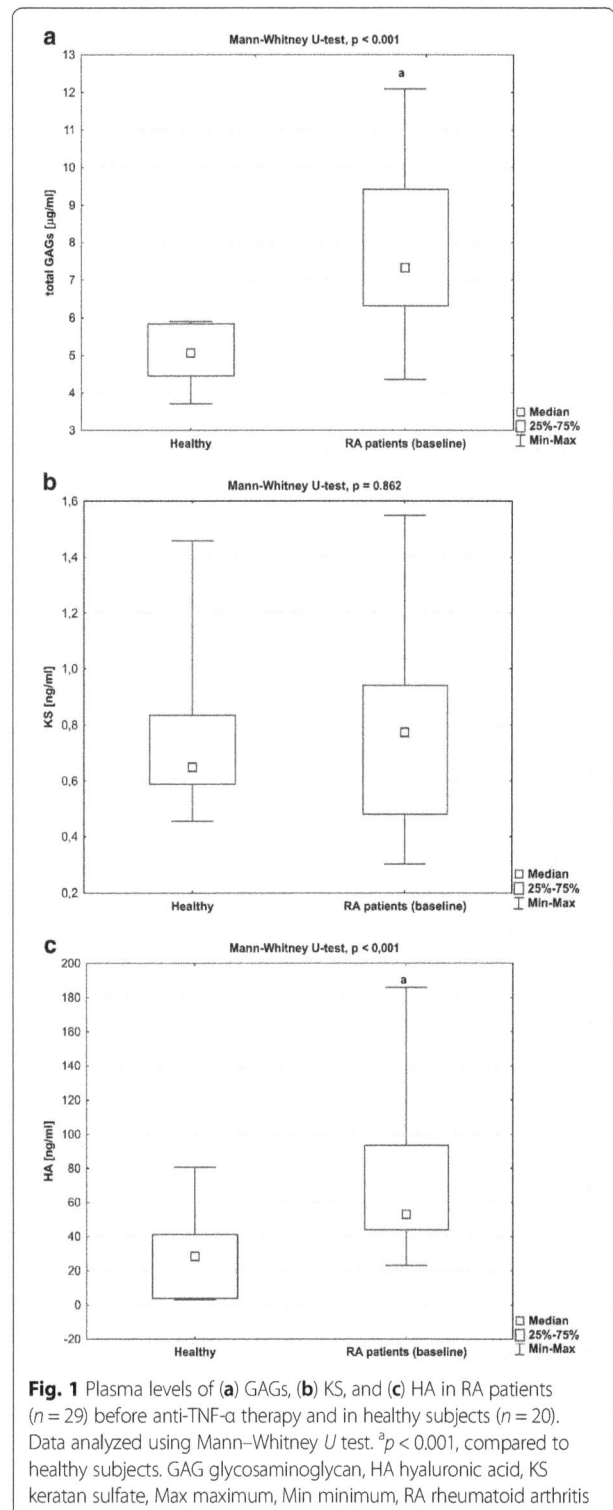

Fig. 1 Plasma levels of (**a**) GAGs, (**b**) KS, and (**c**) HA in RA patients ($n = 29$) before anti-TNF-α therapy and in healthy subjects ($n = 20$). Data analyzed using Mann–Whitney U test. [a]$p < 0.001$, compared to healthy subjects. GAG glycosaminoglycan, HA hyaluronic acid, KS keratan sulfate, Max maximum, Min minimum, RA rheumatoid arthritis

female RA patients. Indeed, a decrease in the total GAGs as well as HA levels toward normal values was observed under anti-TNF-α treatment. Only the plasma concentration of KS in RA women was not affected by the treatment. To the best of our knowledge, this is the first study that

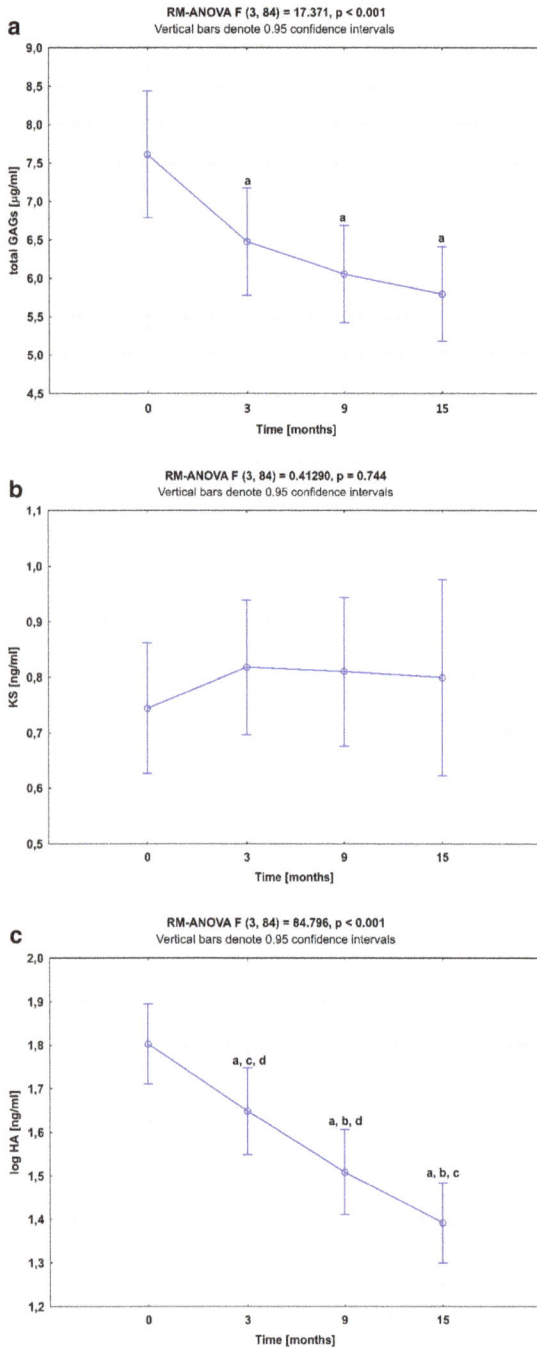

Fig. 2 Temporal course of plasma (**a**) GAGs, (**b**) KS, and (**c**) HA levels in RA patients ($n = 29$) during 15-month anti-TNF-α therapy . Results expressed as mean (SD). Data analyzed using one-way RM-ANOVA, followed by Tukey's multiple comparisons test. [a]$p < 0.001$, compared to baseline (T_0); [b]$p < 0.001$, compared to 3 months after therapy (T_1); [c]$p < 0.001$, compared to 9 months after therapy (T_2); [d]$p < 0.001$, compared to 15 months after therapy (T_3). GAG glycosaminoglycan, HA hyaluronic acid, KS keratan sulfate, RM-ANOVA repeated measures analysis of variance

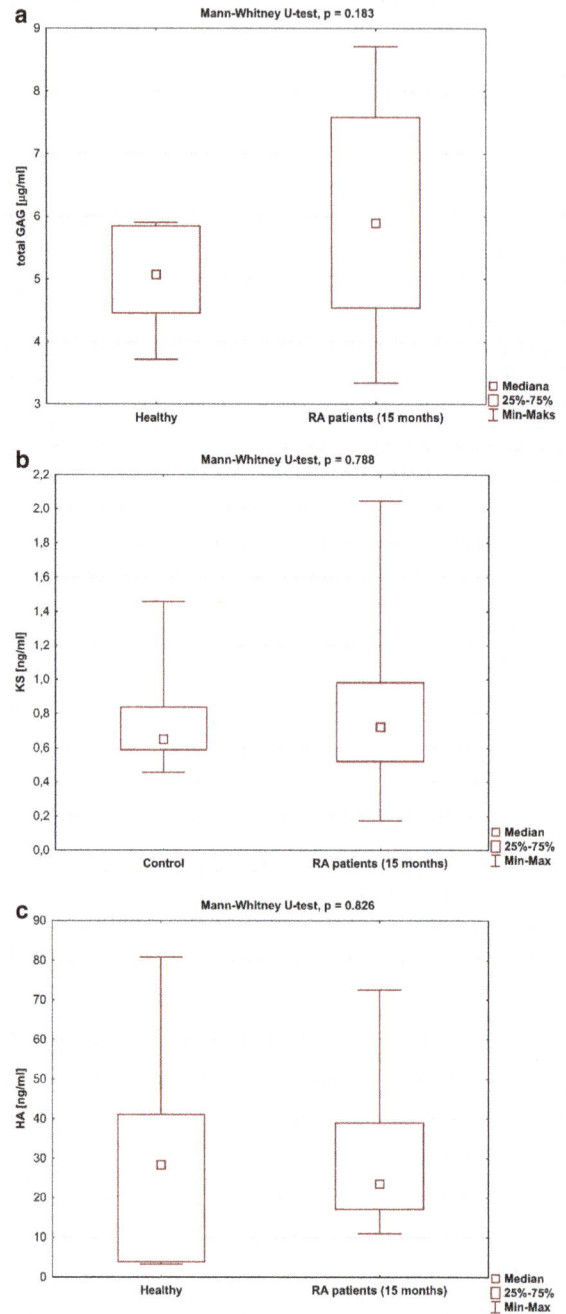

Fig. 3 Plasma levels of (**a**) GAGs, (**b**) KS, and (**c**) HA in RA patients ($n = 29$) after anti-TNF-α therapy and in healthy subjects ($n = 20$). Data analyzed using Mann–Whitney U test. GAG glycosaminoglycan, HA hyaluronic acid, KS keratan sulfate, Max maximum, Min minimum, RA rheumatoid arthritis

reports an association between good clinical response to anti-TNF treatments and the plasma GAGs in RA patients. The quantitative changes in the level of plasma GAGs observed in female RA patients during biological therapy seem to result from an effective inhibition of the key proinflammatory cytokine, TNF-α, rather than from direct impact of TNFαI on the tissue ECM remodeling. This suggestion is supported by the results of Jura-Półtorak et al. [15], who evaluated the plasma GAG profile in relation to disease activity in RA patients treated with conventional synthetic disease-modifying anti-rheumatic drugs (i.e., methotrexate or sulfasalazine). Similarly to our results, they demonstrated a significant increase in the total plasma GAG level in RA patients with a high disease activity (DAS28 > 5.1) in comparison to patients with a low disease activity (DAS28 ≤ 3.2) [15]. Thus, the primary determinant of tissue PG/GAG turnover in RA patients is not the type of medication used for treatment of RA, but the control of disease activity. Moreover, consistent with our results, Jura-Półtorak et al. [15] found that the plasma level of GAGs was significantly elevated in RA patients with a high disease activity in comparison to healthy individuals. On the contrary, Friman et al. [14] showed that the plasma GAG concentrations in female patients with an active, erosive form of RA and in healthy subjects are similar. These discrepancies can result from methodological differences, especially with respect to the binding properties of a bed used in the ion exchange chromatography, that are crucial for the isolation of the plasma GAGs, which are characterized by huge heterogeneity in their electrical charge. In addition, the aforementioned divergences between our results and those of Friman et al. [14] might also be caused by differences in the disease activity of female RA patients, disease duration, as well as a type of anti-rheumatic drugs used. Summarizing, the blood accumulation of the total GAGs in the course of RA observed by us may indicate an increased tissue ECM turnover that is dependent on the disease activity.

Considering our results, we can suppose that decreased levels of total plasma GAGs during 15 months of TNFαI treatment might be due to reduced enzymatic and nonenzymatic catabolic processes. Matrix metalloproteinases (MMPs) and the family of proteins termed a disintegrin and metalloproteinase with a thrombospondin motifs (ADAMTS), as well as reactive oxygen species (ROS), participate in the turnover of tissue PGs/GAGs [9, 27–29]. With regard to the enzymes discussed earlier, the levels of MMP-3 and MMP-1 in serum of RA patients were found to be downregulated by TNFαI therapy [30–33]. Little is known about the effect of TNF-α inhibitors on ADAMTS activity in RA patients. However, inhibition of radiographic progression by TNFαI has been extensively documented through many clinical trials and it can be assumed that this beneficial result is at least partially related to the decreased activity of aggrecanase-1 (ADAMTS-4) and aggrecanase-2 (ADAMTS-5), proteinases responsible for cleavage of the main cartilage matrix PG, aggrecan [28, 34]. Another mechanism of alterations to the plasma GAG level in RA women may be connected with the ability of TNFαI to promote programmed cell death through the inhibition of

nuclear factor-κB (NF-κB) activation. As reported previously, etanercept as well as infliximab induce apoptosis of synovial fluid monocytes/macrophages, which are a constant source of MMPs and ADAMTS [28, 35]. Furthermore, TNF-α blockade normalizes the number of circulating monocytes in RA patients [36].

Besides the proteolytic breakdown of the ECM, oxidative damage plays a very prominent role in postsynthetic modifications of matrix components [29]. It is well known that excessive ROS formation in RA patients leads to peroxidation of the core proteins of PGs as well as the partial cleavage of GAG chains, thereby increasing the plasma GAG content [29, 37]. Thus, it seems that normalization of the total plasma GAG level in RA women found in our study should be partly a reflection of the decreased nonenzymatic free radical degradation of these glycans. Indeed, anti-TNF-α therapy has been shown to suppress ROS generation in RA patients. It is reported that TNF-α blocking drugs reduce serum levels of reactive oxygen metabolites (ROM) as well as serum or urine levels of oxygen stress markers, including pentosidine, 8-hydroxy-2′-dexoyguanosine (8-OHdG), and N^ε-hexanoyl lysine (N^ε-HEL) [38–40]. Inhibition of neutrophil migration into inflamed joints after initiation of anti-TNF-α treatment in RA patients has also been described [41]. The mentioned cells are abundant in RA synovial fluid, and their release of oxygen-derived free radicals and other inflammatory mediators may intensify the catabolism of PGs/GAGs [41].

Because most GAG types are also found in noncartilaginous tissues in significant amounts, their plasma levels do not essentially reflect cartilage PG catabolic activity in RA patients [42]. Keratan sulfate is an exception, in that more than 95% of KS is found in the aggrecan, a large aggregating PG of hyaline, elastic, and fibrous cartilages [42]. Thus, this may indicate that most plasma KS should come from cartilage PG degradation. Elevated levels of plasma KS have been observed in patients with osteoarthritis, as well as in healthy individuals characterized by higher sports activity [43, 44]. In previous studies, the plasma concentrations of KS in RA patients have been shown to increase or decrease [15, 45–47]. In the present study, no significant difference was found in plasma KS levels between female RA patients and controls. We also showed that KS levels in RA women remained unchanged during 15 months of anti-TNF-α therapy. Our findings differ from those of Niki et al. [30], who demonstrated that the infliximab therapy-triggered increase of serum KS levels was more significant in the established RA patients than in the group of early RA patients. The possible explanation for these discrepancies could be connected with methodological differences in measurement of KS. In addition, these divergences might be caused in part by differences in gender of the patients, in the disease activity, and in amount of habitual exercise. In summary, the data presented here suggest that the potential usefulness of plasma antigen KS as an indicator of altered metabolic processes occurring in cartilaginous structures of RA patients during TNFαI therapy needs to be reevaluated.

In contrast to KS, plasma levels of the nonsulfated GAG hyaluronan could be helpful in predicting the efficacy of anti-TNF-α therapy in RA. The circulating levels of HA were greater in female RA patients before anti-TNF-α treatment when compared with age-matched healthy individuals. Similar findings have been reported in previous studies, none of which determined the gender of the patients [15, 48, 49]. In addition, TNFαI therapy led to a significant decrease in HA level, down to the values observed in healthy subjects. The outcomes of this study correspond with the results of Niki et al. [30]. They demonstrated that in the early RA group the serum level of HA gradually decreased during the 54-week infliximab therapy. Moreover, Niki et al. [30] found a strong linear correlation between the blood HA level in patients with early RA and DAS28, as well as inflammatory markers, such as CRP. These results may indicate that HA is an active participant in the inflammatory process accompanying RA. In the systemic circulation and in the synovial fluid of RA patients, the presence of low molecular weight fragments of hyaluronan (LMW-HA) was revealed. Such LMW-HA resulting from tissue HA depolymerization elicit proinflammatory responses by modulating toll-like receptor-4 or by activating NF-κB. NF-κB allows a vicious circle of chronic inflammation in RA by stimulating the expression of several proinflammatory cytokines such as interleukin (IL)-1, IL-6, and TNF-α, which in turn induce alterations in HA metabolism [8, 9, 12, 29, 50]. Since hyaluronan is the most susceptible among all of the GAG types to degradation in the presence of ROS, it may be assumed that suppression of free radical-mediated HA fragmentation may be the main cause of normalization of plasma HA in the course of biological therapy that was observed in our study.

Conclusions

In summary, the results of our study have shown for the first time that anti-TNF-α therapy, which contributes to a clinical improvement in female RA patients, also has a beneficial effect on metabolism of tissue PGs/GAGs. Normalization of plasma levels of total GAGs and HA in RA patients suggests improvement of the ECM remodeling balance, mainly due to a decrease in PG/GAG breakdown. Our observations provide an additional mechanism for explaining cartilage-protective effects associated with anti-TNF-α treatment.

Abbreviations

8-OHdG: 8-Hydroxy-2'-dexoyguanosine; ACR: American College of Rheumatology; ADAMTS: Disintegrin and metalloproteinase with a thrombospondin motifs; BMI: Body mass index; CRP: C-reactive protein; CS/DS: Chondroitin/dermatan sulfate; DAS28: Disease Activity Score based on the evaluation of 28 joints; ECM: Extracellular matrix; ELISA: Enzyme-linked immunosorbent assay; ESR: Erythrocyte sedimentation rate; EULAR: European League Against Rheumatism; GAG: Glycosaminoglycan; HA: Hyaluronic acid; HABP: Hyaluronic acid binding protein; HS/H: Heparan sulfate/heparin; IL: Interleukin; KS: Keratan sulfate; LMW-HA: Low molecular weight fragments of hyaluronan; MMP: Matrix metalloproteinase; NF-κB: nuclear factor-κB; N^ε-HEL: N^ε-hexanoyl lysine; PG: Proteoglycan; RA: Rheumatoid arthritis; RF: Rheumatoid factor; RM-ANOVA: Repeated-measures analysis of variance; ROM: Reactive oxygen metabolites; ROS: Reactive oxygen species; SJC28: Swollen joint count of 28 joints; TJC28: Tender joint count of 28 joints; TNF-α: Tumor necrosis factor alpha; TNFαI: Tumor necrosis factor-alpha inhibitors; VAS: Visual analog scale

Funding

This study was funded by the National Science Centre, Poland (Grant No. 2013/09/N/NZ5/00815).

Authors' contributions

AS and AJ-P were responsible for study conception and design, performing the experiments, acquisition of data, statistical analysis and interpretation of data, writing and revising the article, and final approval of the version of the article to be published. EMK and AG were responsible for study conception and design, performing the experiments, revising the article, and final approval of the version of the article to be published. EJK and MK-M were responsible for study conception and design, including patient recruitment, data collection, and revising the article. KO was responsible for study conception and design, interpretation of data, writing and revising the article, and final approval of the version of the article to be published. All authors read and approved the final manuscript.

Consent for publication

Not applicable.

Competing interests

The authors declare that they have no competing interests.

Author details

[1]Department of Clinical Chemistry and Laboratory Diagnostics, School of Pharmacy with the Division of Laboratory Medicine in Sosnowiec, Medical University of Silesia in Katowice, Jedności 8, 41-200 Sosnowiec, Poland. [2]Department of Internal Medicine and Rheumatology, School of Medicine in Katowice, Medical University of Silesia in Katowice, Ziołowa 45/47, 40-635 Katowice, Poland.

References

1. Smolen JS, Aletaha D, McInnes IB. Rheumatoid arthritis. Lancet. 2016;388: 2023–38.
2. Lauper K, Gabay C. Cardiovascular risk in patients with rheumatoid arthritis. Semin Immunopathol. 2017;39:447–59.
3. Song X, Lin Q. Genomics, transcriptomics and proteomics to elucidate the pathogenesis of rheumatoid arthritis. Rheumatol Int. 2017;37:1257–65.
4. Alam J, Jantan I, Bukhari SNA. Rheumatoid arthritis: recent advances on its etiology, role of cytokines and pharmacotherapy. Biomed Pharmacother. 2017;92:615–33.

5.　Angelotti F, Parma A, Cafaro G, Capecchi R, Alunno A, Puxeddu I. One year in review 2017: pathogenesis of rheumatoid arthritis. Clin Exp Rheumatol. 2017;35:368–78.

6.　Brzustewicz E, Bryl E. The role of cytokines in the pathogenesis of rheumatoid arthritis—practical and potential application of cytokines as biomarkers and targets of personalized therapy. Cytokine. 2015;76:527–36.

7.　Mateen S, Zafar A, Moin S, Khan AQ, Zubair S. Understanding the role of cytokines in the pathogenesis of rheumatoid arthritis. Clin Chim Acta. 2016;455:161–71.

8.　Sorokin L. The impact of the extracellular matrix on inflammation. Nat Rev Immunol. 2010;10:712–23.

9.　Bonnans C, Chou J, Werb Z. Remodelling the extracellular matrix in development and disease. Nat Rev Mol Cell Biol. 2014;15:786–801.

10.　Soares da Costa D, Reis RL, Pashkuleva I. Sulfation of glycosaminoglycans and its implications in human health and disorders. Annu Rev Biomed Eng. 2017;19:1–26.

11.　Mikami T, Kitagawa H. Sulfated glycosaminoglycans: their distinct roles in stem cell biology. Glycoconj J. 2017;34:725–35.

12.　Volpi N, Schiller J, Stern R, Soltés L. Role, metabolism, chemical modifications and applications of hyaluronan. Curr Med Chem. 2009;16: 1718–45.

13.　Gandhi NS, Mancera RL. The structure of glycosaminoglycans and their interactions with proteins. Chem Biol Drug Des. 2008;72:455–82.

14.　Friman C, Juvani M, Skrifvars B. Acid glycosaminoglycans in plasma. II. Findings in rheumatoid arthritis. Scand J Rheumatol. 1977;6:177–82.

15.　Jura-Półtorak A, Komosinska-Vassev K, Kotulska A, Kucharz EJ, Klimek K, Kopec-Medrek M, et al. Alterations of plasma glycosaminoglycan profile in patients with rheumatoid arthritis in relation to disease activity. Clin Chim Acta. 2014;433:20–7.

16.　Smolen JS, Landewé R, Bijlsma J, Burmester G, Chatzidionysiou K, Dougados M, et al. EULAR recommendations for the management of rheumatoid arthritis with synthetic and biological disease-modifying antirheumatic drugs: 2016 update. Ann Rheum Dis. 2017;76:960–77.

17.　Nam JL, Takase-Minegishi K, Ramiro S, Chatzidionysiou K, Smolen JS, van der Heijde D, et al. Efficacy of biological disease-modifying antirheumatic drugs: a systematic literature review informing the 2016 update of the EULAR recommendations for the management of rheumatoid arthritis. Ann Rheum Dis. 2017;76:1113–36.

18.　Szeremeta A, Olczyk K. Tumor necrosis factor α antagonists in the treatment of the patients with rheumatoid arthritis. Reumatologia. 2012;50:438–43.

19.　Arnett FC, Edworthy SM, Bloch DA, McShane DJ, Fries JF, Cooper NS, et al. The American Rheumatism Association 1987 revised criteria for the classification of rheumatoid arthritis. Arthritis Rheum. 1988;31:315–24.

20.　Aletaha D, Neogi T, Silman AJ, Funovits J, Felson DT, Bingham CO, et al. 2010 rheumatoid arthritis classification criteria: an American College of Rheumatology/European League Against Rheumatism collaborative initiative. Ann Rheum Dis. 2010;69:1580–8.

21.　Lu H, McDowell LM, Studelska DR, Zhang L. Glycosaminoglycans in human and bovine serum: detection of twenty-four heparan sulfate and chondroitin sulfate motifs including a novel sialic acid-modified chondroitin sulfate linkage hexasaccharide. Glycobiol Insights. 2010;2010:13–28.

22.　Capobianco G, de Muro P, Cherchi GM, Formato M, Lepedda AJ, Cigliano A, et al. Plasma levels of C-reactive protein, leptin and glycosaminoglycans during spontaneous menstrual cycle: differences between ovulatory and anovulatory cycles. Arch Gynecol Obstet. 2010;282:207–13.

23.　Volpi N, Galeotti F, Yang B, Linhardt RJ. Analysis of glycosaminoglycan-derived, precolumn, 2-aminoacridone-labeled disaccharides with LC-fluorescence and LC-MS detection. Nat Protoc. 2014;9:541–58.

24.　Filisetti-Cozzi TM, Carpita NC. Measurement of uronic acids without interference from neutral sugars. Anal Biochem. 1991;197:157–62.

25.　van den Hoogen BM, van Weeren PR, Lopes-Cardozo M, van Golde LM, Barneveld A, van de Lest CH. A microtiter plate assay for the determination of uronic acids. Anal Biochem. 1998;257:107–11.

26.　Fransen J, van Riel PL. The disease activity score and the EULAR response criteria. Rheum Dis Clin N Am. 2009;35:745–57.

27.　Araki Y, Mimura T. Matrix metalloproteinase gene activation resulting from disordered epigenetic mechanisms in rheumatoid arthritis. Int J Mol Sci. 2017;18. https://doi.org/10.3390/ijms18050905.

28.　García-Hernández MH, González-Amaro R, Portales-Pérez DP. Specific therapy to regulate inflammation in rheumatoid arthritis: molecular aspects. Immunotherapy. 2014;6:623–36.

29.　Fuchs B, Schiller J. Glycosaminoglycan degradation by selected reactive oxygen species. Antioxid Redox Signal. 2014;21:1044–62.

30.　Niki Y, Takeuchi T, Nakayama M, Nagasawa H, Kurasawa T, Yamada H, et al. Clinical significance of cartilage biomarkers for monitoring structural joint damage in rheumatoid arthritis patients treated with anti-TNF therapy. PLoS One. 2012;7:e37447. https://doi.org/10.1371/journal.pone.0037447.

31.　Catrina AI, Lampa J, Ernestam S, af Klint E, Bratt J, Klareskog L, et al. Anti-tumour necrosis factor (TNF)-alpha therapy (etanercept) down-regulates serum matrix metalloproteinase (MMP)-3 and MMP-1 in rheumatoid arthritis. Rheumatology (Oxford). 2002;41:484–9.

32.　den Broeder AA, Joosten LA, Saxne T, Heinegård D, Fenner H, Miltenburg AM, et al. Long term anti-tumor necrosis factor α monotherapy in rheumatoid arthritis: effect on radiological course and prognostic value of markers of cartilage turnover and endothelial activation. Ann Rheum Diss. 2002;61:311–8.

33.　Kawashiri SY, Kawakami A, Ueki Y, Imazato T, Iwamoto N, Fujikawa K, et al. Decrement of serum cartilage oligomeric matrix protein (COMP) in rheumatoid arthritis (RA) patients achieving remission after 6 months of etanercept treatment: comparison with CRP, IgM-RF, MMP-3 and anti-CCP ab. Joint Bone Spine. 2010;77:418–20.

34.　Dancevic CM, McCulloch DR. Current and emerging therapeutic strategies for preventing inflammation and aggrecanase-mediated cartilage destruction in arthritis. Arthritis Res Ther. 2014;16:429. https://doi.org/10.1186/s13075-014-0429-9.

35.　Catrina AI, Trollmo C, af Klint E, Engstrom M, Lampa J, Hermansson Y, et al. Evidence that anti-tumor necrosis factor therapy with both etanercept and infliximab induces apoptosis in macrophages, but not lymphocytes, in rheumatoid arthritis joints: extended report. Arthritis Rheum. 2005;52:61–72.

36.　Chara L, Sánchez-Atrio A, Pérez A, Cuende E, Albarrán F, Turrión A, et al. Monocyte populations as markers of response to adalimumab plus MTX in rheumatoid arthritis. Arthritis Res Ther. 2012;14:R175. https://doi.org/10.1186/ar3928.

37.　Mateen S, Moin S, Khan AQ, Zafar A, Fatima N. Increased reactive oxygen species formation and oxidative stress in rheumatoid arthritis. PLoS One. 2016;11:e0152925. https://doi.org/10.1371/journal.pone.0152925.

38.　Hirao M, Yamasaki N, Oze H, Ebina K, Nampei A, Kawato Y, et al. Serum level of oxidative stress marker is dramatically low in patients with rheumatoid arthritis treated with tocilizumab. Rheumatol Int. 2012;32:4041–5.

39.　Nakajima A, Aoki Y, Sonobe M, Takahashi H, Saito M, Nakagawa K. Serum level of reactive oxygen metabolites (ROM) at 12 weeks of treatment with biologic agents for rheumatoid arthritis is a novel predictor for 52-week remission. Clin Rheumatol. 2017;36:309–15.

40.　Kageyama Y, Takahashi M, Nagafusa T, Torikai E, Nagano A. Etanercept reduces the oxidative stress marker levels in patients with rheumatoid arthritis. Rheumatol Int. 2008;28:245–51.

41.　den Broeder AA, Wanten GJ, Oyen WJ, Naber T, van Riel PL, Barrera P. Neutrophil migration and production of reactive oxygen species during treatment with a fully human anti-tumor necrosis factor-alpha monoclonal antibody in patients with rheumatoid arthritis. J Rheumatol. 2003;30:232–7.

42.　Caterson B, Melrose J. Keratan sulphate, a complex glycosaminoglycan with unique functional capability. Glycobiology 2018 published on 11 January 2018. doi: https://doi.org/10.1093/glycob/cwy003.

43.　Woitge HW, Seibel MJ. Markers of bone and cartilage turnover. Exp Clin Endocrinol Diabetes. 2017;125:454–69.

44.　Roos H, Dahlberg L, Hoerrner LA, Lark MW, Thonar EJ, Shinmei M, et al. Markers of cartilage matrix metabolism in human joint fluid and serum: the effect of exercise. Osteoarthr Cartil. 1995;3:7–14.

45.　Haraoui B, Thonar EJ, Martel-Pelletier J, Goulet JR, Raynauld JP, Ouellet M, et al. Serum keratan sulfate levels in rheumatoid arthritis: inverse correlation with radiographic staging. J Rheumatol. 1994;21:813–7.

46.　Poole AR, Ionescu M, Swan A, Dieppe PA. Changes in cartilage metabolism in arthritis are reflected by altered serum and synovial fluid levels of the cartilage proteoglycan aggrecan. Implications for pathogenesis. J Clin Invest. 1994;94:25–33.

47.　Spector TD, Woodward L, Hall GM, Hammond A, Williams A, Butler MG, et al. Keratan sulphate in rheumatoid arthritis, osteoarthritis, and inflammatory diseases. Ann Rheum Dis. 1992;51:1134–7.

48.　Majeed M, McQueen F, Yeoman S, McLean L. Relationship between serum hyaluronic acid level and disease activity in early rheumatoid arthritis. Ann Rheum Dis. 2004;63:1166–8.

20

Monosodium urate burden assessed with dual-energy computed tomography predicts the risk of flares in gout: a 12-month observational study

MSU burden and risk of gout flare

Tristan Pascart[1,4,5]* (iD), Agathe Grandjean[1,5], Benoist Capon[2,5], Julie Legrand[2,5], Nasser Namane[2,5], Vincent Ducoulombier[1,5], Marguerite Motte[1,5], Marie Vandecandelaere[1,5], Hélène Luraschi[1,5], Catherine Godart[1,5], Eric Houvenagel[1,5], Laurène Norberciak[3,5] and Jean-François Budzik[2,4,5]

Abstract

Background: Predicting the risk of flares in patients with gout is a challenge and the link between urate burden and the risk of gout flare is unclear. The objective of this study was to determine if the extent of monosodium urate (MSU) burden measured with dual-energy computed tomography (DECT) and ultrasonography (US) is predictive of the risk of gout flares.

Methods: This prospective observational study recruited patients with gout to undergo MSU burden assessment with DECT (volume of deposits) and US (double contour sign) scans of the knees and feet. Patients attended follow-up visits at 3, 6 and 12 months. Patients having presented with at least one flare at 6 months were compared to those who did not flare. Odds ratios (ORs) (95% confidence interval) for the risk of flare were calculated.

Results: Overall, 64/78 patients included attended at least one follow-up visit. In bivariate analysis, the number of joints with the double contour sign was not associated with the risk of flare ($p = 0.67$). Multivariate analysis retained a unique variable: DECT MSU volume of the feet. For each 1 cm^3 increase in DECT MSU volume in foot deposits, the risk of flare increased 2.03-fold during the first 6 months after initial assessment (OR 2.03 (1.15–4.38)). The threshold volume best discriminating patients with and without flare was 0.81 cm^3 (specificity 61%, sensitivity 77%).

Conclusions: This is the first study showing that the extent of MSU burden measured with DECT but not US is predictive of the risk of flares.

Keywords: Gout, Flares, Dual-energy computed tomography, Ultrasonography

* Correspondence: tristan.pascart@hotmail.fr
[1]Department of Rheumatology, Lille Catholic Hospitals, University of Lille, 59160 Lomme, France
[4]EA 4490, PMOI, Physiopathologie des Maladies Osseuses Inflammatoires, University of Lille, 59000 Lille, France
Full list of author information is available at the end of the article

Background

Gout is a metabolic condition related to monosodium urate (MSU) crystal deposition in joints and soft tissue leading to NLRP inflammasome-guided recurrent arthritis [1]. Despite the permanent deposition of MSU crystals, flares of inflammatory response are only intercurrent and difficult to predict. Risk factors for gout flares are known or suspected but causality is poorly understood [2, 3].

Initiation and modifications of urate lowering therapy (ULT) are critical times for flares. Prophylaxis of flares with colchicine, non-steroidal anti-inflammatory drugs (NSAIDs) or even oral corticosteroids is recommended by all international guidelines during 6 months following ULT initiation [4–6]. These recommendations are based upon the observation of an increased rate of flares during the first 6 months of ULT in most randomized controlled trials (RCTs) involving ULTs versus placebo [7, 8]. Prophylaxis, especially with colchicine, has been proven effective to decrease the risk of flares [9–11]. It is generally accepted that the reduced serum urate (SU) [12] concentration induces mobilization of the deposited MSU burden, potentially exposing the crystals to the innate immune system [11, 13]. This explanation, however, remains hypothetical.

Ultrasonography (US) and dual-energy computed tomography (DECT) can provide an assessment of the MSU burden [14]. DECT uses two x-ray beams with two different energies allowing to distinguish between urate and calcium in soft tissues surrounding bone, with radiation exposure close to conventional computed tomography (CT) [15]. US, on the other hand, can identify intra-articular cartilage MSU deposition appearing as a double contour (DC) sign, which disappears during urate depletion [16]. The usefulness of US and DECT is now fully recognized for the diagnosis of gout [17]. The clinical relevance of observing and measuring the urate burden by any imaging technique however needs to be determined. Previous data suggest an association between urate burden and past flares [18] but to our knowledge no imaging feature has been associated with the risk of flares [19]. More generally, no data have so far demonstrated that imaging adds to the low cost clinical and biological assessments in the management of gout [19].

The objective of this study was to determine if the extent of urate burden measured with DECT and US predicts the risk of gout flares.

Methods

Patients

This prospective observational study included consecutive patients with a diagnosis of gout according to the American College of Rheumatology (ACR)/European League Against Rheumatism (EULAR) 2015 criteria [17].

They were recruited to undergo quantification of urate deposition of the knees and feet using US and DECT [14, 20] and were subsequently followed in outpatient visits. The study was approved by the institutional review board of the Lille Catholic Hospitals and all participants provided informed consent before inclusion into the study.

Visits

Patients were seen for their follow up as decided by their physician. The initial (M0) visit was contemporary with the US and DECT scans. Demographic characteristics, disease history, treatments and biological data were then collected. Physicians were unaware of the results of the DECT scans results during follow up.

The three follow-up visits examined were those performed at months 3 (M3), 6 (M6) and 12 (M12) (± 1 month allowed). The number of flares since M0 and since the previous timepoint were recorded at each visit. Flare definition was based upon the patient's own assessment according to previous experiences of flares and retrospectively validated by the investigator upon the description of the episode [21]. Data on type and dose of ongoing ULT and flare prophylaxis were collected. Contemporary SU levels were noted when available.

DECT scans

All scans were performed using a single-source CT (Somatom Definition Edge; Siemens, Erlangen, Germany). Knees and feet were scanned axially in two separate acquisitions performed consecutively on the same day. All scans were performed with the same image protocol, with acquisition at 128 × 0.6 mm and pitch at 0.7. Two scans of each body region were acquired with tube potentials of 80 kV and 140 kV. Depending on the scanned body region, quality reference tube currents ranged between 62 and 260 mAs. Automated attenuation-based tube current modulation was used in all examinations.

Axial images with soft (B30f) and bone (B70f) convolution kernels were reconstructed with 1 mm slice thickness and 1 mm increment. Dedicated software (syngo.via VB10B, syngo Dual Energy Gout; Siemens) was used for DECT post-processing, following parameters described elsewhere [22]: HouNsfield unit (HU) threshold, 150; iodine ratio, 1.4; material definition ratio, 1.25; resolution, 4; air distance, 5; bone distance, 10. Two kinds of images were reconstructed for each body region. First, volume-rendered 3D images in which urate crystal deposits coded in green were reconstructed with a bone tissue convolution kernel (B70f). These images allowed a straightforward overview of MSU deposits. Second, multi-planar reformations associating images reconstructed with a soft tissue kernel (B30f) and colored images were reconstructed. The aspect of the final fusion images could be changed by modulating the relative percentages of the morphological and colored images from 0 to 100% with a slider. MSU deposits above 20 cm^3 in patients assessed by DECT were considered extreme and these patients were excluded to avoid over-estimated weight in the OR computations of the risk of flares per unit of MSU volume.

US scans

Examinations were performed by one of four trained musculoskeletal radiologists on an Applio 400 US machine (Toshiba Medical Systems, Tochigi, Japan). High-frequency probes were used: a 12 Mhz probe for the knee examination and an 18 MHz probe for the ankle and foot examination. The patellofemoral joints, talocrural joints and 1st metatarsophalangeal joints were examined by US for the DC sign as defined by Outcome Measures in Rheumatology (OMERACT) [23].

Statistical analysis

All statistical analyses were performed using R version 3.4. Qualitative variables were described as numbers (%) of each response modality; quantitative variables were described as mean ± SD.

Two groups were defined according to the occurrence of flares between M0 and M6: the first group included patients having presented with no flare, the second those having presented with at least one. Group-variable bivariate analysis was applied to search for factors predictive of flaring. Variables assessed were DECT MSU volume in the feet at M0, DECT MSU volume in the knees at M0, SU time course from M0 to M6, use of prophylaxis at M6, number of joints with the DC at M0, use of ULT at M0 and number of flares per year at M0. The chi-square test or Fisher's exact test, as appropriate, was used for comparative analysis of proportions. Continuous variables were compared using Student's t test for normal data, or the Mann-Whitney-Wilcoxon test. Multivariate analysis was then applied to search for factors affecting group assignment: a binary logistic regression model explaining the group and integrating all these data was constructed (a "complete" model). The small sample size required a variable selection procedure. The step by step, backward method, based on the Akaike criterion, was chosen to obtain a "reduced" model. Validation and reduced model performance were assessed by the ROC area under the curve. As they were satisfactory, the odds ratios (ORs) of explanatory variables selected by the automatic selection and their 95% confidence intervals are presented. The cutoff best discriminating between the groups was deduced from the ROC curve. Sensitivity and specificity were calculated according to this threshold. As a single variable was selected by the automatic selection procedure, a further

OR analysis was performed of the ORs of presenting with at least one flare for each period between time points (namely M0–M3, M0–M6, M0–M12 and M6–12) based upon the entire sample of patients attending the analyzed visits with the available number of flares over the considered period of time. These ORs were obtained using a simple binary logistic regression model integrating this unique variable. The significance level was set at 5%.

Results
Patients

Overall, 78 patients were included in the study and had an initial assessment of urate burden with DECT and US scans. Their characteristics and those of the groups of patients who experienced at least one flare or not during the first 6 months of follow up are described in Table 1.

Of these patients, 14 were lost to follow up, 2 were excluded because of extreme volumes of MSU deposits (volumes > 75 cm^3) and the remaining 62 patients attended at least one of the three follow-up visits. Data recorded at each visit are presented in Table 2.

At M6, 27/54 patients (50%) were receiving flare prophylaxis. Of these 27 patients, 10 (38.5%) were receiving 0.5 mg colchicine daily, 12 (46.2%) 1 mg colchicine daily, 1 full dose NSAIDs (3.8%), 1 oral corticosteroids (3.8%) and the last 2 patients were treated with anakinra (7.7%). A total of 47/54 patients were receiving ULT, among whom 27 participants (57.4%) were treated with allopurinol, 17 with febuxostat (36.2%), 2 with benzbromarone (4.3%) and 1 with probenecid (2.1%). At M6, 19 patients (35.2%) had presented with at least one flare since baseline.

Risk factors for flares

Overall, 36 patients without any missing data were seen at M6 and included in the multivariate analysis. The selected potential risk factors for flares during the 6 months following the initial assessment were tested for and presented in Table 3.

The volume of MSU deposition of the feet measured with DECT was the only factor significantly associated with the risk of flares in the bivariate analysis ($p = 0.05$). Moreover, this DECT volume was the only variable retained by the automatic selection procedure in the multivariate analysis (reduced model). The box plot of MSU volumes of the feet in the group of patients having presented with at least one flare between M0 and M6 and the one of those who did not flare are shown in Additional file 1: Figure S1.

The OR obtained in the reduced model was 2.03 with a 95% confidence interval of 1.15–4.38. The risk of developing a flare during the 6 months following initial assessment increased 2.03-fold for each 1 cm^3 increase in

Table 1 Population characteristics and characteristics of patients flaring and not flaring between month 0 (M0) and month 6 (M6) (significance of the p value set at 5%)

Characteristics	Population (n = 78)	Patients without flare between M0 and M6 (n = 33)	Patients with at least 1 flare between M0 and M6 (n = 19)	p value
Demographics				
Age (years)	64.8 ± 13.9	67.4 ± 12.3	67.7 ± 13.8	0.95
Male	68 (87.2%)	26 (78.8%)	17 (89.5%)	0.46
Body mass index (kg/m^2)	28.9 ± 4.3	29.1 ± 4.5	28.7 ± 4	0.62
Current smoking	10 (12.8%)	2 (6.1%)	4 (21.1%)	0.18
Excessive alcohol consumption (n)	38 (48.7%)	16 (48.5%)	8 (42.1%)	0.88
Creatinine clearance (mL/min)	76.8 ± 28.0	70.3 ± 28.2	77.5 ± 32.8	0.51
Comorbidities				
High blood pressure	43 (55.1%)	22 (66.7%)	5 (26.3%)	**0.012**
Coronary heart disease	12 (15.4%)	2 (6.1%)	4 (21.1%)	0.18
Peripheral arterial disease	3 (3.8%)	0 (0%)	0 (0%)	1
Chronic heart disease	18 (23.1%)	8 (24.2%)	2 (10.5%)	0.29
Stroke	8 (10.3%)	5 (15.2%)	0 (0%)	0.15
Dyslipidemia	37 (47.4%)	18 (54.5%)	8 (42.1%)	0.56
Diabetes mellitus	20 (25.6%)	12 (36.4%)	3 (15.8%)	0.21
Obstructive sleep apnea	11 (14.1%)	6 (18.2%)	2 (10.5%)	0.69
Psoriasis	5 (6.4%)	3 (9.1%)	1 (5.3%)	1
Ongoing diuretics	19 (24.4%)	8 (24.2%)	4 (21.1%)	1
Disease characteristics				
Gout duration (years)	11.8 ± 11.9	9.6 ± 11.2	15.8 ± 13.4	0.061
Renal stones	13 (16.7%)	6 (18.2%)	3 (15.8%)	1
Family history of gout	18 (23.1%)	6 (18.2%)	6 (31.6%)	0.32
Declared number of flares over the past year	4.1 ± 5.9	3.2 ± 4.4	4.6 ± 5.8	0.15
Baseline ongoing flare prophylaxis	25 (32.1%)	12 (36.4%)	7 (36.8%)	1
Baseline serum urate (mg/dL)	7.43 ± 2.33	6.93 ± 2.14	7.85 ± 2.12	0.096
Ongoing urate lowering therapy	36 (46.2%)	16 (48.5%)	9 (47.4%)	1
Allopurinol	*18 (50%)*	8 (50%)	5 (55.6%)	0.38
Febuxostat	*16 (44.4%)*	8 (50%)	3 (33.3%)	
Probenecid	*1 (2.8%)*	0 (0%)	1 (11.1%)	
Benzbromarone	*1 (2.8%)*	0 (0%)	0 (0%)	
Subcutaneous tophi	28 (35.9%)	7 (21.2%)	9 (47.4%)	0.098
US tophi	49 (62.8%)	19 (57.6%)	13 (68.4%)	0.63
Number of joints with the US double contour sign (/6)	2.4 ± 1.3	2.2 ± 1	2.8 ± 1.4	0.3
At least one US double contour sign	75 (96.2%)	32 (97%)	19 (100%)	1
DECT MSU volume knees (cm^3)	6.3 ± 28.1	0.6 ± 1.3	1.7 ± 3.4	0.11
DECT MSU volume feet (cm^3)	5.4 ± 16.7	0.9 ± 1.3	2.4 ± 2.1	**0.0064**

US ultrasonography, *DECT* dual-energy computed tomography, *MSU* monosodium urate
Significance of the p value was set at 5% are in bold

MSU volume in deposits in the feet. The threshold volume best discriminating patients with and without flare during the 6 months following initial assessment was 0.81 cm^3, with 61% specificity and 77% sensitivity (Figs. 1 and 2).

Risk of flares between time points according to MSU volume

Having identified the DECT MSU volume of deposits in the feet as the unique significant factor predictive of flares, the ORs of having at least one flare were calculated for

Table 2 Details of the clinical, biological and treatment data collected during each follow-up visit

	Month 0	Month 3	Month 6	Month 12
Patients attending the visit	78 (100%)	42 (65.6%)	54 (84.4%)	38 (59.4%)
Serum urate (mg/dL)	7.43 ± 2.33	6.57 ± 1.9	5.59 ± 1.56	5.63 ± 1.81
Ongoing ULT	36 (46.2%)	33 (78.5%)	47 (87.1%)	34 (89.4%)
Ongoing flare prophylaxis	25 (32.1%)	20 (47.6%)	27 (50%)	16 (42.1%)
Number of flares since M0	N/A	0.6 ± 1.3	0.7 ± 1.4	1.5 ± 3.3
Patients with at least 1 flare since M0	N/A	15 (35.7%)	19 (35.2%)	16 (42.1%)
Number of flares since previous visit	N/A	0.6 ± 1.3	0.3 ± 0.7	0.7 ± 1.6
Patients with at least 1 flare since previous visit	N/A	15 (35.7%)	9 (17%)	12 (31.6%)

M0 month 0, *ULT* urate lowering therapy

periods between time points. All patients with recorded data on the number of flares during each period of time were included in the analysis.

The ORs for risk of flaring between time points are presented in Table 4. The difference in the risk of flaring - associated with increased deposit volume in the feet determined by DECT at M0 - was significant between M0 and M6 and between M0 and M12, but not between M0 and M3 nor between M6 and M12. It is noteworthy that considering all 52 patients who attended the M0 and M6 visits (instead of the 36 patients with all data available who could be included in the multivariate analysis), the OR of flaring between M0 and M6 associated with increased MSU deposit volume was 1.69 (1.17–2.77).

Discussion

This study demonstrates that the extent of the MSU burden measured with DECT but not US predicts the risk of flares. Interestingly, patients with dramatically large volumes of MSU deposition are not necessarily at risk of flare. This is the first study showing the usefulness of DECT for the management of patients with gout, beyond diagnosis. These results also provide proof of concept that urate load is associated with the risk of flares.

With an OR of 2.03, the MSU burden in the feet assessed with DECT is the strongest determinant of

subsequent gout flares identified so far. Some comorbidities, namely hypertension, renal disease and coronary heart disease, have been identified in a population-based study as having hazard ratios of 1.1–1.3 of incident gout flares [3]. Of note, patients with high blood pressure (HBP) were less at risk of flare in our study (Table 1). SU change from baseline has been shown to have an impact on the risk of flares in the febuxostat trials, but the OR was close to 1. This is consistent with our results as changes in SU levels between M0 and M6 were similar between participants experiencing and not experiencing flares. Rapidly obtaining SU levels below the dissolution threshold of MSU was associated with an OR of 1.42 of incident flares in the febuxostat trials and could be related to the mobilization of the MSU burden [13]. Prevalence of the US DC sign provides a different assessment of MSU burden than the one provided with DECT [14] and does not seem to predict the risk of flares. Flare prophylaxis is known to imperfectly prevent gout flares during ULT initiation [11]. The variety of situations included in our study, both in terms of ULT (absence, dose adaptation, initiation) and types of prophylaxis, would probably explain why it did not exhibit a preventive effect.

When the question of introducing or pursuing flare prophylaxis arises, DECT could be a decisive partner in

Table 3 Comparison in bivariate analysis of potential risk factors influencing the risk of presenting with at least one flare during the first 6 months of follow up of patients with all data available

	No flare between M0 and M6	At least 1 flare between M0 and M6	p value
Number of patients	23	13	/
DECT MSU volume knees (cm^3)	0.6 ± 1.2	1.1 ± 1.6	0.24
DECT MSU volume feet (cm^3)	0.9 ± 0.8	2.1 ± 1.9	0.05
Serum urate change between M0 and M6 (mg/dL)	1.51 ± 2.03	1.50 ± 2.48	0.88
Number of joints with the US double contour sign at M0 (/6)	2.5 ± 0.9	2.9 ± 1.5	0.67
Declared number of flares over the past year	3 ± 4.4	4.2 ± 6.2	0.41
Ongoing flare prophylaxis at M6	11 (47.8%)	6 (46.2%)	1
Ongoing urate lowering therapy at M0	13 (56.5%)	6 (46.2%)	0.8

M0 month 0, *M6* month 6, *US* ultrasonography, *DECT* dual-energy computed tomography, *MSU*, monosodium urate

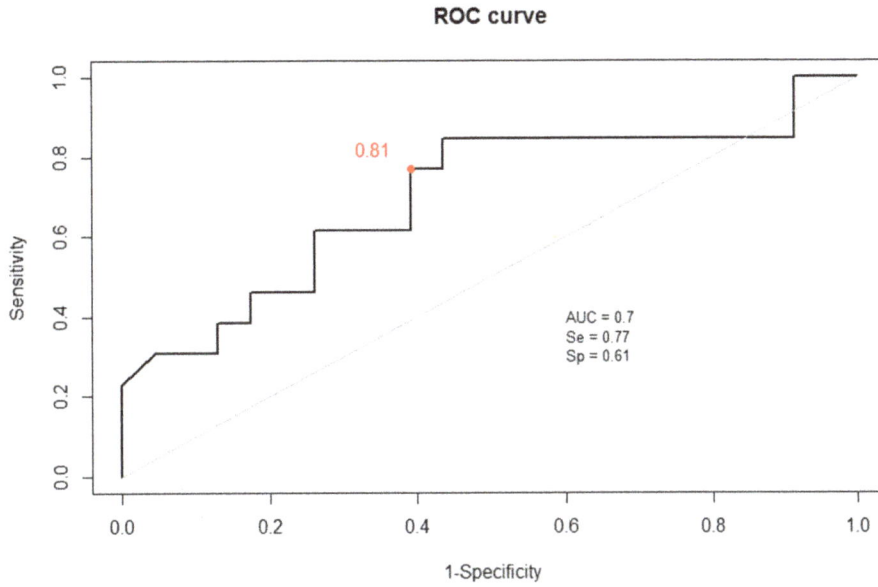

Fig. 1 ROC curve explaining the risk of presenting with at least one flare during the first 6 months of follow up, with the monosodium urate volume deposited in the feet measured with dual-energy computed tomography. The red dot indicates the volume providing the best discrimination between the group of patients presenting with at least one flare and those without flare. The associated predictive values for this volume are shown. AUC, area under the curve; Sp, specificity; Se, sensitivity

the decision-making process. So far, international societies recommend flare prophylaxis during 6 months or until tophus resolution [4–6]. Becker et al. had shown from the febuxostat trials that the presence of subcutaneous tophi was one of the determinants of flare incidence during follow up [13]. Physical examination of tophi can be sufficient to show the presence of a significant MSU burden requiring flare prophylaxis. However, only approximatively 15–30% of patients present with subcutaneous tophi [24, 25]. Our study shows that DECT can provide an assessment of the risk of flares whether subcutaneous tophi are present or not. DECT scanning could be decisive when considering the interruption of flare prophylaxis after 6 months or when tophi are no longer clinically detectable.

MSU burden could be the missing link between ULT and flare reduction. So far, SU has been the primary endpoint in the majority of ULT trials, as observational data consistently show that eventually flare reduction correlates with reduction in SU [26]. In its latest highly debated guidelines, the American College of Physicians has challenged the relevance of targeting SU rather than flares themselves, considering that the evidence linking SU and flares is insufficient in RCTs [26–29]. For instance, the double blind RCTs for the development of febuxostat failed to show flare reduction with febuxostat [30, 31]. Similarly, another RCT of febuxostat versus placebo in early gout showed no reduction after 6 months of treatment [8]. Given that it has already been shown that ULT in its most potent form (pegloticase) decreases the MSU burden assessed with DECT and that our study demonstrates that MSU volumes measured with DECT predict gout flares, DECT could be used as a clinically relevant outcome measure [32]. Depending on the kinetics of MSU depletion with conventional ULTs (hypoxanthine oxidase inhibitors and uricosurics), DECT MSU

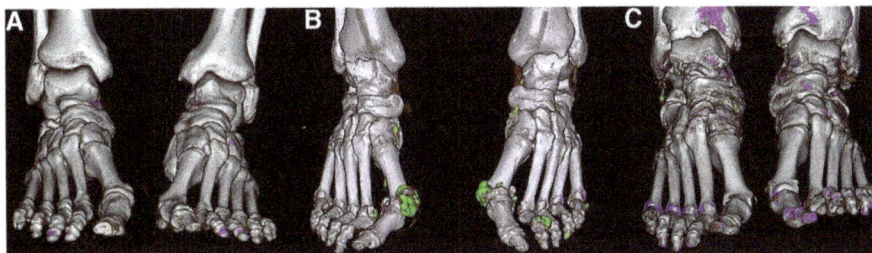

Fig. 2 Dual-energy computed tomography imaging of monosodium urate crystal deposition in the feet. Small (volume 0.17 cm^3) (**a**), large (volume 5.29 cm^3) (**b**) and cutoff (**c**) soft tissue volume of deposits in patients with flare and without flare (volume 0.81 cm^3)

Table 4 Odds ratios for the risk of presenting with at least one flare during follow up between each time point

Time period	Group	Number	M0 DECT MSU volume feet (cm^3)	OR	(95% CI for OR)
M0–M6	0 flares	33	0.9 ± 1.3	**1.69**	**(1.17–2.77)**
	≥ 1 flare	19	2.4 ± 2.1		
M6–M12	0 flares	25	1.4 ± 1.7	1.13	(0.74–1.71)
	≥ 1 flare	12	1.8 ± 1.7		

M month, *DECT* dual-energy computed tomography, *MSU* monosodium urate, *OR* odds ratio, *CI* confidence interval
Significance of the OR with 95% confidence interval not including 1 are in bold

volumes could be considered as a surrogate marker for the risk of flares potentially more efficiently than SU.

We acknowledge that the study design had some limitations, imposing caution while interpreting the results. First, although an effect of volume of the MSU burden measured by DECT on the risk of flares was detected despite the small sample size, the rather small number of patients and the missing data may have underestimated other factors with a smaller effect. Particularly, the study did not detect the expected significant effect of the change in SU levels on the risk of flares [33]. However, the SU change between patients with and without flare was very similar in our study, suggesting that the link between change in SU level itself and the risk of flares may not be as direct as previously hypothesized. For instance, the high risk of flares during pegloticase therapy (and to a lesser extent during less potent ULTs) could be more the reflection of rapid depletion in MSU burden than SU change itself [32, 34, 35]. Second, the study included a panel of treatment initiators, patients already treated needing reinforced therapy and patients remaining under stable ULT treatment, which does not allow us to determine if flare prediction by DECT could be applicable at all stages in gout management. Future studies should assess the relationships operating in each of these subpopulations. Third, the specificity and sensitivity of the 0.81 cm^3 cutoff for MSU deposits in the feet above which there is a significant risk of flaring were probably over-estimated, given the fact that they were calculated based upon the sample that was also used to build the model. Specificity and sensitivity testing in another population is needed. Fourth, 14 patients were lost to follow up which is expected in a population with gout who are known to have compliance issues. In addition, patients did not attend all visits, which may have led to a selection bias towards patients who experienced flare. Fifth, definition of gout flares in this study relied on patient's self-assessment and retrospective confirmation by the physician. Although gout flares are marking painful experiences, the recently published definition of flares was not applied as such and the recollection of having experienced a flare may have been wrong for some patients [21, 36]. Sixth, the accuracy of MSU volume measurement with DECT is still debated, but measurements

were standardized and known artifacts removed [37–39]. Finally, patients were assessed at each visit but there was no assessment of treatment adherence (prophylaxis and ULT) between visits that could potentially have an unmeasured impact on the risk of flares. The same can be said for known triggers for gout attacks such as alcohol intake or intercurrent infection. It can only be assumed that patient behavior was similar between groups.

Conclusions

We believe this study is a step forward in our ability to tailor gout management to individual patients' initial profiles. Particularly, special caution should be given in the prevention of flares in patients with initial high urate burden.

Abbreviations
ACR: American College of Rheumatology; CT: Computed tomography; DC: Double contour; DECT: Dual-energy computed tomography; EULAR: European League Against Rheumatism; M: Month; MSU: Monosodium urate; NSAID: Non-steroidal anti-inflammatory drug; OMERACT: Outcome Measures in Rheumatology; OR: Odds ratio; RCT: Randomized controlled trial; ROC: Receiver operator characteristic; SU: Serum urate; ULT: Urate lowering therapy; US: Ultrasonography

Acknowledgements
We acknowledge the staff of the Department of Medical Research of the Lille Catholic Hospitals for their support.

Authors' contributions
TP designed the study, participated in clinical data collection, analyzed data, and participated in the writing of the manuscript. AG participated in clinical data collection and in the writing of the manuscript. LN performed the statistical analyses. VD, MM, HL, MV, CG and EH contributed to patient recruitment and critical review of the manuscript. NN, JL and BC performed US examinations and read DECT scans. JFB designed the study, performed US examinations, read DECT scans and participated in the writing of the manuscript. All authors read and approved the manuscript.

Consent for publication
Not applicable.

Competing interests
The authors declare that they have no competing interests.

Author details

[1]Department of Rheumatology, Lille Catholic Hospitals, University of Lille, 59160 Lomme, France. [2]Department of Radiology, Lille Catholic Hospitals, University of Lille, 59160 Lomme, France. [3]Department of Medical Research, Biostatistics, Lille Catholic Hospitals, University of Lille, 59160 Lomme, France. [4]EA 4490, PMOI, Physiopathologie des Maladies Osseuses Inflammatoires, University of Lille, 59000 Lille, France. [5]Saint-Philibert Hospital, Rue du Grand But, 59160 Lomme, France.

References

1. Pascart T, Liote F. Gout: state of the art after a decade of developments. Rheumatology (Oxford). 2018. https://doi.org/10.1093/rheumatology/key002.

2. Abhishek A, Valdes AM, Zhang W, Doherty M. Association of serum uric acid and disease duration with frequent gout attacks: a case-control study. Arthritis Care Res (Hoboken). 2016;68:1573–7.

3. Rothenbacher D, Primatesta P, Ferreira A, Cea-Soriano L, Rodriguez LA. Frequency and risk factors of gout flares in a large population-based cohort of incident gout. Rheumatology (Oxford). 2011;50:973–81.

4. Khanna D, Khanna PP, Fitzgerald JD, Singh MK, Bae S, Neogi T, Pillinger MH, Merill J, Lee S, Prakash S, et al. 2012 American College of Rheumatology guidelines for management of gout. Part 2: therapy and antiinflammatory prophylaxis of acute gouty arthritis. Arthritis Care Res (Hoboken). 2012;64: 1447–61.

5. Richette P, Doherty M, Pascual E, Barskova V, Becce F, Castaneda-Sanabria J, Coyfish M, Guillo S, Jansen TL, Janssens H, et al. 2016 Updated EULAR evidence-based recommendations for the management of gout. Ann Rheum Dis. 2017;76:29–42.

6. Hui M, Carr A, Cameron S, Davenport G, Doherty M, Forrester H, Jenkins W, Jordan KM, Mallen CD, McDonald TM, et al. The British Society for Rheumatology Guideline for the management of gout. Rheumatology (Oxford). 2017. https://doi.org/10.1093/rheumatology/kex150.

7. Becker MA, Schumacher HR Jr, Wortmann RL, MacDonald PA, Eustace D, Palo WA, Streit J, Joseph-Ridge N. Febuxostat compared with allopurinol in patients with hyperuricemia and gout. N Engl J Med. 2005;353:2450–61.

8. Dalbeth N, Saag KG, Palmer WE, Choi HK, Hunt B, MacDonald PA, Thienel U, Gunawardhana L. Effects of febuxostat in early gout: a randomized, double-blind, placebo-controlled study. Arthritis Rheumatol. 2017;69:2386–95.

9. Borstad GC, Bryant LR, Abel MP, Scroggie DA, Harris MD, Alloway JA. Colchicine for prophylaxis of acute flares when initiating allopurinol for chronic gouty arthritis. J Rheumatol. 2004;31:2429–32.

10. Poiley J, Steinberg AS, Choi YJ, Davis CS, Martin RL, McWherter CA, Boudes PF, Arhalofenate Flare Study I. A randomized, double-blind, active- and placebo-controlled efficacy and safety study of arhalofenate for reducing flare in patients with gout. Arthritis Rheumatol. 2016;68:2027–34.

11. Latourte A, Bardin T, Richette P. Prophylaxis for acute gout flares after initiation of urate-lowering therapy. Rheumatology (Oxford). 2014;53:1920–6.

12. Bursill D, Taylor WJ, Terkeltaub R, Kuwabara M, Merriman TR, Grainger R, Pineda C, Louthrenoo W, Edwards NL, Andres M, et al. Gout, Hyperuricemia and Crystal-Associated Disease Network (G-CAN) consensus statement regarding labels and definitions for disease elements in gout. Arthritis Care Res (Hoboken). 2018. https://doi.org/10.1002/acr.23607.

13. Becker MA, MacDonald PA, Hunt BJ, Lademacher C, Joseph-Ridge N. Determinants of the clinical outcomes of gout during the first year of urate-lowering therapy. Nucleosides Nucleotides Nucleic Acids. 2008;27:585–91.

14. Pascart T, Grandjean A, Norberciak L, Ducoulombier V, Motte M, Luraschi H, Vandecandelaere M, Godart C, Houvenagel E, Namane N, et al. Ultrasonography and dual-energy computed tomography provide different quantification of urate burden in gout: results from a cross-sectional study. Arthritis Res Ther. 2017;19:171.

15. Choi HK, Al-Arfaj AM, Eftekhari A, Munk PL, Shojania K, Reid G, Nicolaou S. Dual energy computed tomography in tophaceous gout. Ann Rheum Dis. 2009;68:1609–12.

16. Ottaviani S, Gill G, Aubrun A, Palazzo E, Meyer O, Dieude P. Ultrasound in gout: a useful tool for following urate-lowering therapy. Joint Bone Spine. 2015;82:42–4.

17. Neogi T, Jansen TL, Dalbeth N, Fransen J, Schumacher HR, Berendsen D, Brown M, Choi H, Edwards NL, Janssens HJ, et al. 2015 Gout classification criteria: an American College of Rheumatology/European League Against Rheumatism collaborative initiative. Ann Rheum Dis. 2015;74:1789–98.

18. Dalbeth N, Nicolaou S, Baumgartner S, Hu J, Fung M, Choi HK. Presence of monosodium urate crystal deposition by dual-energy CT in patients with gout treated with allopurinol. Ann Rheum Dis. 2018;77:364–70.

19. Dalbeth N, Doyle AJ. Imaging tools to measure treatment response in gout. Rheumatology (Oxford). 2018;57:i27–34.

20. Pascart T, Capon B, Grandjean A, Legrand J, Namane N, Ducoulombier V, Motte M, Vandecandelaere M, Luraschi H, Godart C, et al. The lack of association between the burden of monosodium urate crystals assessed with dual-energy computed tomography or ultrasonography with cardiovascular risk in the commonly high-risk gout patient. Arthritis Res Ther. 2018;20:97.

21. Stamp LK, Morillon MB, Taylor WJ, Dalbeth N, Singh JA, Lassere M, Christensen R. Variability in the reporting of serum urate and flares in gout clinical trials: need for minimum reporting requirements. J Rheumatol. 2018;45:419–24.

22. Finkenstaedt T, Manoliou A, Toniolo M, Higashigaito K, Andreisek G, Guggenberger R, Michel B, Alkadhi H. Gouty arthritis: the diagnostic and therapeutic impact of dual-energy CT. Eur Radiol. 2016;26:3989–99.

23. Gutierrez M, Schmidt WA, Thiele RG, Keen HI, Kaeley GS, Naredo E, Iagnocco A, Bruyn GA, Balint PV, Filippucci E, et al. International consensus for ultrasound lesions in gout: results of Delphi process and web-reliability exercise. Rheumatology (Oxford). 2015;54:1797–805.

24. Liote F, Lancrenon S, Lanz S, Guggenbuhl P, Lambert C, Saraux A, Chiarelli P, Delva C, Aubert JP, Ea HK. GOSPEL: prospective survey of gout in France. Part I: design and patient characteristics (n = 1003). Joint Bone Spine. 2012; 79:464–70.

25. Perez-Ruiz F, Martinez-Indart L, Carmona L, Herrero-Beites AM, Pijoan JI, Krishnan E. Tophaceous gout and high level of hyperuricaemia are both associated with increased risk of mortality in patients with gout. Ann Rheum Dis. 2014;73:177–82.

26. Stamp L, Morillon MB, Taylor WJ, Dalbeth N, Singh JA, Lassere M, Christensen R. Serum urate as surrogate endpoint for flares in people with gout: a systematic review and meta-regression analysis. Semin Arthritis Rheum. 2018. https://doi.org/10.1016/j.semarthrit.2018.02.009.

27. Qaseem A, Harris RP, Forciea MA. Clinical Guidelines Committee of the American College of Physicians: Management of acute and recurrent gout: a clinical practice guideline from the American College of Physicians. Ann Intern Med. 2017;166:58–68.

28. Dalbeth N, Bardin T, Doherty M, Liote F, Richette P, Saag KG, So AK, Stamp LK, Choi HK, Terkeltaub R. Discordant American College of Physicians and international rheumatology guidelines for gout management: consensus statement of the Gout, Hyperuricemia and Crystal-Associated Disease Network (G-CAN). Nat Rev Rheumatol. 2017;13:561–8.

29. Kuehn BM. Chronic disease approaches needed to curb gout's growing burden. JAMA. 2018;319:1307–9.

30. Schumacher HR Jr, Becker MA, Wortmann RL, Macdonald PA, Hunt B, Streit J, Lademacher C, Joseph-Ridge N. Effects of febuxostat versus allopurinol and placebo in reducing serum urate in subjects with hyperuricemia and gout: a 28-week, phase III, randomized, double-blind, parallel-group trial. Arthritis Rheum. 2008;59:1540–8.

31. Becker MA, Schumacher HR, Espinoza LR, Wells AF, MacDonald P, Lloyd E, Lademacher C. The urate-lowering efficacy and safety of febuxostat in the treatment of the hyperuricemia of gout: the CONFIRMS trial. Arthritis Res Ther. 2010;12:R63.

32. Araujo EG, Bayat S, Petsch C, Englbrecht M, Faustini F, Kleyer A, Hueber AJ, Cavallaro A, Lell M, Dalbeth N, et al. Tophus resolution with pegloticase: a prospective dual-energy CT study. RMD Open. 2015;1:e000075.

33. Perez-Ruiz F, Moreno-Lledo A, Urionaguena I, Dickson AJ. Treat to target in gout. Rheumatology (Oxford). 2018;57:i20–6.

34. Sundy JS, Baraf HS, Yood RA, Edwards NL, Gutierrez-Urena SR, Treadwell EL, Vazquez-Mellado J, White WB, Lipsky PE, Horowitz Z, et al. Efficacy and tolerability of pegloticase for the treatment of chronic gout in patients refractory to conventional treatment: two randomized controlled trials. JAMA. 2011;306:711–20.

35. Baraf HS, Becker MA, Gutierrez-Urena SR, Treadwell EL, Vazquez-Mellado J, Rehrig CD, Ottery FD, Sundy JS, Yood RA. Tophus burden reduction with pegloticase: results from phase 3 randomized trials and open-label extension in patients with chronic gout refractory to conventional therapy. Arthritis Res Ther. 2013;15:R137.

36. Gaffo AL, Dalbeth N, Saag KG, Singh JA, Rahn EJ, Mudano AS, Chen YH, Lin CT, Bourke S, Louthrenoo W, et al. Brief Report: Validation of a definition of flare in patients with established gout. Arthritis Rheumatol. 2018;70:462–7.

37. Baer AN, Kurano T, Thakur UJ, Thawait GK, Fuld MK, Maynard JW, McAdams-DeMarco M, Fishman EK, Carrino JA. Dual-energy computed tomography has limited sensitivity for non-tophaceous gout: a comparison study with tophaceous gout. BMC Musculoskelet Disord. 2016;17:91.

38. Coupal TM, Mallinson PI, Gershony SL, McLaughlin PD, Munk PL, Nicolaou S, Ouellette HA. Getting the most from your dual-energy scanner: recognizing, reducing, and eliminating artifacts. AJR Am J Roentgenol. 2016;206:119–28.

39. Chhana A, Doyle A, Sevao A, Amirapu S, Riordan P, Dray M, McGlashan S, Cornish J, Dalbeth N. Advanced imaging assessment of gout: comparison of dual-energy CT and MRI with anatomical pathology. Ann Rheum Dis. 2017. https://doi.org/10.1136/annrheumdis-2017-211343.

21

Potential therapeutic antibodies targeting specific adiponectin isoforms in rheumatoid arthritis

Yeon-Ah Lee[1,2], Dae-Hyun Hahm[3], Jung Yeon Kim[4], Bonjun Sur[5], Hyun Min Lee[6], Chun Jeih Ryu[6], Hyung-In Yang[1,2] and Kyoung Soo Kim[1,7*] [iD]

Abstract

Background: Different adiponectin isoforms appear to be differentially involved in the pathogenesis of various diseases. The purpose of this study was to generate monoclonal antibodies (mAbs) specific to different adiponectin isoforms and investigate whether these mAbs have potential as therapeutic agents for such diseases.

Methods: Hybridoma cells producing monoclonal antibodies were generated and screened using enzyme-linked immunosorbent assay and Western blotting for the production of mAbs recognizing human adiponectin isoforms.

Results: The mAb from hybridoma clone KH7–41 recognized both the middle molecular weight (MMW) (hexamer) and low molecular weight (LMW) (trimer) isoforms of adiponectin in human serum, whereas the KH7–33 mAb detected only MMW (hexamer) adiponectin. The KH4–8 clone recognized both the high molecular weight (HMW) (multimer) and MMW adiponectin isoforms. However, in mouse and rat sera, the abovementioned antibodies recognized only the MMW isomer. These mAbs also recognized adiponectin in various human tissues, such as lung, kidney, and adipose tissues, although the three mAbs had different staining intensities. The mAb from clone KH4–8 effectively inhibited increases in interleukin-6 (IL-6) and IL-8 expression in recombinant adiponectin-stimulated human osteoblasts and human umbilical vein endothelial cells. Also, the mAbs KH7–33 and KH4–8 significantly ameliorated rheumatic symptoms in a collagen-induced arthritis mouse model. This result suggests that these mAb treatments may ameliorate adiponectin-mediated inflammatory response.

Conclusions: mAbs against human adiponectin isomers can potentially be developed as therapeutic antibodies to target specific detrimental isoforms of adiponectin while maintaining the functions of beneficial isoforms.

Keywords: Adiponectin isomer, Monoclonal antibody, Hybridoma, Rheumatoid arthritis, CIA (collagen-induced arthritis) mouse model, Therapeutic antibody

Background

Adipose tissue produces a variety of adipokines (leptin, adiponectin, resistin, and visfatin) as well as pro- and anti-inflammatory cytokines (tumor necrosis factor-alpha (TNF-α), interleukin-4 [IL-4] and IL-6, and others) [1]. Thus, adipose tissue, though once viewed as simply a lipid storage and release depot, is now considered an endocrine tissue [2]. Among adipokines, adiponectin seems to be involved in the pathogenesis of various diseases [3, 4]. In particular, adiponectin levels in synovial fluid and serum are elevated in patients with rheumatoid arthritis (RA) [5, 6]. Adiponectin also induces the production of pro-inflammatory cytokines IL-6, matrix metalloproteinase-1 (MMP-1), and IL-8/CXCL8 by RA synovial fibroblasts *in vitro* [7, 8]. Furthermore, adiponectin stimulates osteopontin production in RA synovial tissue, which is required for osteoclast recruitment and contributes to bone erosion [9]. Expression of a pro-inflammatory cytokine, oncostatin, was also induced by adiponectin in osteoblasts. In a collagen-induced arthritis (CIA) mouse model,

---

* Correspondence: kimks@khu.ac.kr
[1]East-West Bone & Joint Disease Research Institute, Kyung Hee University Hospital at Gangdong, 02447 Seoul, Korea
[7]Department of Clinical Pharmacology and Therapeutics, College of Medicine, Kyung Hee University, 23 Kyung Hee Dae-ro, Dongdaemun-gu, 02447 Seoul, Korea
Full list of author information is available at the end of the article

adiponectin exacerbated arthritis progression through enhancement of the T helper 17 (Th17) response and receptor activator of nuclear factor-kappa B ligand (RANKL) expression [10]. In contrast, adiponectin has been suggested to have anti-inflammatory effects in the context of arthritis [11–13]. Thus, its exact role remains controversial. We recently suggested that adiponectin may contribute to synovitis and joint destruction in RA by stimulating the expression of vascular endothelial growth factor (VEGF) and MMP-1 and MMP-13 in fibroblast-like synoviocytes (FLSs) to a greater extent than do pro-inflammatory mediators [14]. In addition, at physiological concentrations, adiponectin has been suggested to be more important than IL-1β in stimulating the production of mediators that drive synovitis and joint destruction in endothelial cells and osteoblasts [15]. More importantly, we demonstrated that adiponectin in combination with IL-1β may have synergistic effects on the production of pro-inflammatory mediators during arthritic joint inflammation [16]. A recombinant adiponectin monomer produced in *Escherichia coli* was used in most of the above studies.

Adiponectin comprises a carboxyl-terminal globular domain and an amino-terminal collagenous domain [17]. It belongs to the soluble collagen superfamily and is structurally homologous to collagen VIII and X, complement factor C1q [18], and the TNF family [19]. Adiponectin belongs to a family of proteins that form characteristic multimers [20]. Using SDS-PAGE (sodium dodecyl sulfate-polyacrylamide gel electrophoresis) under non-reducing and non-heat-denaturing conditions, Waki et al. showed that adiponectin exists in a wide range of multimeric complexes in plasma and combines via its collagen domain to create three main oligomeric forms: a low-molecular-weight (LMW) trimer, a middle-molecular-weight (MMW) hexamer, and a high-molecular-weight (HMW) 12- to 18-mer [21]. These adiponectin isoforms seem to affect gene expression differently. Frommer et al. showed the differential effects of adiponectin isoforms on effector cells involved in RA pathophysiology: HMW/MMW-enriched and globular adiponectin strongly activated expression of chemokines and pro-inflammatory cytokines in RA synovial fibroblasts (RASFs), while the adiponectin trimer (LMW) led to minimal chemokine and cytokine expression [22]. In addition, adiponectin isoforms differentially affected lipid gene expression in primary human hepatocytes (PHHs) [23]. Population-based studies revealed that HMW adiponectin was negatively associated with low-density lipoprotein cholesterol, triglycerides, apolipoprotein B, and apolipoprotein E and was positively associated with high-density lipoprotein cholesterol [24–26]. Adiponectin isoforms also function as acute-phase reactants influencing inflammation in acute and chronic diseases. In obesity, adiponectin isoform formation is disrupted, leading to the development of pathologic conditions [27]. Given their pathophysiological effects, detrimental adiponectin isoforms could plausibly be targeted as a therapeutic strategy while maintaining the beneficial activities of other adiponectin isoforms. Here, we show that monoclonal antibodies (mAbs) against adiponectin isomers recognize adiponectin isoforms in sera and tissues and we demonstrate anti-arthritic effects in a CIA mouse model.

Methods

Hybridoma production and monoclonal antibody purification

Two BALB/c mice were immunized subcutaneously with 100 μL of complete Freund's adjuvant (CFA) (Difco Laboratories, Detroit, MI, USA) containing 100 μg of recombinant human adiponectin expressed in *E. coli* (ProSpec, Rehovot, Israel). After 2 weeks, the mice were injected with incomplete Freund's adjuvant. The mice were boosted with antigen only (that is, 50 μg of adiponectin intravenously) 2 weeks later. Two days after the last boost, sera were tested for reactivity to recombinant adiponectin using enzyme-linked immunosorbent assay (ELISA). Splenic lymphocytes were fused to FO myeloma cells (ATCC, Manassas, VA, USA) and plated on 96-well plates in Dulbecco's modified Eagle's medium (DMEM) supplemented with 20% fetal bovine serum (FBS) (Invitrogen, Waltham, MA, USA) and HAT component (Sigma-Aldrich Korea, Yongin, Korea) as described previously [28]. The culture supernatants were tested by Western blot and ELISA for reactivity to recombinant human adiponectin. mAbs were purified from culture supernatants of the screened clones by using Protein G-Sepharose column chromatography (GenScript, Piscataway, NJ, USA) in accordance with the protocol of the manufacturer. Studies were conducted in accordance with the National Institutes of Health guidelines and were approved by the Institutional Animal Care and Use Committee of Kyung Hee University.

Collagen-induced arthritis mouse model

Male DBA/1 J mice (4 weeks old) were purchased from Central Lab. Animal Inc. (Seoul, Korea). The animals were kept in a rodent facility and adapted for at least 1 week before CIA induction as previously described [29]. Briefly, the mice (6 weeks old) were immunized at the base of the tail with a 100-μL mixture of chicken collagen type II (CII) 100 μg (Sigma-Aldrich Korea) and CFA. After 14 days, the mice were given a booster injection of 100 μg CII and incomplete Freund's adjuvant. The mice were divided into five groups (n = 8) containing normal, CIA (saline, control), CIA + KH4–8 mAb (6 mg/kg, intraperitoneal injection, three times a week for 6 weeks), CIA + KH7–33 mAb (6 mg/kg, intraperitoneal injection, three times a week for 6 weeks), and CIA + prednisolone (10 mg/kg, intragastric administration, twice a week for 6 weeks). Normal mice and CIA control mice were given an equal volume of normal saline. The treatment antibody concentration was decided on the basis of the treatment dose for therapeutic antibodies in mice [30, 31]. To evaluate the therapeutic effect of mAbs KH4–8 and KH7–33 on the progression of arthritis in CIA mice, body weight, paw volume, squeaking score, and arthritic score were measured [29]. All methods were approved by the Animal Care and Use Committee of Kyung-Hee University (KHUASP[SE]-15–115). All procedures were executed in accordance with the guide for the Care and Use of Laboratory Animals by the Korea National Institute of Health.

Cell culture for *in vitro* functional testing of monoclonal antibodies

Human umbilical vein endothelial cells (HUVECs) and human osteoblasts were obtained from the Korean Cell Line Bank (KCLB, Seoul, Korea) and Cell Applications, Inc. (San Diego, CA, USA), respectively. Endothelial cells and osteoblasts were cultured in T-75 flasks (Nunc, Thermo Fisher Scientific, Waltham, MA, USA) containing EGM-2 (Lonza, Alpharetta, GA, USA) and osteoblast growth medium (Cell Applications, Inc. San Diego, CA, USA), respectively. After the cells had grown to confluence, they were split at a 1:4 ratio. Cell passages 5–6 were used for all experiments. HUVECs (2×10^5 cells per six-well plate in 2 mL of medium) and osteoblasts (1×10^5 cells per six-well plate in 2 mL of medium) were cultured overnight and treated with human recombinant adiponectin, which was produced by using *E. coli* (ProSpec, Rehovot, Israel). To test the ability of the mAb to block adiponectin function, mAb (~120 µg/mL) and adiponectin (2.5 or 5 µg/mL) were mixed and incubated for 1 h before being used to treat cells. After 24-h treatment, the culture supernatants were collected and frozen, and IL-6 and IL-8 were measured by ELISA.

Epitope mapping of monoclonal antibody

Epitope mapping of the KH4–8 mAb was performed by using PEPperMAP° technology (PEPperPRINT GmbH, Heidelberg, Germany) [32]. PEPperMAP° Linear Epitope Mapping of mouse mAb KH4–8 was performed against human adiponectin translated into linear 15–amino acid peptides with a peptide-peptide overlap of 14 amino acids. Human adiponectin peptide microarrays were incubated with the mouse mAb at concentrations of 1 µg/mL, 10 µg/mL, and 100 µg/mL in incubation buffer followed by staining with secondary goat anti-mouse IgG (H + L) DyLight680 antibody. Samples were processed by using an Odyssey Imaging System (LI-COR, Lincoln, NE, USA).

Quantification of spot intensities and peptide annotation were performed using a PepSlide° Analyzer (PEPperPRINT GmbH).

Western blotting

To screen hybridomas for production of mAbs against recombinant human adiponectin, adiponectin (100 ng/well) was resolved via 12% SDS-PAGE and transferred to Hybond-ECL membranes (Amersham, Arlington Heights, IL, USA). The membranes were blocked with 6% non-fat milk dissolved in TBST buffer (10 mM Tris-Cl [pH 8.0], 150 mM NaCl, 0.05% Tween 20). The blots were probed with hybridoma culture supernatants at 4 °C overnight and incubated with a 1:1,000 dilution of horseradish peroxidase–conjugated goat anti-mouse IgG secondary antibody (Sigma-Aldrich Korea). The blots were developed by using the ECL method (Amersham). To detect adiponectin in human, mouse, and rat serum samples, serum was subjected to gradient SDS-PAGE (4–12%) (NuPAGE° Bis-Tris Mini Gels, Invitrogen), blotted, and probed with purified mAb (5 µg/mL) as the primary antibody, as described above. Mouse and rat serum were obtained via heart puncture of male BALB/c mice and Sprague Dawley (SD) rats (8 weeks old), respectively. Human serum was obtained from a male volunteer (55 years old).

Enzyme-linked immunosorbent assay

Culture supernatants from cells treated with mAb plus adiponectin were analyzed with IL-6 and IL-8 ELISA kits (BD Bioscience Korea, Seoul, Korea) in accordance with the protocol of the manufacturer. To screen hybridoma clones for mAbs against adiponectin, 96-well plates were coated with adiponectin (200 ng/well), hybridoma culture supernatants were added after blocking, wells were incubated with a 1:1,000 dilution of horseradish peroxidase–conjugated goat anti-mouse IgG secondary antibody (Sigma-Aldrich Korea), and the ELISA procedure was completed. Sera from CIA were obtained from heart puncture and analyzed for adiponectin, IL-6, TNF-α, and RANKL by using the Luminex° 200™ Total System (Luminex Corporation, Austin, TX, USA) as previously described [33].

Histological assessment of inflammation

Mice were killed after 56 days of CII + CFA treatments. Histochemical staining was performed to determine the degree of immune cell infiltration into the joints. Mice knee joints were dissected, fixed for 3 days in 10% formalin, dehydrated through a graded ethanol series, cleared in xylene, and processed for embedding in paraffin wax with routine protocols.

Coronal sections 8 mm thick were cut through the knee joint by using a manual rotary microtome (Finesse 325, Thermo Shandon Inc., Pittsburgh, PA, USA) and stained with hematoxylin and eosin for routine histological evaluation. Paraffin tissue sections obtained from rat knees were deparaffinized in xylene. The tissue samples were hydrated with ethanol and washed in distilled water, followed by antigen retrieval via heating with 100 mM citrate buffer (pH 6.0) at 65 °C for 1–2 h. The samples were examined with a confocal laser scanning microscope (Olympus BX53, Olympus Corporation, Tokyo, Japan). The degree of inflammation was evaluated on a scale from 0 to 4 by three different experts who were blinded to treatment information. The scale was defined as follows: 0 = no inflammation, 1 = minimal inflammation, 2 = mild inflammation, 3 = moderate inflammation, and 4 = severe inflammation.

Immunohistochemistry

Normal human tissues were obtained from archived paraffin collections at the Department of Pathology, Inje University Sanggye Paik Hospital (Seoul, Korea). Adipose, lung, kidney, and pancreas tissues were obtained from different donors (a 59-year-old woman, a 72-year-old man, a 62-year-old woman, and a 67-year-old man, respectively). Sections (4 μm) of the paraffin blocks were cut and immunohistochemically stained with mAbs (50 μg/mL) by using an automated

system (Vision BioSystems Ltd., Mount Waverley, Australia), as described below. Antigen was retrieved with epitope retrieval solution 1 (Leica Microsystems, Newcastle, UK). Slides were incubated with antibody at room temperature for 20 min and then with a biotinylated secondary antibody for 8 min. The resulting complexes were detected with avidin-peroxidase-conjugated polymer. Color was developed by using 3,3′-diaminobenzidine (DAB) (ScyTek, Logan, UT, USA). Mayer's hematoxylin was used as a counterstain. Positive and negative control stains were used in each run. The study protocol was reviewed and approved by the institutional review board at Inje University Sanggye Paik Hospital. For immunohistochemical staining of adiponectin in the joints of mice using anti-adiponectin antibody (Abcam, Cambridge, MA, USA), moderate nuclear or cell membranous staining was determined as a percentage and scored as follows: 0 = staining in less than 10% of cells, 1 = staining in 10–50% of cells, and 2 = staining in more than 50% of cells. Cases with a score of 1 or 2 were classified as positive.

Statistical analysis

In vitro data are expressed as the mean ± standard error of the mean of quadruplicate samples. The expression levels of the factors were compared between groups by using the Mann–Whitney test. Prism 5.02 software (GraphPad Software, San Diego, CA, USA) was used for

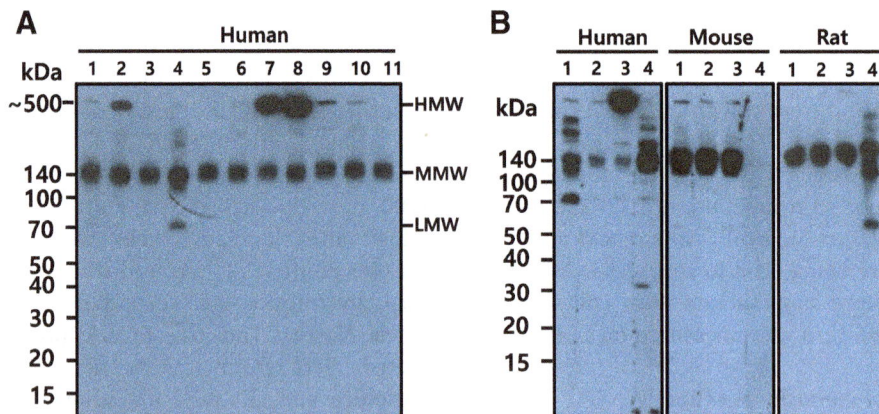

Fig. 1 Detection of serum adiponectin isoforms with monoclonal antibodies (mAbs) against recombinant human adiponectin. **a** Western blot to screen mAbs detecting different adiponectin isoforms. Human serum was loaded into each lane of the gel and resolved by polyacrylamide gel electrophoresis (PAGE) and then transferred to a membrane. Each lane of the membrane was then separately cut and incubated with each mAb from hybridoma culture supernatant. After the secondary antibody was probed, the cut membrane was combined to form one sheet and developed with ECL solution. Eleven different mAbs from culture supernatant were tested to investigate their recognition patterns of adiponectin isoforms in serum. The mAb KH7–33, in lane 3, was selected as a representative recognizing only the middle molecular weight (MMW) isoform of adiponectin. The mAb KH7–41, in lane 4, was selected as a representative recognizing both the MMW and low molecular weight (LMW) isoforms of adiponectin. The mAb KH4–8, in lane 8, was selected as a representative mAb recognizing both the MMW and HMW isoforms of adiponectin. **b** Comparison of the mAb recognition patterns of adiponectin isoforms in human, mouse, and rat sera by Western blot. Human, mouse, and rat sera were separated by sodium dodecyl sulfate–PAGE. All three mAbs (KH7–33, KH7–41, and KH4–8) recognized the rat and mouse adiponectin MMW isoform. Lane 1, KH7–41; lane 2, KH7–33; lane 3, KH4–8; lane 4, commercial antibody against human adiponectin (Boster Immunoleader cat. no. PB9001) or mouse/rat adiponectin (Boster Immunoleader cat. no. PB9011). Mouse and rat serum were obtained via heart puncture of male BALB/c mice and Sprague Dawley rats (8 weeks old), respectively. Human serum was obtained from a male volunteer (55 years old)

statistical analysis and graphing. Statistical differences between CIA mouse groups were identified by using t tests, one-way analysis of variance (ANOVA) with Dunn's Multiple Comparison Test, and two-way ANOVA followed by Bonferroni post-test correction (for multiple comparisons of body weight, squeaking score, paw volume, and arthritis index score). Differences were considered significant at a P value of less than 0.05.

Results

Screening hybridoma clones producing mAb against adiponectin isomers and mAb purification from culture supernatants

Each hybridoma clone generated against recombinant adiponectin was screened by using ELISA performed on its culture supernatant. The optical densities (ODs) of culture supernatants from positive hybridoma clones were 10 times higher than the ODs of negative clones (data not shown). The reactivity of mAb from each clone was confirmed by Western blotting. Hybridomas producing mAb against recombinant human adiponectin were subcloned and screened by using ELISA and Western blotting. To purify mAb from culture supernatants, supernatant (500 mL) from each hybridoma clone was passed through a Protein G-Sepharose column (2-mL bed volume), washed, and eluted with elution buffer in accordance with the protocol of the manufacturer. Approximately 15 mg of mAb was obtained from 500 mL of supernatant. mAb purity was determined by Coomassie staining after PAGE. Purified mAb was detected with anti-mouse IgG-HRP, which suggests that

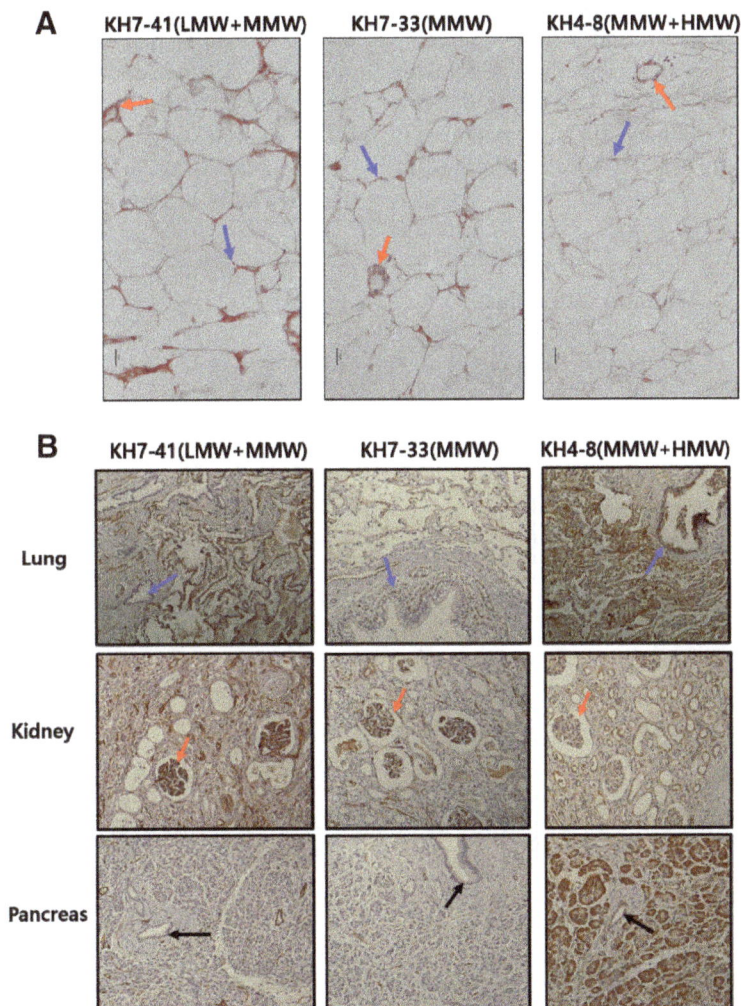

Fig. 2 Immunohistological assays in human tissues with monoclonal antibodies (mAbs). To determine the pattern of recognition of adiponectin isoforms in human tissues by mAbs, **a** normal human adipose tissue was immunostained with mAbs (KH7–41, KH7–33, and KH4–8) (200×, scale bar = 25 μm). mAbs recognized adiponectin in the nucleus of adipocytes (blue arrow) and in vessels and endothelial cells (red arrow). **b** Human lung, kidney, and pancreas were stained with the KH7–41, KH7–33, and KH4–8 mAbs (100×). Abbreviations: *HMW* high molecular weight, *LMW* low molecular weight, *MMW* middle molecular weight

the protein purified from each supernatant was IgG (data not shown).

Differences in patterns of recognition of adiponectin isoforms between the purified mAbs in serum

To determine whether these purified mAbs recognized adiponectin isoforms in human serum, we analyzed the sera by Western blotting following gradient SDS-PAGE (4–12%). As shown in Fig. 1a, different mAbs recognized the various adiponectin isoforms in human serum to differing degrees. In particular, the mAb from KH7–41 (lane 4) recognized the trimeric (LMW) and hexameric (MMW) isoforms of human serum adiponectin. However, the mAb from KH7–33 (lane 3) detected only the hexameric (MMW) isoform whereas the KH4–8 mAb (lane 8) strongly recognized the HMW isoform of human adiponectin but weakly recognized the MMW isoform. The recognition patterns of adiponectin isoforms by these three mAbs in mouse and rat serum were compared with those in human serum (Fig. 1b). Unlike with human serum, the KH7–41 and KH4–8 mAbs did not recognize LMW or HMW adiponectin in mouse or rat serum. These mAbs recognized only MMW adiponectin in mouse and rat serum.

Recognition of adiponectin isoforms in tissues using purified mAbs

To test whether the three mAbs recognized adiponectin isoforms in tissues, human adipose tissue was incubated with each mAb (Fig. 2). All three mAbs stained adipose tissue. The staining patterns of the mAbs were not significantly different from one another. These three antibodies all recognized adiponectin both in the nuclei of adipocytes (blue arrow in Fig. 2a) and in blood vessels (red arrow in Fig. 2a). In contrast, other human tissues were differentially stained by different mAbs (Fig. 2b). In lung tissues, both KH7–41 and KH7–33 recognized adiponectin only in alveoli but not in bronchioles (blue arrow). KH4–8 recognized it in both alveoli and bronchioles, suggesting that the HMW isoform is predominant in bronchioles. In kidney tissue, KH7–33 recognized adiponectin only in glomeruli whereas both KH7–41 and KH4–8 recognized it in glomeruli and tubules. This suggests that the MMW isoform may be absent, or may be present only at a very low level, in tubules. In pancreatic tissue, both KH7–41 and KH7–33 recognized adiponectin only in vessels (yellow arrow) but not in acini or ducts (black arrow). However, KH4–8 recognized adiponectin in vessels, ducts, and acini, suggesting that the HMW isoform is present in all pancreatic tissue.

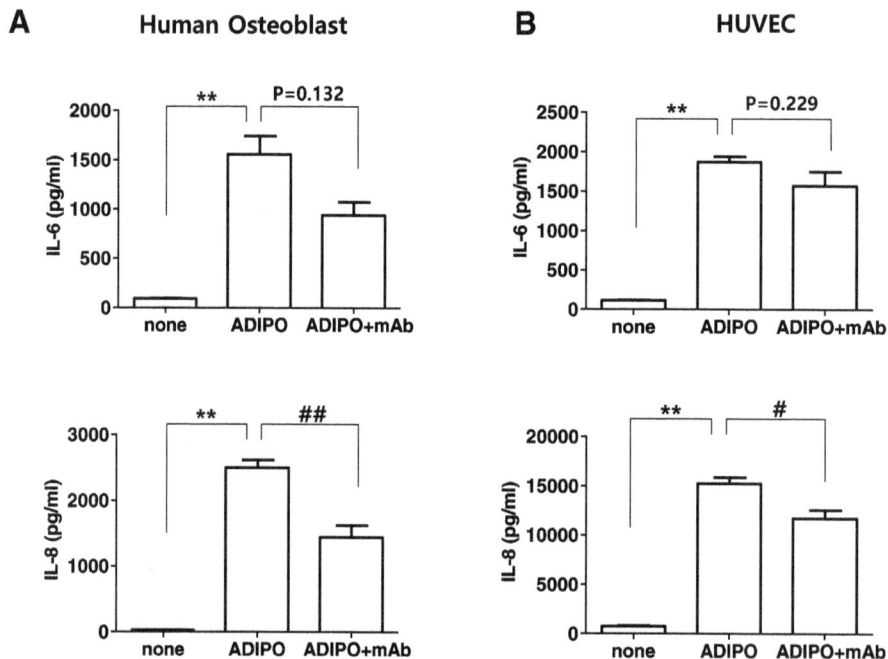

Fig. 3 Inhibition of adiponectin-mediated gene expression *in vitro* by monoclonal antibodies (mAbs). To test the ability of the mAb KH4–8 to block adiponectin function, (**a**) human osteoblasts and (**b**) human umbilical vein endothelial cells (HUVECs) were treated with adiponectin (ADIPO) or KH4–8 mAb (mAb) or both. The mAb (~120 μg/mL) and recombinant adiponectin (2.5 μg/mL) were mixed and incubated for 1 h before being used to treat cells. After 24-h treatment, the culture supernatants were collected and frozen, and interleukin-6 (IL-6) and IL-8 were measured by using enzyme-linked immunosorbent assay (ELISA) (R&D Systems, Minneapolis, MN, USA). The experiments were performed in quadruplicate. The data shown are representative of three independent experiments, and similar results were obtained with all three mAbs. Values are expressed as mean ± standard error of the mean. The expression levels of the factors were compared between groups by using the Mann–Whitney test. *$P < 0.05$, **$P < 0.01$ versus the untreated group, #$P < 0.05$, ##$P < 0.01$ versus the group treated with adiponectin and mAb

Blocking of *in vitro* adiponectin activity by monoclonal antibodies

To test the biological activity of the purified mAbs, HUVECs and human osteoblasts were treated with adiponectin or mAbs or both. As shown in Fig. 3, treating human osteoblasts with adiponectin (2.5 μg/mL) significantly increased IL-6 and IL-8 production compared with levels in the untreated group. Combined administration of KH4–8 mAb (~120 μg/mL) and adiponectin (2.5 μg/mL) significantly inhibited this increase in IL-8 production but did not significantly inhibit the increase in IL-6 production. In addition, as was observed in osteoblasts, treating HUVECs with adiponectin (5 μg/mL) significantly increased IL-6 and IL-8 production compared with levels in the untreated group. Combined administration of KH4–8 mAb (~120 μg/mL) and adiponectin (5 μg/mL) significantly inhibited the increase in IL-8 production but did not significantly inhibit the increase in IL-6 production. Administration of other mAbs yielded inhibition similar to that seen with KH7–33 treatment (data not shown). These results suggest that these mAbs partially inhibit the activity of recombinant adiponectin *in vitro*.

Epitope mapping of monoclonal antibody KH4–8

To further confirm the specific epitope recognized by KH4–8 mAb, epitope mapping was performed as described in the Methods. The epitope recognition site of the KH4–8 mAb was confirmed by peptide microarray (Fig. 4). A six–amino acid sequence (139–144), QQNHYD, from the full 244–amino acid sequence was confirmed to be the epitope of adiponectin. The amino acid sequence (91–97), PRGFPGI, was assumed to be an epitope recognized by contaminant antibody coming from the use of a recycled Protein G-Sepharose column.

Inhibition of arthritic symptoms by monoclonal antibodies in a collagen-induced arthritis mouse model

To test the *in vivo* anti-arthritic effect of our mAbs against adiponectin, mAbs were injected intraperitoneally into a CIA mouse model. As shown in Fig. 5, the injection of mAbs from the KH4–8 and KH7–33 clones inhibited the arthritic symptoms in CIA mice. The anti-arthritic effect of the mAbs was demonstrated by measuring the arthritis index, squeaking index, and paw volume. To further demonstrate the anti-inflammatory effect of mAbs, sera from CIA mice were analyzed for pro-inflammatory cytokines, such as adiponectin, IL-6, TNF-α, and RANKL, by using a Luminex system (Fig. 6). TNF-α and IL-6 were significantly increased in sera of CIA mice compared with that of normal mice and were slightly decreased by treatment with mAb KH4–8 or KH7–33. However, the decrease in adiponectin in CIA mice was not reversed by treatment with mAbs. In contrast, RANKL level in the sera of CIA mice did not vary compared with that of normal mice. The histology of knee joints in CIA mice further

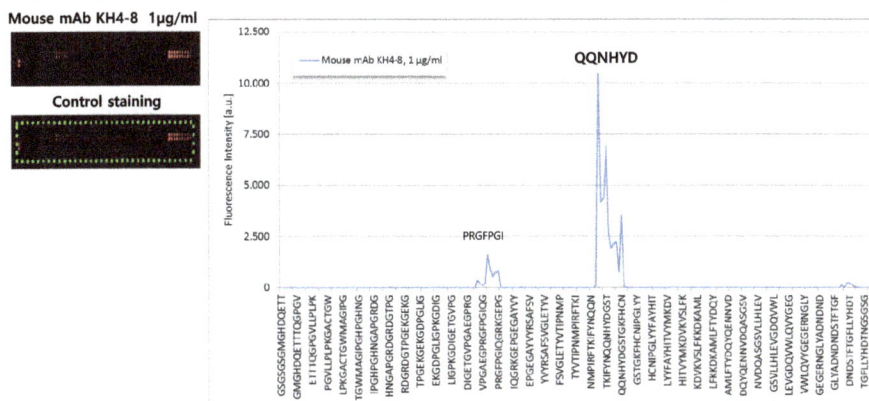

The protein sequence of Adiponectin and mAb KH4-8 recognizing sequence

```
  1 MLLLGAVLLL LALPGHDQET TTQGPGVLLP LPKGACTGWM AGIPGHPGHN GAPGRDGRDG
 61 TPGEKGEKGD PGLIGPKGDI GETGVPGAEG PRGFPGIQGR KGEPGEGAYV YRSAFSVGLE
121 TYVTIPNMPI RFTKIFYNQQ NHYDGSTGKF HCNIPGLYYF AYHITVYMKD VKVSLFKKDK
181 AMLFTYDQYQ ENNVDQASGS VLLHLEVGDQ VWLQVYGEGE RNGLYADNDN DSTFTGFLLY
241 HDTN
```

Fig. 4 Epitope mapping of monoclonal antibody (mAb) KH4–8 against adiponectin. To identify the epitope-recognizing site of the KH4–8 mAb, PEPperMAP® technology was performed as described in the Methods. Human adiponectin was translated into linear 15–amino acid peptides with a peptide-peptide overlap of 14 amino acids. Human adiponectin peptide microarrays were incubated with mouse mAb KH4–8 at different concentrations followed by staining with secondary goat anti-mouse IgG (H + L) DyLight680 antibody. The light intensity was read by a reader. The amino acid sequence QQNHYD (139–144) was confirmed from among the full 244–amino acid sequence to be the epitope of adiponectin

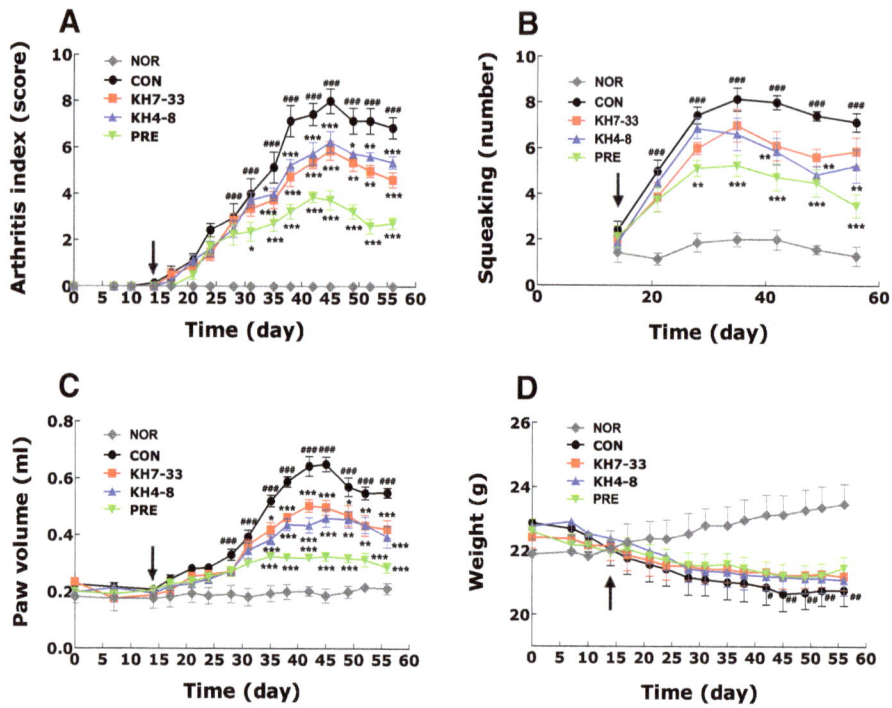

Fig. 5 Anti-arthritic activity of monoclonal antibodies (mAbs) KH4–8 and KH7–33 in a mouse model of collagen-induced arthritis. **a** arthritis index, **b** squeaking score (a value of 0 represents no indication of pain), **c** paw volume, and (**d**) body weight, indicating the severity of arthritis in mouse limbs. The number of arthritic limbs was quantitated, and each limb was assigned a severity score of 0–4. Data indicate the number of arthritic limbs per arthritic mouse and the mean severity score of each arthritic limb. The black arrows indicate the starting day (day 15) of mAb or prednisolone administration. NOR (normal), n = 8; CON (negative control), KH4–8, n = 8; KH7–33, n = 8; PRE (prednisolone, positive control), n = 8. Values are expressed as mean ± standard error of the mean. $^{###}P < 0.001$ versus the NOR group and $^{*}P < 0.05$, $^{**}P < 0.01$, $^{***}P < 0.001$ versus the CON group (two-way analysis of variance followed by Bonferroni correction)

demonstrated the anti-arthritic effect of mAb KH4–8 or KH7–33. As shown in Fig. 7, joint inflammation was increased and the joint cavity was destroyed in CIA mice. Treatment with antibody KH7–33 significantly decreased both the inflammation area and degradation of the joint cavity in arthritic joints compared with those of control CIA mice. Furthermore, we investigated whether adiponectin expression was increased in the joints of CIA mice. The expression of adiponectin was increased in adipose tissue around the joints of CIA mice compared with normal mice on the basis of immunohistochemistry (Fig. 7). However, adiponectin expression increased via induction of inflammation was not decreased by treatment with the mAbs used in this experiment or anti-inflammatory agents.

Discussion

In this study, we developed hybridomas producing mAbs against human adiponectin isoforms as potential therapeutic agents for inflammatory diseases such as RA. These mAbs were shown to recognize human adiponectin isoforms in human sera and tissues by Western blot and immunohistochemistry. Furthermore, these mAbs inhibited

IL-6 and IL-8 production in HUVECs and human osteoblasts stimulated with recombinant adiponectin, suggesting that these mAbs blocked the action of adiponectin in the cells. The *in vivo* anti-arthritic effects of our mAbs were demonstrated in a CIA mouse model on the basis of the arthritis index, squeaking index, and paw volume, in agreement with the observed *in vitro* anti-inflammatory effects of the mAbs. In addition, increased levels of pro-inflammatory cytokines such as TNF-α and IL-6 in the sera of CIA mice were slightly decreased by treatment with mAbs. The anti-arthritic effects of the mAbs were also demonstrated by histology of CIA mouse knee joints. In particular, mAb KH4–8 was found to recognize a six–amino acid sequence (139–144), QQNHYD, from the full 244–amino acid sequence as the epitope of adiponectin. All of these results suggest the potential of mAbs against recombinant adiponectin as a therapeutic antibody in the treatment of RA.

For the development and production of these antibodies, hybridomas producing mAbs against recombinant human adiponectin were screened by ELISA and Western blot. IgGs from culture supernatants were purified by using a Protein G column, and the purity thereof

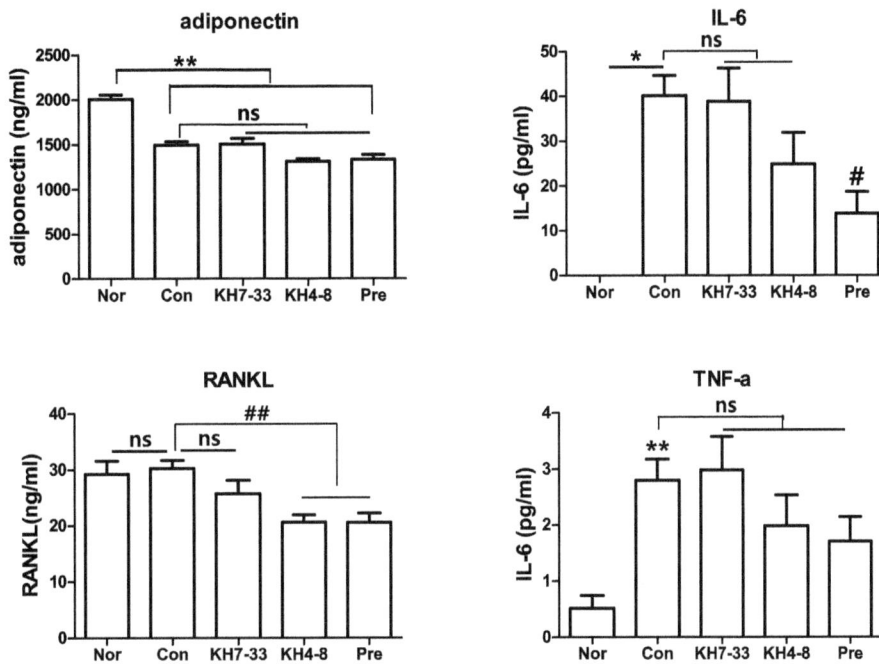

Fig. 6 Anti-inflammatory effect of monoclonal antibodies (mAbs) KH4–8 and KH7–33 on the expression of serum pro-inflammatory cytokines of the collagen-induced arthritis mouse model. The serum levels of adiponectin, interleukin-6 (IL-6), tumor necrosis factor-alpha (TNF-α), and receptor activator of nuclear factor-kappa B ligand (RANKL) were analyzed by using the Luminex system. Values are expressed as mean ± standard error of the mean. The expression levels of the factors were compared between groups ($n = 8$) by using the Mann–Whitney test. **$P < 0.01$, *$P < 0.05$ versus normal (NOR) group, and ##$P < 0.01$, ##$P < 0.05$ versus the control (CON) group. Abbreviations: *ns* not significant, *pre* prednisolone

was determined by Coomassie blue staining. The only proteins detected were the heavy and light chains of mouse IgG. The identities thereof were confirmed by using an anti-mouse IgG secondary antibody coupled to horseradish peroxidase (Additional file 1). To test cross-species reactivity, mAbs purified from three hybridoma clones—KH7–41, KH7–33, and KH4–8—were tested for their ability to detect adiponectin in rat and mouse sera. Western blots employing these mAbs showed different patterns of recognition of adiponectin in human serum, whereas the mAbs had similar recognition patterns in rat and mouse serum. KH7–41 recognized two isoforms of human adiponectin: LMW and MMW. The KH4–8 mAb recognized MMW and HMW, whereas the KH7–33 mAb recognized only one isoform of human adiponectin: MMW. These results indicate that each antibody is molecularly distinct and recognizes a different epitope of human adiponectin.

To generate adiponectin isoform-specific mAbs, adiponectin isoforms purified from serum via gel filtration may be used to immunize mice [34]. This approach can be very labor-intensive. However, this study shows that recombinant adiponectin can also be used to generate mAbs against distinct adiponectin isoforms. Based on our Western blot results, the KH4–8 mAb probably targets HMW/MMW adiponectin isoforms, which are believed to induce higher expression of inflammatory

cytokines than the LMW isoform [35]. In addition, the serum levels of adiponectin isoforms change under disease conditions. For example, in anorexia nervosa, the percentage of HMW relative to total adiponectin (%HMW) is remarkably lower and the percentage of LMW relative to total adiponectin (%LMW) is significantly higher in the anorexia nervosa group compared with the control group [36]. In patients with hypertension, HMW adiponectin has been reported to be significantly lower ($P < 0.05$) and LMW adiponectin significantly higher ($P < 0.01$) than in normotensive persons [37]. The serum level of MMW adiponectin has also been shown to be decreased in endometrial cancer [38]. Adiponectin also plays a central role in obesity-related disease. HMW seems to have the predominant action in metabolic tissues. A recent report demonstrated that an increased LMW/total adiponectin ratio was associated with type 2 diabetes through a relationship to increasing insulin resistance [39]. Adiponectin can be a therapeutic target for obesity, diabetes, and endothelial dysfunction [40]. Thus, it has been suggested that targeting detrimental adiponectin isoforms while maintaining beneficial adiponectin isoforms might prevent or decrease the risk of certain diseases. In addition, mAbs against adiponectin isoforms may be used to study the distribution of adiponectin isoforms in tissues. As shown in Fig. 2, adiponectin isoforms are

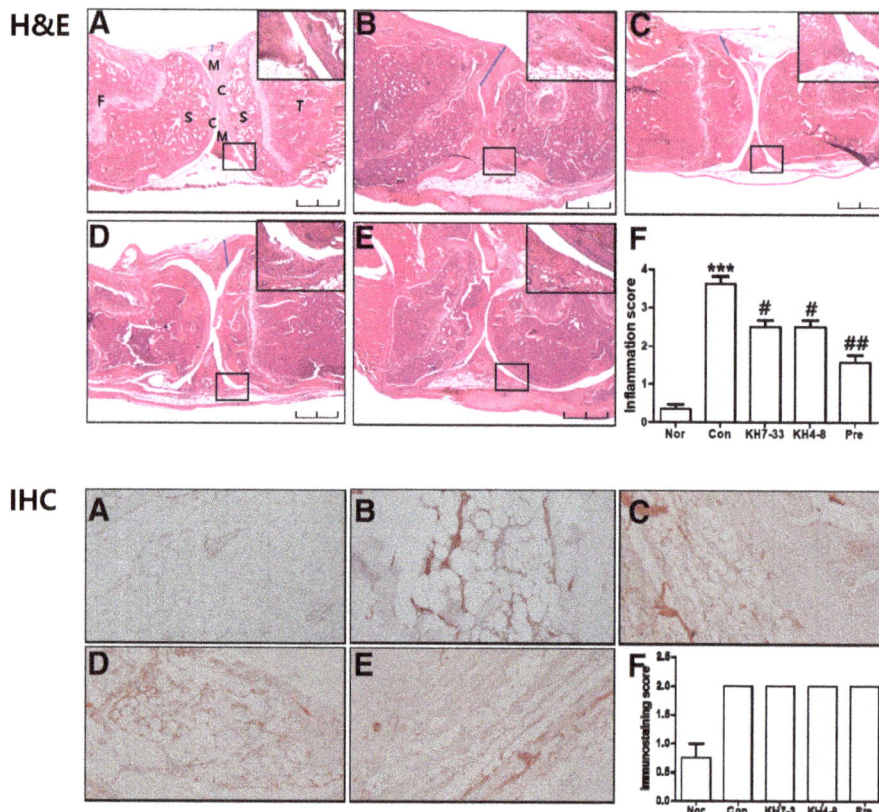

Fig. 7 Anti-adiponectin antibodies reduce the histological signs of inflammation. The upper and lower panels present hematoxylin and eosin (H&E) staining and immunostaining against mouse adiponectin of mouse knee joints (n = 8), respectively. **a** Normal, **b** control, saline-treated arthritic, **c** KH7–33-treated arthritic, **d** KH4–8-treated arthritic, and (**e**) prednisolone-treated arthritic mice. Tissue structure was visualized by using H&E staining (original magnification, 40×). Scale bar = 2 mm. **f** Arthritic symptoms were evaluated by scoring the degree of inflammation on H&E histological sections of knee joints as described in the Methods. Small blue squares on H&E staining are magnified in the upper right corner (400×). Abbreviations: *C* cartilage, *F* femur, *M* meniscus, *S* subchondral bone, *T* tibia. In the lower panel, immunohistochemistry (IHC) reveals adiponectin expression in collagen-induced arthritis mouse joints (200×). The increased adiponectin expression level observed on IHC was not decreased by monoclonal antibody treatment. Adiponectin immunostaining score level was evaluated as described in the Methods. Results are presented as the mean of experiments (± standard error of the mean indicated by error bar) (one-way analysis of variance followed by Dunn's multiple comparison test). ***$P < 0.001$ versus the normal (NOR) group and #$P < 0.05$, ##$P < 0.01$ versus the control (CON) group. Abbreviation: *pre* prednisolone

differentially distributed in tissues. Their differential distribution may also be involved in the pathogenesis of disease or may result from the progression of disease [41, 42]. Moreover, physical exercise induced a 21% decrease in HMW/LMW, whereas diet-induced weight loss shifted the distribution toward a higher molecular weight (42% increase in HMW/MMW) [43]. However, more accurate methods for measuring changes in adiponectin and its isoforms are needed. The mAbs used in this study have potential for measuring adiponectin variation as well as in a variety of clinical diagnostics. For example, KH4–8 mAb can be used for the diagnosis of diet-induced weight loss effects because KH4–8 mAb specifically recognizes the HMW/MMW isoform. These mAbs can also be applied for diagnosis of hypertension or inflammatory disease, which are associated with isoform distribution changes.

Adiponectin level was decreased in the serum of CIA mice, as shown in Fig. 6. However, adiponectin expression was increased in adipose tissue near arthritic joints in CIA mice. In addition, our previous studies demonstrated that adiponectin level in the joint fluid of patients with RA was greatly increased compared with that of patients with osteoarthritis [14]. All of these studies indirectly suggest that adiponectin may be more involved in joint inflammation than other tissues in the CIA mouse model. The mAbs had *in vivo* anti-arthritic effects in a CIA mouse model. In future experiments, the mAbs will be modified to a humanized antibody for human clinical trials, with the goal of using therapeutic antibodies against a specific adiponectin isoform to target specific detrimental isoforms of adiponectin in various diseases while maintaining the function of beneficial isoforms.

Conclusions

The mAbs from hybridomas generated against a recombinant human adiponectin monomer recognized adiponectin isoforms in serum and tissue. These mAbs can potentially be developed as therapeutic or diagnostic antibodies, with the goal of targeting specific detrimental isoforms of adiponectin while maintaining the function of beneficial isoforms. Thus, mAbs against specific adiponectin isoforms could potentially be developed into therapeutic agents to treat RA or inflammatory disease.

Abbreviations

ANOVA: Analysis of variance; CFA: Complete Freund's adjuvant; CIA: Collagen-induced arthritis; CII: Collagen type II; ELISA: Enzyme-linked immunosorbent assay; HMW: High molecular weight; HUVEC: Human umbilical vein endothelial cell; IL: Interleukin; LMW: Low molecular weight; mAb: Monoclonal antibody; MMW: Middle molecular weight; OD: Optical density; RA: Rheumatoid arthritis; RANKL: Receptor activator of nuclear factor-kappa B ligand; SDS-PAGE: Sodium dodecyl sulfate-polyacrylamide gel electrophoresis; TNF: Tumor necrosis factor

Acknowledgments

The present study was supported by a grant from the Korea Health Technology R&D Project through the Korea Health Industry Development Institute (KHIDI) funded by the Ministry of Health and Welfare, Republic of Korea (grant HI17C0658).

Funding

The present study was supported by a grant from the Korea Health Technology R&D Project through the Korea Health Industry Development Institute (KHIDI), funded by the Ministry of Health and Welfare, Republic of Korea (grant HI17C0658).

Authors' contributions

KSK participated in data analysis and design of the study and drafted the manuscript. Y-AL, D-HH, BS, JYK, HML, and CJR performed the experiments. H-IY participated in the design of the study. All authors read and approved the final manuscript.

Consent for publication

Not applicable.

Competing interests

The authors declare that they have no competing interests.

Author details

[1]East-West Bone & Joint Disease Research Institute, Kyung Hee University Hospital at Gangdong, 02447 Seoul, Korea. [2]Division of Rheumatology, Department of Internal Medicine, College of Medicine, Kyung Hee University, 23 Kyung Hee Dae-ro, Dongdaemun-gu, 02447 Seoul, Korea. [3]Department of Physiology, College of Medicine, Kyung Hee University, 23 Kyung Hee Dae-ro, Dongdaemun-gu, 02447 Seoul, Korea. [4]Department of Pathology, Inje University Sanggye Paik Hospital, 1342 Dongil-ro, Nowon-gu, 01757 Seoul, Korea. [5]Acupuncture and Meridian Science Research Center, College of Korean Medicine, Kyung Hee University, 23 Kyung Hee Dae-ro, Dongdaemun-gu, 02447 Seoul, Korea. [6]Department of Integrative Bioscience and Biotechnology, Sejong University, 209 Neungdong-ro, Gwangjin-gu, 05006 Seoul, Korea. [7]Department of Clinical Pharmacology and Therapeutics, College of Medicine, Kyung Hee University, 23 Kyung Hee Dae-ro, Dongdaemun-gu, 02447 Seoul, Korea.

References

1. Lee H, Lee IS, Choue R. Obesity, Inflammation and Diet. Pediatr Gastroenterol Hepatol Nutr. 2013;16:143–52.
2. Ronti T, Lupattelli G, Mannarino E. The endocrine function of adipose tissue: an update. Clin Endocrinol. 2006;64:355–65.
3. Rojas E, Rodriguez-Molina D, Bolli P, Israili ZH, Faria J, Fidilio E, et al. The role of adiponectin in endothelial dysfunction and hypertension. Curr Hypertens Rep. 2014;16:463.
4. Neumann E, Frommer KW, Vasile M, Muller-Ladner U. Adipocytokines as driving forces in rheumatoid arthritis and related inflammatory diseases? Arthritis Rheum. 2011;63:1159–69.
5. Otero M, Lago R, Gomez R, Lago F, Dieguez C, Gomez-Reino JJ, et al. Changes in plasma levels of fat-derived hormones adiponectin, leptin, resistin and visfatin in patients with rheumatoid arthritis. Ann Rheum Dis. 2006;65:1198–201.
6. Schaffler A, Ehling A, Neumann E, Herfarth H, Tarner I, Scholmerich J, et al. Adipocytokines in synovial fluid. JAMA. 2003;290:1709–10.
7. Ehling A, Schaffler A, Herfarth H, Tarner IH, Anders S, Distler O, et al. The potential of adiponectin in driving arthritis. J Immunol. 2006;176:4468–78.
8. Kitahara K, Kusunoki N, Kakiuchi T, Suguro T, Kawai S. Adiponectin stimulates IL-8 production by rheumatoid synovial fibroblasts. Biochem Biophys Res Commun. 2009;378:218–23.
9. Qian J, Xu L, Sun X, Wang Y, Xuan W, Zhang Q, et al. Adiponectin aggravates bone erosion by promoting osteopontin production in synovial tissue of rheumatoid arthritis. Arthritis Res Ther. 2018;20:26.
10. Sun X, Feng X, Tan W, Lin N, Hua M, Wei Y, et al. Adiponectin exacerbates collagen-induced arthritis via enhancing Th17 response and prompting RANKL expression. Sci Rep. 2015;5:11296.
11. Gonzalez-Gay MA, Llorca J, Garcia-Unzueta MT, Gonzalez-Juanatey C, De Matias JM, Martin J, et al. High-grade inflammation, circulating adiponectin concentrations and cardiovascular risk factors in severe rheumatoid arthritis. Clin Exp Rheumatol. 2008;26:596–603.
12. Lee SW, Kim JH, Park MC, Park YB, Lee SK. Adiponectin mitigates the severity of arthritis in mice with collagen-induced arthritis. Scand J Rheumatol. 2008;37:260–8.
13. Wu D, Hua B, Fang Z, Liu J, Liu N, Ma Y. Adiponectin exerts a potent anti-arthritic effect and insulin resistance in collagen-induced arthritic rats. Int J Rheum Dis. 2018;21:1496–503.
14. Choi HM, Lee YA, Lee SH, Hong SJ, Hahm DH, Choi SY, et al. Adiponectin may contribute to synovitis and joint destruction in rheumatoid arthritis by stimulating vascular endothelial growth factor, matrix metalloproteinase-1, and matrix metalloproteinase-13 expression in fibroblast-like synoviocytes more than proinflammatory mediators. Arthritis Res Ther. 2009;11:R161.
15. Lee YA, Ji HI, Lee SH, Hong SJ, Yang HI, Chul Yoo M, et al. The role of adiponectin in the production of IL-6, IL-8, VEGF and MMPs in human endothelial cells and osteoblasts: implications for arthritic joints. Exp Mol Med. 2014;46:e72.
16. Lee YA, Choi HM, Lee SH, Yang HI, Yoo MC, Hong SJ, et al. Synergy between adiponectin and interleukin-1beta on the expression of interleukin-6, interleukin-8, and cyclooxygenase-2 in fibroblast-like synoviocytes. Exp Mol Med. 2012;44:440–7.
17. Yokota T, Oritani K, Takahashi I, Ishikawa J, Matsuyama A, Ouchi N, et al. Adiponectin, a new member of the family of soluble defense collagens, negatively regulates the growth of myelomonocytic progenitors and the functions of macrophages. Blood. 2000;96:1723–32.
18. Yamauchi T, Kamon J, Waki H, Terauchi Y, Kubota N, Hara K, et al. The fat-derived hormone adiponectin reverses insulin resistance associated with both lipoatrophy and obesity. Nat Med. 2001;7:941–6.
19. Maeda K, Okubo K, Shimomura I, Funahashi T, Matsuzawa Y, Matsubara K. cDNA cloning and expression of a novel adipose specific collagen-like factor, apM1 (AdiPose Most abundant Gene transcript 1). Biochem Biophys Res Commun. 1996;221:286–9.
20. McCormack FX, Pattanajitvilai S, Stewart J, Possmayer F, Inchley K, Voelker DR. The Cys6 intermolecular disulfide bond and the collagen-like region of rat SP-A play critical roles in interactions with alveolar type II cells and surfactant lipids. J Biol Chem. 1997;272:27971–9.
21. Waki H, Yamauchi T, Kamon J, Ito Y, Uchida S, Kita S, et al. Impaired multimerization of human adiponectin mutants associated with diabetes. Molecular structure and multimer formation of adiponectin. J Biol Chem. 2003;278:40352–63.
22. Frommer KW, Schaffler A, Buchler C, Steinmeyer J, Rickert M, Rehart S, et al. Adiponectin isoforms: a potential therapeutic target in rheumatoid arthritis? Ann Rheum Dis. 2012;71:1724–32.
23. Wanninger J, Liebisch G, Eisinger K, Neumeier M, Aslanidis C, Voggenreiter L, et al. Adiponectin isoforms differentially affect gene expression and the lipidome of primary human hepatocytes. Metabolites. 2014;4:394 407.

24. Fujimatsu D, Kotooka N, Inoue T, Nishiyama M, Node K. Association between high molecular weight adiponectin levels and metabolic parameters. J Atheroscler Thromb. 2009;16:553–9.

25. Karasek D, Vaverkova H, Halenka M, Jackuliakova D, Frysak Z, Novotny D. Total adiponectin levels in dyslipidemic individuals: relationship to metabolic parameters and intima-media thickness. Biomed Pap Med Fac Univ Palacky Olomouc C zech Repub. 2011;155:55–62.

26. Miyazaki T, Hiki M, Shimada K, Kume A, Kiyanagi T, Sumiyoshi K, et al. The high molecular weight adiponectin level is associated with the atherogenic lipoprotein profiles in healthy Japanese males. J Atheroscler Thromb. 2014; 21:672–9.

27. van Andel M, Heijboer AC, Drent ML. Adiponectin and Its Isoforms in Pathophysiology. Adv Clin Chem. 2018;85:115–47.

28. Kohler G, Milstein C. Continuous cultures of fused cells secreting antibody of predefined specificity. Nature. 1975;256:495–7.

29. Hong R, Sur B, Yeom M, Lee B, Kim KS, Rodriguez JP, et al. Anti-inflammatory and anti-arthritic effects of the ethanolic extract of Aralia continentalis Kitag. in IL-1beta-stimulated human fibroblast-like synoviocytes and rodent models of polyarthritis and nociception. Phytomedicine. 2018;38:45–56.

30. Zhang L, Li P, Song S, Liu Y, Wang Q, Chang Y, et al. Comparative efficacy of TACI-Ig with TNF-alpha inhibitor and methotrexate in DBA/1 mice with collagen-induced arthritis. Eur J Pharmacol. 2013;708:113–23.

31. Hsu YH, Chang MS. Interleukin-20 antibody is a potential therapeutic agent for experimental arthritis. Arthritis Rheum. 2010;62:3311–21.

32. Shukla NM, Salunke DB, Balakrishna R, Mutz CA, Malladi SS, David SA. Potent adjuvanticity of a pure TLR7-agonistic imidazoquinoline dendrimer. PLoS One. 2012;7:e43612.

33. Kim SY, Sy V, Araki T, Babushkin N, Huang D, Tan D, et al. Total adiponectin, but not inflammatory markers C-reactive protein, tumor necrosis factor-alpha, interluekin-6 and monocyte chemoattractant protein-1, correlates with increasing glucose intolerance in pregnant Chinese-Americans. J Diabetes. 2014;6:360–8.

34. Kogan AE, Filatov VL, Kolosova OV, Katrukha IA, Mironova EV, Zhuravleva NS, et al. Oligomeric adiponectin forms and their complexes in the blood of healthy donors and patients with type 2 diabetes mellitus. J Immunoassay Immunochem. 2013;34:180–96.

35. Kontny E, Janicka I, Skalska U, Maśliński W. The effect of multimeric adiponectin isoforms and leptin on the function of rheumatoid fibroblast-like synoviocytes. Scand J Rheumatol. 2015;44:363–8.

36. Amitani H, Asakawa A, Ogiso K, Nakahara T, Ushikai M, Haruta I, et al. The role of adiponectin multimers in anorexia nervosa. Nutrition. 2013;29:203–6.

37. Baumann M, von Eynatten M, Dan L, Richart T, Kouznetsova T, Heemann U, et al. Altered molecular weight forms of adiponectin in hypertension. J Clin Hypertens. 2009;11:11–6.

38. Ohbuchi Y, Suzuki Y, Hatakeyama I, Nakao Y, Fujito A, Iwasaka T, et al. A lower serum level of middle-molecular-weight adiponectin is a risk factor for endometrial cancer. Int J Clin Oncol. 2014;19:667–73.

39. Iwata M, Hara K, Kamura Y, Honoki H, Fujisaka S, Ishiki M, et al. Ratio of low molecular weight serum adiponectin to the total adiponectin value is associated with type 2 diabetes through its relation to increasing insulin resistance. PLoS One. 2018;13:e0192609.

40. Achari AE, Jain SK. Adiponectin, a therapeutic target for obesity, diabetes, and endothelial dysfunction. Int J Mol Sci. 2017;18(6). pii: E1321.

41. Tao T, Wickham EP 3rd, Fan W, Yang J, Liu W. Distribution of adiponectin multimeric forms in Chinese women with polycystic ovary syndrome and their relation to insulin resistance. Eur J Endocrinol. 2010;163:399–406.

42. Haqq AM, Muehlbauer M, Svetkey LP, Newgard CB, Purnell JQ, Grambow SC, et al. Altered distribution of adiponectin isoforms in children with Prader-Willi syndrome (PWS): association with insulin sensitivity and circulating satiety peptide hormones. Clin Endocrinol. 2007;67:944–51.

43. Auerbach P, Nordby P, Bendtsen LQ, Mehlsen JL, Basnet SK, Vestergaard H, et al. Differential effects of endurance training and weight loss on plasma adiponectin multimers and adipose tissue macrophages in younger, moderately overweight men. Am J Physiol Regul Integr Comp Physiol. 2013;305:R490–8.

22

Osteogenic differentiation of fibroblast-like synovial cells in rheumatoid arthritis is induced by microRNA-218 through a ROBO/Slit pathway

Naoki Iwamoto[1]* ⓘ, Shoichi Fukui[1], Ayuko Takatani[1], Toshimasa Shimizu[1], Masataka Umeda[1,2], Ayako Nishino[1,3], Takashi Igawa[1], Tomohiro Koga[1,4], Shin-ya Kawashiri[1,5], Kunihiro Ichinose[1], Mami Tmai[1], Hideki Nakamura[1], Tomoki Origuchi[6], Ko Chiba[7], Makoto Osaki[7], Astrid Jüngel[8], Steffen Gay[8] and Atsushi Kawakami[1]

Abstract

Background: Fibroblast-like synovial cells (FLS) have multilineage differentiation potential including osteoblasts. We aimed to investigate the role of microRNAs during the osteogenic differentiation of rheumatoid arthritis (RA)-FLS.

Methods: RA-FLS were differentiated in osteogenic medium for 21 days. Osteogenic differentiation was evaluated by alkaline phosphatase (ALP) staining and Alizarin Red staining. MicroRNA (miRNA) array analysis was performed to investigate the differentially expressed miRNAs during osteogenic differentiation. Expression of miR-218-5p (miR-218) during the osteogenic differentiation was determined by quantitative real-time PCR. Transfections with an miR-218 precursor and inhibitor were used to confirm the targets of miR-218 and to analyze the ability of miR-218 to induce osteogenic differentiation. Secreted Dickkopf-1 (DKK1) from FLS transfected with miR-218 precursor/inhibitor or roundabout 1 (ROBO1) knockdown FLS established using ROBO1-small interfering RNA (siRNA) were measured by ELISA.

Results: The miRNA array revealed that 12 miRNAs were upregulated and 24 miRNAs were downregulated after osteogenic differentiation. We observed that the level of miR-218 rose in the early phase of osteogenic differentiation and then decreased. Pro-inflammatory cytokines modified the expression of miR-218. The induction of miR-218 in RA-FLS decreased ROBO1 expression, and promoted osteogenic differentiation. Both the overexpression of miR-218 and the knockdown of ROBO1 in RA-FLS decreased DKK1 secretion.

Conclusion: We identified miR-218 as a crucial inducer of the osteogenic differentiation of RA-FLS. MiR-218 modulates the osteogenic differentiation of RA-FLS through the ROBO1/DKK-1 axis. The induction of the osteogenic differentiation of proliferating RA-FLS through the provision of miR-218 into RA-FLS or by boosting the cellular reservoir of miR-218 might thus become a therapeutic strategy for RA.

Keywords: miR-218, Rheumatoid arthritis, Fibroblast-like synovial cells, Osteoblast

* Correspondence: naoki-iwa@nagasaki-u.ac.jp
[1]Department of Immunology and Rheumatology, Division of Advanced Preventive Medical Sciences, Nagasaki University Graduate School of Biomedical Sciences, 1-7-1 Sakamoto, Nagasaki 852-8501, Japan
Full list of author information is available at the end of the article

Background

Rheumatoid arthritis (RA) is a chronic inflammatory disease characterized by marked hyperplasia of the lining layer of the synovium, leading to the destruction of articular cartilage and bone. In RA pathogenesis, fibroblast-like synovial cells (FLS) are pivotal. FLS contribute to the production of pro-inflammatory cytokines, small molecule mediators of inflammation, and proteolytic enzymes that degrade the extracellular matrix [1]. Moreover, FLSs are resistant to programmed cell death [2], resulting in an aggressive, invasive phenotype similar to that of an invasive cancer, and the hyperplastic synovial tissue, also called the pannus, destroys cartilage and bone. Although rapid development of cytokine-targeted therapeutic agents such as tumor necrosis factor (TNF) inhibitors has provided better clinical outcomes including achievement of remission for patients with RA, there are many unfavorable problems such as inadequate response, high cost, and adverse events such as infections [3, 4]. RA-FLS-targeted therapies have thus been explored, and several key mediators that activate cytokine production from FLS [5, 6] or acquire anti-apoptosis property [7] had been elucidated. However, despite the enthusiasm for developing new treatments that directly target FLS, no directly FLS-targeted therapy is available at this time.

In RA, FLS of mesenchymal origin conserve mesenchymal properties. The gene expression pattern of FLS is similar to that of mesenchymal stem cells [8], and in vitro studies have shown that appropriate stimulation in culture induces differentiation of FLS into chondrocytes, adipocytes, muscle cells, and osteoblasts [9–11]. FLS are bone marrow (BM)-derived mesenchymal cells (MSCs) [12], and the multi-linage potential of arthritic FLS is thought to be arrested at the early stage of differentiation by activation of nuclear factor-κB (NF-κB) [13]. Forced cell differentiation might become a candidate therapeutic option for RA; for example, mesenchymal stromal cells showed reduced interleukin-6 (IL-6) production after their differentiation into adipocytes [14]. Until now, there has been no evidence that FLS differentiate into osteoblasts in joints. However, if the induction of intrinsic transdifferentiation of markedly proliferating FLS in the joints causes differentiation of FLS into osteoblasts, it might become a treatment option for RA.

MicroRNAs (miRNAs) are small non-coding RNAs, which regulate gene expression post-transcriptionally by binding to the 5′ untranslated region (UTR), coding regions or 3′ UTR of mRNA [15]. Altered expression of miRNAs has been reported in many diseases such as cancer, infections, and autoimmune diseases including RA, and this might arise from a modulation of diverse biological processes such as cell proliferation, apoptosis, metabolism and cell differentiation by miRNAs [16–18]. There is growing evidence that miRNAs are critical in osteoblast differentiation [19].

Jie et al. reported that miR-145 suppressed the osteogenic differentiation of mouse osteoblastic and myoblastic cell lines (MC3T3 and C2C12) by targeting Sp7 [20]. Other reports revealed that several miRs, e.g., miR-218, miR-34 and miR-195 modulate osteogenic differentiation by suppressing their targets [21–23]. However, the effect of miRNAs on RA-FLS differentiation including osteoblast differentiation had not yet been elucidated.

In the present study, we identified a miRNA (miR-218) that was altered during the osteogenic differentiation of RA-FLS, and we confirmed that this miRNA indeed promoted the osteogenic differentiation of RA-FLS. Our findings also revealed that Wnt/β-catenin signaling is involved in the promotion of the osteogenesis of RA-FLS by miR-218.

Methods

Isolation of FLS and stimulation assays

We obtained synovial tissues from patients with RA who fulfilled the 2010 American College of Rheumatology (ACR)/European League Against Rheumatism (EULAR) classification criteria for RA [24] or the 1987 ACR classification criteria for RA [25] at the time of orthopedic surgery. Each patient provided a signed consent form to participate in the study, which was approved by the Institutional Review Board of Nagasaki University and the Swiss Ethical commission. FLS were isolated from synovial tissues as described previously [26, 27]. Cells were cultivated in Dulbecco's modified Eagle's medium (DMEM) containing 10% heat-inactivated fetal bovine serum (FBS), 100 units/ml penicillin and 100 ng/ml streptomycin (all from Gibco, Basel, Switzerland). FLS from passages 3–8 in monolayer culture were used for the experiments. In the stimulation experiments, FLS were stimulated for 24 h with recombinant TNF-α (10 ng/ml), interleukin-1β (IL-1β) (1 ng/ml) (R&D Systems, Abingdon, UK), recombinant interleukin-6 (IL-6) (100 ng/ml) and recombinant soluble IL-6 receptor (sIL-6R) (100 ng/ml) (Peprotech, Rocky Hill, NJ, USA).

Osteogenic differentiation in vitro

RA-FLSs were plated at a cell density of 1×10^4 in 12-well plates. After they were 70% confluent, medium was replaced with osteogenic differentiation Bulletkit™ medium containing dexamethasone, ascorbate, glycerophosphate, L-Glutamine, Pen/Strep and MCGS (Lonza, Walkersville, MD, USA) to differentiate to osteoblasts. RA-FLS was cultured in the induction medium for up to 21 days. The medium was changed every 3 days. Osteoblast differentiation was evaluated by alkaline phosphatase (ALP) staining and Alizarin Red staining.

ALP staining and Alizarin Red staining

After the osteogenic induction or transfection experiments, cells were fixed in 4% paraformaldehyde and stained with ALP using ALP staining kit (Cosmo Bio, Tokyo). In another set of experiments, we performed Alizarin Red staining to detect the calcification after 21 days of culture in induction medium (late period of induction). Cells were fixed in methanol and stained with Alizarin Red using Calcified Nodule Staining kit (Cosmo Bio). ALP-positive cells were stained blue by ALP staining, and calcium nodules were detected as red bodies by Alizarin Red staining.

Transfection experiments

For a transient transfection approach with the aim to inhibit or enhance the miR-218 function, RA-FLSs were transfected with synthetic precursor miRNA (Pre-miR), with inhibitors of miR-218 (anti-miR), or with scrambled controls (Pre-miR/Anti-miR Negative Control #1; Ambion/Applied Biosystems, Foster City, CA, USA) at a final concentration of 100 nM with the use of Lipofectamine 2000 reagent (Invitrogen, Carlsbad, CA, USA). In another set of experiments, RA-FLSs were transfected with specific small interfering RNA (siRNA) that target ROBO1 mRNA using FlexiTube siRNA Premix (Qiagen, Hilden, Germany) at a final concentration of 25 nM according to the manufacturer's protocol. AllStars Negative control siRNA (siRNA-premix, Qiagen) served as a control. Transfection efficiency of pre/anti-mir-218 and siRNA were controlled by TaqMan-based real-time polymerase chain reaction (PCR).

RNA isolation and quantitative real-time PCR analysis

A *mir*Vana miRNA Isolation kit was used for isolation of total RNA (Ambion/Applied Biosystems). Specific single TaqMan miRNA assays (Ambion/Applied Biosystems) were used to measure the expression levels of selected miRNA in a model light cycler 1.5 (Roche Diagnostics). Expression of the U6B small nuclear RNA (RNU6B) was used as endogenous control to normalize the data. In the analysis of the expression of specific mRNA, gene expression was quantified using SYBR Green Real-time PCR, as previously described [27]. The primers were obtained from Takara Bio (Tokyo) and Integrated DNA Technologies (Coraville, IA, USA). The primer sequences are shown in Table 1. The amounts of loaded complementary DNA (cDNA) were normalized using glyceraldehyde-3-phosphate dehydrogenase (GAPDH) as an endogenous control. For relative quantification, the comparative threshold cycle (Ct) method was used.

In silico prediction analysis of miRNA targeting genes

MiRecords (http://c1.accurascience.com/miRecords/) was used to predict miRNA transcript targets. MiRecords is a database that combines the following miRNA target prediction tools: DIANA-microT, Micro inspector, miRanda, Mir Target2, mi Target, NB miRTar, Pic Tar, PITA, RNA hybrid, and TargetScan. Results were filtered based on the observation that a given miRNA targeted a transcript present in a minimum of five of these miRNA target prediction tools.

ELISA

Protein in cell supernatant was detected by ELISA with an ELISA kit specific for Dickkopf-1 (DKK1) according to the manufacturer's instructions (R&D Systems). Absorption was measured at 450 nm.

miRNA and DNA microarray assay analyses

miRNA expression profiles during osteogenic differentiation were established by applying SurePrint G3 Human miRNA, 8 × 60 K (release 18.0) microarrays containing 1887 human miRNA oligonucleotide probes (Agilent Technologies, Santa Clara, CA, USA). DNA microarray analysis was performed using whole human genome DNA microarray SurePrint G3 Human Gene Expression, 8 × 60 K (ver. 2) microarrays (Agilent Technologies). All procedures were carried out according to the manufacturer's recommendations. Microarray data were analyzed by GeneSpring software ver. 12.5.0 or 12.6.1 (Agilent Technologies). The raw signals were log2 transformed and normalized using the percentile shift normalization method: the value was set at the 90th percentile for miRNA microarray and the 75th percentile for DNA microarray.

Table 1 SYBR green primers used for real-time PCR

ALP forward	5'-AGCTCAACACCAACGTGGCTAA-3'
ALP reverse	5'-TTGTCCATCTCCAGCCTGGTC-3'
RUNX2 forward	5'-CTTTGTAGCACAAACATTGCTGGA-3'
RUNX2 reverse	5'-AAAGCTGTGGTACCTGTTCTGGA-3'
CTNNB1 forward	5'-CATCCTAGCTCGGGATGTTCAC-3'
CTNNB1 reverse	5'-TCCTTGTCCTGAGCAAGTTCAC-3'
CDH11 forward	5'-CAGGTGCTACAGCGCTCCAA-3'
CDH11 reverse	5'-TTAATGTTCCCATCACCAGAGTCAA-3'
ROBO1 forward	5'-CGGCAGAGTATGCTGGTCTGAA-3'
ROBO1 reverse	5'-CTAGGGCACTGAGACGCATGAA-3'
DKK1 forward	5'-CCAGACCATTGACAACTACCAG-3'
DKK1 reverse	5'-AGGCGAGACAGATTTGCAC-3'
GAPDH forward	5'-GCACCGTCAAGGCTGAGAAC-3'
GAPDH reverse	5'-TGGTGAAGACGCCAGTGGA-3'

CDH11 cadherin 11, *ALP* alkaline phosphatase, *RUNX2* runt related transcription factor 2, *CTNNB* catenin beta 1, *ROBO1* roundabout 1, DKK1 dickkopf-1, *GAPDH* glyceraldehyde-3-phosphate dehydrogenase

Statistical analyses

GraphPad Prism software (GraphPad, San Diego, CA, USA) was used for statistical analyses. Normal distributions of the data were confirmed using the Kolmogorov-Smirnov test. Statistical significance was evaluated by Student's paired t test (for parametric data) or the Wilcoxon matched-pairs signed rank test (non-parametric data) for related data. All data are expressed as the mean ± standard error of the mean (SEM). p values < 0.05 were considered significant.

Results

RA-FLS osteogenic differentiation

We first investigated whether RA-FLS can differentiate into osteoblasts. To induce the differentiation of RA-FLS, the medium was replaced with osteogenic induction medium. Osteoblasts were then evidenced by ALP staining (Fig. 1a, b) and Alizarin Red staining for matrix mineralization (Fig. 1a, c). ALP and runt related transcription factor 2 (RUNX2) were used as phenotypic markers of osteogenic differentiation, and as shown in

Fig. 1d, the expression of those mRNAs was significantly increased at day 21 after osteogenic induction.

Expression of miR-218 during osteogenic differentiation of RA-FLS

To explore miRNAs involved in the osteogenic differentiation of RA-FLS, we started by examining the miRNA expression profiles by microarrays. Our microarray analysis of three pairs (RA-FLS cultured in osteogenic induction medium versus an untreated control) identified 36 differentially expressed miRNAs among all three pairs. Of these, 12 miRNAs were upregulated miRNA s and 24 were downregulated miRNAs (Additional file 1: Figure S1).

Among these miRNAs, miR-218-5p (miR-218) was one of the most significantly and consistently downregulated miRNAs after osteogenic induction. To validate the microarray findings, quantitative real-time PCR with additional RA-FLS cultured in osteogenic induction medium was performed. In agreement with the microarray analysis results, there was significant downregulation in the expression of

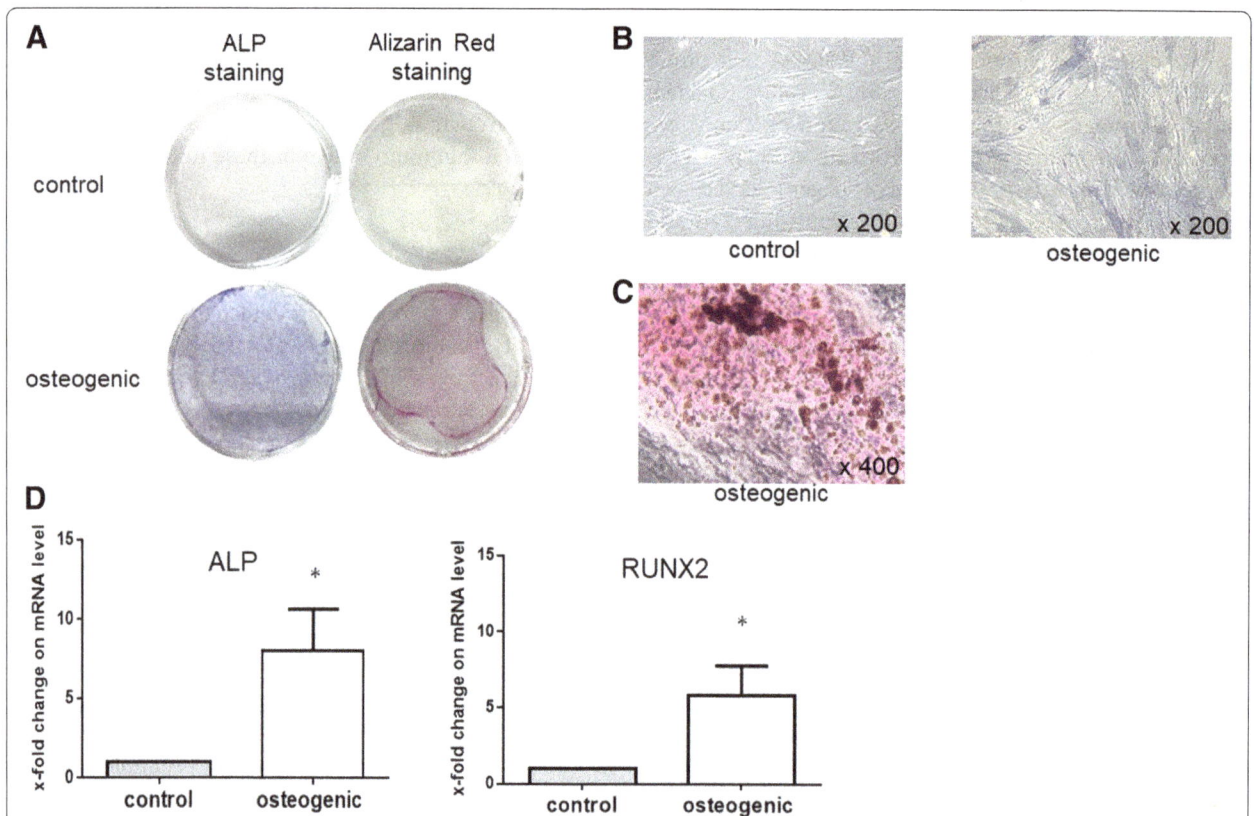

Fig. 1 Osteogenic differentiation of rheumatoid arthritis (RA)-fibroblast-like synovial cells (FLS) cultured in osteogenic induction medium. **a** Representative images of alkaline phosphatase (ALP) staining (right) and Alizarin Red staining (left). RA-FLS ($n = 6$) were cultured in osteogenic induction medium or control medium. After 21 days, cells were stained with ALP and Alizarin Red. **b** Representative image of the morphology of RA-FLS with ALP staining. Right: RA-FLS were cultured in control medium. Left: RA-FLS were cultured in osteogenic induction medium (magnification × 200). **c** Visualization of calcified nodules by Alizarin Red staining. RA-FLS were cultured in osteogenic induction medium (magnification × 400). **d** RA-FLS ($n = 5$) were cultured in osteogenic induction medium or control medium for 21 days. Expression of ALP, runt related transcription factor 2 (RUNX2) was determined by quantitative real-time PCR. Values are presented as means ± SEM: *$p < 0.05$ versus control, as determined by Student's paired t test or Wilcoxon matched-pairs signed rank test

mir-218 after osteogenic induction. The miR-218 decreased with fold-change of 0.203 ± 0.026 ($p < 0.0001$) at day 21 after osteogenic induction compared with the untreated control (Fig. 2a). We next investigated the time course of miR-218 expression during osteogenic differentiation. In response to osteogenic differentiation, miR-218 rose until 12 h and then decreased at 7 days, and remained decreased at 21 days (Fig. 2b).

miR-218 promotes osteogenesis of RA-FLS

To determine the role of miR-218 in the osteogenic differentiation of RA-FLS, RA-FLS were transfected with pre-miR-218 or anti-miR-218 and the respective negative control. In RA-FLS, transfection with pre-miR-218 increased the levels of miR-218 with fold-change of 1.34 $\times 10^5 \pm 1.70 \times 10^5$ compared to the scrambled control. Knockdown with anti-miR-218 reduced the expression of miR-218 with fold-change of 0.098 ± 0.058 indicating successful transfection. At 14 days after transfection, osteogenesis ability was examined. Strong ALP staining was observed (Fig. 3a, b). Interestingly, in addition to ALP and RUNX2 mRNA, other osteogenesis-associated genes such as catenin beta 1 (CTNNB1) and cadherin 11 (CDH11) were also significantly upregulated in pre-miR-218 transfected RA-FLS compared to the scrambled control from 72 h after transfection (Fig. 3c). In contrast, in the anti-miR-218 transfected RA-FLS, no ALP staining was observed (Fig. 3a), and osteogenic specific markers were not upregulated. Moreover, the transfection of anti-miR-218 did not attenuate the osteogenic differentiation induced by osteogenic induction medium (please contact author for data requests). This gain-and-loss of function assays with miR-218 showed miR-218 solely induced the osteogenic differentiation of RA-FLS without osteogenic induction medium.

The expression of miR-218 is modulated by pro-inflammatory cytokines

We next investigated whether miR-218 is modulated in the physiopathological condition of RA. To simulate the inflammatory conditions present in RA in vivo, we stimulated RA-FLS with TNF-α and IL-1β or IL-6. Although the difference was not statistically significant, the stimulation of these cytokines downregulated the expression of miR-218 numerically (Additional file 2: Figure S2). This result suggests that the conditions in which inflammation occurs in RA, which is a bone erosion-progressive state, also presents a disadvantage for the osteogenic differentiation of RA-FLS.

ROBO1 is targeted by miR-218 in RA-FLS

To elucidate the functional consequences of upregulation of miR-218, we searched for potential gene targets of miR-218 that might contribute to the osteogenesis of RA-FLS. We performed a DNA microarray using gain-and-loss of function assays with miR-218, and we also conducted an in silico identification of potential gene targets of miR-218 using the MiRecords (http://c1.accurascience.com/miRecords/). From the microarray result, the genes increased by knockdown of miR-218 and decreased by overexpression of miR-218 were considered as potential targets (microarray data are available from Gene Expression Omnibus (GEO, http://www.ncbi.nlm.nih.gov/geo/) [GEO:GSE 111946]. Among the candidates that were predicted by both in silico and microarray analyses, we focused on roundabout 1 (ROBO1), a transmembrane receptor proteins implicated in the Slit-ROBO pathway with an established relationship to osteogenesis [28], and we further analyzed ROBO1. Overexpression of miR-218 reduced the expression of ROBO1 with fold-change of 0.29 ± 0.07 ($p < 0.05$)

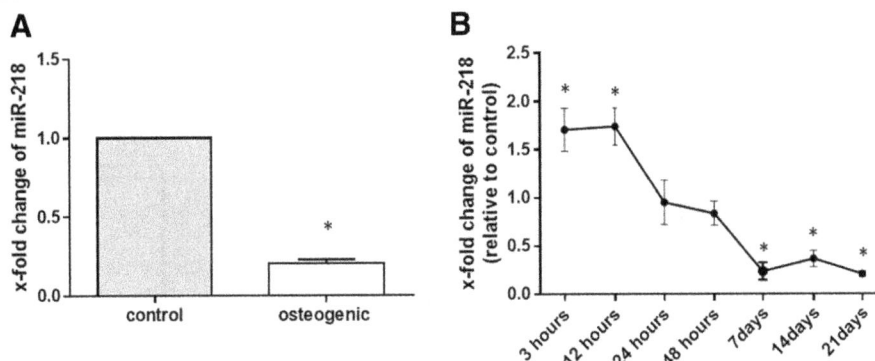

Fig. 2 Expression of microRNA-218-5p (miR-218) during osteogenic differentiation of rheumatoid arthritis (RA)-fibroblast-like synovial cells (FLS), as determined by TaqMan-based Real-time polymerase chain reaction analysis. Expression of miR-218 in osteogenic differentiation was determined relative to the controls, which was defined as 1. **a** miR-218 was markedly reduced in RA-FLS ($n = 5$) at 21 days after culture in osteogenic induction medium compared to culture in control medium. Values are presented as means $\pm$ SEM: $*p < 0.0001$ versus control, as determined by Student's paired t test. **b** The time course of expression of miR-218 during osteogenic differentiation ($n = 4$–5). Points and bars represent means and SEM respectively: $*p < 0.05$ versus control, as determined by Student's paired t test

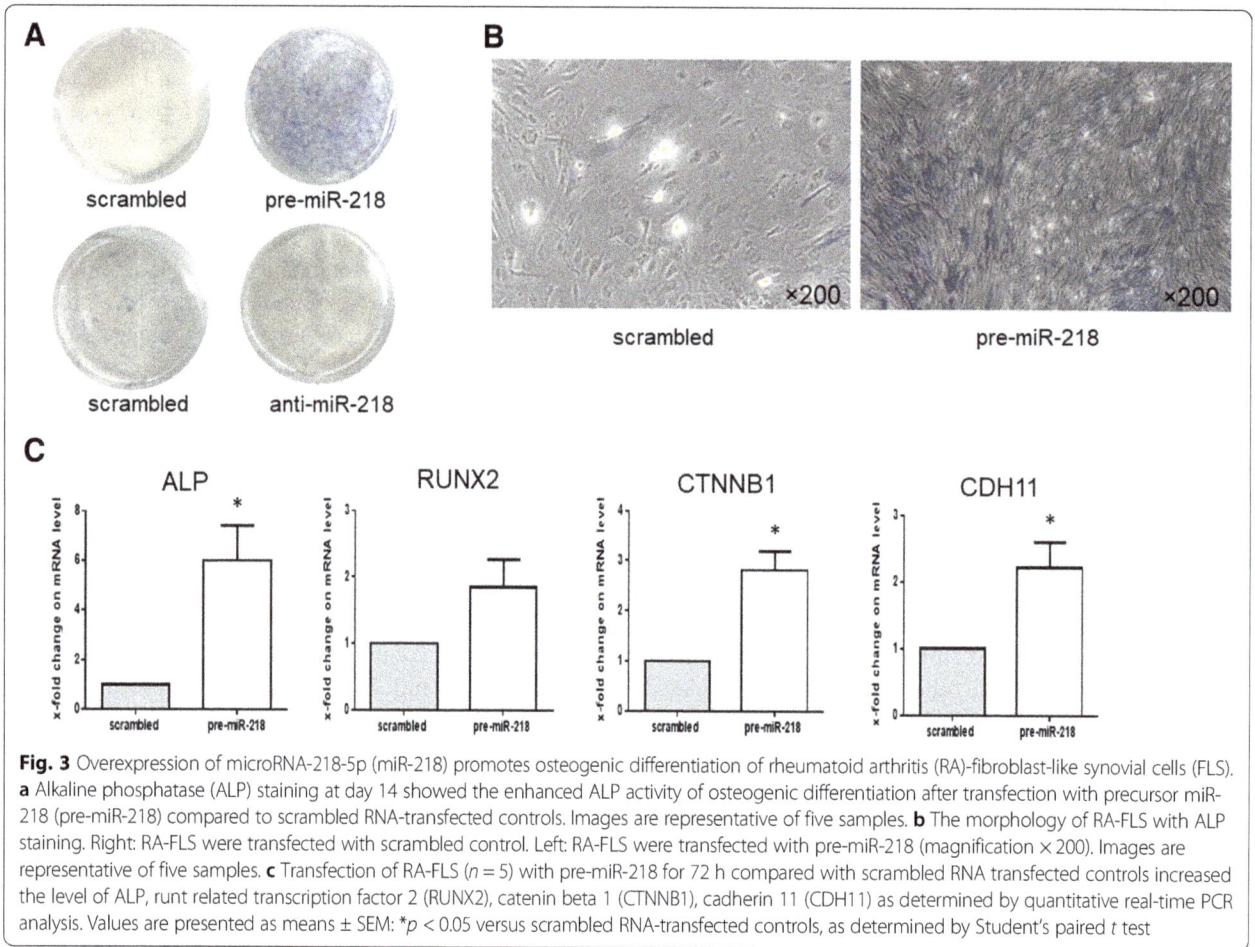

Fig. 3 Overexpression of microRNA-218-5p (miR-218) promotes osteogenic differentiation of rheumatoid arthritis (RA)-fibroblast-like synovial cells (FLS). **a** Alkaline phosphatase (ALP) staining at day 14 showed the enhanced ALP activity of osteogenic differentiation after transfection with precursor miR-218 (pre-miR-218) compared to scrambled RNA-transfected controls. Images are representative of five samples. **b** The morphology of RA-FLS with ALP staining. Right: RA-FLS were transfected with scrambled control. Left: RA-FLS were transfected with pre-miR-218 (magnification ×200). Images are representative of five samples. **c** Transfection of RA-FLS (n = 5) with pre-miR-218 for 72 h compared with scrambled RNA transfected controls increased the level of ALP, runt related transcription factor 2 (RUNX2), catenin beta 1 (CTNNB1), cadherin 11 (CDH11) as determined by quantitative real-time PCR analysis. Values are presented as means ± SEM: *$p < 0.05$ versus scrambled RNA-transfected controls, as determined by Student's paired t test

at the mRNA level. Conversely, knockdown of miR-218 increased the expression of ROBO1 with fold-change of 1.34 ± 0.10 ($p < 0.05$) (Fig. 4a, b). Taken together, these findings confirmed ROBO1 as a target of miR-218 in RA-FLS.

miR-218 and the suppression of ROBO1 promote osteogenesis through DKK1 suppression

Wnt/β-catenin signaling plays a crucial role in osteogenesis [29], therefore we next investigated whether miR-218 affects inhibitor of Wnt/β-catenin signaling. The level of

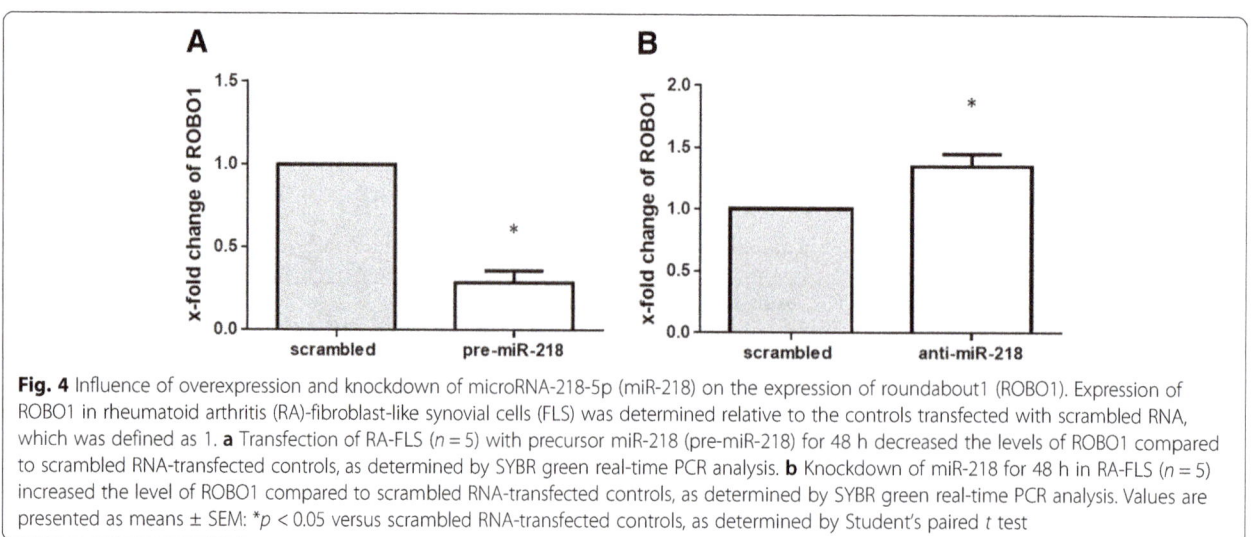

Fig. 4 Influence of overexpression and knockdown of microRNA-218-5p (miR-218) on the expression of roundabout1 (ROBO1). Expression of ROBO1 in rheumatoid arthritis (RA)-fibroblast-like synovial cells (FLS) was determined relative to the controls transfected with scrambled RNA, which was defined as 1. **a** Transfection of RA-FLS (n = 5) with precursor miR-218 (pre-miR-218) for 48 h decreased the levels of ROBO1 compared to scrambled RNA-transfected controls, as determined by SYBR green real-time PCR analysis. **b** Knockdown of miR-218 for 48 h in RA-FLS (n = 5) increased the level of ROBO1 compared to scrambled RNA-transfected controls, as determined by SYBR green real-time PCR analysis. Values are presented as means ± SEM: *$p < 0.05$ versus scrambled RNA-transfected controls, as determined by Student's paired t test

DKK1 (which has been shown to be a potent inhibitor of Wnt/β-catenin signaling) that we detected in RA-FLS transfected with pre-miR-218-conditioned medium was significantly reduced compared to that detected in scrambled control-conditioned medium (Fig. 5a). These findings were confirmed at the mRNA level by quantitative real-time PCR. Overexpression of miR-218 reduced the expression of DKK-1 with fold-change of 0.33 ± 0.08 ($p < 0.005$) (Fig. 5b).

To mimic the promotion of the osteogenic condition of RA-FLS by miR-218 as we observed, we silenced the expression of ROBO1 with siRNA. After transfection with ROBO1-specific siRNA, the expression of ROBO1 was decreased with fold-change of 0.30 ± 0.08, indicating successful transfection. Similar to the effect of miR-218 overexpression, silencing of ROBO1 reduced DKK1 secretion from RA-FLS (Fig. 5c). These results suggest that miR-218 promote osteogenic differentiation of RA-FLS through ROBO1 suppression and inhibition of DKK1 secretion, therefore activation of Wnt/β-catenin signaling is presumed to be the possible mechanism of miR-218-induced osteogenesis of RA-FLS.

Discussion

This is the first study to show that a miRNA could induce the osteogenic differentiation of FLS from RA, a bone-erosive disease. Our findings demonstrated that the expression of miR-218 was altered during osteogenic induction and most interestingly, miR-218 directly promoted the osteogenic differentiation of RA-FLS through the suppression of DKK1.

Skeletal homeostasis is a continuous process that is maintained by a balance between bone resorption by osteoclasts and bone formation by osteoblasts. In RA, bone erosion is considered to be the result of a disruption of this balance, inadequate bone formation, and an enhancement of osteoclast activity [30]. Inadequate bone formation in RA was recently elucidated. Two studies reported that IL-6, a key pro-inflammatory cytokine of RA, decreased osteoblast proliferation and induced osteoblast apoptosis [31, 32]. IL-6 inhibited the formation of mineralized bone nodules in an in vitro rat osteogenesis model [32]. Another study focused on DKK1, which we observed to be a key regulator of the promotion of osteogenesis by miR-218. DKK1 expression was

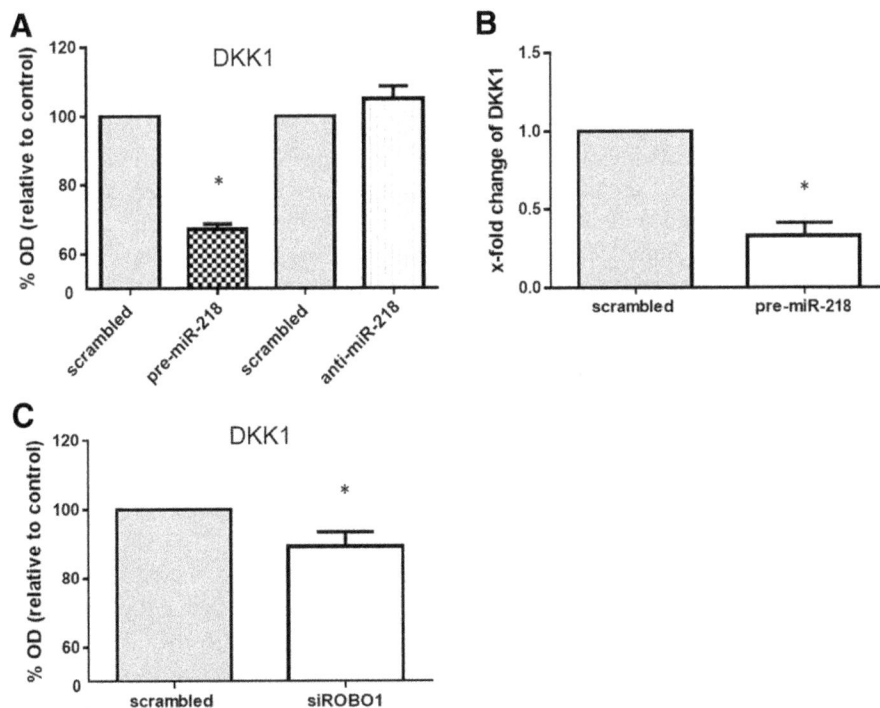

Fig. 5 Suppression of Dickkopf-1 (DKK1) by overexpression of microRNA-218-5p (miR-218) or silencing of roundabout1 (ROBO1). **a** At the protein level, transfection of rheumatoid arthritis (RA)-fibroblast-like synovial cells (FLS) ($n = 4$) with precursor miR-218 (pre-miR-218) for 48 h decreased DKK1 protein production in the culture supernatant compared to scrambled RNA transfected controls, as determined by ELISA. Graphs represent optical density (OD) value; each mean amount of DDK1 protein are as follows; scrambled control: pre-miR-218 1.17 ng/ml:0.76 ng/ml, scrambled control: anti-miR-218 1.58 ng/ml:1.65 ng/ml, respectively. **b** At the mRNA level, transfection of RA-FLS ($n = 4$) with pre-miR-218 for 48 h decreased DKK1 expression compared to scrambled RNA transfected controls, as determined by SYBR green real-time PCR analysis. **c** Secretion of DKK1 from RA-FLS ($n = 4$) was decreased after transfection with ROBO1-specific small interfering RNA (siRNA) compared to the scrambled RNA transfected controls, as determined by ELISA. Graphs represent OD value; each mean amount of DDK1 protein are as follows; scrambled control: siROBO1.28 ng/ml:1.09 ng/ml, respectively. Values are presented as means ± SEM: *$p < 0.05$ versus scrambled RNA-transfected controls, as determined by Student's paired t test

increased in FLS and endothelial cells in an animal model of arthritis, and TNF markedly increased the production of DKK1 from cultured FLS. In addition, serum DKK1 was elevated in patients with RA [33].

An in vivo study by Walsh et al. using an animal model of RA demonstrated that the presence of inflammation modified osteoblast-lineage cell function, resulting in impaired osteoblast maturation and significant reduction of mineralized bone formation within the site of arthritic erosion [34]. In clinical practice, the repair of bone erosion is uncommon but it has been demonstrated to occur. For example, 6% of patients with RA treated with adalimumab were shown to have bone repair [35], and 1-year treatment with TNF inhibitor was shown to reduce the mean depth of erosion detected by high-resolution computed tomography [36]. Although the mechanisms underlying the repair of bone erosion in RA have been not elucidated, the possible main mechanism might be the correction of the imbalance of bone remodeling that arises from inflammation. It is not elucidated that the osteogenic differentiation of RA-FLS, which we showed in an in vitro study, occurs in the joints in RA. However, if it does occur in the joints in RA, it is possible that proliferation of FLS contributes to bone repair by induction of osteogenic differentiation by miR-218.

Although the role of miR-218 in human disease and cell physiology has not been widely addressed, several studies of miR-218 have been reported. For example, miR-218 suppresses gastric cancer cell proliferation via regulation of angiopoietin-2 [37], and miR-218 inhibits proliferation of glioma cells by targeting ROBO1 [38]. Two studies revealed that miR-218 promotes osteogenic differentiation of mesenchymal stem cells through regulation of Wnt/β-catenin signaling, targeting DKK2, sclerostin, and secreted frizzled related protein 2 [22, 39]. The difference in targets compared to our present study might be due to the difference in the types of cells examined, because miRNA may have different effects depending on cell type.

Our study suggests that the ROBO1-DKK1 axis is important for osteogenesis in RA-FLS. ROBO1 is a member of the ROBO family; it serves as a transmembrane receptor of Slit, and emerging evidence has indicated that a ROBO/Slit signaling pathway is crucial in axon guidance [40]. In addition to axon guidance, the ROBO/Slit pathway is also involved in cell processes such as cell proliferation, cell motility, and angiogenesis [41, 42]. The effect of the ROBO/Slit signaling pathway in osteogenesis remains unknown, but Sun et al. reported that slit2 reduced ALP expression and osteoblastic gene expression in the osteoblastic cell line MC3T3-E1 [28]. Our present findings also showed that knockdown of ROBO1 significantly reduced DKK1 secretion from RA-FLS.

Wnt/β-catenin signaling is known as one of the important molecular cascades and is central to osteogenesis, and DKK1 is a potent inhibitor of this signaling pathway, causing deregulation of bone formation [43]. As described above, in vivo and in vitro studies have shown an increase of DKK1 in both an arthritic animal model and in patients with RA. In fact, patients with RA with radiological progression within 2 years have been shown to have higher baseline levels of serum DKK1 compared to the patients without radiological progression [44]. Wang et al. reported that serum DKK1 is significantly correlated with bone erosion, and that treatment with a TNF-α inhibitor or IL-1 receptor antagonist decreased serum DKK1 levels [45]. Considering these results, the reduction of DKK1 secretion by miR-218 might provide a protective effect against RA bone erosion besides the effect of miR218 toward RA-FLS osteogenesis.

In the present study, miR-218 promoted osteogenic differentiation despite a significant decrement of miR-218 after osteoblast differentiation. A negative and positive feedback loop between microRNA and its target gene or cellular response have been observed [46–48]. This crosstalk was also seen in the Wnt/β-catenin signaling pathway; miR-122 inhibits the Wnt/β-catenin signaling pathway, which negatively regulates the expression of miR-121 in glioma cells [49]. miR-372 and miR-373 activate the Wnt/β-catenin signaling pathway by targeting Wnt/β-catenin signaling inhibitors including DKK1, and these miRs are induced by Wnt/β-catenin signaling-dependent transcription [50]. Such crosstalk with miR-218 might be implicated in RA-FLS osteogenesis.

Conclusions

In conclusion, our study showed that the expression of miR-218 was altered during the osteogenic differentiation of RA-FLS, and that miR-218 promoted the osteogenic differentiation of RA-FLS by targeting ROBO1 and suppressing DKK1. The induction of the osteogenic differentiation of proliferated FLS in RA synovial tissue has two potential effects; the attenuation of RA disease progression derived from FLS as effector cells, and the repair of destruction of bone. Therefore, strategies to provide miR-218 to RA-FLS or to boost the cellular reservoir of miR-218 might become a therapeutic strategy for RA. This attractive hypothesis should be further tested in animal models. At the least, overexpression of miR-218 might contribute to bone repair and suppression of bone erosion by the inhibition of DKK1 secretion, which we observed herein as an effect of miR-218 in RA-FLS, and modification of the inflammatory and invasive phenotype of RA-FLS.

Abbreviations

ACR: American College of Rheumatology; ALP: Alkaline phosphatase; BM: Bone marrow; CDH11: Cadherin 11; Ct: Comparative threshold cycle; CTNNB1: Catenin beta 1; DKK1: Dickkopf-1; DMEM: Dulbecco's modified Eagle's medium; ELISA: Enzyme-linked immunosorbent assay; EULAR: European League Against Rheumatism; FBS: Fetal bovine serum; FLS: Fibroblast-like synovial cells; GAPDH: Glyceraldehyde-3-phosphate dehydrogenase; IL-1β: Interleukin-1β; IL-6: Interleukin-6; miR-218: miR-218-5p; miRNA: MicroRNA; MSCs: Mesenchymal cells; NF-κB: Nuclear factor-κB; PCR: Polymerase chain reaction; pre-miR: Precursor miRNA; RA: Rheumatoid arthritis; RNU6B: U6B small nuclear RNA; ROBO1: Roundabout 1; RUNX2: Runt related transcription factor 2; SEM: Standard error of the mean; siRNA: Small interfering RNA; TNF: Tumor necrosis factor; UTR: Untranslated region

Acknowledgements

We thank Kaori Furukawa and Yoshiko Takahashi for the excellent technical support.

Funding

This work was supported by grants from the Japan Society for the Promotion of Science (Grants-in-Aid for Scientific Research 16 K19605 to Dr Iwamoto).

Authors' contributions

NI, AK: conception and design of the study, analysis and interpretation of data, and drafting the article. AJ, SG: experimental conception and design, stimulation experiment, miR-expression experiment. SF: partly performed cell culture experiment. KT, MO: supplied clinical samples. SF, AT, TS, MU, AN, TI, TK, SK, KI, MT, HN, TO, AJ, SG, AK: analysis and interpretation of data, critical revision the manuscript. All authors have given their final approval of the manuscript to be published as presented.

Consent for publication

Not applicable.

Competing interests

The authors declare that they have no competing interests.

Author details

[1]Department of Immunology and Rheumatology, Division of Advanced Preventive Medical Sciences, Nagasaki University Graduate School of Biomedical Sciences, 1-7-1 Sakamoto, Nagasaki 852-8501, Japan. [2]Medical Education Development Center, Nagasaki University School Hospital, Nagasaki, Japan. [3]Center for Comprehensive Community Care Education, Nagasaki University Graduate School of Biomedical Sciences, Nagasaki, Japan. [4]Center for Bioinformatics and Molecular Medicine, Nagasaki University Graduate School of Biomedical Sciences, Nagasaki, Japan. [5]Departments of Community Medicine, Division of Advanced Preventive Medical Sciences, Nagasaki University Graduate School of Biomedical Sciences, Nagasaki, Japan. [6]Department of Physical Therapy, Nagasaki University Graduate School of Biomedical Sciences, Nagasaki, Japan. [7]Department of Orthopedic Surgery, Nagasaki University Graduate School of Biomedical Sciences, Nagasaki, Japan. [8]Center of Experimental Rheumatology, University Hospital Zurich and University of Zurich, Schlieren, Zurich, Switzerland.

References

1. Stanczyk J, Ospelt C, Gay RE, Gay S. Synovial cell activation. Curr Opin Rheumatol. 2006;18:262–7.
2. Korb A, Pavenstadt H, Pap T. Cell death in rheumatoid arthritis. Apoptosis. 2009;14:447–54.
3. Ianculescu I, Weisman MH. Infection, malignancy, switching, biosimilars, antibody formation, drug survival and withdrawal, and dose reduction: what have we learned over the last year about tumor necrosis factor inhibitors in rheumatoid arthritis? Curr Opin Rheumatol. 2016;28:303–9.
4. Joensuu JT, Huoponen S, Aaltonen KJ, Konttinen YT, Nordstrom D, Blom M. The cost-effectiveness of biologics for the treatment of rheumatoid arthritis: a systematic review. PLoS One. 2015;10:e0119683.
5. McInnes IB, Schett G. The pathogenesis of rheumatoid arthritis. N Engl J Med. 2011;365:2205–19.
6. Tian J, Chen JW, Gao JS, Li L, Xie X. Resveratrol inhibits TNF-alpha-induced IL-1beta, MMP-3 production in human rheumatoid arthritis fibroblast-like synoviocytes via modulation of PI3kinase/Akt pathway. Rheumatol Int. 2013;33:1829–35.
7. Bartok B, Firestein GS. Fibroblast-like synoviocytes: key effector cells in rheumatoid arthritis. Immunol Rev. 2010;233:233–55.
8. Choi HS, Ryu CJ, Choi HM, Park JS, Lee JH, Kim KI, Yang HI, Yoo MC, Kim KS. Effects of the pro-inflammatory milieu on the dedifferentiation of cultured fibroblast-like synoviocytes. Mol Med Rep. 2012;5:1023–6.
9. Yamasaki S, Nakashima T, Kawakami A, Miyashita T, Tanaka F, Ida H, Migita K, Origuchi T, Eguchi K. Cytokines regulate fibroblast-like synovial cell differentiation to adipocyte-like cells. Rheumatology (Oxford). 2004;43:448–52.
10. Zvaifler NJ, Tsai V, Alsalameh S, von Kempis J, Firestein GS, Lotz M. Pannocytes: distinctive cells found in rheumatoid arthritis articular cartilage erosions. Am J Pathol. 1997;150:1125–38.
11. De Bari C, Dell'Accio F, Tylzanowski P, Luyten FP. Multipotent mesenchymal stem cells from adult human synovial membrane. Arthritis Rheum. 2001;44:1928–42.
12. Marinova-Mutafchieva L, Williams RO, Funa K, Maini RN, Zvaifler NJ. Inflammation is preceded by tumor necrosis factor-dependent infiltration of mesenchymal cells in experimental arthritis. Arthritis Rheum. 2002;46:507–13.
13. Li X, Makarov SS. An essential role of NF-kappaB in the "tumor-like" phenotype of arthritic synoviocytes. Proc Natl Acad Sci USA. 2006;103:17432–7.
14. Okada A, Yamasaki S, Koga T, Kawashiri SY, Tamai M, Origuchi T, Nakamura H, Eguchi K, Kawakami A. Adipogenesis of the mesenchymal stromal cells and bone oedema in rheumatoid arthritis. Clin Exp Rheumatol. 2012;30:332–7.
15. Axtell MJ. Evolution of microRNAs and their targets: are all microRNAs biologically relevant? Biochim Biophys Acta. 2008;1779:725–34.
16. Churov AV, Oleinik EK, Knip M. MicroRNAs in rheumatoid arthritis: altered expression and diagnostic potential. Autoimmun Rev. 2015;14:1029–37.
17. Lee CH, Kim JH, Lee SW. The role of microRNA in pathogenesis and as markers of HCV chronic infection. Curr Drug Targets. 2017;18:756–765.
18. Yang G, Wu D, Zhu J, Jiang O, Shi Q, Tian J, Weng Y. Upregulation of miR-195 increases the sensitivity of breast cancer cells to Adriamycin treatment through inhibition of Raf-1. Oncol Rep. 2013;30:877–89.
19. Kim KM, Lim SK. Role of miRNAs in bone and their potential as therapeutic targets. Curr Opin Pharmacol. 2014;16:133–41.
20. Jia J, Tian Q, Ling S, Liu Y, Yang S, Shao Z. miR-145 suppresses osteogenic differentiation by targeting Sp7. FEBS Lett. 2013;587:3027–31.
21. Grunhagen J, Bhushan R, Degenkolbe E, Jager M, Knaus P, Mundlos S, Robinson PN, Ott CE. MiR-497 approximately 195 cluster microRNAs regulate osteoblast differentiation by targeting BMP signaling. J Bone Miner Res. 2015;30:796–808.
22. Hassan MQ, Maeda Y, Taipaleenmaki H, Zhang W, Jafferji M, Gordon JA, Li Z, Croce CM, van Wijnen AJ, Stein JL, Stein GS, Lian JB. miR-218 directs a Wnt signaling circuit to promote differentiation of osteoblasts and osteomimicry of metastatic cancer cells. J Biol Chem. 2012;287:42084–92.
23. Wei J, Shi Y, Zheng L, Zhou B, Inose H, Wang J, Guo XE, Grosschedl R, Karsenty G. miR-34s inhibit osteoblast proliferation and differentiation in the mouse by targeting SATB2. J Cell Biol. 2012;197:509–21.
24. Aletaha D, Neogi T, Silman AJ, Funovits J, Felson DT, Bingham CO 3rd, Birnbaum NS, Burmester GR, Bykerk VP, Cohen MD, Combe B, Costenbader KH, Dougados M, Emery P, Ferraccioli G, Hazes JM, Hobbs K, Huizinga TW, Kavanaugh A, Kay J, Kvien TK, Laing T, Mease P, Menard HA, Moreland LW, Naden RL, Pincus T, Smolen JS, Stanislawska-Biernat E, Symmons D, Tak PP, Upchurch KS, Vencovsky J, Wolfe F, Hawker G. 2010 Rheumatoid arthritis classification criteria: an American College of Rheumatology/European league against rheumatism collaborative initiative. Ann Rheum Dis. 2010;69:1580–8.
25. Arnett FC, Edworthy SM, Bloch DA, McShane DJ, Fries JF, Cooper NS, Healey LA, Kaplan SR, Liang MH, Luthra HS, et al. The American rheumatism association 1987 revised criteria for the classification of rheumatoid arthritis. Arthritis Rheum. 1988;31:315–24.
26. Ospelt C, Kurowska-Stolarska M, Neidhart M, Michel BA, Gay RE, Laufer S, Gay S. The dual inhibitor of lipoxygenase and cyclooxygenase ML3000 decreases the expression of CXCR3 ligands. Ann Rheum Dis. 2008;67:524–9.
27. Suzuki T, Iwamoto N, Yamasaki S, Nishino A, Nakashima Y, Horai Y, Kawashiri SY, Ichinose K, Arima K, Tamai M, Nakamura H, Origuchi T, Miyamoto C, Osaki M, Ohyama K, Kuroda N, Kawakami A. Upregulation of thrombospondin 1 expression in synovial tissues and plasma of rheumatoid arthritis: role of transforming growth factor-beta1 toward fibroblast-like synovial cells. J Rheumatol. 2015;42:943 7.

28. Sun H, Dai K, Tang T, Zhang X. Regulation of osteoblast differentiation by slit2 in osteoblastic cells. Cells Tissues Organs. 2009;190:69–80.

29. Lerner UH, Ohlsson C. The WNT system: background and its role in bone. J Intern Med. 2015;277:630–49.

30. Deal C. Bone loss in rheumatoid arthritis: systemic, periarticular, and focal. Curr Rheumatol Rep. 2012;14:231–7.

31. Li Y, Backesjo CM, Haldosen LA, Lindgren U. IL-6 receptor expression and IL-6 effects change during osteoblast differentiation. Cytokine. 2008; 43:165–73.

32. Malaval L, Liu F, Vernallis AB, Aubin JE. GP130/OSMR is the only LIF/IL-6 family receptor complex to promote osteoblast differentiation of calvaria progenitors. J Cell Physiol. 2005;204:585–93.

33. Diarra D, Stolina M, Polzer K, Zwerina J, Ominsky MS, Dwyer D, Korb A, Smolen J, Hoffmann M, Scheinecker C, van der Heide D, Landewe R, Lacey D, Richards WG, Schett G. Dickkopf-1 is a master regulator of joint remodeling. Nat Med. 2007;13:156–63.

34. Walsh NC, Reinwald S, Manning CA, Condon KW, Iwata K, Burr DB, Gravallese EM. Osteoblast function is compromised at sites of focal bone erosion in inflammatory arthritis. J Bone Miner Res. 2009;24:1572–85.

35. Dohn UM, Ejbjerg B, Boonen A, Hetland ML, Hansen MS, Knudsen LS, Hansen A, Madsen OR, Hasselquist M, Moller JM, Ostergaard M. No overall progression and occasional repair of erosions despite persistent inflammation in adalimumab-treated rheumatoid arthritis patients: results from a longitudinal comparative MRI, ultrasonography, CT and radiography study. Ann Rheum Dis. 2011;70:252–8.

36. Finzel S, Rech J, Schmidt S, Engelke K, Englbrecht M, Stach C, Schett G. Repair of bone erosions in rheumatoid arthritis treated with tumour necrosis factor inhibitors is based on bone apposition at the base of the erosion. Ann Rheum Dis. 2011;70:1587–93.

37. Tang S, Wang D, Zhang Q, Li L. miR-218 suppresses gastric cancer cell proliferation and invasion via regulation of angiopoietin-2. Exp Ther Med. 2016;12:3837–42.

38. Gu JJ, Gao GZ, Zhang SM. MiR-218 inhibits the tumorgenesis and proliferation of glioma cells by targeting Robo1. Cancer Biomark. 2016;16:309–17.

39. Zhang WB, Zhong WJ, Wang L. A signal-amplification circuit between miR-218 and Wnt/beta-catenin signal promotes human adipose tissue-derived stem cells osteogenic differentiation. Bone. 2014;58:59–66.

40. Brose K, Bland KS, Wang KH, Arnott D, Henzel W, Goodman CS, Tessier-Lavigne M, Kidd T. Slit proteins bind Robo receptors and have an evolutionarily conserved role in repulsive axon guidance. Cell. 1999;96:795–806.

41. Dickinson RE, Duncan WC. The SLIT-ROBO pathway: a regulator of cell function with implications for the reproductive system. Reproduction. 2010;139:697–704.

42. Rama N, Dubrac A, Mathivet T, Ni Charthaigh RA, Genet G, Cristofaro B, Pibouin-Fragner L, Ma L, Eichmann A, Chedotal A. Slit2 signaling through Robo1 and Robo2 is required for retinal neovascularization. Nat Med. 2015;21:483–91.

43. Wang Y, Li YP, Paulson C, Shao JZ, Zhang X, Wu M, Chen W. Wnt and the Wnt signaling pathway in bone development and disease. Front Biosci (Landmark Ed). 2014;19:379–407.

44. Seror R, Boudaoud S, Pavy S, Nocturne G, Schaeverbeke T, Saraux A, Chanson P, Gottenberg JE, Devauchelle-Pensec V, Tobon GJ, Mariette X, Miceli-Richard C. Increased Dickkopf-1 in recent-onset rheumatoid arthritis is a new biomarker of structural severity. Data from the ESPOIR cohort. Sci Rep. 2016;6:18421.

45. Wang SY, Liu YY, Ye H, Guo JP, Li R, Liu X, Li ZG. Circulating Dickkopf-1 is correlated with bone erosion and inflammation in rheumatoid arthritis. J Rheumatol. 2011;38:821–7.

46. Cui H, Ge J, Xie N, Banerjee S, Zhou Y, Antony VB, Thannickal VJ, Liu G. miR-34a inhibits lung fibrosis by inducing lung fibroblast senescence. Am J Respir Cell Mol Biol. 2017;56:168–78.

47. Han X, Zhen S, Ye Z, Lu J, Wang L, Li P, Li J, Zheng X, Li H, Chen W, Li X, Zhao L. A feedback loop between miR-30a/c-5p and DNMT1 mediates cisplatin resistance in ovarian Cancer cells. Cell Physiol Biochem. 2017;41:973–86.

48. Kim HY, Kwon HY, Ha Thi HT, Lee HJ, Kim GI, Hahm KB, Hong S. MicroRNA-132 and microRNA-223 control positive feedback circuit by regulating FOXO3a in inflammatory bowel disease. J Gastroenterol Hepatol. 2016;31:1727–35.

49. Wang G, Zhao Y, Zheng Y. MiR-122/Wnt/beta-catenin regulatory circuitry sustains glioma progression. Tumour Biol. 2014;35:8565–72.

50. Zhou AD, Diao LT, Xu H, Xiao ZD, Li JH, Zhou H, Qu LH. Beta-catenin/LEF1 transactivates the microRNA-371-373 cluster that modulates the Wnt/beta-catenin-signaling pathway. Oncogene. 2012;31:2968–78.

23

Knee pain as a predictor of structural progression over 4 years: data from the Osteoarthritis Initiative, a prospective cohort study

Yuanyuan Wang[1*] (iD), Andrew J. Teichtahl[1], François Abram[2], Sultana Monira Hussain[1], Jean-Pierre Pelletier[3], Flavia M. Cicuttini[1†] and Johanne Martel-Pelletier[3†]

Abstract

Background: There is evidence that knee pain not only is a consequence of structural deterioration in osteoarthritis (OA) but also contributes to structural progression. Clarifying this is important because targeting the factors related to knee pain may offer a clinical approach for slowing the progression of knee OA. The aim of this study was to examine whether knee pain over 1 year predicted cartilage volume loss, incidence and progression of radiographic osteoarthritis (ROA) over 4 years.

Methods: Osteoarthritis Initiative participants with no ROA (Kellgren-Lawrence grade $\leq$ 1) ($n = 2120$) and with ROA (Kellgren-Lawrence grade $\geq$ 2) ($n = 2249$) were examined. Knee pain was assessed at baseline and 1 year using the Western Ontario and McMaster Universities Osteoarthritis Index (WOMAC). Knee pain patterns were categorised as no pain (WOMAC pain < 5 at baseline and 1 year), fluctuating pain (WOMAC pain $\geq$ 5 at either time point) and persistent pain (WOMAC pain $\geq$ 5 at both time points). Cartilage volume, incidence and progression of ROA were assessed using magnetic resonance imaging and x-rays at baseline and 4-years.

Results: In both non-ROA and ROA, greater baseline WOMAC knee pain score was associated with increased medial and lateral cartilage volume loss ($p \leq 0.001$), incidence (OR 1.07, 95% CI 1.01–1.13) and progression (OR 1.07, 95% CI 1.03–1.10) of ROA. Non-ROA and ROA participants with fluctuating and persistent knee pain had increased cartilage volume loss compared with those with no pain (p for trend ≤ 0.01). Non-ROA participants with fluctuating knee pain had increased risk of incident ROA (OR 1.62, 95% CI 1.04–2.54), corresponding to a number needed to harm of 19.5. In ROA the risk of progressive ROA increased in participants with persistent knee pain (OR 1.82, 95% CI 1.28–2.60), corresponding to a number needed to harm of 9.6.

Conclusions: Knee pain over 1 year predicted accelerated cartilage volume loss and increased risk of incident and progressive ROA. Early management of knee pain and controlling knee pain over time by targeting the underlying mechanisms may be important for preserving knee structure and reducing the burden of knee OA.

Keywords: Pain, Knee osteoarthritis, Cartilage, Incidence, Progression, Magnetic resonance imaging

* Correspondence: yuanyuan.wang@monash.edu
†Flavia M. Cicuttini and Johanne Martel-Pelletier contributed equally to this work.
[1]Department of Epidemiology and Preventive Medicine, School of Public Health and Preventive Medicine, Monash University, 553 St Kilda Road, Melbourne, VIC 3004, Australia
Full list of author information is available at the end of the article

Background

Pain and structural articular degeneration are major clinical manifestations of knee osteoarthritis (OA). Although previous studies have predominantly focussed on whether structural disease progression predicts knee pain in people with knee OA [1–4], there have been relatively few studies examining whether knee pain is a predictor of structural progression of knee OA [5, 6]. There is increasing evidence for an important interplay between joint structures such as cartilage, bone, muscle and other soft tissues in maintaining joint health [7]. Pain through mechanisms such as inflammation and reduced mobility can adversely affect these joint structures, resulting in structural progression [8, 9]. Thus it is plausible that knee pain not only is a consequence of structural deterioration in OA but also contributes to structural progression. Clarifying this is important, because if this is the case, targeting the factors related to knee pain may offer a potential strategy for slowing disease progression of OA.

The major structural outcomes commonly examined in the development and progression of knee OA include cartilage volume loss assessed by magnetic resonance imaging (MRI) and incidence and progression of radiographic osteoarthritis (ROA). The findings of prospective cohort studies examining whether knee pain is a predictor of structural progression are summarised in Table 1. Inconsistent results have emerged regarding whether knee pain predicts cartilage volume/thickness loss [1, 5, 10–14]. This may be attributable to small to moderate sample sizes, different study populations, subgroup analyses and varied outcome measures. Although some studies found no association between baseline knee pain and subsequent cartilage volume loss in symptomatic knee OA [1, 10, 13] or asymptomatic [11] individuals, other studies showed relationships of baseline knee pain [14], frequent knee pain [5] and change in knee pain [1, 12, 13] with cartilage volume/thickness loss. In terms of studies with radiographic outcomes, some studies have suggested no association between baseline knee pain and progression of ROA [6, 15–17], whereas other studies have reported associations of baseline knee pain with incident ROA [16, 18], incident accelerated knee OA [19] and progressive ROA [18]. Differences in study population, assessment of knee pain, duration of follow-up and definition of incidence and progression of knee ROA may provide potential explanations of the inconclusive results. Larger cohort studies with longer follow-up have shown significant associations between knee pain and incidence and/or progression of knee ROA [16, 18, 19].

The National Institutes of Health Osteoarthritis Initiative (OAI) is the largest observational cohort of knee OA [20] and offers the opportunity to examine whether knee pain predicts structural progression. The aim of the present study was to examine whether baseline knee pain and knee pain patterns over 1 year are predictors of cartilage volume loss, incidence and progression of ROA over 4 years in a large cohort of individuals with and without knee ROA.

Methods

Osteoarthritis Initiative

Data were extracted from the OAI database, which holds data derived from a publicly available, multicentre, population-based cohort study of knee OA (https://oai.nih.gov). The OAI comprises data of 4796 participants aged 45–79 years with or at risk for knee OA at baseline. OAI exclusion criteria were inflammatory arthritis, severe joint space narrowing in both knees, unilateral knee replacement and severe joint space narrowing in the contralateral knee, inability to undergo MRI or provide a blood sample, use of walking aids except a single straight cane ≤ 50% of the time, or unwillingness to provide informed consent. Participants were recruited at four clinical sites, and the study was approved by the institutional review board at each of the sites. All participants gave informed consent.

Participants of the current study

Bilateral standing posteroanterior fixed-flexion knee radiographs [21] were assessed for baseline Kellgren-Lawrence (K-L) grading (0–4) ($n = 4369$). If both knees had no evidence of ROA, the dominant knee was selected for analyses. If only one knee had evidence of ROA, this was the selected knee for analyses. If both knees had evidence of ROA, the most severe knee was selected for analyses. When the severity was equal between sides, the most painful knee was selected for analyses. In the case of equal pain in both knees, the dominant knee was selected for analyses. Participants had been categorized into two groups based on their baseline K-L grade as part of their participation in the study: non-ROA (incidence cohort) defined by a baseline K-L grade ≤ 1 ($n = 2120$) and ROA (progression cohort) defined by a baseline K-L grade ≥ 2 ($n = 2249$).

Knee pain assessment

Knee pain was assessed yearly using the Western Ontario and McMaster Universities Osteoarthritis Index (WOMAC) pain subscale [22], Likert scale version. It consists of five items with scores ranging 0 to 20 and 20 being the worst pain. "Symptomatic" was defined as a WOMAC pain score ≥ 5 based on the Low-Intensity Symptom State-Attainment Index cut-off [23]. This definition has been used in a previous OAI study in which WOMAC knee pain score ≥ 5 represented the upper tertile of all participants with any pain in the

Table 1 Prospective cohort studies examining knee pain as a predictor of knee structural outcomes

Author, year	Participants	Exposure	Outcome measure	Main results
Outcome: change in cartilage volume or thickness				
Raynauld et al., 2004 [10]	40 patients with symptomatic knee OA 2-year follow-up ($N = 32$)	WOMAC pain	Cartilage volume loss; slow (< 2% global cartilage loss) and rapid (> 15% global cartilage loss) progressors	Trend for higher baseline knee pain in rapid progressors than in slow progressors (49.9 ± 6.1 vs. 34.0 ± 4.4, $p = 0.05$)
Wluka et al., 2004 [11]	81 healthy post-menopausal women 2.5-year follow-up ($N = 57$)	WOMAC pain	Change in tibial cartilage volume	Baseline knee pain not associated with change in tibial cartilage volume (data not shown)
Wluka et al., 2004 [1]	132 people with symptomatic knee OA 2-year follow-up ($N = 117$)	WOMAC pain	Change in tibial cartilage volume	The severity of baseline knee pain did not predict subsequent tibial cartilage volume loss ($r = 0.13$, $p = 0.14$) There was a weak association between worsening of knee pain and increased tibial cartilage volume loss ($r = 0.28$, $p = 0.002$)
Raynauld et al., 2006 [12]	110 patients with symptomatic knee OA 2-year follow-up ($N = 107$)	WOMAC pain	Change in cartilage volume for the entire knee (global) and medial and lateral knee compartments	Medial compartment cartilage volume loss was associated with simultaneous knee pain change at 2 years (β coefficient − 0.45, $p = 0.03$)
Pelletier et al., 2007 [13]	110 patients with symptomatic knee OA 2-year follow-up ($N = 107$)	WOMAC pain	Change in knee cartilage volume from subregions	Baseline WOMAC pain not associated cartilage volume loss in medial central femoral condyle or medial central tibial plateau An increase in WOMAC pain score associated with cartilage volume loss in medial central tibial plateau (β coefficient − 0.26, $p = 0.007$)
Eckstein et al., 2011 [5]	718 participants with radiographic knee OA (K-L grades 2–4) 12-month follow-up	Questionnaire categorized as no, infrequent or frequent pain	Change in cartilage thickness in the central subregion of medial weight-bearing femoral condyle	Change in cartilage thickness − 12 μm in knees without pain vs − 54 μm in those with frequent pain at baseline, $p = 0.01$ The percentage of "progressors" (knees with cartilage thinning) was greater in knees with frequent pain than in those without pain for total joint (29% vs 16%, $p = 0.004$) and medial compartment (23% vs 13%, $p = 0.015$), but not for lateral compartment (20% vs 16%, $p = 0.29$)
Saunders et al., 2012 [14]	912 randomly selected individuals, 53% had radiographic OA in the medial compartment, 24% had radiographic OA in the lateral compartment 2.9-year follow-up ($N = 399$)	WOMAC pain	Change in tibial cartilage volume	Pain independently predicted lateral tibial cartilage volume loss. WOMAC knee pain: B − 0.14 (95% CI, − 0.22, − 0.05); knee pain yes/no: B − 0.96 (95% CI, − 1.91, − 0.00). No significant associations for medial tibial cartilage volume loss
Outcome: radiographic incidence or progression of OA				
Spector et al., 1992 [15]	169 patients with OA of the hands or knees 11-year follow-up ($N = 63$)	VAS pain	Radiographic progression defined by > 10% reduction in joint space width or a K-L grade increase ≥ 1	9 of 15 people with knee pain at baseline had radiographic progression, compared with 6 of 16 without knee pain at baseline ($p = 0.20$)
Cooper et al., 2000 [16]	583 people from a population	Have you had pain in or	Incident and progressive OA defined	Knee pain associated with incident OA when

Table 1 Prospective cohort studies examining knee pain as a predictor of knee structural outcomes *(Continued)*

Author, year	Participants	Exposure	Outcome measure	Main results
	cohort 5.1-year follow-up (N = 354)	around your knee on most days for at least 1 month, at some time during the last year?	using thresholds of both K-L grade 2 and K-L grade 1	defined by K-L ≥ 1 (OR 2.9, 95% CI 1.2–6.7) but not K-L ≥ 2 (OR 1.3, 95% CI 0.6–2.7) No association between knee pain and progressive OA defined by either K-L ≥ 1 (OR 0.8, 95% CI 0.4–1.7) or K-L ≥ 2 (OR 2.4, 95% CI 0.7–8.0)
Wolfe et al., 2002 [17]	1507 patients with symptomatic knee OA	VAS pain	Joint space narrowing score = 3	Knee pain not associated with progression to maximum joint space narrowing (data not shown)
Miyazaki et al., 2002 [6]	106 patients with medial compartment knee OA 6-year follow-up (N = 74)	Knee rating system of the Hospital for Special Surgery	Radiographic progression defined as ≥ 1 grade increase in narrowing of joint space width of the medial compartment	Baseline knee pain not associated with radiographic progression (OR 0.93, 95% CI 0.78–1.11, p = 0.43)
Mazzuca et al., 2005 [46]	174 obese women with unilateral knee OA 16- and 30-month follow-up	WOMAC pain	Joint space narrowing ≥ 0.50 mm	Baseline WOMAC pain > 11 as a predictor of joint space narrowing ≥ 0.50 mm: Month 16 (n = 73): sensitivity 77%, positive predictive value 36%, specificity 59%, negative predictive value 89% Month 30 (n =70): sensitivity 65%, positive predictive value 45%, specificity 62%, negative predictive value 78%
Muraki et al., 2012 [18]	3040 people from a population-based cohort 3.3-year follow-up (N = 2262)	Have you experienced right/ left knee pain on most days in the past month, in addition to now?	Incident radiographic knee OA; progressive radiographic knee OA	Knee pain at baseline associated with incident K-L grade ≥ 3 knee OA (OR 2.53, 95% CI 1.59–4.00) and progressive radiographic knee OA (OR 2.63, 95% CI 1.81–3.81), but not incident K-L grade ≥ 2 knee OA
Driban et al., 2016 [19]	1930 participants with no radiographic knee OA in either knee 4-year follow-up	WOMAC pain	Incident accelerated knee OA: at least one knee progressed to end-stage knee OA (K-L grade ≥ 3)	Individuals with accelerated knee OA had greater WOMAC pain (OR 2.00, 95% CI 1.33–3.00)

Abbreviations: K-L Kellgren Lawrence, OA Osteoarthritis, VAS Visual analogue scale, WOMAC Western Ontario and McMaster Universities Osteoarthritis Index

cohort [24]. The knee pain patterns from baseline to 1-year follow-up were categorised as follows: no knee pain (WOMAC pain < 5 at both baseline and 1 year), fluctuating knee pain (WOMAC pain ≥ 5 at either baseline or 1 year) and persistent knee pain (WOMAC pain ≥ 5 at both baseline and 1 year).

Cartilage volume assessment

Knee MRI was performed for the target knee using a 3-T apparatus (Magnetom Trio; Siemens, Erlangen, Germany). Cartilage volume was measured by sagittal double-echo steady-state imaging for medial and lateral tibiofemoral compartments (condyle and plateau) using an automatic human cartilage segmentation (ArthroLab, Montreal, QC, Canada) as previously described and validated [25, 26]. The test-retest revealed an excellent measurement error of 0.3 ± 1.6%, corresponding to a measurement error of 30.3 ± 126.2 mm^3 [26]. The annual rate of cartilage volume loss over 4 years was obtained by calculating (4-year follow-up volume – baseline volume)/baseline volume/4, expressed as a percentage.

Assessment of incidence and progression of ROA

Incidence of ROA was defined by a baseline K-L grade of 0 or 1 and a K-L grade ≥ 2 at 4-year follow-up. Progression of ROA was defined by a baseline K-L grade of 2 or 3 and an increase in K-L grade ≥ 1 at 4-year follow-up.

Statistical analyses

Demographic, clinical, radiological and MRI data were systematically entered into a computerized database. Participant characteristics were compared between participants with and without ROA using independent samples t tests or chi-square tests when appropriate. With 2120 non-ROA participants, our study had 80% power to detect a regression coefficient as low as 0.006 between baseline knee pain and cartilage volume loss with five predictors, and a relative risk as low as 1.41 between baseline knee pain and incidence of ROA, α error of 0.05, two-sided significance. With 2249 participants with ROA, our study had 80% power to detect a regression coefficient as low as 0.0057 between baseline knee pain and cartilage volume loss with five predictors, and a relative risk as low as 1.27 between baseline knee pain and progression of ROA, α error of 0.05, two-sided significance. The association between baseline knee pain and cartilage volume loss was examined using multiple linear regression. The association between knee pain patterns over 1 year and cartilage volume loss was examined using the F-test (generalised linear model) with estimated marginal means (SE), and linear trend was assessed using multiple linear regression. The

associations of baseline knee pain and knee pain patterns over 1 year with incidence and progression of ROA were examined using binary logistic regression. The attributable risk and number needed to harm (NNH) were calculated. NNH is a measure of how many people need to be exposed to a risk factor in order for one person to have a particular adverse effect. All the analyses were adjusted for gender, baseline age, body mass index (BMI) and K-L grade. All tests were two-sided, and $p < 0.05$ was considered statistically significant. Statistical analyses were performed using the IBM SPSS Statistics software package (version 24; IBM, Armonk, NY, USA).

Results

Participant characteristics at baseline, as well as knee pain and structure changes over time, are shown in Table 2. Compared with non-ROA participants, participants with ROA were older, had higher BMIs and WOMAC pain scores, were more likely to have fluctuating and persistent knee pain, and had a greater rate of cartilage volume loss (all $p < 0.001$). The incidence and progression of ROA were 9.6% and 17.8%, respectively. There was no significant difference in age, gender or BMI between those who completed ($n = 3395$) and those who did not complete ($n = 974$) the 4-year follow-up. The non-completers had higher K-L grade and worse knee pain and were more likely to have ROA than the completers (all $p < 0.05$).

Associations between baseline knee pain and structural progression over 4 years

In non-ROA, a greater baseline WOMAC pain score was associated with increased rate of cartilage volume loss in medial (regression coefficient 0.04%, 95% CI 0.02–0.06%) and lateral (0.04%, 0.02–0.06%) compartments by MRI, adjusted for age, gender, BMI and K-L grade. A higher baseline WOMAC pain score was also associated with increased incidence of ROA (OR 1.07, 95% CI 1.01–1.13) (top half of Table 3). In ROA, a greater baseline WOMAC pain score was associated with increased rate of cartilage volume loss in medial (regression coefficient 0.04%, 95% CI 0.02–0.07%) and lateral (0.05%, 0.03–0.07%) compartments by MRI. A higher baseline WOMAC pain score was also associated with increased progression of ROA (OR 1.07, 95% CI 1.03–1.10) (bottom half of Table 3).

Associations between knee pain patterns over 1 year and structural progression over 4 years

In non-ROA, the annual rate of cartilage volume loss in the medial compartment was 0.63% (SE 0.03%) in participants with no knee pain, 0.81% (0.08%) in those with fluctuating knee pain, and 0.93% (0.12%) in those with

Table 2 Characteristics of study participants

	Non-ROA n = 2120	ROA n = 2249	p Value
Baseline characteristics			
Age, years	59.9 (9.1)	62.7 (8.9)	< 0.001
Female, n (%)	1224 (57.7)	1311 (58.3)	0.71
Body mass index, kg/m^2	27.6 (4.5)	29.8 (4.8)	< 0.001
Kellgren-Lawrence grade, n (%)			–
0	1432 (67.5)	–	
1	688 (32.5)	–	
2	–	1173 (52.2)	
3	–	787 (35.0)	
4	–	289 (12.8)	
WOMAC pain score (range 0–20)	1.9 (2.7)	3.7 (3.8)	< 0.001
WOMAC pain score ≥ 5, n (%)	307 (14.5)	760 (33.8)	< 0.001
Change in knee pain and structure			
Knee pain pattern over 1 year, n (%)			< 0.001
No knee pain at both baseline and 1 year	1669 (80.5)	1265 (57.8)	
Fluctuating knee pain (pain at either baseline or 1 year)	274 (13.2)	464 (21.2)	
Persistent knee pain (pain at both baseline and 1 year)	131 (6.3)	459 (21.0)	
Annual percentage cartilage volume loss over 4 years			
Medial compartment	0.68 (1.13)	1.36 (1.95)	< 0.001
Lateral compartment	0.73 (1.03)	1.21 (1.41)	< 0.001
Incidence of ROA over 4 years, n (%)	165 (9.6)	–	–
Progression of ROA over 4 years, n (%)	–	272 (17.8)	–

ROA Radiographic osteoarthritis, WOMAC Western Ontario and McMaster Universities Osteoarthritis Index
Data displayed as mean (SD) or number (%)

Table 3 Associations of baseline Western Ontario and McMaster Universities Osteoarthritis Index knee pain score with annual percentage cartilage volume loss and incidence and progression of radiographic knee osteoarthritis over 4 years

	Univariable analysis		Multivariable analysis[a]	
Non-ROA				
	Regression coefficient (95% CI)	p Value	Regression coefficient (95% CI)	p Value
Annual percentage cartilage volume loss in medial compartment	0.04 (0.01, 0.06)	0.001	0.04 (0.02, 0.06)	0.001
Annual percentage cartilage volume loss in lateral compartment	0.04 (0.02, 0.06)	< 0.001	0.04 (0.02, 0.06)	< 0.001
	OR (95% CI)	p Value	OR (95% CI)	p Value
Incidence of radiographic knee osteoarthritis	1.10 (1.05, 1.16)	< 0.001	1.07 (1.01, 1.13)	0.02
ROA				
	Regression coefficient (95% CI)	p Value	Regression coefficient (95% CI)	p Value
Annual percentage cartilage volume loss in medial compartment	0.06 (0.03, 0.08)	< 0.001	0.04 (0.02, 0.07)	0.001
Annual percentage cartilage volume loss in lateral compartment	0.06 (0.04, 0.08)	< 0.001	0.05 (0.03, 0.07)	< 0.001
	OR (95% CI)	p Value	OR (95% CI)	p Value
Progression of radiographic knee osteoarthritis	1.08 (1.05, 1.12)	< 0.001	1.07 (1.03, 1.10)	< 0.001

ROA Radiographic osteoarthritis
[a]Adjusted for age, gender, body mass index and Kellgren-Lawrence grade

persistent knee pain (p for trend = 0.003), adjusted for age, gender, BMI, and K-L grade (Table 4). The rate was greater in participants with fluctuating ($p = 0.04$) and persistent ($p = 0.02$) knee pain than in those without knee pain. Similar results were found in the lateral compartment. Although persistent knee pain was not significantly associated with the incidence of ROA (OR 1.57, 95% CI 0.85–2.90), fluctuating knee pain was associated with increased incidence of ROA (OR 1.62, 95% CI 1.04–2.54; p for trend = 0.03) (Table 4). The attributable risk of fluctuating knee pain for incident ROA was 35% (4–55%), with an NNH of 19.5.

In ROA, the annual rate of cartilage volume loss in the medial compartment was 1.26% (SE 0.06%) in participants with no knee pain, 1.47% (0.11%) in those with fluctuating knee pain, and 1.60% (0.12%) in those with persistent knee pain (p for trend = 0.01), adjusted for age, gender, BMI and K-L grade (Table 5). The rate was greater in participants with persistent ($p = 0.02$) knee pain than in those without knee pain. Similar results were shown in the lateral compartment. Although fluctuating knee pain was not significantly associated with the progression of ROA (OR 1.34, 95% CI 0.94–1.89), persistent knee pain was associated with increased progression of ROA (OR 1.82, 95% CI 1.28–2.60; p for trend = 0.001) (Table 5). The attributable risk of persistent knee pain for progressive ROA was 37% (18–50%), corresponding to the NNH of 9.6.

Similar results were observed for the association between knee pain patterns over 2 and 3 years and structural progression over 4 years (Additional file 1: Tables S1 and S2).

Discussion

In this large prospective cohort study, greater baseline knee pain, as well as fluctuating and persistent knee pain over 1 year, predicted structural progression over 4 years in participants with and without knee ROA, as evidenced by accelerated cartilage volume loss and increased incidence and progression of ROA. Among non-ROA participants with fluctuating knee pain over 1 year, 35% of the incident ROA risk over 4 years could be attributed to fluctuating knee pain, corresponding to an NNH of 19.5. In participants with ROA with persistent knee pain over 1 year, 37% of the progressive ROA risk over 4 years could be attributed to persistent knee pain, corresponding to an NNH of 9.6. These data suggest that knee pain is an important predictive factor for the deterioration of knee structural outcomes and highlight the significant adverse impact of persistent knee

Table 4 Associations of knee pain patterns over 1 year with annual percentage cartilage volume loss and incidence of radiographic knee osteoarthritis over 4 years in participants without radiographic knee osteoarthritis at baseline

	Univariable analysis		Multivariable analysis[a]	
	Estimated marginal mean (SE)	p Value	Estimated marginal mean (SE)	p Value
Annual percentage cartilage volume loss in medial compartment				
No knee pain at both baseline and 1 year	0.63 (0.03)		0.63 (0.03)[b,c]	
Fluctuating knee pain (pain at either time point)	0.80 (0.08)	0.01[d]	0.81 (0.08)[b]	0.01[d]
Persistent knee pain (pain at both time points)	0.94 (0.12)		0.93 (0.12)[c]	
Trend		0.004		0.003
Annual percentage cartilage volume loss in lateral compartment				
No knee pain at both baseline and 1 year	0.68 (0.03)		0.68 (0.03)[e,f]	
Fluctuating knee pain (pain at either time point)	0.88 (0.08)	0.008[d]	0.89 (0.08)[e]	0.005[d]
Persistent knee pain (pain at both time points)	0.92 (0.11)		0.93 (0.11)[f]	
Trend		0.003		0.002
	OR (95% CI)	p Value	OR (95% CI)	p Value
Incidence of radiographic knee osteoarthritis				
No knee pain at both baseline and 1 year	1.00		1.00	
Fluctuating knee pain (pain at either time point)	1.96 (1.29, 2.99)	0.002	1.62 (1.04, 2.54)	0.03
Persistent knee pain (pain at both time points)	2.07 (1.16, 3.72)	0.01	1.57 (0.85, 2.90)	0.15
Trend		< 0.001		0.03

[a]Adjusted for age, gender, body mass index and Kellgren-Lawrence grade
[b]$p = 0.04$ for between-group difference
[c]$p = 0.02$ for between-group difference
[d]For difference in annual percentage cartilage volume loss in medial/lateral compartment among the three knee pain pattern groups
[e]$p = 0.01$ for between-group difference
[f]$p = 0.03$ for between-group difference

Table 5 Associations of knee pain patterns over 1 year with annual percentage cartilage volume loss and progression of radiographic knee osteoarthritis over 4 years in participants with radiographic knee osteoarthritis at baseline

	Univariable analysis		Multivariable analysis[a]	
	Estimated marginal mean (SE)	p Value	Estimated marginal mean (SE)	p Value
Annual percentage cartilage volume loss in medial compartment				
No knee pain at both baseline and 1 year	1.22 (0.06)		1.26 (0.06)[b]	
Fluctuating knee pain (pain at either time point)	1.52 (0.11)	0.001[c]	1.47 (0.11)	0.03[c]
Persistent knee pain (pain at both time points)	1.68 (0.12)		1.60 (0.12)[b]	
Trend		< 0.001		0.01
Annual percentage cartilage volume loss in lateral compartment				
No knee pain at both baseline and 1 year	1.06 (0.05)		1.08 (0.05)[d,e]	
Fluctuating knee pain (pain at either time point)	1.41 (0.08)	< 0.001[c]	1.38 (0.08)[d]	< 0.001[c]
Persistent knee pain (pain at both time points)	1.46 (0.09)		1.39 (0.09)[e]	
Trend		< 0.001		< 0.001
	Odds ratio (95% CI)	p Value	Odds ratio (95% CI)	p Value
Progression of radiographic knee osteoarthritis				
No knee pain at both baseline and 1 year	1.00		1.00	
Fluctuating knee pain (pain at either time point)	1.46 (1.04, 2.06)	0.03	1.34 (0.94, 1.89)	0.10
Persistent knee pain (pain at both time points)	2.13 (1.53, 2.97)	< 0.001	1.82 (1.28, 2.60)	0.001
Trend		< 0.001		0.001

*Adjusted for age, gender, body mass index and Kellgren-Lawrence grade
[b]$p = 0.02$ for between-group difference
[c] For difference in annual percentage cartilage volume loss in medial/lateral compartment among the three knee pain pattern groups
[d]$p = 0.001$ for between-group difference
[e]$p = 0.002$ for between-group difference

pain on knee structures. The findings suggest that treating patients with knee pain both early in the disease course and over time is important for preserving knee structure and is likely to have a significant impact on reducing disease burden.

There have been conflicting data on the association between knee pain and structural progression of knee OA [1, 5, 6, 10, 12–19]. This may have resulted from limited sample sizes and durations of follow-up in both MRI and radiological studies. Cohort studies with larger sample sizes and/or longer durations of follow-up have shown significant associations of knee pain with MRI [5, 14] and radiographic [16, 18, 19] outcomes. One cohort study analysing baseline and 12-month follow-up data in a large subsample of 718 participants with K-L grades 2–4 from the OAI showed knees with frequent pain had greater rates of cartilage thickness loss in the central subregion of the medial femoral condyle than knees without pain [5]. Our study of a large knee ROA cohort with 4 years of follow-up showed that higher levels of baseline knee pain predicted increased structural progression over 4 years assessed by both MRI (cartilage volume loss) and x-ray (progression of ROA). Our study extended the previous OAI study [5] by examining baseline knee pain as a continuous variable, thus indicating a dose-response relationship;

by investigating knee pain pattern over time and its association with structural outcomes, showing associations for cartilage volume loss of both medial and lateral tibiofemoral compartments and consistent results for MRI and radiographic outcomes; and by examining participants with and without knee ROA simultaneously. The effect sizes for some of the associations appeared small, particularly for those between baseline WOMAC knee pain score and annual percentage cartilage volume loss (Table 3). However, it is important to put them in context. For example, in those with no ROA, even small changes in the annual rate of cartilage volume loss for small changes in knee pain will have significant impacts over many years. Only three studies have examined the relationship between knee pain and structural changes in non-OA populations [11, 16, 19]. Although one study found no association between baseline knee pain and tibial cartilage volume loss over 2.5 years [11], the other reported baseline knee pain being associated with incident ROA defined by K-L ≥ 1 but not K-L ≥ 2 over 5.1 years [16] and incident accelerated knee OA over 4 years [19]. We defined incident ROA using the more stringent K-L grade ≥ 2 at follow-up. Our large 4-year follow-up study of participants with no ROA demonstrated that baseline knee pain predicted cartilage volume loss and incidence of ROA, suggesting a predictive role of knee pain in adverse structural outcomes, even in people without knee ROA.

Given the fluctuating nature of knee pain, we examined the association between knee pain patterns over 1 year and structural progression over 4 years. We found that fluctuating and persistent knee pain over 1 year predicted increased cartilage volume loss as well as incidence and progression of ROA over 4 years in participants with and without ROA, with positive linear relationships observed between the frequency of knee pain over 1 year and structural progression over 4 years. Previous studies reported that worsening of knee pain was associated with increased cartilage volume loss simultaneously (i.e., over the same time period) [1, 12, 13]. The adverse effect of ongoing (fluctuating or persistent) knee pain on knee structure has not previously been examined. We found that fluctuating and persistent knee pain over 1 year contributed substantially to the incidence and progression of ROA over 4 years. For every 20 non-ROA participants with fluctuating knee pain over 1 year, 1 developed incident ROA in 4 years. For every ten ROA participants with persistent knee pain over 1 year, one had progressive ROA in 4 years. These findings support the importance of controlling knee pain over time and that targeting people with fluctuating or persistent knee pain for early intervention will be important for preserving knee structure and delaying structural progression.

The mechanism of knee pain and structural change is likely to be multifactorial. Optimal knee function requires a complex interplay of structural and biomechanical factors, including supporting musculature. It has been shown that increased size and decreased fat content of the vastus medialis predict reduced cartilage volume loss, and the most significant predictor of increased muscle size is an improvement in knee pain [27–29]. Nonetheless, the causes of knee pain are complex and heterogeneous and include structural factors [30], inflammatory hyperalgesia [31], central mechanisms incorporating brain areas processing fear, emotions and in aversive conditioning [32], and genetic predispositions toward peripheral pain sensitisation [33]. There is evidence that inflammation [8, 9] and other structural abnormalities, such as bone marrow lesions and effusion-synovitis [34–36], are associated with greater knee pain and structural progression. Greater K-L grade is associated with higher levels of knee pain [30] and accelerated cartilage loss [37]. However, it is less likely that our findings are explained by disease severity, because all the analyses were adjusted for baseline K-L grade, and the outcome of annual percentage loss in cartilage volume took into account the baseline amount of cartilage volume. Understanding and appropriately targeting

the factors related to knee pain in an individual may be particularly important for modifying disease trajectory, such as targeting quadriceps strengthening, bone marrow lesions, synovitis, central sensitisation, or weight loss.

This study has limitations. The selection of target knee for each participant was based on radiographic severity. It is more likely that this target knee is the one contributing to pain, but it is also possible that knee pain originates from the other knee and that there has been switching. This would have underestimated the magnitude of observed associations. There is also evidence that pain in one knee has adverse effects on the other knee through compensatory gait mechanisms that shift the load distribution from the affected limb to the healthy contralateral limb during weight-bearing activities [38, 39]. We did not adjust our results for medications that may influence pain over time, because the information was obtained by questionnaire, and the answers were limited. However, any symptoms experienced by the participants, including fluctuating symptoms, would have been present despite any therapies, so the notion of pain predicting structural progression remains valid. Furthermore, knee pain was analysed prior to the assessment of structural outcomes, thus it is unlikely that these results can be explained simply by structural changes causing pain. Although there was potential selection bias in the study, in which the non-completers had higher K-L grade and worse knee pain than the completers, this would not affect the interpretation of our results. We did not examine other structural abnormalities associated with pain, such as bone marrow lesions and effusion-synovitis [40–42], but this does not affect the interpretation of our findings, because such structural alterations are likely to be on the causal pathway from knee pain to structural outcomes [43–45]. There was an issue of multiple testing in our analyses. For each of the incidence cohort and the progression cohort, we examined two knee pain variables and three outcome variables, and thus we performed six tests. If we performed the Bonferroni correction, the significance level should be $0.05/6 = 0.008$. Most of our results remained significant after applying the Bonferroni correction. However, it is important to consider that we did not perform completely independent, unrelated analyses, because both cartilage volume loss and radiographic changes are on the same disease pathway. We found consistent results for incidence and progression of ROA, as well as for MRI and radiographic outcomes, after adjustment for potential confounders, suggesting a true association rather than a chance association. There is also the possibility of residual confounding that knee pain could be a biomarker of other unmeasured factors which are associated with structural progression.

The present study has several strengths. The OAI offered a unique opportunity to study the disease profile of a large number of participants and explore the impact of knee pain on structural progression. Until now, the assessment of cartilage volume change by quantitative MRI has mostly been done using manual or semi-automated technologies, which have the intrinsic limitation of variability in results with respect to human intervention. This imposed limitations on a complete analysis of the OAI cohort. The validation of fully automated technology to assess cartilage volume and its change over time [26] has greatly improved the capacity and reliability of the analysis of the OAI MRI dataset. We examined whether knee pain predicted structural endpoints in people with and without ROA. The OAI intentionally recruited participants at risk of knee OA. This enriched the population for the outcome of interest and thus increased the power of the study to detect significant associations between knee pain and structural outcomes. Knee pain was assessed at baseline and 1 year later using a valid questionnaire, from which knee pain patterns were investigated with a positive linear relationship observed between the frequency of knee pain over 1 year and structural progression over 4 years. This is important because knee pain can fluctuate with time, and thus an isolated baseline assessment may have limited effect on predicting structural progression many years later.

Conclusions

Greater baseline knee pain, as well as fluctuating and persistent knee pain over 1 year, predicted increased cartilage volume loss and incidence of ROA in people with no ROA and increased cartilage volume loss and progression of ROA in those with ROA over 4 years. With its large cohort, this study provides evidence that knee pain is an important predictor of structural disease progression in population-based individuals with and without knee OA. This study suggests that controlling knee pain early in the disease course as well as over time by targeting the underlying mechanisms may be important for preserving knee structure and reducing the burden of knee OA. Further studies are needed to determine if this is the case.

Abbreviations
BMI: Body mass index; K-L: Kellgren-Lawrence; MRI: Magnetic resonance imaging; NNH: Number needed to harm; OA: Osteoarthritis; OAI: Osteoarthritis Initiative; ROA: Radiographic osteoarthritis; VAS: Visual analogue scale; WOMAC: Western Ontario and McMaster Universities Osteoarthritis Index

Acknowledgements
We thank the OAI participants and coordinating centre for their work in generating the clinical and radiological data of the OAI cohort and making them publicly available.

Funding
The OAI is a public-private partnership comprised of five contracts (NO1-AR-2-2258, NO1-AR-2-2259, NO1-AR-2-2260, NO1-AR-2-2261, NO1-AR-2-2262) funded by the National Institutes of Health, a branch of the U.S. Department of Health and Human Services, in four clinical sites (University of Maryland School of Medicine and The Johns Hopkins University, Baltimore, MD, USA; The Ohio State University, Columbus, OH, USA; University of Pittsburgh, Pittsburgh, PA, USA; and Memorial Hospital of Rhode Island, Pawtucket, RI, USA) and conducted by the OAI study investigators. Private funding partners include Merck Research Laboratories, Novartis Pharmaceuticals Corporation, GlaxoSmithKline, and Pfizer Inc. Private sector funding for the OAI is managed by the Foundation for the National Institutes of Health. For the current study, the image reading was funded by the Osteoarthritis Research Unit, University of Montreal Hospital Research Centre, Montreal, QC, Canada, and the statistical analyses were funded in part by Medibank (Australia). The funders had no role in study design; collection, analysis and interpretation of data; preparation of the manuscript; or the decision to submit the manuscript for publication. YW is a recipient of a National Health and Medical Research Council (NHMRC) Career Development Fellowship (Clinical Level 1, APP1065464). SMH is a recipient of an NHMRC Early Career Fellowship (APP1142198).

Authors' contributions
All authors contributed substantially to the conception and design of the work. FA, JPP and JMP contributed to data acquisition. YW and AJT performed statistical analysis and drafted the manuscript. All authors contributed to analysis and interpretation of data for the work and reviewed the manuscript critically for important intellectual content. JMP and MFC had equal contributions as senior authors. All authors had full access to all the data and take responsibility for the integrity of the data and the accuracy of the data analysis. JMP and FMC are the guarantors of the article. All authors read and approved the final manuscript.

Consent for publication
Not applicable.

Competing interests
YW, AJT, SMH and FMC have no competing interests and are not part of the OAI investigative team. JPP, JMP and FA are not part of the OAI investigative team. JPP and JMP are shareholders in ArthroLab Inc. FA is an employee of ArthroLab Inc.

Author details
[1]Department of Epidemiology and Preventive Medicine, School of Public Health and Preventive Medicine, Monash University, 553 St Kilda Road, Melbourne, VIC 3004, Australia. [2]Medical Imaging Research & Development, ArthroLab Inc., Montreal, QC, Canada. [3]Osteoarthritis Research Unit, University of Montreal Hospital Research Centre (CRCHUM), Montreal, QC, Canada.

References
1. Wluka AE, Wolfe R, Stuckey S, Cicuttini FM. How does tibial cartilage volume relate to symptoms in subjects with knee osteoarthritis? Ann Rheum Dis. 2004;63:264–8.
2. Sharma L, Chmiel JS, Almagor O, Dunlop D, Guermazi A, Bathon JM, Eaton CB, Hochberg MC, Jackson RD, Kwoh CK, et al. Significance of preradiographic magnetic resonance imaging lesions in persons at increased risk of knee osteoarthritis. Arthritis Rheumatol. 2014;66:1811–9.
3. Urish KL, Keffalas MG, Durkin JR, Miller DJ, Chu CR, Mosher TJ. T2 texture index of cartilage can predict early symptomatic OA progression: data from the osteoarthritis initiative. Osteoarthritis Cartilage. 2013;21:1550–7.
4. Sowers MF, Hayes C, Jamadar D, Capul D, Lachance L, Jannausch M, Welch G. Magnetic resonance-detected subchondral bone marrow and cartilage defect characteristics associated with pain and X-ray-defined knee osteoarthritis. Osteoarthritis Cartilage. 2003;11:387–93.
5. Eckstein F, Cotofana S, Wirth W, Nevitt M, John MR, Dreher D, Frobell R. Greater rates of cartilage loss in painful knees than in pain-free knees after adjustment for radiographic disease stage: data from the osteoarthritis initiative. Arthritis Rheum. 2011;63:2257–67.
6. Miyazaki T, Wada M, Kawahara H, Sato M, Baba H, Shimada S. Dynamic load at baseline can predict radiographic disease progression in medial compartment knee osteoarthritis. Ann Rheum Dis. 2002;61:617–22.

7. Loeser RF, Goldring SR, Scanzello CR, Goldring MB. Osteoarthritis: a disease of the joint as an organ. Arthritis Rheum. 2012;64:1697–707.

8. Wang X, Hunter D, Xu J, Ding C. Metabolic triggered inflammation in osteoarthritis. Osteoarthritis Cartilage. 2015;23:22–30.

9. Neogi T, Guermazi A, Roemer F, Nevitt MC, Scholz J, Arendt-Nielsen L, Woolf C, Niu J, Bradley LA, Quinn E, Frey Law L. Association of joint inflammation with pain sensitization in knee osteoarthritis: the Multicenter Osteoarthritis Study. Arthritis Rheumatol. 2016;68:654–61.

10. Raynauld JP, Martel-Pelletier J, Berthiaume MJ, Labonte F, Beaudoin G, de Guise JA, Bloch DA, Choquette D, Haraoui B, Altman RD, et al. Quantitative magnetic resonance imaging evaluation of knee osteoarthritis progression over two years and correlation with clinical symptoms and radiologic changes. Arthritis Rheum. 2004;50:476–87.

11. Wluka AE, Wolfe R, Davis SR, Stuckey S, Cicuttini FM. Tibial cartilage volume change in healthy postmenopausal women: a longitudinal study. Ann Rheum Dis. 2004;63:444–9.

12. Raynauld JP, Martel-Pelletier J, Berthiaume MJ, Beaudoin G, Choquette D, Haraoui B, Tannenbaum H, Meyer JM, Beary JF, Cline GA, Pelletier JP. Long term evaluation of disease progression through the quantitative magnetic resonance imaging of symptomatic knee osteoarthritis patients: correlation with clinical symptoms and radiographic changes. Arthritis Res Ther. 2006;8:R21.

13. Pelletier JP, Raynauld JP, Berthiaume MJ, Abram F, Choquette D, Haraoui B, Beary JF, Cline GA, Meyer JM, Martel-Pelletier J. Risk factors associated with the loss of cartilage volume on weight-bearing areas in knee osteoarthritis patients assessed by quantitative magnetic resonance imaging: a longitudinal study. Arthritis Res Ther. 2007;9:R74.

14. Saunders J, Ding C, Cicuttini F, Jones G. Radiographic osteoarthritis and pain are independent predictors of knee cartilage loss: a prospective study. Intern Med J. 2012;42:274–80.

15. Spector TD, Dacre JE, Harris PA, Huskisson EC. Radiological progression of osteoarthritis: an 11 year follow up study of the knee. Ann Rheum Dis. 1992; 51:1107–10.

16. Cooper C, Snow S, McAlindon TE, Kellingray S, Stuart B, Coggon D, Dieppe PA. Risk factors for the incidence and progression of radiographic knee osteoarthritis. Arthritis Rheum. 2000;43:995–1000.

17. Wolfe F, Lane NE. The longterm outcome of osteoarthritis: rates and predictors of joint space narrowing in symptomatic patients with knee osteoarthritis. J Rheumatol. 2002;29:139–46.

18. Muraki S, Akune T, Oka H, Ishimoto Y, Nagata K, Yoshida M, Tokimura F, Nakamura K, Kawaguchi H, Yoshimura N. Incidence and risk factors for radiographic knee osteoarthritis and knee pain in Japanese men and women: a longitudinal population-based cohort study. Arthritis Rheum. 2012;64:1447–56.

19. Driban JB, Price LL, Eaton CB, Lu B, Lo GH, Lapane KL, McAlindon TE. Individuals with incident accelerated knee osteoarthritis have greater pain than those with common knee osteoarthritis progression: data from the Osteoarthritis Initiative. Clin Rheumatol. 2016;35:1565–71.

20. Peterfy CG, Schneider E, Nevitt M. The osteoarthritis initiative: report on the design rationale for the magnetic resonance imaging protocol for the knee. Osteoarthritis Cartilage. 2008;16:1433–41.

21. Nevitt MC, Peterfy C, Guermazi A, Felson DT, Duryea J, Woodworth T, Chen H, Kwoh K, Harris TB. Longitudinal performance evaluation and validation of fixed-flexion radiography of the knee for detection of joint space loss. Arthritis Rheum. 2007;56:1512–20.

22. Bellamy N, Buchanan WW, Goldsmith CH, Campbell J, Stitt LW. Validation study of WOMAC: a health status instrument for measuring clinically important patient relevant outcomes to antirheumatic drug therapy in patients with osteoarthritis of the hip or knee. J Rheumatol. 1988;15:1833–40.

23. Bellamy N, Bell MJ, Pericak D, Goldsmith CH, Torrance GW, Raynauld JP, Walker V, Tugwell P, Polisson R. BLISS index for analyzing knee osteoarthritis trials data. J Clin Epidemiol. 2007;60:124–32.

24. Ruhdorfer A, Wirth W, Hitzl W, Nevitt M, Eckstein F. Association of thigh muscle strength with knee symptoms and radiographic disease stage of osteoarthritis: data from the osteoarthritis initiative. Arthritis Care Res (Hoboken). 2014;66:1344–53.

25. Martel-Pelletier J, Roubille C, Abram F, Hochberg MC, Dorais M, Delorme P, Raynauld JP, Pelletier JP. First-line analysis of the effects of treatment on progression of structural changes in knee osteoarthritis over 24 months: data from the osteoarthritis initiative progression cohort. Ann Rheum Dis. 2015;74:547–56.

26. Dodin P, Pelletier JP, Martel-Pelletier J, Abram F. Automatic human knee cartilage segmentation from 3D magnetic resonance images. IEEE Trans Biomed Eng. 2010;57:2699–711.

27. Wang Y, Wluka AE, Berry PA, Siew T, Teichtahl AJ, Urquhart DM, Lloyd DG, Jones G, Cicuttini FM. Increase in vastus medialis cross-sectional area is associated with reduced pain, cartilage loss, and joint replacement risk in knee osteoarthritis. Arthritis Rheum. 2012;64:3917–25.

28. Raynauld JP, Pelletier JP, Roubille C, Dorais M, Abram F, Li W, Wang Y, Fairley J, Cicuttini FM, Martel-Pelletier J. Magnetic resonance imaging-assessed vastus medialis muscle fat content and risk for knee osteoarthritis progression: relevance from a clinical trial. Arthritis Care Res (Hoboken). 2015;67:1406–15.

29. Teichtahl AJ, Wluka AE, Wang Y, Wijethilake PN, Strauss BJ, Proietto J, Dixon JB, Jones G, Forbes A, Cicuttini FM. Vastus medialis fat infiltration – a modifiable determinant of knee cartilage loss. Osteoarthritis Cartilage. 2015;23:2150–7.

30. Neogi T, Felson D, Niu J, Nevitt M, Lewis CE, Aliabadi P, Sack B, Torner J, Bradley L, Zhang Y. Association between radiographic features of knee osteoarthritis and pain: results from two cohort studies. BMJ. 2009; 339:b2844.

31. Schaible HG, Richter F, Ebersberger A, Boettger MK, Vanegas H, Natura G, Vazquez E, Segond von Banchet G. Joint pain. Exp Brain Res. 2009; 196:153–62.

32. Kulkarni B, Bentley DE, Elliott R, Julyan PJ, Boger E, Watson A, Boyle Y, El-Deredy W, Jones AK. Arthritic pain is processed in brain areas concerned with emotions and fear. Arthritis Rheum. 2007;56:1345–54.

33. Valdes AM, De Wilde G, Doherty SA, Lories RJ, Vaughn FL, Laslett LL, Maciewicz RA, Soni A, Hart DJ, Zhang W, et al. The Ile585Val *TRPV1* variant is involved in risk of painful knee osteoarthritis. Ann Rheum Dis. 2011;70:1556–61.

34. Xu L, Hayashi D, Roemer FW, Felson DT, Guermazi A. Magnetic resonance imaging of subchondral bone marrow lesions in association with osteoarthritis. Semin Arthritis Rheum. 2012;42:105–18.

35. Yusuf E, Kortekaas MC, Watt I, Huizinga TW, Kloppenburg M. Do knee abnormalities visualised on MRI explain knee pain in knee osteoarthritis? A systematic review. Ann Rheum Dis. 2011;70:60–7.

36. Atukorala I, Kwoh CK, Guermazi A, Roemer FW, Boudreau RM, Hannon MJ, Hunter DJ. Synovitis in knee osteoarthritis: a precursor of disease? Ann Rheum Dis. 2016;75:390–5.

37. Eckstein F, Benichou O, Wirth W, Nelson DR, Maschek S, Hudelmaier M, Kwoh CK, Guermazi A, Hunter D. Magnetic resonance imaging-based cartilage loss in painful contralateral knees with and without radiographic joint space narrowing: Data from the osteoarthritis initiative. Arthritis Rheum. 2009;61:1218–25.

38. Mundermann A, Dyrby CO, Andriacchi TP. Secondary gait changes in patients with medial compartment knee osteoarthritis: increased load at the ankle, knee, and hip during walking. Arthritis Rheum. 2005;52:2835–44.

39. Jones RK, Chapman GJ, Findlow AH, Forsythe L, Parkes MJ, Sultan J, Felson DT. A new approach to prevention of knee osteoarthritis: reducing medial load in the contralateral knee. J Rheumatol. 2013;40:309–15.

40. Felson DT, Niu J, Guermazi A, Roemer F, Aliabadi P, Clancy M, Torner J, Lewis CE, Nevitt MC. Correlation of the development of knee pain with enlarging bone marrow lesions on magnetic resonance imaging. Arthritis Rheum. 2007;56:2986–92.

41. Zhang Y, Nevitt M, Niu J, Lewis C, Torner J, Guermazi A, Roemer F, McCulloch C, Felson DT. Fluctuation of knee pain and changes in bone marrow lesions, effusions, and synovitis on magnetic resonance imaging. Arthritis Rheum. 2011;63:691–9.

42. Felson DT, Chaisson CE, Hill CL, Totterman SM, Gale ME, Skinner KM, Kazis L, Gale DR. The association of bone marrow lesions with pain in knee osteoarthritis. Ann Intern Med. 2001;134:541–9.

43. Hunter DJ, Zhang Y, Niu J, Goggins J, Amin S, LaValley MP, Guermazi A, Genant H, Gale D, Felson DT. Increase in bone marrow lesions associated with cartilage loss: a longitudinal magnetic resonance imaging study of knee osteoarthritis. Arthritis Rheum. 2006;54:1529–35.

44. Tanamas SK, Wluka AE, Pelletier JP, Pelletier JM, Abram F, Berry PA, Wang Y, Jones G, Cicuttini FM. Bone marrow lesions in people with knee osteoarthritis predict progression of disease and joint replacement: a longitudinal study. Rheumatology (Oxford). 2010;49:2413–9.

45. Wang X, Blizzard L, Jin X, Chen Z, Zhu Z, Halliday A, Cicuttini F, Jones G, Ding C. Quantitative assessment of knee effusion-synovitis in older adults: association with knee structural abnormalities. Arthritis Rheumatol. 2016;68: 837–44.

24

Persistence and adverse events of biological treatment in adult patients with juvenile idiopathic arthritis: results from BIOBADASER

Juan José Bethencourt Baute[1], Carlos Sanchez-Piedra[2], Dolores Ruiz-Montesinos[3], Marta Medrano San Ildefonso[4], Carlos Rodriguez-Lozano[5], Eva Perez-Pampin[6], Ana Ortiz[7], Sara Manrique[8], Rosa Roselló[9], Victoria Hernandez[10], Cristina Campos[11], Agustí Sellas[12], Walter Alberto Sifuentes-Giraldo[13], Javier García-González[14], Fernando Sanchez-Alonso[2], Federico Díaz-González[15], Juan Jesús Gómez-Reino[6], Sagrario Bustabad Reyes[15*] and on behalf of the BIOBADASER study group

Abstract

Background: Biologic therapy has changed the prognosis of patients with juvenile idiopathic arthritis (JIA). The aim of this study was to examine the pattern of use, drug survival, and adverse events of biologics in patients with JIA during the period from diagnosis to adulthood.

Methods: All patients included in BIOBADASER (Spanish Registry for Adverse Events of Biological Therapy in Rheumatic Diseases), a multicenter prospective registry, diagnosed with JIA between 2000 and 2015 were analyzed. Proportions, means, and SDs were used to describe the population. Incidence rates and 95% CIs were calculated to assess adverse events. Kaplan-Meier analysis was used to compare the drug survival rates.

Results: A total of 469 patients (46.1% women) were included. Their mean age at diagnosis was 9.4 ± 5.3 years. Their mean age at biologic treatment initiation was 23.9 ± 13.9 years. The pattern of use of biologics during their pediatric years showed a linear increase from 24% in 2000 to 65% in 2014. Biologic withdrawal for disease remission was higher in patients who initiated use biologics prior to 16 years of age than in those who were older (25.7% vs 7.9%, $p < 0.0001$). Serious adverse events had a total incidence rate of 41.4 (35.2–48.7) of 1000 patient-years. Patients younger than 16 years old showed significantly increased infections ($p < 0.001$).

Conclusions: Survival and suspension by remission of biologics were higher when these compounds were initiated in patients with JIA who had not yet reached 16 years of age. The incidence rate of serious adverse events in pediatric vs adult patients with JIA treated with biologics was similar; however, a significant increase of infection was observed in patients under 16 years old.

Keywords: Juvenile idiopathic arthritis, Biologic treatment, Safety therapy, Clinical practice

* Correspondence: sagrario.bustabad@gmail.com
[15]Servicio de Reumatología, Hospital Universitario de Canarias, c/Ofra s/n 38320, La Laguna, Santa Cruz de Tenerife, Spain
Full list of author information is available at the end of the article

Background

Juvenile idiopathic arthritis (JIA) comprises a group of diseases of unknown etiology that have in common arthritis in at least one joint persisting for at least 6 weeks in patients younger than 16 years of age [1]. JIA is the most frequent chronic rheumatic disease in childhood [2–4] and is classified into seven categories: systemic, persistent or extended oligoarthritis, rheumatoid Factor (RF) positive polyarthritis, RF-negative polyarthritis, enthesitis-related arthritis, psoriatic arthritis, and undifferentiated arthritis [1]. When uncontrolled, JIA leads to severe joint damage and impairment in skeletal maturation [5–7]. Fortunately, during the last decade, the arrival of biologics has dramatically changed the prognoses for these patients [8, 9]. A number of well-designed clinical trials, as well as cohort studies, have demonstrated that biologics are an effective option for patients with JIA who do not respond to or who cannot tolerate treatment with synthetic disease-modifying antirheumatic drugs (DMARDs) [10–12]. Some studies have shown that the sooner treatment is begun for JIA and the more aggressive it is, the better the outcomes obtained [13–16]. The ReACCh-Out cohort studied remission in patients with JIA in Canada and concluded that the probability of attaining remission with contemporary treatments within 5 years of diagnosis averaged about 50%, except for children with polyarthritis [17].

JIA is not confined to childhood, and 41% of patients require medication in their thirties, with some 28% maintaining high disease activity [18]. The transition period from pediatric- to adult-focused health care for adolescents with chronic conditions is attracting growing attention [19]. A recent study assessing the importance of transition to adult rheumatologic care in young people with JIA concluded that the maintenance of JIA diagnosis and DMARD therapy depended on the use of specialized care services [20]. Nowadays, young people with rheumatic diseases have a greater rate of survival, although high morbidity persists that could be avoided, in part, with multidisciplinary management [21]. Recently, several professional groups and international agencies have attempted to create consensus recommendations and guidelines trying to improve this situation [22, 23]. Data from the British Society for Rheumatology Biologics Register shows that tumor necrosis factor inhibitor (TNFi) therapies are an effective treatment option for adults with JIA, with a safety profile similar to that seen in rheumatoid arthritis (RA) [24]. However, because adults with JIA comprise a heterogeneous group of patients whose clinical evolution, need for, and response to treatments are not well studied, follow-up and monitoring of these patients are required [25]. The aim of the present study was to evaluate the pattern of use, the survival, and the safety of biologic agents in patients with JIA during the period from diagnosis to adulthood who are included in the BIOBADASER registry.

Methods

Study design

BIOBADASER (Spanish Registry for Adverse Events of Biological Therapy in Rheumatic Diseases) is a multicenter prospective observational study monitored annually, the main objective of which is long-term safety assessments of patients who undergoing biologic therapies [26, 27]. Established in February 2000, BIOBADASER is based on clinical practice. The quality of the database is ensured by a clear definition of its aim, an optimized number of variables, and an easy method of data collection that allows for consistency checks. Incompleteness and agreement of data with patient charts are assessed by online monitoring of the entire included population and by on-site annual audits of 10% of the patients registered. All detected errors and inconsistencies are corrected on the basis of results of said monitoring. The BIOBADASER registry is supported by the Spanish Medicines Agency, and the clinical studies were approved by the ethics committee of Hospital Clinic Barcelona. All patients included in the BIOBADASER registry, or their legal representatives, signed a written informed consent prior to inclusion.

Population

For this analysis, we selected all adult patients included in the database diagnosed with JIA. Owing to the initial design of the registry (BIOBADASER was not initially designed as a specific registry for JIA), patients with JIA were classified into systemic/oligoarthritis/polyarticular JIA, JIA related to enthesitis, or psoriatic JIA. Patients were enrolled in the registry when biologic treatment was initiated, and they were followed prospectively and evaluated if an adverse event (AE) occurred or if a change in the biologic therapy was decided either owing to an AE or because of inefficacy. The analysis of this study includes data from 2000 to December 2015, and only those patients still under active follow-up at the end of the study period were included.

Variables

The following data were collected: (1) patient data, including gender, date of birth, diagnosis, date of diagnosis, and comorbidities; (2) data on treatment, including types of biologics and dates of initiation and discontinuation, reason for discontinuation, concomitant antirheumatic treatment and tuberculosis (TB) prophylaxis; and (3) data on AEs, including date of occurrence, type and classification of AE according to the Medical Dictionary for Regulatory Activities [MedDRA]) v13 [28], severity, and outcome.

Statistical analysis

The patients included were described using descriptive statistics indicated by the type and distribution of variables. Proportions, means, and SDs or IQRs were used to describe our population and the use of treatments. The incidence rate (IR) per 1000 patient-years with 95% CI was estimated by group. Results were expressed as IR with the 95% CI. Survival rates were defined as end of treatment for any reason. IR comparisons between age groups were obtained by Poisson regression. Log-rank tests were used to assess the equality of survivor functions across age groups, monotherapy vs combined therapy, and treatment groups. All analyses were performed using Stata version 13.1 software (StataCorp, College Station, TX, USA).

Results

A total of 469 patients from the BIOBADASER registry, 46.1% of them women ($n = 216$), were classified as systemic/oligoarthritis/polyarticular JIA (70.5%), JIA related to enthesitis (25%), and psoriatic JIA (4.5%). The mean age was 34.5 years (SD = 15.3). The mean age at diagnosis was 9.4 years (SD = 5.3), and the mean evolution years was 24.1 (SD = 14.1). Uveitis was recorded in 12.6% of patients (50% of them antinuclear antibody [ANA]-positive). Overall, the ANA test result was positive in 30.2% of patients with systemic/oligoarthritis/polyarticular JIA, 14.3% of patients with psoriatic JIA, and 6.8% of patients with enthesitis. HLA-B27 was determined in 42.9% of patients, with 22% testing positive (59.8% in enthesitis-related arthritis, 23.8% in psoriatic arthritis, and 8.5% in systemic/oligoarthritis/polyarticular JIA). The mean age at the beginning of biologic treatment was 23.9 years (SD = 13.9), and the mean number of years that patients were treated with these compounds was 9.6 (SD = 3.8). Table 1 shows the baseline characteristics of patients included in this analysis.

Table 2 shows the biologics and concomitant treatments. The most frequently used biologics as first-line treatments were etanercept (43.5%), infliximab (30.5%), and adalimumab (19%). Almost half of the patients included in the registry (42.4%) were receiving monotherapy with biologics, and corticoids were used in 32.3% of patients with JIA. With respect to the pattern of use, Fig. 1 shows the annual percentage of patients diagnosed of JIA from 2000 to 2015 whose treatment with biologics began at age 16 years or younger ($n = 137$). In 2000, 25% of patients received the first biologic at a pediatric age, with this percentage increasing linearly until reaching 65% in 2015. The mean age of patients who started biologic treatment before 16 years of age was 8.06 years (SD = 4.3).

Table 3 shows the type of biologic used in the initial treatment of patients younger vs older than 16 years old. Etanercept was the most frequently prescribed drug as a first-line treatment in patients under 16 years old (59.1%), whereas infliximab was the most often biologic used in those aged 16 years or older (40.4%). Maintaining this division, the reasons for suspension in both groups of ages were inefficiency (37.1% and 37.4%, respectively), followed by adverse effects (28.6% and 28%, respectively). The

Table 1 Baseline characteristics of patients included in the study

Variable	Median (IQR) (Years)	No. (%)
Total number of patients		469
Sex, female		216 (46.1)
Age[a]	32.8 [22.8–43.6]	
Age at diagnosis	10.3 [4.4–14.3]	
Age at the beginning of biological treatment, median [IQR]**	22.1 [13.9–32.5]	
Years of disease progression	22.5 [12.3–33.9]	
Time in treatment with biologic	9.7 [6.8–12.6]	
JIA categories:		
- Oligoarticular, polyarticular, and systemic		331(70.5)
- Enthesitis-related arthritis		117 (25)
- Psoriatic arthritis		21 (4.5)
Positive RF		32 (6.8)
ANA-positive		111 (23.7)
HLA-B27-positive:		
- Positive		103 (22)
- Negative		98 (20.9)
- Not done		268 (57.1)
Uveitis:		
- Without uveitis		410 (87.4)
- Uveitis, ANA-negative		30 (6.4)
- Uveitis, ANA-positive		29 (6.2)

Abbreviations: ANA Antinuclear antibodies, *HLA* Human leukocyte antigen, *JIA* Juvenile idiopathic arthritis, *RF* Rheumatoid factor
[a]Age at the end of BIOBADASER phase II (December 2015)

suspension rate due to disease remission was higher in patients who initiated biologic treatment before 16 years old (25.7%) than in those who began it at 16 years old or later (7.9%; $p < 0.0001$). A total of 266 (56.7%) patients received only one biologic, and 7.5% were treated with five or more such compounds.

With respect to survival rates by age groups, retention of the first biologic was higher when it was started before 16 years of age ($p = 0.02$) (Fig. 2a). However, when survival rates were analyzed in patients who had received biologics as monotherapy or in combination, no significant differences were observed in terms of biologic retention ($p = 0.52$) (Fig. 2b). Regarding the therapeutic target, a nonsignificant tendency toward a better retention of TNFi compounds with respect to non-TNFi was observed ($p = 0.06$) (Fig. 2c) when they were analyzed as a first- or second-line treatment.

Table 4 shows that the most frequent AEs were infections, gastrointestinal disorders, skin and subcutaneous tissue disorders, and site-of-administration reactions. Regarding serious AEs, no differences were observed if the biologic therapy was initiated before age 16 years vs

Table 2 Biologics as first-line and subsequently, and concomitant therapy in patients with juvenile idiopathic arthritis

Drug	First-line	Second-line or later	Total
Etanercept	204 (43.5)	119 (25.8)	323 (34.7)
Infliximab	143 (30.5)	58 (12.6)	201 (21.6)
Adalimumab	89 (19.0)	108 (23.4)	197 (21.2)
Anakinra	8 (1.7)	15 (3.3)	23 (2.5)
Rituximab	0 (0.0)	72 (15.6)	72 (7.7)
Abatacept	5 (1.1)	28 (6.1)	33 (3.6)
Tocilizumab	16 (3.4)	40 (8.7)	56 (6.0)
Golimumab	2 (0.4)	13 (2.8)	15 (1.6)
Certolizumab	2 (0.4)	5 (1.1)	7 (0.8)
Canakinumab	0 (0.0)	2 (0.4)	2 (0.2)
Ustekinumab	0 (0.0)	1 (0.2)	1 (0.1)
Use of concomitant drugs			
- Monotherapy	177 (37.7)	217 (47.1)	394 (42.4)
- Methotrexate	225 (48.0)	184 (39.9)	409 (44.0)
- Glucocorticoids	155 (33.1)	145 (31.5)	300 (32.3)
- Leflunomide	29 (6.2)	26 (5.7)	55 (5.9)
- Sulfasalazine	26 (5.5)	13 (2.8)	39 (4.2)
- Gold salts	1 (0.2)	–	1 (0.1)
- Azathioprine	3 (0.6)	5 (1.1)	8 (0.9)
- Hydroxychloroquine	4 (0.9)	5 (1.1)	9 (1.0)

Data are expressed as number of patients (%)

Table 3 Characteristics of patients by age at the beginning of biologic treatment according to biologic compound, number of biologic drugs, and reasons for suspension

	< 16 Years	≥16 Years	p Value
Number of patients	137 (29.2)	332 (70.8)	
Age at the beginning of biological treatment	9.0 [4.2]	30.2 [11.4]	< 0.001
Years of disease progression	2.7 [3.1]	19.5 [2.1]	< 0.001
Biologic compound			
Etanercept	81 (59.1)	123 (37.1)	< 0.001
Adalimumab	31 (21.6)	58 (17.5)	
Infliximab	9 (6.6)	134 (40.4)	
Tocilizumab	8 (5.8)	8 (2.4)	
Abatacept	–	5 (1.5)	
Anakinra	6 (4.4)	2 (0.6)	
Certolizumab	2 (1.5)	–	
Golimumab	–	2 (0.6)	
Reason for suspension			
Inefficacy	26 (37.1)	80 (37.4)	< 0.001
Remission	18 (25.7)	17 (7.9)	
Adverse event	20 (28.6)	60 (28.0)	
Loss of tracking	4 (5.7)	20 (9.4)	
Pregnancy or gestational desire	–	13 (6.1)	
Other reasons	2 (2.9)	22 (10.3)	
Unknown	–	2 (0.9)	
Number of biologic drugs			
1 drug	83 (60.6)	183 (55.1)	0.244
> 1 drug	54 (39.4)	149 (44.9)	
2	27 (19.7)	67 (20.2)	
3	13 (9.5)	38 (11.5)	
4	11 (8.0)	12 (3.6)	
5 or more	3 (2.2)	32 (9.6)	

Data are expressed as mean [SD] or as number of patients (%). Chi-squared tests were used to compare distributions for categorical variables, and Student's t tests were used for numerical variables

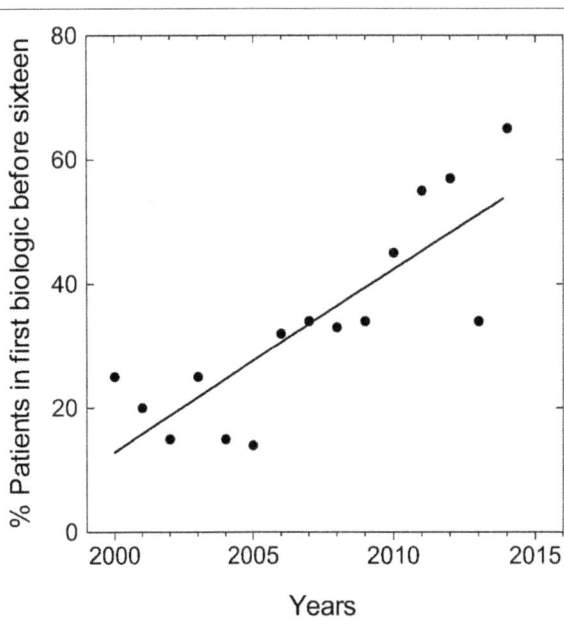

Fig. 1 Dot plot showing the variations in the percentage of patients with juvenile idiopathic arthritis included in BIOBADASER annually who received their first biologic before age 16 since years 2000 to 2015

later. Conversely, the analysis of infections showed a significant increase in the IR in patients under 16 years of age: 253.2 (221.4–289.6) vs 136.0 (122.8–150.6) ($p < 0.001$). A total of 37.2% of infections occurred during the first year of treatment (only 4.0% in the first month). Additional file 1: Table S1 shows the frequency of infections classified by type in patients younger or older than 16 years old. Only one fatal event (mycoplasma pneumonia in a patient treated with anakinra) was recorded. The IRs of total AEs in the three categories in which BIOBADASER classified patients with JIA were as follows: 424.9 (399.8–451.7) for systemic/oligoarthritis/polyarticular JIA, 262.8 (232–297.9) in cases of enthesitis, and 252.9 (188.8–338.8) for psoriatic JIA ($p < 0.001$). Regarding serious AEs, the

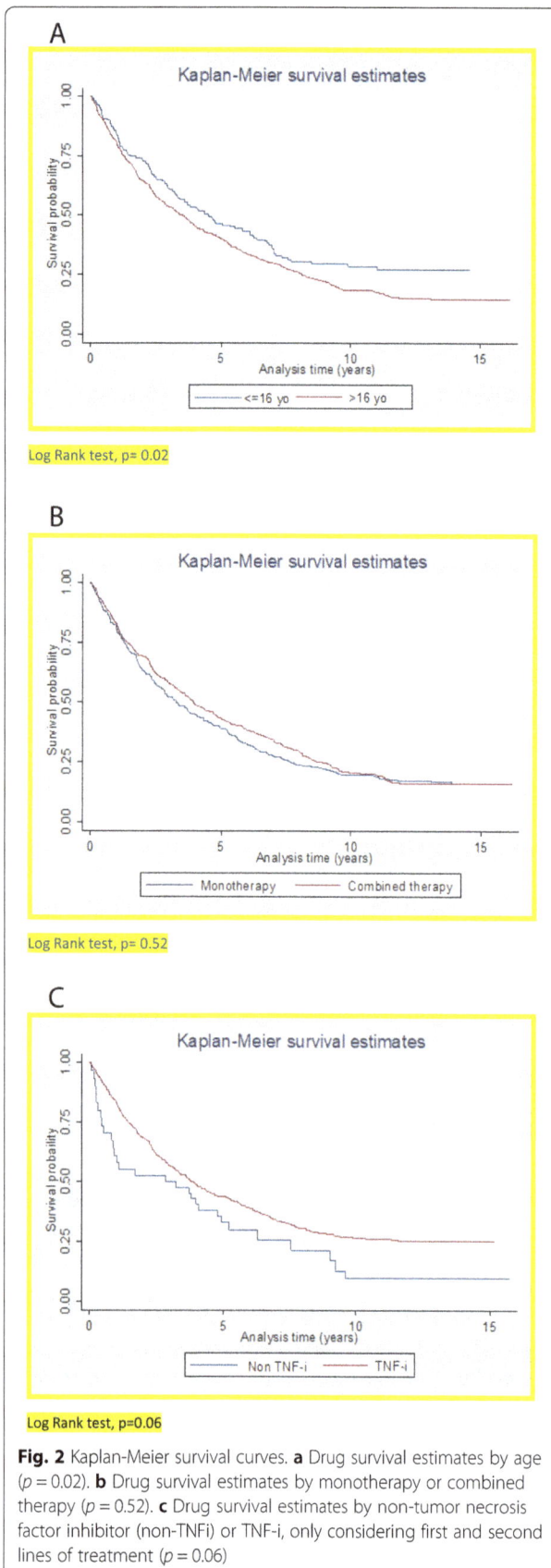

Fig. 2 Kaplan-Meier survival curves. **a** Drug survival estimates by age ($p = 0.02$). **b** Drug survival estimates by monotherapy or combined therapy ($p = 0.52$). **c** Drug survival estimates by non-tumor necrosis factor inhibitor (non-TNFi) or TNF-i, only considering first and second lines of treatment ($p = 0.06$)

IRs were 44.1 (36.5–53.3), 36 (25.7–50.4), and 33.7 (15.2–75.1), respectively ($p = 0.36$). When patients with JIA were classified on the basis of biologic therapy with TNFi or non-TNFi, the IRs for total AEs were 345.0 (325.1–366.0) and 617 (541.7–702.8), respectively ($p = 0.009$). Regarding serious AEs, the IRs were 78.8 (54.8–113.4) and 37.1 (30.9–44.4), respectively ($p = 0.924$).

With respect to opportunistic infections, three cases of pulmonary TB and one case of disseminated TB were recorded; these patients had received chemoprophylaxis with isoniazid, except in one case owing to a negative Mantoux test result.

Discussion

The most important findings of this work can be summarized as follows:

1. The use of biologics for the management of JIA during the pediatric years has consistently increased during the last 15 years.

2. In patients with JIA treated with biologics before 16 years of age, both the survival and drug withdrawal due to disease remission are higher than when these compounds are started during adulthood.

3. The safety of biologics in JIA is similar when used before or after 16 years of age in cases of serious AEs; however, in patients younger than 16 years old, infections are more frequent.

During the last 15 years, the advent of biologic drugs has changed the prognosis of and therapeutic approach to many rheumatic diseases, including JIA. As in adults, early initiation of biologic therapy in pediatric patients with JIA is important when control of the disease with conventional DMARDs is not achievable [29–31]. Patients with active JIA refractory to DMARDs and steroids are currently treated with TNFi or interleukin-6 antagonists or T-cell activation inhibitors in order to maintain inactive disease and the remission of JIA. Biologic drugs are typically well tolerated by children, and that—combined with early and aggressive therapy—yields optimal outcomes [9]. In this regard, in our present study, the pattern of biologic use showed that the annual percentage of patients with JIA who began treatment with these compounds before reaching 16 years of age increased almost threefold from 2000 to 2015. The biologics used in our registry of patients were, in order of frequency: etanercept, infliximab, and adalimumab. Infliximab was the second most used biologic in our series, with 30.5% of patients receiving this compound as the first biologic drug. Similarly, previous studies have reported the use of infliximab as a first biologic in patients with JIA ranged between 20.6% and 32% [24, 32]. When differentiating whether the treatment was started before or after 16 years old, it was found than 93% of patients ($n = 134$) initiated infliximab in adulthood. The reason for the significant use of infliximab, a TNFi

Table 4 Incidence of adverse events recorded in patients with juvenile idiopathic arthritis

	By age		p Value	Total
	< 16 years	≥16 years		
Total adverse events	457.6 (414.1–505.7)	346.9 (325.4–369.8)	< 0.001	373.2 (353.6–393.8)
Serious adverse events	35.7 (24.9–51.0)	43.2 (36.1–51.8)	0.347	41.4 (35.2–48.7)
Fatal adverse events	1.2 (0.2–8.4)	–	0.999	0.3 (0.0–2.0)
By system/organ class				
Infections and infestations	253.2 (221.4–289.6)	136.0 (122.8–150.6)	< 0.001	163.8 (151–177.6)
Gastrointestinal disorders	30.9 (21.0–45.4)	18.1 (13.7–24.0)	0.028	21.1 (16.9–26.5)
Skin and subcutaneous tissue disorders	17.8 (10.7–29.6)	21.1 (16.2–27.3)	0.797	20.3 (16.1–25.6)
General disorders and administration site conditions	21.4 (13.5–34.0)	20.0 (15.3–26.0)	0.566	20.3 (16.1–25.6)
Eye disorders	23.8 (15.3–36.8)	13.3 (9.6–18.4)	0.037	15.8 (12.1–20.5)
Musculoskeletal and connective tissue disorders	11.9 (6.4–22.1)	11.8 (8.4–16.7)	0.988	11.8 (8.7–16)
Surgical and medical procedures	3.6 (1.2–11.1)	13.7 (9.9–18.9)	0.025	11.3 (8.3–15.4)
Nervous system disorders	10.7 (5.6–20.6)	11.5 (8.1–16.3)	0.857	11.3 (8.3–15.4)
Blood and lymphatic system disorders	10.7 (5.6–20.6)	8.9 (5.9–13.2)	0.631	9.3 (6.6–13.1)
Renal and urinary disorders	3.6 (1.2–11.1)	11.1 (7.7–15.9)	0.061	9.3 (6.6–13.1)
Reproductive system and breast disorders	4.8 (1.8–12.7)	9.6 (6.5–14.1)	0.190	8.5 (5.9–12.1)
Injury, poisoning, and procedural complications	8.3 (4.0–17.5)	8.1 (5.4–12.3)	0.957	8.2 (5.7–11.8)
Respiratory, thoracic, and mediastinal disorders	11.9 (6.4–22.1)	5.9 (3.6–9.6)	0.083	7.3 (5–10.8)
Neoplasms: benign, malignant, and unspecified (including cysts and polyps)	3.6 (1.2–11.1)	5.9 (3.6–9.6)	0.422	5.4 (3.4–8.4)
Hepatobiliary disorders	2.4 (0.6–9.5)	5.9 (3.6–9.6)	0.225	5.1 (3.2–8.1)
Metabolism and nutrition disorders	1.2 (0.2–8.4)	5.9 (3.6–9.6)	0.120	4.8 (3–7.7)
Pregnancy, puerperium, and perinatal conditions	0.0	5.5 (3.3–9.2)	0.997	4.2 (2.5–7)
Vascular disorders	1.2 (0.2–8.4)	4.8 (2.8–8.3)	0.178	3.9 (2.3–6.7)
Psychiatric disorders	5.9 (2.5–14.3)	3.3 (1.7–6.4)	0.298	3.9 (2.3–6.7)
Ear and labyrinth disorders	2.4 (0.6–9.5)	3.0 (1.5–5.9)	0.783	2.8 (1.5–5.2)
Immune system disorders	2.4 (0.6–9.5)	2.6 (1.2–5.4)	0.916	2.5 (1.3–4.9)
Cardiac disorders	3.6 (1.2–11.1)	1.8 (0.8–4.4)	0.368	2.3 (1.1–4.5)
Endocrine disorders	2.4 (0.6–9.5)	1.5 (0.6–3.9)	0.583	1.7 (0.8–3.8)
Congenital, familial, and genetic disorders	0.0	1.8 (0.8–4.4)	0.403	1.4 (0.6–3.4)

Data represent the incidence (95% CI) × 1000 patients/yr

without indication in any category of JIA, in patients with JIA in adulthood may be due to different factors. These might be that infliximab and etanercept were the first TNFi available, and for a period of time they were the only biologic available, to treat DMARD-resistant inflammatory arthritis, as well as the tendency of many rheumatologists to reclassify adult JIA as RA [20], where infliximab is indicated.

The variable course of JIA and the passage from adolescence to adulthood constitutes an important challenge for the physician. According to a study conducted by the American College of Rheumatology, 45% of pediatric rheumatologists are reluctant to treat patients aged 18 years and older, and 28% of adult rheumatologists are treating patients younger than 17 years old [33]. Various

studies have reported that one-third of patients with JIA continue to present clinical disease activity into adulthood [34–36]. In addition, most patients with JIA who start biologic therapy during childhood reach adulthood with little evidence to support the benefits of continuing these treatments [37–39] or even of their long-term safety. This scenario implies a greater complexity in monitoring the safety of those drugs than is currently acknowledged. Studies based on routine clinical practice, as presented in this work, allow the assessment of treatment effectiveness and long-term adverse reactions in daily practice.

In our study, those patients who started treatment with biologics before the age 16 years presented with a percentage of drug suspension, owing to disease remission, greater than that in those who initiated these compounds at a later age (25.7% vs 7.9%, respectively). Different European cohorts have reported that male sex and earlier initiation of biologic therapy increased the likelihood of halting treatment owing to the onset of clinical remission [40]. With respect to drug survival, we found a significantly better retention rate when biologics were started before age 16 than in adulthood. The gap between diagnosis and biologic treatment initiation in the group of patients younger than 16 was 2.7 ± 3.1 years. A previous report [41] found no differences in the retention rates of the biologic therapy based on the age of treatment initiation in patients with JIA. In this study, the median age of patients who started biologic therapy was 16.2 ± 9.4 years old, with a gap between initiation of biologic treatment and diagnosis of 7.5 ± 4.9 years. This difference in start time of biologic treatment with respect to diagnosis might explain, at least in part, the divergent results in retention rates vis-à-vis age of biologic initiation between the two studies. In terms of drug survival, we found no differences between the use of biologics in monotherapy vs in combination, and when differentiated by age, our results were similar to those previously reported [42].

The aim of this study was to collect long-term outcome data on children receiving biologic agents for JIA, not only to assess drug survival but also to explore the reasons why biologic therapies had been discontinued. In our group of patients, inefficacy was the main reason for biologic therapy discontinuation regardless of age at drug onset, followed by AE and remission. In this regard, other series have found dissimilar results. Verazza et al. [43], in a series of 1038 patients with JIA treated with etanercept, found that the main cause of treatment discontinuation was disease remission, followed by inefficacy and AEs. Nevertheless, in a cohort of 301 patients with JIA, the most common reasons for stopping biologic treatment were AEs, with infusion reactions being the most frequently reported [44]. In a comparative study of adult and juvenile populations with inflammatory arthritis [42], the same biologic therapy profile as in our study was observed (infliximab vs etanercept) in both adults and children. Inefficacy was the most frequent reason for discontinuation of biologic therapy in both groups, being neuropsychiatric, gastrointestinal, and ocular complications, but not infections, as the most frequents AEs in the juvenile population. Although it may seem interesting to compare incidences of AEs and survival curves head-to-head for biologic treatments in adult patients, this would involve analyzing two different populations with clearly differentiated baseline pathologies and characteristics.

Regarding the limitations of our study, BIOBADASER was not specifically designed for JIA, and the categorization of these patients differs from the most currently used classification [1]. Because correct classification in categories is important in terms of therapeutic indications and prognosis, the new 2016 version of BIOBADASER classifies patients with JIA as systemic, persistent, or extended oligoarthritis; RF-positive polyarthritis; RF-negative polyarthritis; enthesitis-related arthritis; psoriatic arthritis; and undifferentiated arthritis [1]. Another limitation of our study is that we did not compare drugs individually. Nevertheless, our results included a safety comparison between TNFi and other biologic therapies. With respect to strengths of BIOBADASER, this registry allows the possibility of studying safety information in biologic treatments in a large cohort of patients with JIA followed in routine clinical practice by rheumatologists during a relevant period. BIOBADASER adds to the limitations of randomized clinical trials, which typically include a relatively low number of subjects followed for a short period of time, which hampers the ability of such studies to detect rare events and/or long-term side effects [45].

Conclusions

In summary, thus far, there are few studies based on general clinical practice that focus on the safety of biologic treatments in patients with JIA. The prospective records of these adult patients with JIA treated with biologic therapy can contribute to improving knowledge about the behavior of this disease in adulthood. In our study, survival and suspension by remission of biologics were higher when these compounds were initiated in patients with JIA who had not yet reached 16 years of age. The IR of serious AE in child vs adult patients with JIA treated with biologics was similar.

Abbreviations

AE: Adverse event; ANA: Antinuclear antibody; BIOBADASER: Spanish Registry for Adverse Events of Biological Therapy in Rheumatic Diseases; DMARD: Disease-modifying antirheumatic drug; FER: Spanish Society of Rheumatology; HLA: Human leukocyte antigen; IR: Incidence rate; JIA: Juvenile idiopathic arthritis; RA: Rheumatoid arthritis; RF: Rheumatoid factor; TB: Tuberculosis; TNFi: Tumor necrosis factor inhibitor

Acknowledgements

The authors thank Jesús Sánchez-Costa and Cristina Oliva, clinical research associates, for their dedication to BIOBADASER.

Funding

BIOBADASER is supported by the Research Unit of the Spanish Society of Rheumatology (FER) and the Spanish Agency for Medicines and Medical Devices (AEMyPS). Grants in approximately equal amounts were received from Biogen, Bristol-Myers Squibb, Pfizer, Roche, Samsung Bioepis, Lilly, Regeneron, Novartis, Janssen, Celgene, and MSD. These pharmaceutical companies had no role in this study. All researchers in this work are independent from the funders. In the collaboration contracts signed by the Spanish Society of Rheumatology, independence of the BIOBADASER registry has been affirmed with respect to the analyses as well as the diffusion of data and results.

Authors' contributions

JJBB and CSP wrote the initial draft of the manuscript. All authors had access to the data, contributed to its interpretation, and collaborated in the development of the manuscript. All authors critically reviewed and provided feedback on subsequent versions. All authors made the decision to submit the manuscript for publication and vouch for the accuracy and completeness of the data and fidelity of this report to the study protocol. All authors read and approved the final manuscript.

Consent for publication

Not applicable.

Competing interests

The authors declare that they have no competing interests.

Author details

[1]Servicio de Reumatología, Hospital Universitario de Canarias, Tenerife, Spain. [2]Research Unit, Sociedad Española de Reumatología, Madrid, Spain. [3]Servicio de Reumatología, Hospital Universitario del Virgen Macarena, Sevilla, Spain. [4]Servicio de Reumatología Hospital Universitario Miguel Servet, Zaragoza, Spain. [5]Servicio de Reumatología, Hospital Universitario de Gran Canaria Dr. Negrín, Las Palmas, Spain. [6]Servicio de Reumatología, Hospital Clínico Universitario de Santiago, A Coruña, Spain. [7]Servicio de Reumatología, Hospital de La Princesa, Madrid, Spain. [8]UGC de Reumatología, Instituto de Investigación Biomédica de Málaga (IBIMA), Hospital Regional Universitario de Málaga, Universidad de Málaga, Málaga, Spain. [9]Servicio de Reumatología, Hospital San Jorge, Huesca, Spain. [10]Servicio de Reumatología, Hospital Clinic de Barcelona, Barcelona, Spain. [11]Servicio de Reumatología, Hospital General Universitario Valencia, Valencia, Spain. [12]Servicio de Reumatología, Hospital Vall d'Hebron, Barcelona, Spain. [13]Servicio Reumatología, Hospital Ramón y Cajal, Madrid, Spain. [14]Servicio de Reumatología, Hospital 12 de Octubre, Madrid, Spain. [15]Servicio de Reumatología, Hospital Universitario de Canarias, c/Ofra s/n 38320, La Laguna, Santa Cruz de Tenerife, Spain.

References

1. Petty RE, Southwood TR, Manners P, Baum J, Glass DN, Goldenberg J, He X, Maldonado-Cocco J, Orozco-Alcala J, Prieur AM, et al. International League of Associations for Rheumatology classification of juvenile idiopathic arthritis: second revision, Edmonton, 2001. J Rheumatol. 2004;31(2):390–2.

2. Thierry S, Fautrel B, Lemelle I, Guillemin F. Prevalence and incidence of juvenile idiopathic arthritis: a systematic review. Joint Bone Spine. 2014;81(2):112–7.

3. Martinez Mengual L, Fernandez Menendez JM, Solis Sanchez G, Fernandez Diaz M, Fernandez Gonzalez N, Malaga Guerrero S: Epidemiological study of juvenile idiopathic arthritis in the last sixteen years in Asturias (Spain) [in Spanish]. An Pediatr (Barc) 2007, 66(1):24–30.

4. Modesto C, Anton J, Rodriguez B, Bou R, Arnal C, Ros J, Tena X, Rodrigo C, Rotes I, Hermosilla E, et al. Incidence and prevalence of juvenile idiopathic arthritis in Catalonia (Spain). Scand J Rheumatol. 2010;39(6):472–9.

5. Bowyer SL, Roettcher PA, Higgins GC, Adams B, Myers LK, Wallace C, Rennebohm R, Moore TL, Pepmueller PH, Spencer C, et al. Health status of patients with juvenile rheumatoid arthritis at 1 and 5 years after diagnosis. J Rheumatol. 2003;30(2):394–400.

6. Magni-Manzoni S, Rossi F, Pistorio A, Temporini F, Viola S, Beluffi G, Martini A, Ravelli A. Prognostic factors for radiographic progression, radiographic damage, and disability in juvenile idiopathic arthritis. Arthritis Rheum. 2003; 48(12):3509–17.

7. Mason T, Reed AM, Nelson AM, Thomas KB. Radiographic progression in children with polyarticular juvenile rheumatoid arthritis: a pilot study. Ann Rheum Dis. 2005;64(3):491–3.

8. Otten MH, Anink J, Prince FH, Twilt M, Vastert SJ, ten Cate R, Hoppenreijs EP, Armbrust W, Gorter SL, van Pelt PA, et al. Trends in prescription of biological agents and outcomes of juvenile idiopathic arthritis: results of the Dutch national Arthritis and Biologics in Children Register. Ann Rheum Dis. 2015;74(7):1379–86.

9. Stoll ML, Cron RQ. Treatment of juvenile idiopathic arthritis: a revolution in care. Pediatr Rheumatol Online J. 2014;12:13.

10. Shenoi S, Wallace CA. Tumor necrosis factor inhibitors in the management of juvenile idiopathic arthritis: an evidence-based review. Paediatr Drugs. 2010;12(6):367–77.

11. De Benedetti F, Brunner HI, Ruperto N, Kenwright A, Wright S, Calvo I, Cuttica R, Ravelli A, Schneider R, Woo P, et al. Randomized trial of tocilizumab in systemic juvenile idiopathic arthritis. N Engl J Med. 2012; 367(25):2385–95.

12. Lovell DJ, Ruperto N, Mouy R, Paz E, Rubio-Perez N, Silva CA, Abud-Mendoza C, Burgos-Vargas R, Gerloni V, Melo-Gomes JA, et al. Long-term safety, efficacy, and quality of life in patients with juvenile idiopathic arthritis treated with intravenous abatacept for up to seven years. Arthritis Rheumatol. 2015;67(10):2759–70.

13. Albers HM, Wessels JA, van der Straaten RJ, Brinkman DM, Suijlekom-Smit LW, Kamphuis SS, Girschick HJ, Wouters C, Schilham MW, le Cessie S, et al. Time to treatment as an important factor for the response to methotrexate in juvenile idiopathic arthritis. Arthritis Rheum. 2009;61(1):46–51.

14. Beukelman T, Patkar NM, Saag KG, Tolleson-Rinehart S, Cron RQ, DeWitt EM, Ilowite NT, Kimura Y, Laxer RM, Lovell DJ, et al. 2011 American College of Rheumatology recommendations for the treatment of juvenile idiopathic arthritis: initiation and safety monitoring of therapeutic agents for the treatment of arthritis and systemic features. Arthritis Care Res (Hoboken). 2011;63(4):465–82.

15. Otten MH, Prince FH, Armbrust W, ten Cate R, Hoppenreijs EP, Twilt M, Koopman-Keemink Y, Gorter SL, Dolman KM, Swart JF, et al. Factors associated with treatment response to etanercept in juvenile idiopathic arthritis. JAMA. 2011;306(21):2340–7.

16. Wallace CA, Giannini EH, Spalding SJ, Hashkes PJ, O'Neil KM, Zeft AS, Szer IS, Ringold S, Brunner HI, Schanberg LE, et al. Trial of early aggressive therapy in polyarticular juvenile idiopathic arthritis. Arthritis Rheum. 2012;64(6):2012–21.

17. Guzman J, Oen K, Tucker LB, Huber AM, Shiff N, Boire G, Scuccimarri R, Berard R, Tse SM, Morishita K, et al. The outcomes of juvenile idiopathic arthritis in children managed with contemporary treatments: results from the ReACCh-Out cohort. Ann Rheum Dis. 2015;74(10):1854–60.

18. Selvaag AM, Aulie HA, Lilleby V, Flato B. Disease progression into adulthood and predictors of long-term active disease in juvenile idiopathic arthritis. Ann Rheum Dis. 2016;75(1):190–5.

19. Sharma N, O'Hare K, Antonelli RC, Sawicki GS. Transition care: future directions in education, health policy, and outcomes research. Acad Pediatr. 2014;14(2):120–7.

20. Luque Ramos A, Hoffmann F, Albrecht K, Klotsche J, Zink A, Minden K. Transition to adult rheumatology care is necessary to maintain DMARD therapy in young people with juvenile idiopathic arthritis. Semin Arthritis Rheum. 2017;47(2):269–75.

21. Castrejón I: Transitional care programs for patients with rheumatic diseases: review of the literature [in Spanish]. Reumatol Clin 2012, 8(1):20–26.

22. Calvo I, Anton J, Bustabad S, Camacho M, de Inocencio J, Gamir ML, Grana J, La Cruz L, Robledillo JC, Medrano M, et al. Consensus of the Spanish Society of Pediatric Rheumatology for transition management from pediatric to adult care in rheumatic patients with childhood onset. Rheumatol Int. 2015;35(10):1615–24.

23. Foster HE, Minden K, Clemente D, Leon L, McDonagh JE, Kamphuis S, Berggren K, van Pelt P, Wouters C, Waite-Jones J, et al. EULAR/PReS standards and recommendations for the transitional care of young people with juvenile-onset rheumatic diseases. Ann Rheum Dis. 2017;76(4):639–46.

24. McErlane F, Foster HE, Davies R, Lunt M, Watson KD, Symmons DP, Hyrich KL. Biologic treatment response among adults with juvenile idiopathic arthritis: results from the British Society for Rheumatology Biologics Register. Rheumatology (Oxford). 2013;52(10):1905–13.

25. Hilderson D, Eyckmans L, Van der Elst K, Westhovens R, Wouters C, Moons P. Transfer from paediatric rheumatology to the adult rheumatology setting: experiences and expectations of young adults with juvenile idiopathic arthritis. Clin Rheumatol. 2013;32(5):575–83.

26. Carmona L, de la Vega M, Ranza R, Casado G, Titton DC, Descalzo MÁ, Gómez-Reino J. BIOBADASER, BIOBADAMERICA, and BIOBADADERM: safety registers sharing commonalities across diseases and countries. Clin Exp Rheumatol. 2014;32(5 Suppl 85):S163–7.

27. Sanchez-Piedra C, Hernández Miguel MV, Manero J, Roselló R, Sánchez-Costa JT, Rodríguez-Lozano C, Campos C, Cuende E, Fernández-Lopez JC, Bustabad S, Martín Domenech R, Pérez-Pampín E, Del Pino-Montes J, Millan-Arciniegas AM, Díaz-González F, Gómez-Reino JJ; en representación del Grupo de trabajo BIOBADASER Fase III. Objectives and methodology of BIOBADASER phase iii. Reumatol Clin. 2017. https://doi.org/10.1016/j.reuma.2017.08.001. [Epub ahead of print] English, Spanish.

28. Brown EG, Wood L, Wood S. The medical dictionary for regulatory activities (MedDRA). Drug Saf. 1999;20(2):109–17.

29. Lovell DJ, Ruperto N, Goodman S, Reiff A, Jung L, Jarosova K, Nemcova D, Mouy R, Sandborg C, Bohnsack J, et al. Adalimumab with or without methotrexate in juvenile rheumatoid arthritis. N Engl J Med. 2008;359(8):810–20.

30. Lovell DJ, Reiff A, Ilowite NT, Wallace CA, Chon Y, Lin SL, Baumgartner SW, Giannini EH. Safety and efficacy of up to eight years of continuous etanercept therapy in patients with juvenile rheumatoid arthritis. Arthritis Rheum. 2008;58(5):1496–504.

31. Ruperto N, Lovell DJ, Quartier P, Paz E, Rubio-Perez N, Silva CA, Abud-Mendoza C, Burgos-Vargas R, Gerloni V, Melo-Gomes JA, et al. Abatacept in children with juvenile idiopathic arthritis: a randomised, double-blind, placebo-controlled withdrawal trial. Lancet. 2008;372(9636):383–91.

32. Dimopoulou D, Trachana M, Pratsidou-Gertsi P, Sidiropoulos P, Kanakoudi-Tsakalidou F, Dimitroulas T, Garyfallos A. Predictors and long-term outcome in Greek adults with juvenile idiopathic arthritis: a 17-year continuous follow-up study. Rheumatology. 2017;56(11):1928–38.

33. Harnett T. Who will treat arthritis in 2005? Rheumatologist. 2007;(1). https://www.the-rheumatologist.org/article/who-will-treat-arthritis-in-2005/.

34. Foster HE, Marshall N, Myers A, Dunkley P, Griffiths ID. Outcome in adults with juvenile idiopathic arthritis: a quality of life study. Arthritis Rheum. 2003;48(3):767–75.

35. Minden K, Niewerth M, Listing J, Biedermann T, Bollow M, Schontube M, Zink A. Long-term outcome in patients with juvenile idiopathic arthritis. Arthritis Rheum. 2002;46(9):2392–401.

36. Packham JC, Hall MA. Long-term follow-up of 246 adults with juvenile idiopathic arthritis: functional outcome. Rheumatology (Oxford). 2002;41(12):1428–35.

37. Anink J, Prince FH, Dijkstra M, Otten MH, Twilt M, ten Cate R, Gorter SL, Koopman-Keemink Y, van Rossum MA, Hoppenreijs EP, et al. Long-term quality of life and functional outcome of patients with juvenile idiopathic arthritis in the biologic era: a longitudinal follow-up study in the Dutch Arthritis and Biologicals in Children Register. Rheumatology (Oxford). 2015; 54(11):1964–9.

38. Kearsley-Fleet L, McErlane F, Foster HE, Lunt M, Watson KD, Symmons DP, Hyrich KL. Effectiveness and safety of TNF inhibitors in adults with juvenile idiopathic arthritis. RMD Open. 2016;2(2):e000273.

39. Minden K, Niewerth M, Zink A, Seipelt E, Foeldvari I, Girschick H, Ganser G, Horneff G. Long-term outcome of patients with JIA treated with etanercept, results of the biologic register JuMBO. Rheumatology (Oxford). 2012;51(8): 1407–15.

40. Papsdorf V, Horneff G. Complete control of disease activity and remission induced by treatment with etanercept in juvenile idiopathic arthritis. Rheumatology (Oxford). 2011;50(1):214–21.

41. Mourão AF, Santos MJ, Melo Gomes JA, Martins FM, Mendonça SC, Oliveira Ramos F, Fernandes S, Salgado M, Guedes M, Carvalho S. Effectiveness and long-term retention of anti-tumour necrosis factor treatment in juvenile and adult patients with juvenile idiopathic arthritis: data from Reuma.pt. Rheumatology. 2015;55(4):697–703.

42. Favalli EG, Pontikaki I, Becciolini A, Biggioggero M, Ughi N, Romano M, Crotti C, Gattinara M, Gerloni V, Marchesoni A, et al. Real-life 10-year retention rate of first-line anti-TNF drugs for inflammatory arthritides in adult- and juvenile-onset populations: similarities and differences. Clin Rheumatol. 2017;36(8):1747–55.

43. Verazza S, Davi S, Consolaro A, Bovis F, Insalaco A, Magni-Manzoni S, Nicolai R, Marafon DP, De Benedetti F, Gerloni V, et al. Disease status, reasons for discontinuation and adverse events in 1038 Italian children with juvenile idiopathic arthritis treated with etanercept. Pediatr Rheumatol Online J. 2016;14(1):68.

44. Romano M, Pontikaki I, Gattinara M, Ardoino I, Donati C, Boracchi P, Meroni PL, Gerloni V. Drug survival and reasons for discontinuation of the first course of biological therapy in 301 juvenile idiopathic arthritis patients. Reumatismo. 2014;65(6):278–85.

45. Pincus T, Stein CM. Why randomized controlled clinical trials do not depict accurately long-term outcomes in rheumatoid arthritis: some explanations and suggestions for future studies. Clin Exp Rheumatol. 1997;15(Suppl 17):S27–38.

Permissions

All chapters in this book were first published in AR&T, by BioMed Central; hereby published with permission under the Creative Commons Attribution License or equivalent. Every chapter published in this book has been scrutinized by our experts. Their significance has been extensively debated. The topics covered herein carry significant findings which will fuel the growth of the discipline. They may even be implemented as practical applications or may be referred to as a beginning point for another development.

The contributors of this book come from diverse backgrounds, making this book a truly international effort. This book will bring forth new frontiers with its revolutionizing research information and detailed analysis of the nascent developments around the world.

We would like to thank all the contributing authors for lending their expertise to make the book truly unique. They have played a crucial role in the development of this book. Without their invaluable contributions this book wouldn't have been possible. They have made vital efforts to compile up to date information on the varied aspects of this subject to make this book a valuable addition to the collection of many professionals and students.

This book was conceptualized with the vision of imparting up-to-date information and advanced data in this field. To ensure the same, a matchless editorial board was set up. Every individual on the board went through rigorous rounds of assessment to prove their worth. After which they invested a large part of their time researching and compiling the most relevant data for our readers.

The editorial board has been involved in producing this book since its inception. They have spent rigorous hours researching and exploring the diverse topics which have resulted in the successful publishing of this book. They have passed on their knowledge of decades through this book. To expedite this challenging task, the publisher supported the team at every step. A small team of assistant editors was also appointed to further simplify the editing procedure and attain best results for the readers.

Apart from the editorial board, the designing team has also invested a significant amount of their time in understanding the subject and creating the most relevant covers. They scrutinized every image to scout for the most suitable representation of the subject and create an appropriate cover for the book.

The publishing team has been an ardent support to the editorial, designing and production team. Their endless efforts to recruit the best for this project, has resulted in the accomplishment of this book. They are a veteran in the field of academics and their pool of knowledge is as vast as their experience in printing. Their expertise and guidance has proved useful at every step. Their uncompromising quality standards have made this book an exceptional effort. Their encouragement from time to time has been an inspiration for everyone.

The publisher and the editorial board hope that this book will prove to be a valuable piece of knowledge for researchers, students, practitioners and scholars across the globe.

Contributors

Timothy R. D. J. Radstake
Laboratory of Translational Immunology and Department of Rheumatology and Clinical Immunology, University Medical Center Utrecht, Utrecht, The Netherlands

Chiara Angiolilli, Pawel A. Kabala and Kris A. Reedquist
Laboratory of Translational Immunology and Department of Rheumatology and Clinical Immunology, University Medical Center Utrecht, Utrecht, The Netherlands
Amsterdam Rheumatology and Immunology Center, Department of Clinical Immunology and Rheumatology and Department of Experimental Immunology, Academic Medical Center/ University of Amsterdam, Amsterdam, The Netherlands

Marzia Rossato
Laboratory of Translational Immunology and Department of Rheumatology and Clinical Immunology, University Medical Center Utrecht, Utrecht, The Netherlands
Functional Genomics Center, University of Verona, Verona, Italy

Dominique L. Baeten
Amsterdam Rheumatology and Immunology Center, Department of Clinical Immunology and Rheumatology and Department of Experimental Immunology, Academic Medical Center/ University of Amsterdam, Amsterdam, The Netherlands

Aleksander M. Grabiec
Amsterdam Rheumatology and Immunology Center, Department of Clinical Immunology and Rheumatology and Department of Experimental Immunology, Academic Medical Center/ University of Amsterdam, Amsterdam, The Netherlands
Department of Microbiology, Faculty of Biochemistry, Biophysics and Biotechnology, Jagiellonian University, Kraków, Poland

Wi S. Lai and Perry J. Blackshear
Signal Transduction Laboratory, National Institute of Environmental Health Sciences, Research Triangle Park, NC 27709, USA

Gianluca Fossati, Paolo Mascagni and Christian Steinkühler
Italfarmaco Research and Development, Cinisello Balsamo, Italy

Qian Niu, Zhuo-chun Huang, Xiao-juan Wu, Ya-xiong Jin, Yun-fei An, Ya-mei Li, Huan Xu, Bin Yang and Lan-lan Wang
Department of Laboratory Medicine, West China Hospital, Sichuan University, 37#, Guoxue Alley, Chengdu 610041, China

Sang-Heon Park, Seul-Ki Kim, Jung-Ah Kang, Ji-Sun Kwak, Young-Ok Son, Wan-Su Choi, Sung-Gyoo Park and Jang-Soo Chun
School of Life Sciences, Gwangju Institute of Science and Technology, Gwangju 61005, Republic of Korea

Jinseol Rhee
Keimyung University Dongsan Medical Center, Daegu 41931, Republic of Korea

Tanja Alexandra Stamm
Section for Outcomes Research, Center for Medical Statistics, Informatics, and Intelligent Systems, Medical University of Vienna, Spitalgasse 23, 1090 Vienna, Austria
Department of Medicine III, Division of Rheumatology, Medical University of Vienna, Waehringer Guertel 18-20, 1090 Vienna, Austria

Klaus Peter Machold, Daniel Aletaha and Farideh Alasti
Department of Medicine III, Division of Rheumatology, Medical University of Vienna, Waehringer Guertel 18-20, 1090 Vienna, Austria

Josef Smolen
Department of Medicine III, Division of Rheumatology, Medical University of Vienna, Waehringer Guertel 18-20, 1090 Vienna, Austria
Department of Internal Medicine, Centre for Rheumatic Diseases, Hietzing Hospital, Wolkersbergenstraße 1, 1130 Vienna, Austria

Peter Lipsky
RILITE Research Institute, 250 W Main Street, Charlottesville, Virginia 22902,USA

David Pisetsky
Medical Research Service Durham VA Medical Center, and Duke University Medical Center, 151G Durham VA Medical Center, 508 Fulton Street, Durham, North Carolina 27705, USA.

Robert Landewe
Department of Medicine, Division of Rheumatology, Academic Medical Center Amsterdam, Amsterdam, The Netherlands

Desiree van der Heijde, Alexandre Sepriano Tom Huizinga
Department of Rheumatology, Leiden University Medical Centre, Albinusdreef 2, 2300 RC Leiden, The Netherlands

Martin Aringer
Division of Rheumatology, Department of Medicine III, University Medical Center and Faculty of Medicine Carl Gustav Carus at the TU Dresden, Fetscherstrasse 74, 01309 Dresden, Germany

Dimitri Boumpas
8Rheumatology Medical School University of Crete, Heraklion and Joint Rheumatology Program, National and Kapodestrian University of Athens, Athens, Greece

Gerd Burmester
Department of Rheumatology and Clinical Immunology, Charité – University Medicine Berlin, Free University and Humboldt University Berlin, Berlin, Germany

Maurizio Cutolo
Research Laboratory and Division of Rheumatology, Department of Internal Medicine, University of Genova, Viale Benedetto XV, 6, 16132 Genoa, Italy

Wolfgang Ebner
Department of Internal Medicine, Centre for Rheumatic Diseases, Hietzing Hospital, Wolkersbergenstraße 1, 1130 Vienna, Austria

Winfried Graninger
Department of Rheumatology, Medical University of Graz, Auenbruggerplatz 15, 8036 Graz, Styria, Austria

Georg Schett
Department of Internal Medicine 3, Rheumatology and Immunology, Friedrich-Alexander-University Erlangen-Nürnberg (FAU) and Universitätsklinikum Erlangen, Ulmenweg 18, 91054 Erlangen, Germany

Hendrik Schulze-Koops
Division of Rheumatology and Clinical Immunology, Department of Internal Medicine IV, Ludwig Maximilians University of Munich, Pettenkoferstraße 8a, 80336 Munich, Germany

Paul-Peter Tak
Amsterdam Rheumatology and Immunology Center, Academic Medical Centre, University of Amsterdam, Amsterdam, the Netherlands
Department of Medicine, Cambridge University, Cambridge, UK
Department of Rheumatology, Ghent University, Ghent, Belgium
GlaxoSmithKline Research and Development, Stevenage, UK

Emilio Martin-Mola
Hospital Universitario La Paz, Paseo de la Castellana 261, 28046 Madrid, Spain

Ferdinand Breedveld
Leiden University Medical Center, Albinusdreef 2, 2300 RC Leiden, The Netherlands

Janine Schniering, Matthias Brunner, Oliver Distler and Britta Maurer
Center of Experimental Rheumatology, Department of Rheumatology, University Hospital Zurich, Gloriastrasse 25, 8091 Zurich, Switzerland

Li Guo
Center of Experimental Rheumatology, Department of Rheumatology, University Hospital Zurich, Gloriastrasse 25, 8091 Zurich, Switzerland
Department of Rheumatology, Renji Hospital, Shanghai Jiao Tong University, Shanghai, China

Shuang Ye
Department of Rheumatology, Renji Hospital, Shanghai Jiao Tong University, Shanghai, China

Martin Béhé
Center for Radiopharmaceutical Sciences, Villigen-PSI, Switzerland

Roger Schibli
Center for Radiopharmaceutical Sciences, Villigen-PSI, Switzerland Institute of Pharmaceutical Sciences, Department of Chemistry and Applied Biosciences, Zurich, Switzerland

Jonathan Aldridge, Jayesh M. Pandya, Linda Meurs, Kerstin Andersson, Inger Nordström, Anna-Carin Lundell and Anna Rudin
Department of Rheumatology and Inflammation Research, Institute of Medicine, Sahlgrenska Academy of University of Gothenburg, S-405 30 Gothenburg, Sweden

Elke Theander
Department of Rheumatology, Skåne University Hospital Lund and Malmö, Lund University, Lund, Sweden

David Simon, Arnd Kleyer, Francesca Faustini, Matthias Englbrecht, Andreas Berlin, Sebastian Kraus, Axel J. Hueber, Juergen Rech and Georg Schett
Friedrich-Alexander-University Erlangen-Nürnberg (FAU), Department of Internal Medicine 3 – Rheumatology and Immunology, Universitätsklinikum Erlangen, Ulmenweg 18, D-91054 Erlangen, Germany

Judith Haschka and Roland Kocijan
St. Vincent Hospital, Medical Department II, the VINFORCE Study Group, Academic Teaching Hospital of Medical University of Vienna, Vienna, Austria

Michael Sticherling
Department of Dermatology, University of Erlangen-Nuremberg, Erlangen, Germany

Zoe E. Betteridge
Department of Pharmacy and Pharmacology, University of Bath, Bath, UK

Neil J. McHugh
Department of Pharmacy and Pharmacology, University of Bath, Bath, UK
Royal National Hospital for Rheumatic Diseases, Royal United Hospitals Foundation Trust, Bath, UK

Lynsey Priest
Division of Molecular and Clinical Cancer Sciences, University of Manchester, Manchester, UK

Fiona Blackhall
Division of Molecular and Clinical Cancer Sciences, University of Manchester, Manchester, UK
CRUK Lung Cancer Centre of Excellence, The Christie NHS Foundation Trust, Wilmslow Road, Manchester, UK

Robert G. Cooper
MRC/ARUK Centre for Integrated Research into Musculoskeletal Ageing, University of Liverpool, Liverpool, UK

Janine A. Lamb
Centre for Epidemiology, Faculty of Biology, Medicine and Health, Manchester Academic Health Science Centre, University of Manchester, Manchester, UK

Ursula Schulte-Wrede, Heike Hirseland and Andreas Grützkau
German Rheumatism Research Center Berlin (DRFZ), an Institute of the Leibniz-Association, Immune Monitoring Core Facility, Charitéplatz 1, 10117 Berlin, Germany

Joachim R. Grün
German Rheumatism Research Center Berlin (DRFZ), an Institute of the Leibniz-Association, Immune Monitoring Core Facility, Charitéplatz 1, 10117 Berlin, Germany
German Rheumatism Research Center Berlin (DRFZ), an Institute of the Leibniz-Association, Bioinformatics Group, Berlin, Germany

Andreas Radbruch
German Rheumatism Research Center Berlin (DRFZ), an Institute of the Leibniz-Association, Immune Monitoring Core Facility, Charitéplatz 1, 10117 Berlin, Germany
German Rheumatism Research Center Berlin (DRFZ), an Institute of the Leibniz-Association, Cell Biology Group, Berlin, Germany

Till Sörensen and Thomas Häupl
Department of Rheumatology and Clinical Immunology, Charité - Universitätsmedizin Berlin, Berlin, Germany

Marta Steinbrich-Zöllner, Peihua Wu, Denis Joachim Sieper and Uta Syrbe
Department of Gastroenterology, Infectiology and Rheumatology, Charité -Universitätsmedizin Berlin, Berlin, Germany

Poddubnyy
Department of Gastroenterology, Infectiology and Rheumatology, Charité -Universitätsmedizin Berlin, Berlin, Germany
German Rheumatism Research Center Berlin (DRFZ), an Institute of the Leibniz-Association, Epidemiology Unit, Berlin, Germany

Huantian Zhang and Zhengang Zha
Institute of Orthopedic Diseases and Center for Joint Surgery and Sports Medicine, the First Affiliated Hospital, Jinan University, Guangzhou, People's Republic of China

Yuanfeng Chen
Institute of Orthopedic Diseases and Center for Joint Surgery and Sports Medicine, the First Affiliated Hospital, Jinan University, Guangzhou, People's Republic of China
Department of Orthopaedics and Traumatology, Li Ka Shing Institute of Health Sciences and Lui Che Woo Institute of Innovative Medicine, Faculty of Medicine, The Chinese University of Hong Kong, Prince of Wales Hospital, Shatin, Hong Kong SAR, People's Republic of China
The CUHK-ACC Space Medicine Centre on Health Maintenance of Musculoskeletal System, The Chinese University of Hong Kong Shenzhen Research Institute, Shenzhen, People's Republic of China

Dan Zhang and Po Sing Leung
School of Biomedical Sciences, Faculty of Medicine, The Chinese University of Hong Kong, Hong Kong, Hong Kong SAR, People's Republic of China

Ki Wai Ho
Department of Orthopaedics and Traumatology, Li Ka Shing Institute of Health Sciences and Lui Che Woo Institute of Innovative Medicine, Faculty of Medicine, The Chinese University of Hong Kong, Prince of Wales Hospital, Shatin, Hong Kong SAR, People's Republic of China

Sien Lin and Gang Li
Department of Orthopaedics and Traumatology, Li Ka Shing Institute of Health Sciences and Lui Che Woo Institute of Innovative Medicine, Faculty of Medicine, The Chinese University of Hong Kong, Prince of Wales Hospital, Shatin, Hong Kong SAR, People's Republic of China
The CUHK-ACC Space Medicine Centre on Health Maintenance of Musculoskeletal System, The Chinese University of Hong Kong Shenzhen Research Institute, Shenzhen, People's Republic of China

Wade Chun-Wai Suen
Department of Orthopaedics and Traumatology, Li Ka Shing Institute of Health Sciences and Lui Che Woo Institute of Innovative Medicine, Faculty of Medicine, The Chinese University of Hong Kong, Prince of Wales Hospital, Shatin, Hong Kong SAR, People's Republic of China
Department of Haematology, University of Cambridge, Cambridge CB2 0PT, UK

Yoshiya Tanaka, Yoshihisa Fujino and Shinya Matsuda
University of Occupational and Environmental Health, 1-1 Iseigaoka, Yahatanishi-ku, Kitakyushu, Fukuoka 807-0804, Japan

Kazuyoshi Saito
University of Occupational and Environmental Health, 1-1 Iseigaoka, Yahatanishi-ku, Kitakyushu, Fukuoka 807-0804, Japan
Tobata General Hospital, 1-3-33 Fukuryugi, Tobata-ku, Kitakyushu, Fukuoka 804-0025, Japan

Hideto Kameda
Toho University, 2-22-36 Ohashi, Meguro-ku, Tokyo 153-8515, Japan

Yuko Kaneko
Keio University School of Medicine, 35 Shinanomachi, Shinjuku-ku, Tokyo 160-8582, Japan

Eiichi Tanaka
Tokyo Women's Medical University, 10-22 Kawada-cho, Shinjuku-ku, Tokyo 162-0054, Japan

Shinsuke Yasuda
Hokkaido University, N15, W7, Kita-ku, Sapporo, Hokkaido 060-8638, Japan

Naoto Tamura
Juntendo University School of Medicine, 2-1-1 Hongo, Bunkyo-ku, Tokyo 113-8421, Japan

Keishi Fujio
The University of Tokyo, 7-3-1 Hongo, Bunkyo-ku, Tokyo 113-8654, Japan

Takao Fujii
Wakayama Medical University, 811-1 Kimiidera, Wakayama 641-8509, Japan

Toshihisa Kojima
Nagoya University Graduate School of Medicine, 65 Tsurumai-cho, Showa-ku, Nagoya, Aichi 466-8550, Japan

Tatsuhiko Anzai
EPS Corporation, 6-29 Shinogawamachi, Shinjuku-ku, Tokyo 162-0814, Japan

Chikuma Hamada
Tokyo University of Science, 6-3-1 Niijuku, Katsuhika-ku, Tokyo 125-8585, Japan

Hitoshi Kohsaka
Tokyo Medical and Dental University, 1-5-45 Yushima, Bunkyo-ku, Tokyo 113-8510, Japan

Dimitrios Chanouzas , Michael Sagmeister, Phoebe Sharp and Serena Johal
Institute of Inflammation and Ageing, College of Medical and Dental Sciences, University of Birmingham, Birmingham B15 2TT, UK
Renal Unit, University Hospitals Birmingham NHS Foundation Trust, Mindelsohn Way, Edgbaston, Birmingham B15 2TH, UK

Lucy Powley, Jessica Bowen and Lovesh Dyall
Renal Unit, University Hospitals Birmingham NHS Foundation Trust, Mindelsohn Way, Edgbaston, Birmingham B15 2TH, UK

Charles J. Ferro
Renal Unit, University Hospitals Birmingham NHS Foundation Trust, Mindelsohn Way, Edgbaston, Birmingham B15 2TH, UK

Institute of Translational Medicine Birmingham, Heritage Building, Mindelsohn Way, Edgbaston, Birmingham B15 2TH, UK

Matthew D. Morgan
Renal Unit, University Hospitals Birmingham NHS Foundation Trust, Mindelsohn Way, Edgbaston, Birmingham B15 2TH, UK
Institute of Clinical Sciences, College of Medical and Dental Sciences, University of Birmingham, Birmingham B15 2TT, UK

Lorraine Harper
Renal Unit, University Hospitals Birmingham NHS Foundation Trust, Mindelsohn Way, Edgbaston, Birmingham B15 2TH, UK
Institute of Translational Medicine Birmingham, Heritage Building, Mindelsohn Way, Edgbaston, Birmingham B15 2TH, UK
Institute of Clinical Sciences, College of Medical and Dental Sciences, University of Birmingham, Birmingham B15 2TT, UK

Peter Nightingale
Institute of Translational Medicine Birmingham, Heritage Building, Mindelsohn Way, Edgbaston, Birmingham B15 2TH, UK

Paul Moss
Institute of Immunology and Immunotherapy, College of Medical and Dental Sciences, University of Birmingham, Birmingham B15 2TT, UK

Carlo Marchetti, Benjamin Swartzwelter, Tania Azam and Nick Powers
Department of Medicine, University of Colorado Denver, Aurora, CO, USA

Isak W. Tengesdal, Dennis M. de Graaf, Charles A. Dinarello and Leo A. B. Joosten
Department of Medicine, University of Colorado Denver, Aurora, CO, USA
Department of Internal Medicine and Radboud Institute of Molecular Life Sciences (RIMLS), Radboud University Medical Center, Geert Grooteplein Zuid 8, 6525, GA, Nijmegen, The Netherlands

Marije I. Koenders
Department of Rheumatology, Radboud University Medical Center, Nijmegen, The Netherlands

Rekha Narasimhan, David Boyle and Arthur Kavanaugh
Division of Rheumatology, University of California, San Diego, 9500 Gilman Drive, San Diego, CA 92093, USA

Roxana Coras and Monica Guma
Division of Rheumatology, University of California, San Diego, 9500 Gilman Drive, San Diego, CA 92093, USA
Department of Medicine, Autonomous University of Barcelona, Plaça Cívica, 08193 Bellaterra, Barcelona, Spain

Sara B. Rosenthal
Center for Computational Biology and Bioinformatics, University of California, San Diego, 9500 Gilman Drive, San Diego, CA 92093, USA

Shannon R. Sweeney, Alessia Lodi and Stefano Tiziani
Department of Nutritional Sciences and Dell Pediatric Research Institute, Dell Medical School, University of Texas at Austin, 1400 Barbara Jordan Blvd, Austin, TX, USA

Yan He, Yan Li, Chunlian Zhong, Yuan Liu, Hongyan Qian, Jingxiu Xuan, Lihua Duan and Guixiu Shi
Department of Rheumatology and Clinical Immunology, The First Affiliated Hospital of Xiamen University, Xiamen, China

Xiaoqing Yuan
Department of Rheumatology and Clinical Immunology, The First Affiliated Hospital of Xiamen University, Xiamen, China
Ningbo City Medical Treatment Center Lihuili Hospital, No. 57 Xingning Road, Ningbo 315000, China

Marc Dorais
StatSciences Inc., Notre-Dame-de-l'Île-Perrot, Quebec, Canada

Johanne Martel-Pelletier, Jean-Pierre Raynauld, Philippe Delorme and Jean-Pierre Pelletier
Osteoarthritis Research Unit, University of Montreal Hospital Research Centre (CRCHUM), Montreal, Quebec, Canada

Meliha C. Kapetanovic
Department of Clinical Sciences Lund, Section of Rheumatology, Lund University and Skåne University Hospital, Kioskgatan 5, SE-221 85 Lund, Sweden

Peter Nilsson
Department of Clinical Sciences, Lund University, Malmö, Sweden
Department of Emergency and Internal Medicine, Skåne University Hospital, Malmö, Sweden

Carl Turesson
Department of Clinical Sciences, Malmö, Lunds University and Skåne University Hospital, Malmö, Sweden

Martin Englund
Clinical Epidemiology Unit, Orthopaedics, Department of Clinical Sciences, Lund University, Lund, Sweden

Nicola Dalbeth
Department of Medicine, University of Auckland, Auckland, New Zealand

Lennart Jacobsson
Department of Rheumatology and Inflammation Research, Sahlgrenska Academy at University of Gothenburg, Gothenburg, Sweden

Tanja A. Stamm
Section for Outcomes Research, Center for Medical Statistics, Informatics, and Intelligent Systems, Medical University of Vienna, Spitalgasse 23, 1090 Vienna, Austria

Michaela A. Stoffer-Marx
Section for Outcomes Research, Center for Medical Statistics, Informatics, and Intelligent Systems, Medical University of Vienna, Spitalgasse 23, 1090 Vienna, Austria
Division of Rheumatology, Department of Medicine 3, Medical University of Vienna, Vienna, Austria

Kurt Redlich and Josef S. Smolen
Division of Rheumatology, Department of Medicine 3, Medical University of Vienna, Vienna, Austria

Meike Klinger and Simone Luschin
Division of Rheumatology, Department of Medicine 3, Medical University of Vienna, Vienna, Austria

Department of Health Sciences, University of Applied Sciences FH Campus Wien, Favoritenstraße 226, 1100 Vienna, Austria

Monika Zettel-Tomenendal
Department of Health Sciences, University of Applied Sciences FH Campus Wien, Favoritenstraße 226, 1100 Vienna, Austria

Silvia Meriaux-Kratochvila
Department of Health Sciences, University of Applied Sciences FH Campus Wien, Favoritenstraße 226, 1100 Vienna, Austria
Physio Austria, Lange Gasse 30/1, Vienna, Austria

Valerie Nell-Duxneuner
Klinikum Peterhof of NOEGKK with Ludwig Boltzmann Department of Epidemiology of Rheumatic Diseases, Sauerhofstraße 9-15, Baden bei Wien, Austria

Jochen Zwerina
Ludwig Boltzmann Institute of Osteology, 1st Medical Department at Hanusch Hospital, Hanusch Hospital of the WGKK and AUVA Trauma Center, Heinrich Collin Str. 30, 1140 Vienna, Austria

Ingvild Kjeken
National advisory unit on rehabilitation in rheumatology, Department of rheumatology, Diakonhjemmet Hospital, Oslo, Norway
Program of Occupational Therapy, Prosthetics and Orthotics, Oslo Metropolitan University, Oslo, Norway

Marion Hackl
Ergotherapie Austria, Bundesverband der Ergotherapeutinnen und Ergotherapeuten Österreichs, Holzmeistergasse 7-9/2/1, Vienna, Austria

Sylvia Öhlinger
University of Applied Sciences for Health Professions Upper Austria, Semmelweisstraße 34, Linz, Austria

Anthony Woolf
Bone and Joint Research Group, Royal Cornwall Hospital, Truro, UK

Anna Szeremeta, Agnieszka Jura-Półtorak, Ewa Maria Koźma, Andrzej Głowacki and Krystyna Olczyk
Department of Clinical Chemistry and Laboratory Diagnostics, School of Pharmacy with the Division of Laboratory Medicine in Sosnowiec, Medical University of Silesia in Katowice, Jedności 8, 41-200 Sosnowiec, Poland

Eugeniusz Józef Kucharz and Magdalena Kopeć-Mędrek
Department of Internal Medicine and Rheumatology, School of Medicine in Katowice, Medical University of Silesia in Katowice, Ziołowa 45/47, 40-635 Katowice, Poland

Agathe Grandjean, Vincent Ducoulombier, Marguerite Motte, Marie Vandecandelaere, Hélène Luraschi, Catherine Godart and Eric Houvenagel
Department of Rheumatology, Lille Catholic Hospitals, University of Lille, 59160 Lomme, France
Saint-Philibert Hospital, Rue du Grand But, 59160 Lomme, France

Tristan Pascart
Department of Rheumatology, Lille Catholic Hospitals, University of Lille, 59160 Lomme, France
EA 4490, PMOI, Physiopathologie des Maladies Osseuses Inflammatoires, University of Lille, 59000 Lille, France

Saint-Philibert Hospital, Rue du Grand But, 59160 Lomme, France

Benoist Capon, Julie Legrand and Nasser Namane
Department of Radiology, Lille Catholic Hospitals, University of Lille, 59160 Lomme, France
Saint-Philibert Hospital, Rue du Grand But, 59160 Lomme, France

Jean-François Budzik
Department of Radiology, Lille Catholic Hospitals, University of Lille, 59160 Lomme, France
EA 4490, PMOI, Physiopathologie des Maladies Osseuses Inflammatoires, University of Lille, 59000 Lille, France
Saint-Philibert Hospital, Rue du Grand But, 59160 Lomme, France

Laurène Norberciak
Department of Medical Research, Biostatistics, Lille Catholic Hospitals, University of Lille, 59160 Lomme, France
Saint-Philibert Hospital, Rue du Grand But, 59160 Lomme, France

Yeon-Ah Lee and Hyung-In Yang
East-West Bone and Joint Disease Research Institute, Kyung Hee University Hospital at Gangdong, 02447 Seoul, Korea
Division of Rheumatology, Department of Internal Medicine, College of Medicine, Kyung Hee University, 23 Kyung Hee Dae-ro, Dongdaemun-gu, 02447 Seoul, Korea

Kyoung Soo Kim
East-West Bone and Joint Disease Research Institute, Kyung Hee University Hospital at Gangdong, 02447 Seoul, Korea
Department of Clinical Pharmacology and Therapeutics, College of Medicine, Kyung Hee University, 23 Kyung Hee Dae-ro, Dongdaemun-gu, 02447 Seoul, Korea

Dae-Hyun Hahm
Department of Physiology, College of Medicine, Kyung Hee University, 23 Kyung Hee Dae-ro, Dongdaemun-gu, 02447 Seoul, Korea

Jung Yeon Kim
Department of Pathology, Inje University Sanggye Paik Hospital, 1342 Dongil-ro, Nowon-gu, 01757 Seoul, Korea

Bonjun Sur
Acupuncture and Meridian Science Research Center, College of Korean Medicine, Kyung Hee University, 23 Kyung Hee Dae-ro, Dongdaemun-gu, 02447 Seoul, Korea

Hyun Min Lee and Chun Jeih Ryu
Department of Integrative Bioscience and Biotechnology, Sejong University, 209 Neungdong-ro, Gwangjin-gu, 05006 Seoul, Korea

Naoki Iwamoto, Shoichi Fukui, Ayuko Takatani, Toshimasa Shimizu, Takashi Igawa, Kunihiro Ichinose, Mami Tmai, Hideki Nakamura and Atsushi Kawakami
Department of Immunology and Rheumatology, Division of Advanced Preventive Medical Sciences, Nagasaki University Graduate School of Biomedical Sciences, 1-7-1 Sakamoto, Nagasaki 852-8501, Japan

Masataka Umeda
Department of Immunology and Rheumatology, Division of Advanced Preventive Medical Sciences, Nagasaki University Graduate School of Biomedical Sciences, 1-7-1 Sakamoto, Nagasaki 852-8501, Japan
Medical Education Development Center, Nagasaki University School Hospital, Nagasaki, Japan

Ayako Nishino
Department of Immunology and Rheumatology, Division of Advanced Preventive Medical Sciences, Nagasaki University Graduate School of Biomedical Sciences, 1-7-1 Sakamoto, Nagasaki 852-8501, Japan
Center for Comprehensive Community Care Education, Nagasaki University Graduate School of Biomedical Sciences, Nagasaki, Japan

Tomohiro Koga
Department of Immunology and Rheumatology, Division of Advanced Preventive Medical Sciences, Nagasaki University Graduate School of Biomedical Sciences, 1-7-1 Sakamoto, Nagasaki 852-8501, Japan
Center for Bioinformatics and Molecular Medicine, Nagasaki University Graduate School of Biomedical Sciences, Nagasaki, Japan

Shin-ya Kawashiri
Department of Immunology and Rheumatology, Division of Advanced Preventive Medical Sciences, Nagasaki University Graduate School of Biomedical Sciences, 1-7-1 Sakamoto, Nagasaki 852-8501, Japan
Departments of Community Medicine, Division of Advanced Preventive Medical Sciences, Nagasaki University Graduate School of Biomedical Sciences, Nagasaki, Japan

Tomoki Origuchi
Department of Physical Therapy, Nagasaki University Graduate School of Biomedical Sciences, Nagasaki, Japan

Ko Chiba and Makoto Osaki
Department of Orthopedic Surgery, Nagasaki University Graduate School of Biomedical Sciences, Nagasaki, Japan

Astrid Jüngel and Steffen Gay
Center of Experimental Rheumatology, University Hospital Zurich and University of Zurich, Schlieren, Zurich, Switzerland

Yuanyuan Wang, Andrew J. Teichtahl, Sultana Monira Hussain and Flavia M. Cicuttini
Department of Epidemiology and Preventive Medicine, School of Public Health and Preventive Medicine, Monash University, 553 St Kilda Road, Melbourne, VIC 3004, Australia

François Abram
Medical Imaging Research and Development ArthroLab Inc., Montreal, QC, Canada

Jean-Pierre Pelletier and Johanne Martel-Pelletier
Osteoarthritis Research Unit, University of Montreal Hospital Research Centre (CRCHUM), Montreal, QC, Canada

Juan José Bethencourt Baute
Servicio de Reumatología, Hospital Universitario de Canarias, Tenerife, Spain

Carlos Sanchez-Piedra and Fernando Sanchez-Alonso
2Research Unit, Sociedad Española de Reumatología, Madrid, Spain

Dolores Ruiz-Montesinos
Servicio de Reumatología, Hospital Universitario del Virgen Macarena, Sevilla, Spain

Marta Medrano San Ildefonso
Servicio de Reumatología Hospital Universitario Miguel Servet, Zaragoza, Spain

Carlos Rodriguez-Lozano
Servicio de Reumatología, Hospital Universitario de Gran Canaria Dr. Negrín, Las Palmas, Spain

Eva Perez-Pampin and Juan Jesús Gómez-Reino
Servicio de Reumatología, Hospital Clínico Universitario de Santiago, A Coruña, Spain

Ana Ortiz
Servicio de Reumatología, Hospital de La Princesa, Madrid, Spain

Sara Manrique
UGC de Reumatología, Instituto de Investigación Biomédica de Málaga (IBIMA), Hospital Regional Universitario de Málaga, Universidad de Málaga, Málaga, Spain

Rosa Roselló
Servicio de Reumatología, Hospital San Jorge, Huesca, Spain

Victoria Hernandez
Servicio de Reumatología, Hospital Clinic de Barcelona, Barcelona, Spain

Cristina Campos
Servicio de Reumatología, Hospital General Universitario Valencia, Valencia, Spain

Agustí Sellas
Servicio de Reumatología, Hospital Vall d'Hebron, Barcelona, Spain

Walter Alberto Sifuentes-Giraldo
Servicio Reumatología, Hospital Ramón y Cajal, Madrid, Spain

Javier García-González
Servicio de Reumatología, Hospital 12 de Octubre, Madrid, Spain

Federico Díaz-González and Sagrario Bustabad Reyes
Servicio de Reumatología, Hospital Universitario de Canarias, c/Ofra s/n 38320, La Laguna, Santa Cruz de Tenerife, Spain

Index